Sports Science and Health Management

Sports Science and Health Management

Edited by Jacob Meyer

SYRAWOOD
PUBLISHING HOUSE
New York

Published by Syrawood Publishing House,
750 Third Avenue, 9th Floor,
New York, NY 10017, USA
www.syrawoodpublishinghouse.com

Sports Science and Health Management
Edited by Jacob Meyer

International Standard Book Number: 978-1-68286-562-0 (Hardback)

Cataloging-in-Publication Data

Sports science and health management / edited by Jacob Meyer.
p. cm.
Includes bibliographical references and index.
ISBN 978-1-68286-562-0
1. Sports sciences. 2. Health. 3. Health services administration.
4. Physical education and training. I. Meyer, Jacob.
GV558 .S66 2018
613.71--dc23

Printed in China.

Table of Contents

PREFACE

Sports science and health management studies the effect exercise has on the human body. Physical training is goal oriented with training programs that help in the development of skills and improve the athletic performance of an individual. While understanding the long-term perspectives of the topics, the book makes an effort in highlighting their impact as a modern tool for the growth of the discipline. It explores all the important aspects of sports science and health management in the present day scenario. With state-of-the-art inputs by acclaimed experts of this field, this book targets students and professionals.

Various studies have approached the subject by analyzing it with a single perspective, but the present book provides diverse methodologies and techniques to address this field. This book contains theories and applications needed for understanding the subject from different perspectives. The aim is to keep the readers informed about the progresses in the field; therefore, the contributions were carefully examined to compile novel researches by specialists from across the globe.

Indeed, the job of the editor is the most crucial and challenging in compiling all chapters into a single book. In the end, I would extend my sincere thanks to the chapter authors for their profound work. I am also thankful for the support provided by my family and colleagues during the compilation of this book.

Editor

1

Comparing Continuous and Intermittent Exercise: An "Isoeffort" and "Isotime" Approach

Andrea Nicolò, Ilenia Bazzucchi, Jonida Haxhi, Francesco Felici, Massimo Sacchetti*

Department of Human Movement, Social and Health Sciences, "Foro Italico" University, Rome, Italy

Abstract

The present study proposes an alternative way of comparing performance and acute physiological responses to continuous exercise with those of intermittent exercise, ensuring similar between-protocol overall effort (isoeffort) and the same total duration of exercise (isotime). This approach was expected to overcome some drawbacks of traditional methods of comparison. Fourteen competitive cyclists (20±3 yrs) performed a preliminary incremental test and four experimental 30-min self-paced protocols, i.e. one continuous and three passive-recovery intermittent exercise protocols with different work-to-rest ratios (2 = 40:20s, 1 = 30:30s and 0.5 = 20:40s). A "maximal session effort" prescription was adopted for this experimental design. As expected, a robust perceived exertion template was observed irrespective of exercise protocol. Similar between-protocol pacing strategies further support the use of the proposed approach in competitive cyclists. Total work, oxygen uptake and heart rate mean values were significantly higher ($P<0.05$) in the continuous compared to intermittent protocols, while lactate values were lower. Manipulating the work-to-rest ratio in intermittent exercise, total work, oxygen uptake and heart rate mean values decreased with the decrease in the work-to-rest ratio, while lactate values increased. Despite this complex physiological picture, all protocols showed similar ventilatory responses and a nearly perfect relationship between respiratory frequency and perceived exertion. In conclusion, our data indicate that overall effort and total duration of exercise are two critical parameters that should both be controlled when comparing continuous with intermittent exercise. On an isoeffort and isotime basis, the work-to-rest ratio manipulation affects physiological responses in a different way from what has been reported in literature with traditional methods of comparison. Finally, our data suggest that during intermittent exercise respiratory frequency reflects physiological strain better than oxygen uptake, heart rate and blood lactate.

Editor: Conrad P. Earnest, University of Bath, United Kingdom

Funding: This study received no external funding. The study was supported by the University of Rome "Foro Italico", Italy. The funders had no role in study design, data collection and analysis, decision to publish, or preparation of the manuscript.

Competing Interests: The authors have declared that no competing interests exist.

* E-mail: massimo.sacchetti@uniroma4.it

Introduction

The comparison of continuous (CON) with intermittent (INT) exercise is a central issue in sport science and exercise physiology. When low-volume INT is compared with CON, as well as when the two modes of exercise are compared on a work-matched basis, INT induces similar or even superior adaptations in a range of physiological, performance-related and health-related markers [1]. Moreover, INT is considered as being superior to CON in inducing further adaptations in already highly-trained endurance athletes [2].

Acute physiological responses to INT vs. CON have been extensively studied and traditionally compared on a work-matched basis [3–5]. However, work matching of training bouts when comparing CON and INT is highly inconsistent with descriptive data quantifying the actual training characteristics of successful endurance athletes across a broad range of sports [6]. Moreover, it induces unequal overall effort among different exercise protocols [7,8]. Indeed, using this kind of comparison, previous studies have reported that INT is more physiologically demanding than CON, as indicated by higher values of oxygen uptake (VO_2), heart rate (HR), minute ventilation (V_E), blood lactate (La^-) and rate of perceived exertion (RPE) [3–5]. Therefore, in order to ensure maximal physical stress in different exercise protocols (thus a comparable physiological demand), many authors have used time to exhaustion (TTE) protocols [9–13]. Nonetheless, apart from concerns about validity and reliability [14], a TTE protocol has the disadvantage of inducing high between-subject variability in TTE and hence heterogeneous physiological responses, both in CON [15] and in INT protocols [9–13]. Moreover, when comparing exercise protocols to exhaustion, considerably different total durations of exercise can be found [9,11–13], which can mask the real between-protocol differences in physiological responses.

As a solution to the above-mentioned problems, Seiler and colleagues [8,16,17] introduced a novel approach, called "iso-effort", for comparing various INT exercise protocols. This modality, extensively used to prescribe INT in athletic training [16,17], requires athletes to self-pace their exercise intensity in response to a prescription of "maximal session effort" [8], ensuring similar between-protocol overall effort [17]. They used this approach to investigate performance and physiological responses to INT protocols with different work durations [17], with different recovery time [16], as well as adaptations to different intensity and total work duration training regimens [8].

However, to the best of our knowledge, the "isoeffort" approach has never been used to compare either CON to INT exercise, or various INT protocols with different work-to-rest ratios. This was the aim of the present study. We compared performance and physiological responses in four cycling protocols, one CON and three INT with different work-to-rest ratios. The protocols were designed on an "isoeffort" basis and matched for total duration of exercise ("isotime"). We expected this matching modality to overcome some drawbacks of traditionally used methods of comparison, and thus provide novel insight into acute physiological responses to CON vs. INT.

Materials and Methods

Ethics Statement

All participants gave their written informed consent according to the declaration of Helsinki. For minors enrolled in the study, we obtained written informed consent from the next of kin. The experimental protocols were approved by the Ethics Committee of the University of Rome La Sapienza.

Subjects

Fourteen male subjects (mean ± SD: age 20±3 years, stature 1.76±0.07 m, body mass 64±7 kg) volunteered to participate in this study. All the subjects were well-trained [18] competitive cyclists with a minimum of 3 years' cycling experience and 350 km training per week. The subjects were asked to refrain from strenuous exercise, consumption of alcohol and caffeine for at least 24 h before each test.

Experimental Overview

All testing was completed in the laboratory with a room temperature of 20–21°C and at the same time of day (±2 h). Participants visited the laboratory on 5 occasions over a four-week period, with visits separated by at least 48 hours. In the first visit, subjects performed a preliminary ramp incremental exercise test. In the following visits, they performed four experimental cycling protocols, one CON and three INT protocols differing in the work-to-rest ratio. The experimental protocols were performed in a random order. All the cycling protocols were performed on an electromagnetically-braked cycle ergometer (Lode Excalibur Sport, Groningen, the Netherlands), whose settings were adjusted and recorded for each subject during the first visit to be reproduced in the following visits. Performance, physiological and perceptual responses were recorded during all the tests.

Preliminary Test

Before the ramp incremental test, the Borg 6–20 Rating of Perceived Exertion (RPE) scale was presented to subjects, and appropriate instructions about the interpretation and use of the scale were given according to established recommendations [19]. During the test, subjects were asked to express an RPE value every minute during exercise and immediately after exhaustion. RPE data from this test served for familiarization purposes and were not used for further analysis.

A 5 min warm-up at 100W, 2 min of rest and 3 min of unloaded pedaling preceded the incremental ramp exercise test to exhaustion, which consisted of a continuous ramped increase in work rate of 30 $W \cdot min^{-1}$, starting from 0W. Preferred pedaling cadence (94±3 rpm) was selected by each subject and was kept constant throughout the test, which terminated when cadence fell by more than 10 rpm, despite strong verbal encouragement. During the test, pulmonary gas exchange was measured breath-by-breath as described below. VO_2max was defined as the highest value of a 30-s average and the maximum power output of the test (Pmax) as the highest power output achieved at exhaustion, registered to the nearest 1 W. Breath-by-breath data were averaged over 10s and the first ventilatory threshold (VT1) was determined from a cluster of measures including 1) the first disproportionate increase in carbon dioxide output (VCO_2) from visual inspection of individual plots of VCO_2 versus VO_2, 2) an increase in V_E/VO_2 with no increase in V_E/VCO_2, and 3) an increase in end-tidal O_2 tension with no fall in end-tidal CO_2 tension. The second ventilatory threshold (VT2) was determined from a cluster of measurements including 1) the first disproportionate increase in minute ventilation (V_E) from visual inspection of individual plots of V_E versus VCO_2, 2) the first systematic increase in V_E/VCO_2, and 3) the first systematic decrease in end-tidal CO_2 tension [20]. The power output values corresponding to VT1 (PVT1) and VT2 (PVT2) were estimated with account taken of the mean response time of the VO_2 response, which was assumed to approximate 40s [20].

After recovering from exercise, subjects were familiarized with the linear mode of the ergometer used in the experimental protocols. In this modality, also called rpm-dependent mode, torque is linearly related to cadence, while power output is exponentially related to cadence. Subjects were required not to increase pedaling cadence excessively (keeping it at about 100 rpm) immediately before starting the work phase of INT protocols, so as to avoid rpm-dependent artifacts in power output.

Experimental Protocols

The experimental protocols, consisting of a CON and three INT protocols with different work-to-rest ratios (2 = 40:20s, 1 = 30:30s and 0.5 = 20:40s), were matched for total duration of exercise (30 min). In all the protocols, subjects were required to self-select their exercise intensity in response to a prescription of "maximal session effort" [8]. This approach was used to ensure similar between-protocol overall effort [17]. Recovery in INT protocols consisted of unloaded pedaling (with the ergometer in the hyperbolic mode). In line with previous studies adopting the linear mode in cycling [21], the α linear factor (indicating the slope of the relationship between torque and cadence) was set for each subject considering the 50% Δ (the power output halfway between PVT1 and Pmax, expressed in W) and the preferred cadence, according to the formula: $\alpha = 50\%\ \Delta/\text{preferred cadence}^2$. The linear factor was kept constant for each subject in the 4 experimental protocols. Given the fact that power output was rpm-dependent, this would allow subject to pedal at higher cadences during INT protocols compared to CON exercise. The fact that the freely chosen cadence adopted by competitive cyclists during INT formats similar to those investigated in the present study [11] is higher than the cadence reported during a 30-min CON time trial [22], supports our decision to keep the linear factor constant for each subject.

Prior to the experimental protocols, participants performed a standardized warm up consisting of 3 min at 100 W, 6 min at 50% Pmax, 1 min at 60% Pmax, two self-paced 10s submaximal sprints with 40 s recovery in between, and finishing with 1 min of pedaling at 100W. The experimental protocols were preceded by 3 min of unloaded pedaling and started with the work phase.

With the exception of elapsed time, no feedback on performance or physiological measurements and no encouragement, either during or after the cycling protocol, was given to participants to minimize external factor influence [14]. Power output, heart rate (HR), gas exchange parameters, minute ventilation (V_E) and respiratory frequency (f_R) were registered continuously during the cycling experimental protocols, while La^- and RPE were collected every three minutes. Blood lactate was also collected before the experimental protocols and 3 min post exercise.

Cardiopulmonary Parameters and Blood Lactate

Pulmonary gas exchange and ventilatory parameters were measured breath-by-breath using open-circuit indirect calorimetry (Quark b2, Cosmed, Rome, Italy). Appropriate calibration procedures were performed following the manufacturer's instructions.

Capillary blood samples were drawn from the earlobe and lactate was measured by a portable lactate analyzer (Lactate Pro, Arkray KDK, Japan).

Data Analysis

With the exception of power output, physiological parameters were averaged continuously during the intermittent exercise bouts and summarized as 3 min time epochs. Average power was calculated from work period only.

The maximum value of respiratory frequency (f_R) was defined as the highest 60s average (including rest periods in INT) for all the five protocols performed in this study.

The relationship between RPE and f_R was calculated for all the experimental protocols. A correlation between these two parameters was also obtained pooling together data from the 4 experimental protocols. Using the regression equation of this correlation, f_R (expressed as a % of the $f_R$max) was associated with the 15-point RPE scale.

Statistical Analysis

Statistical analyses were carried out with PASW statistics 18 (SPSS Inc, Chicago, Illinois, USA). A one-way repeated-measures ANOVA was used to analyze mean values of performance and physiological parameters. A two-way repeated-measures ANOVA was used to analyze performance and physiological parameters as a function of time. When the sphericity assumption was violated, the Greenhouse-Geisser adjustment was performed. When significant differences were found, the Bonferroni test was used to determine the origin of such differences. Linear regressions with Pearson's coefficient were used to establish the relationship between RPE/f_R, RPE/elapsed time and f_R/elapsed time respectively. Descriptors recommended by Hopkins [23] were used to express the magnitude of correlations. Alpha level was set at $P<0.05$ for all the statistical analyses performed. The results are expressed as mean (±SD).

Results

The VO_2max and the Pmax measured during the ramp incremental test were 4.3±0.3 L min^{-1} (67±6 ml kg^{-1} min^{-1}) and 434±34 W, respectively. PVT1 and VO_2 at VT1 were 213±24 W and 2.9±0.2 L min^{-1}, respectively. PVT2 and VO_2 at VT2 were 308±24 W and 3.7±0.2 L min^{-1}, respectively.

Table 1 reports mean values of several performance and physiological parameters for the 4 experimental protocols. Mean power output (considering only the work phase in INT protocols) was significantly different ($P<0.05$) in all cases (CON = 307±36, 40:20s = 400±35, 30:30s = 464±51 and 20:40s = 573±66 W). Total work was higher in CON compared to all INT protocols ($P<0.05$). In the INT protocols, total work decreased with the decrease in the work-to-rest ratio, with differences observed in all cases ($P<0.05$). Values expressed relative to CON total work were 87±3%, 76±3% and 62±3% for 40:20s, 30:30s and 20:40s, respectively (figure 1). Mean VO_2 was higher in CON and lower in INT, particularly for INT protocols with a lower work-to-rest ratio, and all the protocols differed to one another ($P<0.05$), with the exception of the comparison between CON and 40:20s, where a trend ($P=0.056$) was observed (table 1). Conversely, an opposite situation was observed for La^-, with the lowest values found in CON (5.8±2.5 mmol·L^{-1}) and the highest values in the 20:40s (9.5±2.2 mmol·L^{-1}). Significant differences ($P<0.05$) were observed for CON and 40:20s (7.2±2.7 mmol·L^{-1}) compared to 20:40s, and for 30:30s (8.5±2.4 mmol·L^{-1}) compared to CON. No between-protocol differences were found for mean values of f_R and V_E (table 1).

Figures 2 and 3 depict power output (considering only the work phase in INT), VO_2, La^-, VCO_2, RPE, f_R, HR and V_E as a function of time for the 4 experimental protocols. A significant protocol by time interaction was found for La^-, where a more rapid increase of La^- at the onset of exercise was observed for the three INT protocols compared to CON. A main effect of time was observed for all the parameters investigated, and a main effect of protocol was found for power output, VO_2, VCO_2, La^- and HR, but not for f_R, RPE and V_E. In particular, power output data showed a similar pacing strategy among the 4 protocols, and a robust, almost linear growth over time was found for RPE and f_R. Moreover, a significant ($P<0.01$), nearly perfect relationship was found between f_R and RPE for the 4 experimental protocols, as indicated by the correlation coefficients (CON = 0.91±0.08, 40:20s = 0.92±0.05, 30:30s = 0.93±0.07 and 20:40s = 0.91±0.08). The relationship between f_R and RPE was also nearly perfect when pooling together values of the 4 protocols (figure 4). In addition, a significant ($P<0.01$) nearly perfect relationship was found between RPE and elapsed time for the 4 protocols (CON = 0.93±0.04, 40:20s = 0.95±0.04, 30:30s = 0.96±0.04 and 20:40s = 0.93±0.04) and a significant ($P<0.01$) very large/nearly perfect correlation between f_R and elapsed time (CON = 0.87±0.11, 40:20s = 0.89±0.10, 30:30s = 0.92±0.05 and 20:40s = 0.87±0.19). No differences in f_R maximum values were found between the 5 protocols performed in this study (ramp = 54.8±7.4, CON = 57.6±5.8, 40:20s = 56.7±4.4, 30:30s = 57.8±5.9 and 20:40s = 54.8±5 breaths·min^{-1}).

Discussion

The present investigation proposes a new modality of comparing performance and physiological responses to continuous with those of intermittent exercise protocols, and highlights the importance of matching these protocols for both total duration of exercise and overall effort. On an "isoeffort" and "isotime" basis, the higher total work found in CON compared to INT indicates that in order to ensure similar between-protocol overall effort, the total work should be different in the two exercise modes. In addition, when manipulating the work-to-rest ratio with this approach we obtained a complex physiological picture that differs from the responses reported in literature with traditional methods of comparison [11,24–26]. Within this physiological framework, similar between-protocol responses of respiratory frequency, as well as a nearly perfect relationship with RPE in all the experimental protocols indicate that, during INT exercise, respiratory frequency reflects physiological strain better than the physiological parameters traditionally used.

In order to remove both between-subject and between-protocol variability in time to exhaustion, typical of TTE protocols [9–13], in the present study the total duration of exercise was fixed for all the protocols investigated. We also required athletes to self-select their exercise intensity in response to a prescription of "maximal session effort" [8]. This approach, called "isoeffort" [8], has the great advantage of ensuring similar overall effort among exercise

Table 1. Total work and mean values of several performance and physiological parameters for the four experimental protocols.

	CON	40:20s	30:30s	20:40s
Total work (kJ)	552±65	480±42 a	418±46 ab	344±40 abc
Power output (W)	307±36	267±23 a	232±25 ab	191±22 abc
Power output of work phase (W)	307±36	400±35 a	464±51 ab	573±66 abc
Pedaling cadence (rpm)	90±4	101±4 a	104±5 ab	109±5 abc
VO_2 (ml·min^{-1})	3655±382	3443±263	3147±234 ab	3000±307 abc
VO_2 (%VO_{2max})	85±6	80±5	75±6 ab	69±5 abc
HR (beats·min^{-1})	174±4	173±7	169±5 ab	164±7 abc
HR (%HR_{max})	91±3	90±3	88±3 ab	85±4 abc
La^- (mmol·L^{-1})	5.8±2.5	7.2±2.7	8.5±2.4 a	9.5±2.2 ab
f_R (breaths·min^{-1})	46±4	46±5	45±6	45±6
V_T (L)	2.52±0.44	2.50±0.41	2.56±0.49	2.53±0.46
V_E (L·min^{-1})	115±23	115±17	113±17	112±19

VO_2 = oxygen uptake; HR = heart rate; La^- = blood lactate; f_R = respiratory frequency; V_T = tidal volume; V_E = minute ventilation.
Values are expressed as mean ± SD. If not otherwise specified, recovery phases in INT are included. (a) $P<0.05$ vs. CON. (b) $P<0.05$ vs. 40:20s. (c) $P<0.05$ vs. 30:30s.

protocols [17], differently from the traditionally employed work-matching modality [8]. Developed on the basis of how INT exercise is prescribed in athletic training, the "isoeffort" approach has been adopted in only a few of the investigations focusing on INT [7,8,16,17]. In particular, to the best of our knowledge, it had never been used to compare either CON to INT exercise, or INT protocols differing in the work-to-rest ratio, as we have done in the present study.

Since we constrained the total duration of exercise to 30 min, the mean exercise intensity during the CON protocol approximated the VT2 intensity. It should be acknowledged that this is generally not representative of continuous training sessions, which are often performed by athletes at lower exercise intensities [6]. However, the unique design used in our study provides novel insights into physiological responses to continuous and intermittent exercise protocols, with important implications for exercise prescription. It could be argued that the comparison of different self-paced "isotime" protocols can be influenced by the pacing strategy adopted, but our data add the novel finding that competitive cyclists adopt a similar pacing strategy with a robust RPE template, irrespective of exercise protocol. This confirms the effectiveness of this approach in inducing similar between-protocol overall effort in well-trained athletes. In this perspective, the reason why the study that first proposed the term "isoeffort" [8] did not show similar between-protocol RPE values, is probably due to the adoption of considerably different total durations of exercise in various INT protocols. Nevertheless, Seiler et al. [8] demonstrated that the "isoeffort" approach allows for targeting

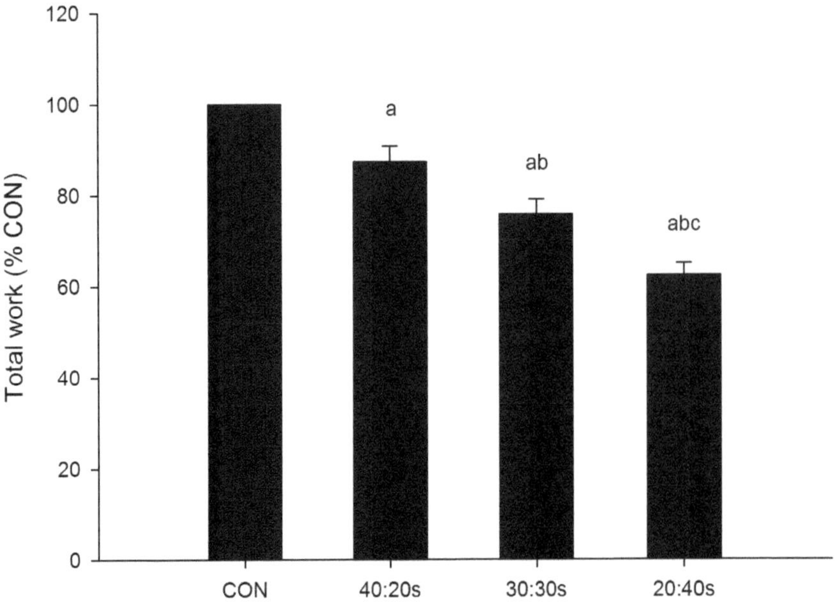

Figure 1. Total work. Total work expressed as a % of CON value, for the 4 experimental protocols. (a) $P<0.05$ vs. CON. (b) $P<0.05$ vs. 40:20s. (c) $P<0.05$ vs. 30:30s.

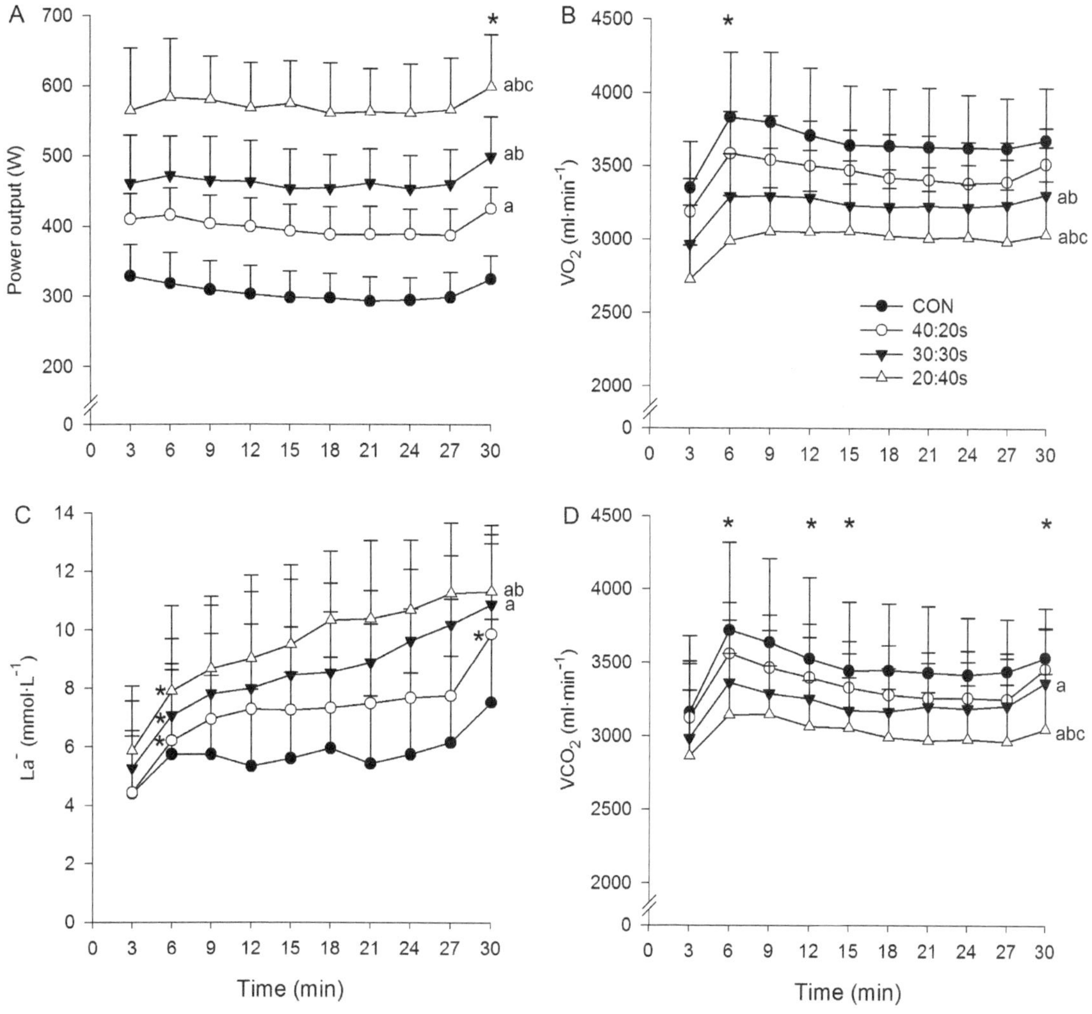

Figure 2. Power output, blood lactate and gas exchange parameters. Power output (work phase only in INT) (A), VO_2 (B), blood lactate (C) and VCO_2 (D) for CON (closed circles), 40:20s (open circles), 30:30s (closed triangles) and 20:40s (open triangles). Data points for gas exchange parameters result from a three minute average, including also the recovery periods in INT. Letters (a, b and c) report main effect of protocol. (a) $P<0.05$ vs. CON. (b) $P<0.05$ vs. 40:20s. (c) $P<0.05$ vs. 30:30s. Asterisks in the upper part of each graph report main effect of time, while asterisks near a data point indicate protocol by time interaction (found for La^-). *$P<0.05$ vs. the previous value.

specific physiological responses, contrasting previous observations [27].

On an "isoeffort" and "isotime" basis, our data demonstrate that CON enables athletes to accumulate considerably greater total work compared to INT. This is direct evidence that in order to provide similar between-protocol effort, total work should be higher in CON than in INT. In other words, this suggests that, when comparing different exercise protocols on a work-matched basis, researchers should be aware that they are comparing a more demanding INT protocol with a less demanding CON protocol. This is of particular importance, considering that the large body of evidence demonstrating similar or even superior adaptations after INT compared to CON training, mainly arises from studies that compare the two modalities on a work-matched basis [1].

Our data showed higher VO_2 values, but lower La^- values in CON compared to INT. In intermittent protocols, as the work-to-rest ratio decreased, the VO_2 decreased as well, while the La^- increased. In contrast, previous studies that investigated the effect of work-to-rest ratio manipulation on physiological responses [11,24–26] did not reveal an opposite trend in VO_2 and La^- responses (high VO_2– low La^- and viceversa). In fact, Ballor and Volovsek [24] compared three INT protocols with the same work and rest durations to those adopted in our study, with the difference that both the absolute work intensity and the total duration of exercise were fixed. They found that HR,V_E,VO_2 and blood lactate responses were higher in the 40:20s, lower in the 20:40s and in-between in the 30:30s. The discrepancy with our results can therefore be explained by the fact that they matched for total duration of exercise but not for overall effort, comparing a highly demanding 40:20s with a less demanding 30:30s and an even less demanding 20:40s. In a previous investigation [11], we also compared a 40:20s with a 30:30s INT with the same absolute exercise intensity, but the exercise was prolonged to exhaustion. In line with what is reported by Ballor and Volovsek [24], that study showed higher values of HR,V_E,VO_2 and blood lactate in the 40:20s compared to the 30:30s. On that occasion we matched for overall effort (maximal at the end of exercise), but the total duration of exercise was considerably longer in the 30:30s. Collectively, the differences between the previous and the present data indicate that overall effort and total duration of exercise are

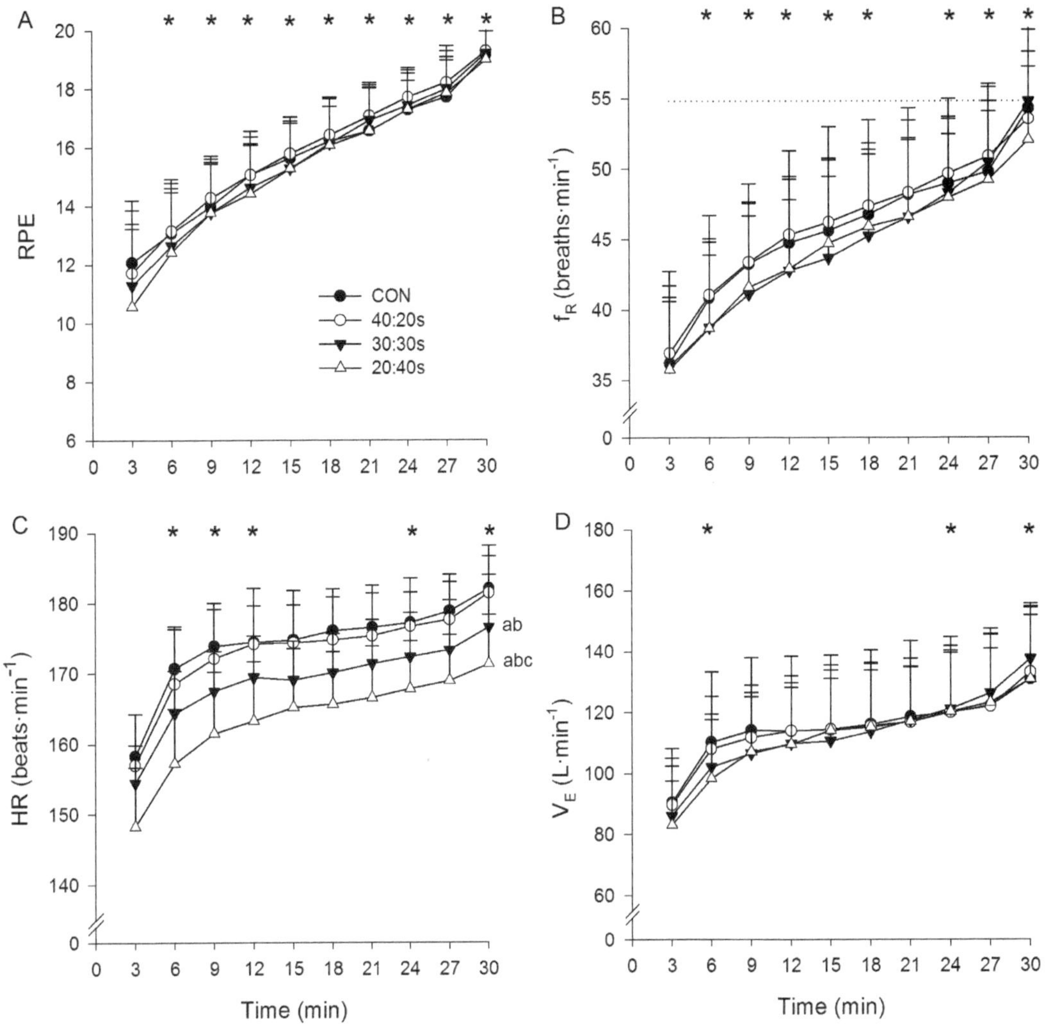

Figure 3. Perceived exertion, heart rate and respiratory parameters. RPE (A), f_R (B), HR (C) and V_E (D) for CON (closed circles), 40:20s (open circles), 30:30s (closed triangles) and 20:40s (open triangles). Data points for f_R, HR and V_E result from a three minute average, including also the recovery periods in INT. Dotted line in panel B indicate the f_R maximum value reached in the incremental ramp exercise test. Letters (a, b and c) report main effect of protocol. (a) $P<0.05$ vs. CON. (b) $P<0.05$ vs. 40:20s. (c) $P<0.05$ vs. 30:30s. Asterisks in the upper part of each graph report main effect of time. No protocol by time interaction was observed for the 4 variables. *$P<0.05$ vs. the previous value.

two crucial variables that have to be both controlled when investigating acute physiological responses.

From a practical viewpoint, it is interesting to note that the parameters generally used to monitor exercise intensity or physiological strain during CON exercise, i.e. power output, HR, VO_2 and La^- showed contrasting responses during INT exercise. Based on HR response alone which is the most used physiological parameter in the field [27], it could be concluded that as the work-to-rest ratio decreases the physiological demand of an exercise protocol decreases as well. Conversely, the analysis of the La^- response alone could lead coaches and researchers to exactly the opposite conclusion. It would therefore seem evident that none of the single cited parameters effectively reflects physiological strain during intermittent exercise. Despite this complex physiological picture, ventilatory parameters showed similar responses in the four investigated exercise protocols. While it is beyond the scope of this study to speculate on the mechanisms underlying such response, it is interesting to note that the common denominator between the protocols investigated seems to be a similar overall effort. In this view, it is even more interesting to consider that, beyond showing similar between-protocol responses, respiratory frequency showed an almost linear increase over time, as well as a nearly perfect relationship with RPE in all the experimental protocols. These data suggest that respiratory frequency reflects physiological strain irrespective of the CON or INT nature of the exercise.

Together with V_E, f_R is the physiological parameter that accounts for the greatest source of variance in RPE during continuous exercise [28]. In addition, f_R and RPE respond in a similar way to some experimental interventions such as prior exercise-induced muscle damage or fatigue [29,30] and exposure to a hot environment [31]. However, to the best of our knowledge, this is the first study that shows a strong relationship between the two parameters during intermittent exercise. While RPE is a widely recognized marker of intensity and homeostatic disturbance during exercise [32], the practice of using f_R as an exercise monitoring tool is not common, although promising. As a matter of fact, the linear relationship between f_R and RPE obtained in this study allowed us to put f_R values into an effort perspective (Figure 4). For instance, values of 80% and 88% of the f_R

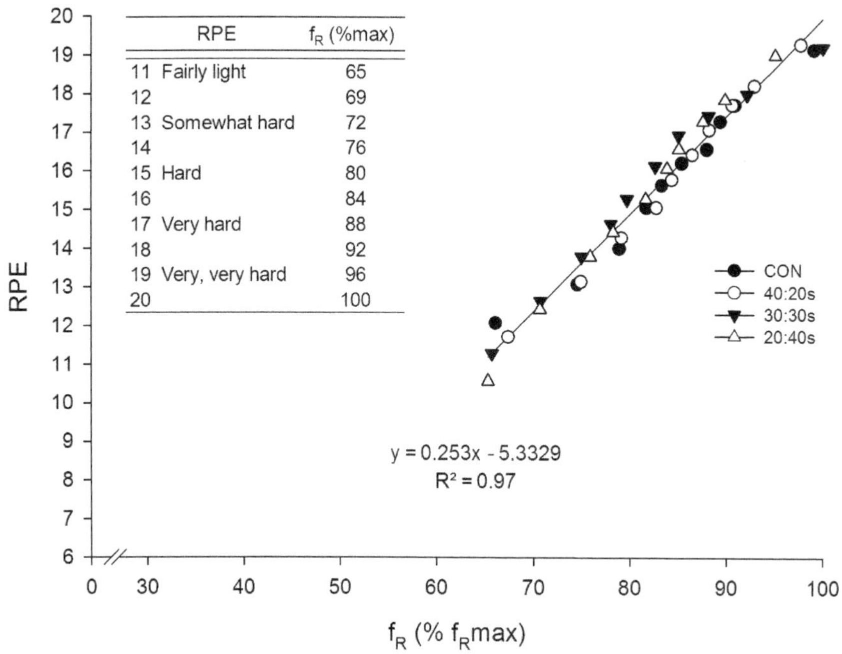

Figure 4. Relationship between perceived exertion and respiratory frequency. Relationship between RPE values and 3-min average values of f_R, expressed as a % of the f_R maximum value reached in the ramp incremental exercise test, for CON (closed circles), 40:20s (open circles), 30:30s (closed triangles) and 20:40s (open triangles). The linear regression results from pooling together data from the 4 experimental protocols. The regression equation of the relationship has been used to associate f_R with the 15-point RPE scale for the RPE range registered in this study (from 11 to 20), as shown in the upper left corner of the chart.

maximum value would correspond to an exercise effort perceived as hard and very hard, respectively. While it could be worthwhile obtaining an individualized relationship for each athlete, the association provided here can be used as a general guide for monitoring exercise sessions of both continuous and intermittent nature. Despite the similarities between RPE and f_R responses, they are two distinct parameters that could be used together for a psychophysiological understanding of exercise-induced fatigue. Nevertheless, one of the advantages in monitoring f_R over RPE is that it is an objective physiological parameter that can be measured continuously during exercise. RPE, on the other hand, is collected at discrete points in time and requires subjects to report their perception of effort, which is less practical, especially during competitions. Given the accuracy of relatively unobtrusive portable devices registering f_R [33], data provided in this study pave the way to possible utilization of f_R as a monitoring tool for physiological strain in the field, both during training and competition. This could be of particular value for exercises of an intermittent nature.

Conclusions

The present study indicates that overall effort and total duration of exercise are two critical parameters that should both be controlled when comparing continuous with intermittent exercise protocols. On an "isoeffort" and "isotime" basis, the work-to-rest ratio manipulation affects physiological responses in a different way from what previous studies with traditional methods of comparison report [11,24–26]. Despite a complex physiological framework, ventilatory parameters showed similar between-protocol responses. In particular, respiratory frequency showed an almost linear increase over time as well as a nearly perfect relationship with RPE in all the experimental protocols. These data suggest that, during intermittent exercise, respiratory frequency reflects physiological strain better than VO_2, HR and blood lactate.

Acknowledgments

The authors wish to thank Alessandra Conti for her skillful technical support.

Author Contributions

Conceived and designed the experiments: AN IB FF MS. Performed the experiments: AN IB JH MS. Analyzed the data: AN IB FF. Contributed reagents/materials/analysis tools: AN MS. Wrote the paper: AN IB JH FF MS.

References

1. Gibala MJ, Little JP, Macdonald MJ, Hawley JA (2012) Physiological adaptations to low-volume, high-intensity interval training in health and disease. J Physiol 590: 1077–1084.
2. Laursen PB, Jenkins DG (2002) The scientific basis for high-intensity interval training: optimising training programmes and maximising performance in highly trained endurance athletes. Sports Med 32: 53–73.
3. Astrand I, Astrand PO, Christensen EH, Hedman R (1960) Intermittent muscular work. Acta Physiol Scand 48: 448–453.
4. Edwards RH, Ekelund LG, Harris RC, Hesser CM, Hultman E, et al. (1973) Cardiorespiratory and metabolic costs of continuous and intermittent exercise in man. The Journal of physiology 234: 481–497.
5. Edwards RH, Melcher A, Hesser CM, Wigertz O, Ekelund LG (1972) Physiological correlates of perceived exertion in continuous and intermittent exercise with the same average power output. European journal of clinical investigation 2: 108–114.
6. Seiler S (2010) What is best practice for training intensity and duration distribution in endurance athletes? Int J Sport Physiol Perform 5: 276–291.

7. Sandbakk O, Sandbakk SB, Ettema G, Welde B (2013) Effects of intensity and duration in aerobic high-intensity interval training in highly trained junior cross-country skiers. J Strength Cond Res 27: 1974–1980.
8. Seiler S, Joranson K, Olesen BV, Hetlelid KJ (2013) Adaptations to aerobic interval training: interactive effects of exercise intensity and total work duration. Scand J Med Sci Sports 23: 74–83.
9. Billat VL, Slawinksi J, Bocquet V, Chassaing P, Demarle A, et al. (2001) Very short (15s-15s) interval-training around the critical velocity allows middle-aged runners to maintain VO2 max for 14 minutes. Int J Sports Med 22: 201–208.
10. Midgley AW, McNaughton LR, Carroll S (2007) Physiological determinants of time to exhaustion during intermittent treadmill running at vVO_2max. Int J Sports Med 28: 273–280.
11. Nicolò A, Bazzucchi I, Lenti M, Haxhi J, Scotto di Palumbo A, et al. (2014) Neuromuscular and Metabolic Responses to High-Intensity Intermittent Cycling Protocols with Different Work-to-Rest Ratios. Int J Sport Physiol Perform 9: 151–160.
12. Thevenet D, Tardieu-Berger M, Berthoin S, Prioux J (2007) Influence of recovery mode (passive vs. active) on time spent at maximal oxygen uptake during an intermittent session in young and endurance-trained athletes. Eur J Appl Physiol 99: 133–142.
13. Zafeiridis A, Sarivasiliou H, Dipla K, Vrabas IS (2010) The effects of heavy continuous versus long and short intermittent aerobic exercise protocols on oxygen consumption, heart rate, and lactate responses in adolescents. Eur J Appl Physiol 110: 17–26.
14. Currell K, Jeukendrup AE (2008) Validity, reliability and sensitivity of measures of sporting performance. Sports Med 38: 297–316.
15. Mann T, Lamberts RP, Lambert MI (2013) Methods of Prescribing Relative Exercise Intensity: Physiological and Practical Considerations. Sports Med 43: 613–625.
16. Seiler S, Hetlelid KJ (2005) The impact of rest duration on work intensity and RPE during interval training. Med Sci Sports Exerc 37: 1601–1607.
17. Seiler S, Sjursen JE (2004) Effect of work duration on physiological and rating scale of perceived exertion responses during self-paced interval training. Scand J Med Sci Sports 14: 318–325.
18. De Pauw K, Roelands B, Cheung SS, de Geus B, Rietjens G, et al. (2013) Guidelines to Classify Subject Groups in Sport-Science Research. Int J Sport Physiol Perform 8: 111–122.
19. Borg G (1970) Perceived exertion as an indicator of somatic stress. Scandinavian journal of rehabilitation medicine 2: 92–98.
20. Whipp BJ (2007) Physiological mechanisms dissociating pulmonary CO2 and O-2 exchange dynamics during exercise in humans. Experimental Physiology 92: 347–355.
21. Burnley M, Doust JH, Vanhatalo A (2006) A 3-min all-out test to determine peak oxygen uptake and the maximal steady state. Med Sci Sports Exerc 38: 1995–2003.
22. Foss O, Hallen J (2005) Cadence and performance in elite cyclists. Eur J Appl Physiol 93: 453–462.
23. Hopkins W (2002) A scale of magnitudes for effect statistics. Available: http://www.sportsci.org/resource/stats/effectmag.html. Accessed 10 January 2014.
24. Ballor DL, Volovsek AJ (1992) Effect Of Exercise To Rest Ratio On Plasma Lactate Concentration At Work Rates Above And Below Maximum Oxygen-Uptake. Eur J Appl Physiol Occup Physiol 65: 365–369.
25. Gosselin LE, Kozlowski KF, Devinney-Boymel L, Hambridge C (2012) Metabolic response of different high-intensity aerobic interval exercise protocols. Journal of strength and conditioning research/National Strength & Conditioning Association 26: 2866–2871.
26. Rozenek R, Funato K, Kubo J, Hoshikawa M, Matsuo A (2007) Physiological responses to interval training sessions at velocities associated with Vo_2max. J Strength Cond Res 21: 188–192.
27. Buchheit M, Laursen PB (2013) High-Intensity Interval Training, Solutions to the Programming Puzzle Part I: Cardiopulmonary Emphasis. Sports Med 43: 313–338.
28. Hampson DB, Gibson ASC, Lambert MI, Noakes TD (2001) The influence of sensory cues on the perception of exertion during exercise and central regulation of exercise performance. Sports Med 31: 935–952.
29. Davies RC, Rowlands AV, Eston RG (2009) Effect of exercise-induced muscle damage on ventilatory and perceived exertion responses to moderate and severe intensity cycle exercise. Eur J Appl Physiol 107: 11–19.
30. Marcora SM, Bosio A, de Morree HM (2008) Locomotor muscle fatigue increases cardiorespiratory responses and reduces performance during intense cycling exercise independently from metabolic stress. American Journal Of Physiology-Regulatory Integrative And Comparative Physiology 294: R874–R883.
31. Hayashi K, Honda Y, Ogawa T, Kondo N, Nishiyasu T (2006) Relationship between ventilatory response and body temperature during prolonged submaximal exercise. J Appl Physiol 100: 414–420.
32. Eston R (2012) Use of Ratings of Perceived Exertion in Sports. Int J Sport Physiol Perform 7: 175–182.
33. Kim JH, Roberge R, Powell JB, Shafer AB, Williams WJ (2013) Measurement Accuracy of Heart Rate and Respiratory Rate during Graded Exercise and Sustained Exercise in the Heat Using the Zephyr BioHarness (TM). Int J Sports Med 34: 497–501.

2

Prevalence of Different Head-Neck Positions in Horses Shown at Dressage Competitions and Their Relation to Conflict Behaviour and Performance Marks

Kathrin Kienapfel[1]*, Yvonne Link[2], Uta König v. Borstel[3]*

1 Department of Animal Ecology, Evolution and Biodiversity, Ruhr Universität Bochum, Bochum, Germany, **2** Institute of Animal Breeding and Husbandry, Christian-Albrechts University of Kiel, Kiel, Germany, **3** Department of Animal Breeding and Genetics, Georg-August-Universität Göttingen, Göttingen, Germany

Abstract

Much controversy exists among riders, and in particular among those practicing dressage, regarding what can be considered an "appropriate" Head-Neck-Position (HNP). The objective was to assess the prevalence of different HNPs in the field, the behavioural reactions of horses during warm-up and competition rides in relation to HNP and the relation between HNP and marks achieved in the competition. Horses (n = 171) were selected during dressage competitions according to their HNP (3 categories based on the degree of flexion), and their behaviour was recorded during 3 minutes each of riding in the warm-up area and in the competition. Scans were carried out on an additional 355 horses every 15 minutes to determine the proportion of each HNP in the warm-up area. Sixty-nine percent of the 355 horses were ridden with their nasal planes behind the vertical in the warm-up area, 19% were ridden at or behind the vertical and only 12% were ridden with their nasal plane in front of the vertical. Horses carrying their nasal plane behind the vertical exhibited significantly ($P<0.0001$) more conflict behaviours than horses with their nose held in front of the vertical. Horses were commonly presented with a less flexed HNP during competition compared to warm-up ($P<0.05$). A HNP behind the vertical was penalised with lower marks in the lower ($P = 0.0434$) but not in the higher ($P = 0.9629$) competition levels. Horses in higher classes showed more ($P = 0.0015$) conflict behaviour than those in lower classes. In conclusion, dressage horses are commonly ridden during warm-up for competitions with their nasal plane behind the vertical, and this posture seems to cause significantly more conflict behaviour than HNPs in front of the vertical.

Editor: Kim A. Bard, University of Portsmouth, United Kingdom

Funding: The authors acknowledge support by German Research Foundation and the Open Access Publication Funds of the Göttingen University. The funders had no role in study design, data collection and analysis, decision to publish, or preparation of the manuscript.

Competing Interests: The authors have declared that no competing interests exist.

* Email: Kathrin.Kienapfel@rub.de (KK); koenigvb@gwdg.de (UK)

Introduction

Riding styles, and in particular horses' postures during riding commonly are subject to welfare debates. While there is little doubt that riding horses with extremely elevated heads entails welfare issues [1], in the past years there has been much discussion regarding the so-called "classical" and the "modern" riding style. With regard to the HNP the "modern" riding technique is also referred to as rollkur, hyperflexion or LDR (Low, Deep and Round). It has been practiced at least as early as in the 17th century [2]. The "classical" riding style was summarized and codified in the German military regulations from 1912 [3]. These regulations include the rule that the horses' nasal plane should be slightly in front of the vertical.

Today both riding techniques are used. However, especially the "modern" technique is a controversial issue and there is an urgent need for an objective assessment of its implications. Pfeil-Rotermund & Zeeb emphasized in their study the expression and conflict behaviour of show jumping horses [4]. They showed that recording the influence of the rider on the horse with ethological methods is possible. Caanitz studied the horses' expressive behaviour at the beginning of their training as a result of the interaction between horse and rider [5]. She found, that horses which hold the nasal plane behind the vertical express more defensive behaviour than those carrying their nasal planes in front of the vertical. These results were confirmed by other studies [6,7,8]. Horses ridden in rollkur or LDR showed more signs of discomfort, such as tail-swishing, abnormal oral behaviour and ears fixed back, than horses ridden in "normal" poll flexion with the nasal plane mostly in front of the vertical, a posture also termed as "competition frame" [6,7]. Horses not only express higher levels of discomfort when ridden in rollkur-posture, they also avoided rollkur, if given the opportunity [6]. One study suggested that a reason for increased discomfort during rollkur may be the restricted vision [9]. The latter has also been held responsible for more pronounced fear reactions due to higher levels of arousal or anxiety in horses ridden in rollkur-positions compared with normal poll flexion [6].

The aim of the present study was to quantify behaviour patterns in horses competing at dressage competitions, and to assess potential differences between HNPs and competition levels. Of particular interest was the influence of HNP on the achieved mark in the competition. In view of the study of Pfeil-Rotermund & Zeeb, we expected a difference in conflict behaviours between levels of dressage [4].

Material and Methods

Ethics statement

This type of non-invasive, behavioural research is approved under the German animal protection act and does not require a study-specific permission. The authors did not manage or handle the horses in any way. Riders of the horses were not informed about the study as this information might have biased results. Researchers did not interfere in any way with riding styles, horses or riders, and all riding corresponded to the routine competition procedures. No additional activity was undertaken for the purpose of this study.

Pilot study

In order to assess the potential influence of bias in the observer from the main study, a pilot study was conducted on 29 horses from one dressage competition not included in the main study, using two different observers: one of these observers was familiar with horses, while the other was entirely unfamiliar with horses. However, as students of biology both were familiar with taking behavioural observations. The two observers were recruited in class at university, they provided written consent for the use of their observations in this study, and they thus knew that they were participating in research. Methods for behavioural observations were the same as described below, but observations were made only in the warm-up area. Also in contrast to the main study, but in accordance with an earlier study [7] HNPs were grouped only into two categories: the horse carries the nasal plane in front of the vertical or the horse carries the nasal plane behind the vertical. Due to data loss, observations from this pilot study could not be traced back to individual observers. Therefore, an additional part of pilot study was conducted. It included as observer the person from the main experiment as well as an additional observer unfamiliar with horses, who likewise provided written consent and knew that he was participating in research. Both persons observed the videos of 5 different horses during dressage competitions unrelated to those involved in the main experiment, but selected to include the full range of HNPs observed in the main study. Both observers used the same HNP classifications and ethogram as described for the main experiment. Inter-observer reliability for the total number of conflict behaviours as well as for the individual conflict behaviours tail-swishing, abnormal oral behaviour and change in gait was calculated based on variance components of a generalized linear mixed model analysis [7] using observer as a fixed factor and horse as a random factor. Inter-observer agreement for the categorical variable HNP, as well as for the behaviours with rare occurrence (all other behavioural variables) were assessed as percentage of agreement between the two observers.

Main study

During a total of 180 rides, dressage horses (n = 171) were observed at eleven local, national and international dressage events. Due to the convenience sampling, nine horses were observed twice during two independent rides. Horses varied in sex, age and breed, but were mostly warmbloods. They took part in different types of dressage classes at German levels A, L, M and S (approximately corresponding to novice, elementary, medium and advanced levels e.g. in the New Zealand classification system). Levels were combined into two groups with lower (A–L) and higher (M–S) dressage performance level. Observed rides were selected for the study based on horses' HNP during warm-up, with 30 horses each per HNP-class as described below within each of the two performance level groups (A–L and M–S). Horses were subjectively categorised into one of three possible HNPs:

- Nasal plane mostly in front of the vertical ("IV") (maximum flexion within a ride such that the nasal plane is at the vertical)
- Nasal plane slightly behind the vertical up to ten degrees ("AV") (minimum flexion within a ride such that the nasal plane is at the vertical)
- Nasal plane more than ten degrees behind the vertical ("BV")

Compared to the pilot study, the HNPs behind the vertical were further distinguished into two categories, to allow for a more accurate differentiation between different degrees of flexion.

The observation of the conflict behaviour and the HNPs was carried out during the phases of active riding, when the reins were short and the horse did not stand relaxed. In order to be assigned to one of the above categories, horses had to spend an approximate minimum of 95 percent of the three-minute interval in the respective HNP. Horses that were ridden less than three minutes continuously or with an unsteady, variable HNP, that did not fit clearly into one of the categories above, were excluded. The horses were observed live for 3 minutes in the warm-up area and again for the first 3 minutes of the test (starting immediately after the start signal). According to a previously validated method [8], during both observation periods, the frequency of individual behaviour patterns (table 1) potentially indicative of discomfort or conflict was recorded, and in addition the sum of all behaviour patterns calculated. From here on in the current text, these responses will be referred to as "conflict behaviour".

In a second part of the experiment, for a total of 26.25 hours, scan sampling every 15 minutes (105 times) was conducted on eight days of three dressage events. All horses (N = 355 in total) present at that time in the warm-up area were classified according to their HNP. These scans were made only during warm-up before the tests at the levels L, M and S.

Marks at the levels A and L are given on a scale from 1 to 10, while most of the marks given at levels M and S are reported in percent. Therefore, marks reported in percent were transformed (i.e. divided by ten) to obtain marks that are displayed on a comparable scale, and thus to allow for a combined analysis. All statistical analyses were conducted with SAS 9.2 (SAS Institute Inc., Cary, North Carolina, USA, 2009). With the exception of these marks (Kolmogorov-Smirnov: $P = 0.1110$), data were not normally distributed ($P < 0.05$). Therefore, marks were analysed with a mixed model accounting for repeated observations per horse. Frequencies of conflict behaviour were analysed with a generalized linear mixed model, assuming either an underlying Poisson (total number of conflict behaviour and tail-swishing), binary (head-tossing and bucking) or overdispersed Poisson (all other variables) distribution. Model fit was verified based on scaled Pearson statistics. In all cases, the effect of the fixed factors HNP (in front, at or behind the vertical) as well as the situation (warm-up or test; except for the analysis of marks), the level group (A/L and M/S) and their interactions were tested. The tukey-adjustment was used to adjust for multiple comparisons. With the analysis of the marks, in addition the numbers of behaviours observed during warm-up (total number only) and during the test (total number and individual conflict behaviour) were each considered in a separate analysis as a covariate. Fisher's exact test was used to assess separately by competition level group the

Table 1. Ethogram of the observed behaviour acts (adapted from [6], [8]).

Behaviours	Description
Tail-swishing	Fast movements of the tail
Ears fixed back	Ears are >5 sec fixed back
Head tossing	Fast up and down movement of the head
Mouth wide opened	The mouth is >3 sec. as wide open as the noseband permits
Showing teeth	Lips pulled back showing teeth for >3 sec.
Abnormal oral behaviour	Chewing with an open mouth, showing tongue
Nose tilting	The horse tilts its nose to one side
Going-against-reins	The horse pulls against the reins and breaks the line between elbow of the rider and rings of the bit
Change in gait	The horse changes the gait
Crabbing	Hind legs of the horse do not follow the track of the front legs
Attempts to buck	The horse shifts its weight on the front legs and moves the hind legs upwards

significance of deviations from expected percentages of HNPs during test situation in relation to HNP during warm-up.

Results

Pilot study

The independent observers classified 43.4% of the 29 observed horses to be ridden with an HNP in front of the vertical and 58.6% with the nasal plane behind the vertical. According to their observations, the horses ridden with an HNP in front of the vertical showed on average 10.6 behavioural acts as listed in table 1 per three minutes in the warm-up area, while the horses ridden with an HNP behind the vertical showed on average 23.3 behavioural acts. Inter-observer reliability for the total number of conflict behaviours was 0.99±0.01. For tail-swishing, abnormal oral behaviour and gait change it was 0.99±0.01, 0.90±0.10 and 0.43±0.46, respectively. Inter-observer agreement for head-tossing was 80%, and for the remaining conflict behaviours as well as HNP it was 100%.

Main study

Marks. The interaction between group level and HNP was significant ($P = 0.0002$) such that riders using a more flexed HNP were awarded lower marks in the lower levels (A/L), but not in the higher (M/S) levels (Figure 1). The total number of conflict behaviours shown during warm-up ($P = 0.2438$) or during the test ($P = 0.4236$) did not influence the marks. Of the individual conflict behaviours shown during the test, only the frequency of "going against the reins" tended to influence marks (−0.16±0.08 marks per additional occurrence of the behaviour pattern; $P = 0.0504$), and horses that bucked (5.8±0.52) tended to receive lower scores than horses that did not buck (6.7±0.09) during the test ($P = 0.0675$).

Behaviour. The total number of conflict behaviours was significantly influenced by the HNP ($P<0.0001$) and the level ($P = 0.0015$), but not by the situation (warm-up or test; $P = 0.5907$). Horses ridden "IV" showed significantly fewer conflict behaviours, compared to those in the categories "AV" or "BV" ($P<0.05$) (Figure 2). Horses in the higher levels (re-transformed least-square mean frequency of conflict behaviours per three minutes of riding: 12.5) showed significantly ($P = 0.0014$) more conflict behaviours compared to horses in the lower levels (9.3 behaviours). The interaction between HNP and level was not significant ($P = 0.2776$), indicating that the effect of the different HNPs was similar at both the lower and higher levels.

When considering the individual behaviour acts, the same trend of higher frequencies of conflict behaviour in more flexed HNPs can be observed (Figure 3). Only for mouth-opening, no significant ($P>0.1$) overall effect of HNP on frequencies of behavioural acts could be found. Head-tossing could not be statistically compared, because it was only observed in the category "BV". In addition to HNP, the situation influenced a number of individual behaviour acts. Loss of rhythm ($P = 0.0570$) and unusual oral behaviour ($P = 0.0240$) occurred more frequently during the test compared to the warm-up. Head-tilting ($P = 0.0243$) and ears pointed backwards ($P<0.0001$) occurred more frequently during warm-up compared to the test. Going against the reins was shown more often ($P<0.0001$) in the lower level (A/L: re-transformed least square mean frequency: 0.7 times/ride) compared to the higher level (M/S: 0.3 times/ride) horses, while tail-swishing was

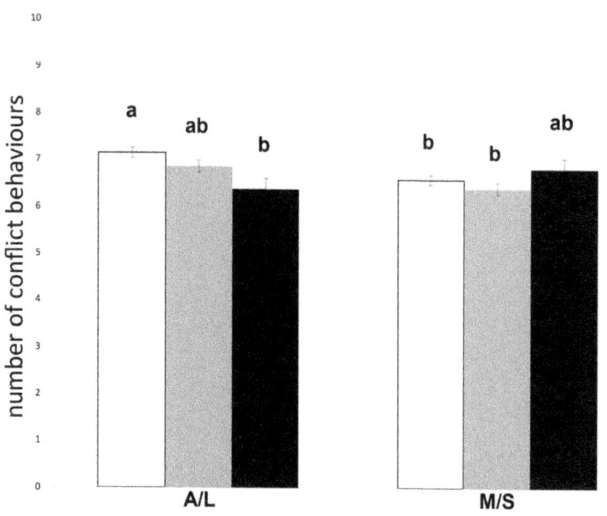

Figure 1. Marks: least square means (± SE) of dressage marks by level group (lower levels A and L versus higher levels M and S) and by head-neck position (white = nasal plane in front of the vertical, grey = nasal plane at the vertical, black = nasal plane behind the vertical). Different letters a,b indicate statistically significant differences at P<0.05.

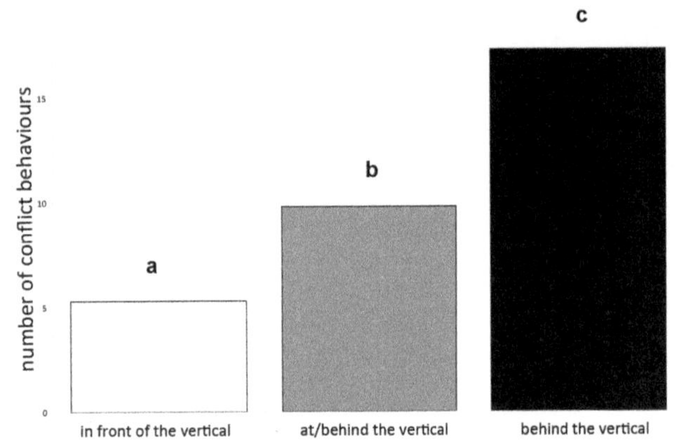

Figure 2. Behaviour: mean (re-transformed least square means) total frequency of conflict behaviour per 3-min. ride depending on the head-neck position (white = nasal plane in front of the vertical, grey = nasal plane at the vertical, black = nasal plane behind the vertical). Different letters a,b,c indicate significant differences at P<0.0001.

shown approximately twice as often in the higher-level horses (10.1) compared to the lower level horses (5.8; P<0.0001).

Change in head-neck position from warm-up to competition. Both for lower (Fisher's exact test: P<0.0001) and higher (Fisher's exact test: P=0.0479) level horses, the distribution of HNPs during competition deviated significantly from that expected by chance (i.e. an equal distribution). Regardless of the HNP used during warm-up, riders rarely (A/L: 11%; M/S: 3% of the observed rides) presented their horses during competition with a HNP BV (Figure 4). Instead, in more than half of the rides (A/L: 53%; M/S: 54% of the observed rides) horses were presented during competition with an HNP in front of the vertical. In particular, those riders who warmed-up their horses with an HNP in front of the vertical, rarely made changes to this HNP when entering the competition (in 87% (A/L) and 80% (M/S) of these rides the HNP remained unchanged in front of the vertical).

Scans, frequency of hyperflexion. Of the 355 horses observed during warm-up, 11.9% were ridden with their nasal planes in front of the vertical. Only 18.7% of the horses were ridden with an HNP at the vertical, and 69.4% of the horses were ridden with an HNP behind the vertical (Figure 5).

Discussion

Regardless of the competition level, horses exhibited more conflict behaviours the more the head was kept behind the vertical. Other studies obtained similar results, supporting the assumption that a strongly flexed HNP is perceived by horses as uncomfortable [6,8,9,11]. Contrary to claims by some practitioners and/or scientists (e.g [30]), the lack of an interaction between HNP and level indicates that a strongly flexed HNP has similar effects on the horse, regardless of whether it is achieved by a more or a less proficient rider.

Tail-swishing may be due to different reasons. In a completely "natural" environment it is a defense reaction to flies. But an unusual infestation of flies as an explanation for tail-swishing in certain horses can be ruled out, because all horses were exposed to the same conditions. Tail-swishing can also be a reaction to the use of spurs and a whip [12]. Therefore its increased frequency in horses ridden with an HNP more strongly behind the vertical can be an indication that these horses are exposed more often to the forceful actions of legs, spurs and whips, as also observed in the study by von Borstel *et al.* [6]. Taken together, these findings indicate that horses with a more strongly flexed HNP may be ridden in a more aggressive fashion [8]. In addition tail-swishing is linked to situations of fear and pain [12]. Another study showed that a very low, deep, round HNP induces a state of heightened arousal or anxiety, and in that study tail-swishing also occurred more frequently during hyperflexion [6]. According to McGreevy tail-swishing seems to be a typical response to a conflict [10]. Generally, shortening the reins (as required to achieve a hyperflexed HNP) leads to higher rein tensions [11]. Since increases in rein tension are used as a stop signal the simultaneous increase in the use of whip and spurs, which are mainly used as "go" signals, are likely to induce such a state of conflict in the horse [13]. Kienapfel found "mouth wide open" to be the second most frequent behaviour [8]. This result could not be confirmed in the present study. Potentially the routine use of tight nosebands prevented the horses from showing this behavioural act more frequently [14,15]. In another study, 47% of jumping horses had the nosebands fastened so tight, that no finger fitted between the leather and the nasal bone [16], i.e. considerably tighter than the allowed minimum of two fingers. For dressage horses, unfortunately no comparable data are available yet.

The increase of gait changes and loss of rhythm and regularity of gait could likewise be an indicator for dissonant riding aids. Another explanation may be found in the principles of locomotor mechanics of the horses. A flexion of the horse's neck modifies the gaits [17,18,19]. This may be because of or in addition to the higher physiological "workload" in hyperflexion [20]. Whether the workload is so high, that changes in gait and loss of rhythm and regularity are correlated, remains to be examined.

Becker-Birck et al. found no differences in the behaviour of lunged horses without riders in different HNPs, where the HNPs were achieved with draw reins [21]. The same pattern occurred in the study of Kienapfel [22]. Horses, which were lunged in different HNPs showed subjectively few signs of discomfort in the hyperflexed position. In our study and other studies without draw reins, the opposite effect could be seen [6,8,9]. Becker-Birch's observation is possibly an effect of "learned helplessness" [21]; all horses were used to draw reins at lunging and had possibly learned that there is no way to avoid the adjusted HNP.

Many riders prepared their horses with the nasal plane "BV", but the prevalence was significantly lower during competition, indicating that the majority of riders might be aware of what is the correct HNP according to the guidelines. Apparently the riders pay more attention to HNP of their horses when under the eyes of the judges. Potentially, riders also perceive their horse to be more relaxed or willing during competition, when they release their horse from a more flexed HNP during warm-up to a less flexed HNP just before the start of the test. In particular when horses were ridden with the head "BV" in the warm-up area, riding style changed markedly in competition. Only 23.3% of the horses at levels A and L were ridden during competition in the same way as in the warm-up area. This group of less advanced riders might not have the feeling for the right head position, or their teachers do not correct this way of riding. At levels M and S, 6.7% of the riders presented their horses in the competition with the horse's head "BV". Riders at these levels supposedly know that riding in a HNP behind the vertical should, according to the FEI-guidelines ("The head should remain in a steady position, as a rule slightly in front of the vertical, with a supple poll as the highest point of the neck, and no resistance should be offered to the Athlete." [22]) lead to lower marks for their performance, which may be the reason for

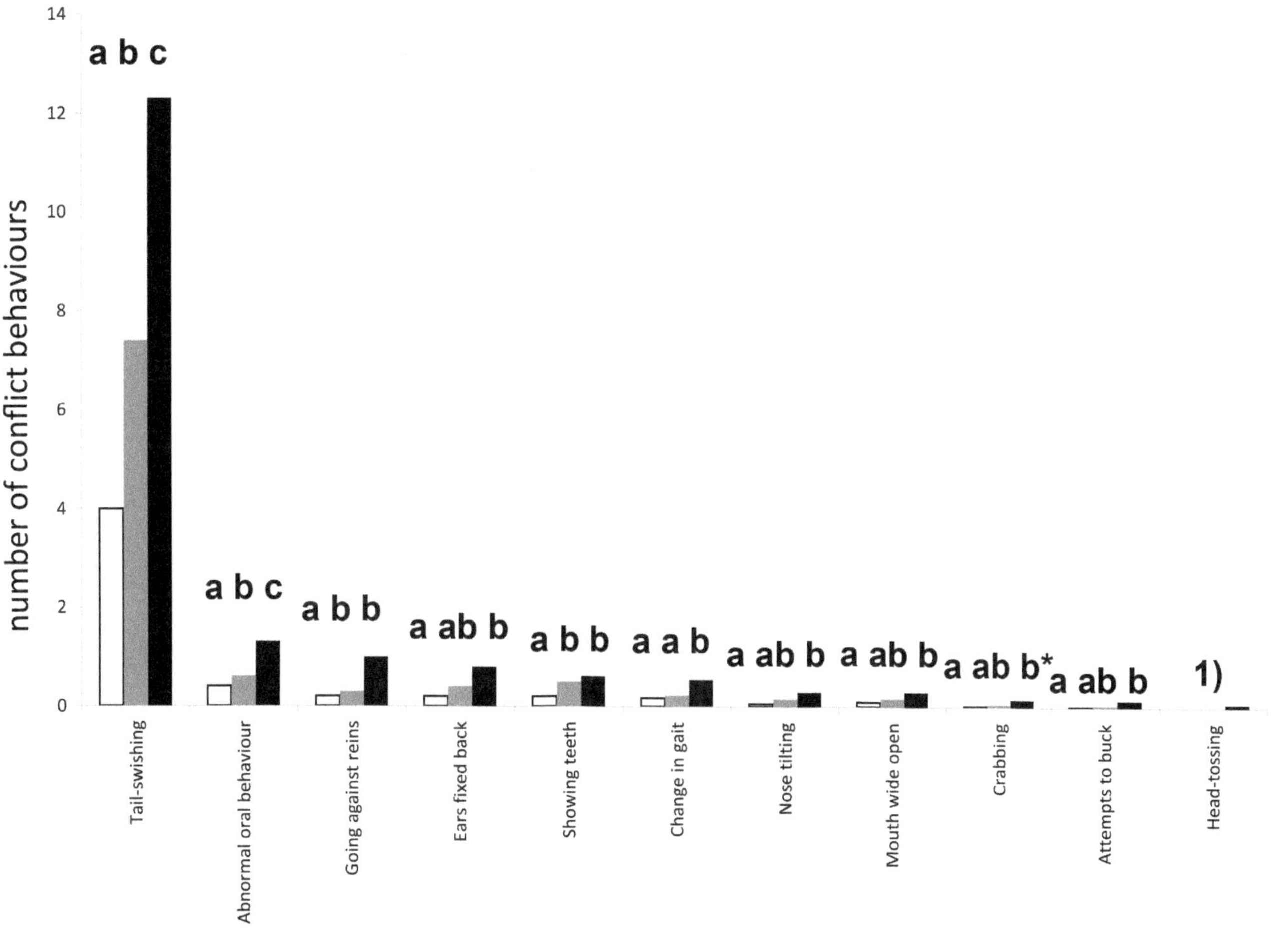

Figure 3. Individual conflict behaviour: mean (re-transformed least square means) frequency of individual conflict behaviour per 3-min. ride depending on the head-neck position with the nasal planes in the respective categories. Different letters a,b,c indicate statistically significant differences at P<0.05 (*P<0.1). 1) Effect not estimable due occurrence in just one category (HNP behind the vertical).

them to change the HNP in the competition. Interestingly, according to our results judges appeared to penalize deviations in the HNP from the ideal with lower marks in the lower, but not in the higher classes according to the guidelines. Although the low proportion of strongly flexed HNPs during competition in the higher levels may partially bias results, these findings raise the question whether judges potentially pay less attention to such aspects in the higher classes. Considering that riders in the higher levels serve as examples, if not idols, for riders of the lower classes, these findings are rather alarming. It seems difficult to justify, why rules are applied differently to riders of higher and lower levels.

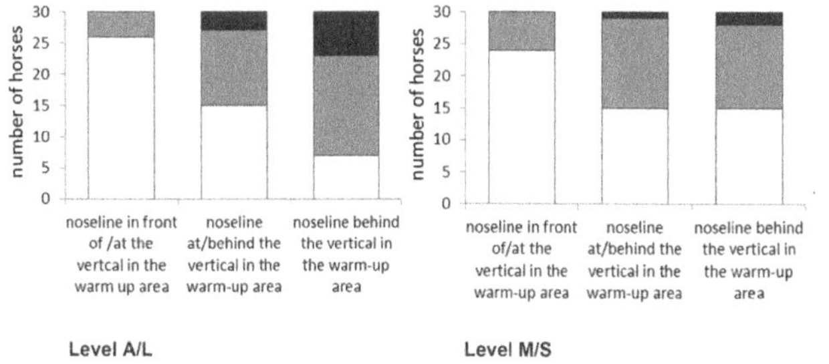

Figure 4. Distribution of head-neck-positions: distribution (number of horses) of head-neck positions (HNP) in competition by HNP in the warm-up area. HNP in competition: white = nasal plane in front of the vertical, grey = nasal plane at the vertical, black = nasal plane behind the vertical. At both group levels, HNP distributions deviated significantly from chance, with more riders than expected presenting their horses in competition with an HNP in front of the vertical (A/L: P<0.0001, M/S: P = 0.0479).

Marks

Riding style in the warm-up area did not influence marks obtained in competition. Therefore, a warm-up with a HNP BV either does not lead to lasting tensions in the horses that would compromise performance in competition, even if the riders then changed to a less restrictive HNP, or judges do not penalize this potential tension. Plewa explained that a short and tight neck resulting in a lack of relaxation, change in gaits and the horse's behaviour can influence the mark [23]. However, this influence on marks could not be detected in the present study. The general lack of influence of the frequency of conflict behaviour on marks is likewise an alarming finding. Either, judges ignored these behavioural signs of discomfort or horses' discomfort is associated antagonistically with other parameters of performance.

In competitions at level S the marks for "suppleness" (how the horse reacts to the rider aids) and "contact" (connection to the horses' mouth) are the most variable marks in the final grading [24]. Suppleness is thought to be a sign of a content horse and

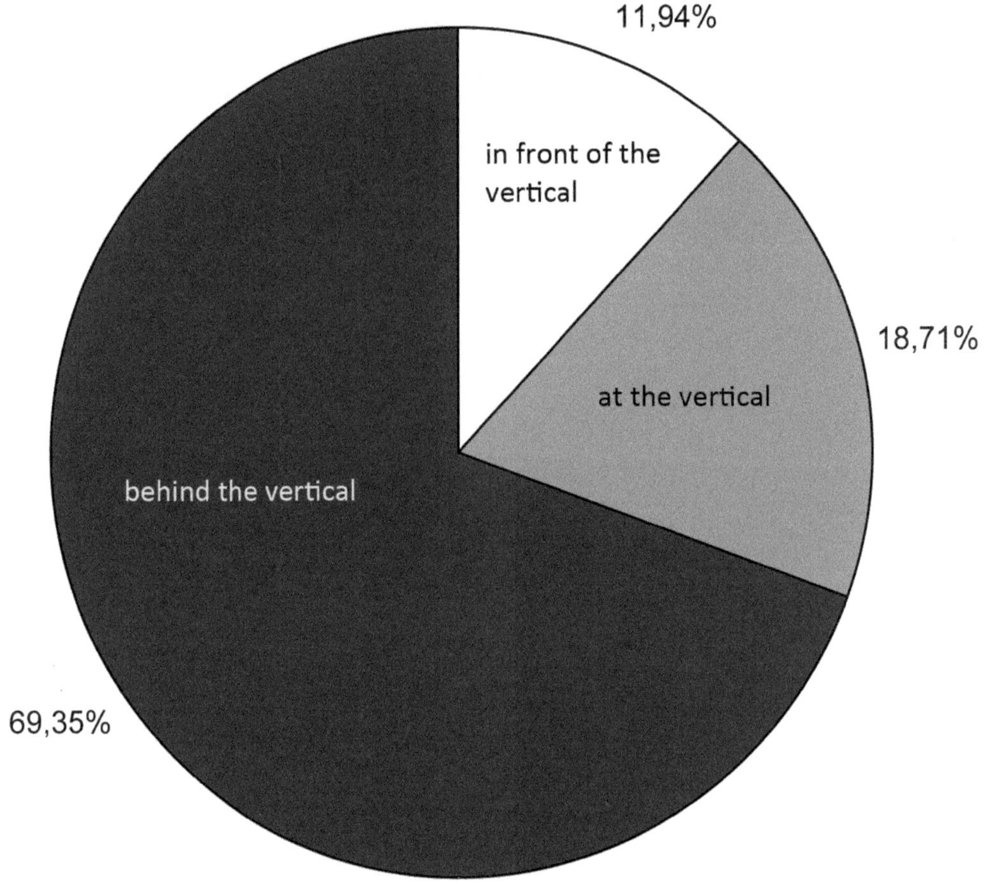

Figure 5. Behavioural Scans: proportions of horses ridden with the different Head-Neck-Positions with the nasal planes in the respective categories at the warm-up area.

therefore should be connected with low levels of discomfort, so assessing these relationships based on detailed marks would be interesting for future studies.

Also, overall marks improve with a longer preparation time [25]. Specifically which aspects are affected by preparation time, and if there is a relationship between the specific marks for suppleness and preparation time has yet to be studied.

Levels

According to earlier studies, in show-jumping [4], as well as in dressage and western [26] horses in lower classes show more conflict behaviour than horses in higher classes. In contrast, in the present study as well as in the dressage horses observed by Pfeil-Rotermund & Zeeb [4], the frequency of conflict behaviour increased with higher levels. The assumption that incorrect riding aids [4] and thereby the less correct application of learning theory [26] in lower level riders induced the defensive behaviour, does not seem to be applicable for the competition context as studied in the present study as well as in the study by Pfeil-Rothermund and Zeeb [4]. Rather, it seemed to be that during competitions, the riders in higher classes rode much more aggressively, thus outweighing any beneficial effects of an improved seat and a more controlled application of riding aids. Measures of spur and whip use could be included in future research to investigate these aspects further.

Scans

Although in an earlier study, Kienapfel used only two different HNPs to group horses in warm-up areas, her results are comparable and in agreement with the present study [8]. She observed that 92.8% of the horses belonged in the group "BV". Comparable to this group are all horses with the nasal plane "BV" and "AV" of the present study, which comprised 88.06% of all horses in the warm-up areas.

These results are backed by studies showing that photographs of horses advertised for sale in magazines or trading websites, were presented in 68% [27] and 70% [28] of the cases, respectively, with their nasal planes behind the vertical. Presumably, these horses were presented at their best according to the vendors' point of view [28].

In summary, approximately 90% of all dressage horses are ridden in the warm-up area with the nasal plane BV, i.e. a style which does not conform with the rules of the FEI (FEI-Rules, Chapter 1, Article 401, 5).

Method

As there was only one observer in the present study and because the observer was not blinded to the HNP group, observer bias might have been present, posing some constraints to the present study. On the other hand, results from the pilot study suggest that other observers, including two entirely unfamiliar with horses, obtain similar results. With the exception of gait change, which may be difficult to recognize for people unfamiliar with horses, inter-observer reliability and inter-observer agreement was very high, and indeed generally higher than inter-observer reliabilities from other behavioural research in horses [29,30,31]. Therefore, these results suggest that any observer bias, if present, was of limited extent. However, in future studies that include observations of the conflict behaviour "gait change", particular attention should be paid to this behaviour, which may require a more thorough definition to allow also laypersons to identify it correctly.

Conclusions

Results of the present study indicate that horses are frequently ridden at dressage competitions with an HNP behind the vertical, although more commonly so during warm-up compared to the competition itself. Such a flexed HNP is penalized with lower marks in the lower, but not in the higher competition levels. Furthermore, the current results indicate that horses show conflict behaviour more frequently when ridden with an HNP behind the vertical rather than at or in front of the vertical. Since this effect was observed regardless of the competition level, it is suggested that the flexed posture itself rather than the rider's skills or the training level of the horse is the main factor inducing conflict behaviour.

Acknowledgments

Sincere thanks to Prof. Holger Preuschoft for his tireless support and advice for this study ! Many thanks to Lisa Eschner, Jonas Henske and Dennis Henseleit for their time and effort in taking the behavioural observations for the pilot study. Finally we would also like to express our gratitude to the reviewers who considerably helped with their comments to improve the manuscript!

Author Contributions

Conceived and designed the experiments: KK YL. Performed the experiments: YL. Analyzed the data: YL UK KK. Contributed reagents/materials/analysis tools: YL KK. Contributed to the writing of the manuscript: YL KK UK.

References

1. Lesimple C, Fureix C, Menguy H, Hausberger M (2010) Correction: Human Direct Actions May Alter Animal Welfare, a Study on Horses (*Equus caballus*). PLoS ONE 5 (4): e10257. doi:10.1371
2. Cavendish W (1667) A new Method, and extraordinary invention, to dress horses, and work them according to nature. London: Tho. Milbourn.
3. HDV (1937) Heeresdienstvorschrift. Herford: Mittler.
4. Pfeil-Rotermund S, Zeeb K (1994) Zum Ausdruckverhalten von Springpferden. In: KTBL-Schriften Vertrieb, editors. KTBL-Schrift 281 Arbeiten zur artgemäβen Tierhaltung 1994: Münster-Hiltrup. p. 231–239.
5. Caanitz H (1996) Ausdrucksverhalten von Pferden und Interaktion zwischen Pferd und Reiter zu Beginn der Ausbildung. Dissertation Tierärztliche Hochschule Hannover
6. von Borstel UU, Duncan IJH, Shoveller AK, Merkies K, Keeling LJ, et al. (2009) Impact of riding in a coercively obtained Rollkur posture onwelfare and fear of performance horses. Applied Animal Behaviour Science 116: 228–236.
7. König von Borstel U, Glißmann C (2014) Alternatives to conventional evaluation of rideability in horse performance tests: suitability of rein tenions and behavioural parameters. PLoS ONE 9: e87285.
8. Kienapfel K (2011) Und was meinen die Pferde dazu? Über das Ausdrucksverhalten von Pferden bei verschiedenen Halsstellungen. Pferdeheilkunde 27: 372–380.
9. van Dierendonck M, van Dalum M, Beekmans M, Christensen JW (2012) Acute stress response of dressage horses ridden in three different head and neck positions. In: Randle H, Waran N, Williams J, editors. 8th International Equitation Science Conference: Edinburgh.p 62.
10. McGreevy P (2004) Equine Behaviour: A guide for veterinarians and equine scientists. Edinburg, London, New York, Oxford, Philadelphia, St Louis, Sydney, Toronto: Saunders.
11. Ludewig AK, Gauly M, König v Borstel, U (2011) Effect of shortened reins on rein tension, stress and discomfort behaviour in dressage horses. In: Van Dierendonck M, de Cocp P, Visser K, editors. Proceedings of the 7th International Equitation Science Conference, Hooge Mierde, Netherlands: Wageningen Academic Publishers.
12. Zeitler-Feicht MH (2008) Handbuch Pferdeverhalten. Stuttgart: Eugen Ulmer.
13. McLean A, McGreevy PD (2010) Horse-training techniques that may defy the principles of learning theory and compromise welfare. Journal of Veterinary Behavior: Clinical Applications and Research 5: 187–195.
14. McGreevy P, Warren-Smith A, Guisard Y (2012) The effect of double bridles and jaw-clamping crank nosebands on temperature of eyes and facial skin of horses. Journal of Veterinary Behavior: Clinical Applications and Research 7: 142–148.
15. Kienapfel K, Preuschoft H (2010) Viel zu eng! Über die Verschnallung der Nasenriemen. Pferdeheilkunde 26: 178–185.
16. Doherty O, Casey V, McGreevy P, Conwa R, O'Muiris E, et al. (2013) Two methods of measuring in- vivo pressures applied by a cavesson noseband. In: Heleski C, Wickens C, editors. 9th International Equitation Science Conference Proceedings. Newark: University of Delaware. p. 38.
17. Gómez Álvarez CB, Rhodin M, Bobbert M F, Meyer H, Weishaupt MA, et al. (2006) The effect of head and neck position on the thoracolumbar kinematics in the unridden horse. Equine Veterinary Journal 38: 445–451.
18. Weishaupt MA, Wiestner T, von Peinen K, Waldern N M, Roepstorff L, et al. (2006) Effect of head and neck position on vertical ground reaction forces and interlimb coordination in the dressage horse ridden at walk and trot on a treadmill. Equine veterinary Journal 36: 387–392.
19. Waldner NM, Wiestner T, von Peinen K, Gómez Álvarez CG, Roepstorff L, et al. (2009) Influence of different head-neck positions on vertical ground reaction forces, linear and time parameters in the unridden horse walking and trotting on a treadmill. Equine veterinary Journal 41: 268–273.
20. Wijnberg ID, Slentjens J, van der Kolk JH, Back W (2010) Effect of head and neck position on outcome of quantative neuromuscular diagnostic techniques in warmblood riding horses directly following moderate exercise. Equine veterinary Journal 42: 261–267.
21. Becker-Birck M, Schmidt A, Wulf M, Aurich J, von der Wense A, et al. (2013) Cortisol release, heart rate and heart rate variability, and superficial body temperature, in horses lunged either with hyperflexion of the neck or with an extended head and neck position. Journal of Animal Physiology and Animal Nutrition 97: 322–330.
22. Kienapfel K (2014) The effect of three different head–neck positions on the average EMG activity of three important neck muscles in the horse. Journal of Animal Physiology and Animal Nutrition (in print) Fédération Equestre Internationale Reproduction (2011) FEI Dressage Rules, Switzerland, pp. 10.
23. Plewa D (2006) Der Einfluss der Beizäumung auf die Bewertung durch den Dressurrichter. Progress in Equine Sports Medicine. Pferdeheilkunde 22: 700–702.
24. Hawson LA, McLean AN, McGreevy PD (2010) Variability of scores in the Olympic dressage competition and implications for horse training and welfare. Journal of Veterinary Behaviour 5: 170–176.
25. Murray RC, Mann S, Parkin TDH (2006) Warm-up in dressage competions: association with level, completion type and final score. Equine Comparative Exercise Physiology 3: 185–189.
26. König von Borstel U, Kassebaum L, Gauly M (2011) Effect of discipline (Western vs Dressage) and skill level on learning and discomfort behaviour of riding horses. In: Van Dierendonck M, de Cocp P, Visser K, editors. Proceedings of the 7th International Equitation Science Conference, Hooge Mierde, Netherlands: Wageningen Academic Publishers, p 75.
27. McGreevy PD, Harman A, McLean A, Hawson L (2010) Over-flexing the horse's neck: A modern Equestrian obsession? Journal of Veterinary Behaviour: Clinical Applications and Research 5: 180–186.
28. Hutchings K, Randle H (2013) Is horse head position used as an indicator of training in advertisements? In: Heleski C, Wickens C, editors. 9th International Equitation Science Conference Proceedings. Newark, USA: University of Delaware, p 79.
29. McGrogan C, Hutchison MD, King JE (2008) Dimensions of horse personality based on owner and trainer supplied personality traits. Applied Animal Behavior Science 113: 206–14.
30. McDonnell SM, Diehl NK (1990) Computer-assisted recording of live and videotaped horse behavior: reliability studies. Applied Animal Behavior Science 27: 1–7.
31. König v Borstel U, Pirsich W, Gauly M, Bruns E (2012) Repeatability and reliability of scores from ridden temperament tests conducted during performance tests. Applied Animal Behavior Science 2012;139: 251–63.

3

Numerical Relations and Skill Level Constrain Co-Adaptive Behaviors of Agents in Sports Teams

Pedro Silva[1]*, Bruno Travassos[2], Luís Vilar[3,4], Paulo Aguiar[5], Keith Davids[6,7], Duarte Araújo[4], Júlio Garganta[1]

1 CIFI2D - Centre for Research, Education, Innovation and Intervention in Sport, Faculdade de Desporto, Universidade do Porto, Porto, Portugal, **2** CIDESD, Department of Sport Sciences, Universidade da Beira Interior, Covilhã, Portugal, **3** Faculty of Physical Education and Sports, Lusófona University of Humanities and Technologies, Lisboa, Portugal, **4** CIPER, Faculdade de Motricidade Humana, Universidade de Lisboa, Cruz Quebrada Dafundo, Lisboa, Portugal, **5** Centre for Mathematics, Faculdade de Ciências, Universidade do Porto, Porto, Portugal, **6** Centre for Sports Engineering Research, Sheffield Hallam University, Sheffield, United Kingdom, **7** FiDiPro Programme, University of Jyväskylä, Jyväskylä, Finland

Abstract

Similar to other complex systems in nature (e.g., a hunting pack, flocks of birds), sports teams have been modeled as social neurobiological systems in which interpersonal coordination tendencies of agents underpin team swarming behaviors. Swarming is seen as the result of agent co-adaptation to ecological constraints of performance environments by collectively perceiving specific possibilities for action (affordances for self and shared affordances). A major principle of invasion team sports assumed to promote effective performance is to outnumber the opposition (creation of numerical overloads) during different performance phases (attack and defense) in spatial regions adjacent to the ball. Such performance principles are assimilated by system agents through manipulation of numerical relations between teams during training in order to create artificially asymmetrical performance contexts to simulate overloaded and underloaded situations. Here we evaluated effects of different numerical relations differentiated by agent skill level, examining emergent inter-individual, intra- and inter-team coordination. Groups of association football players (national – NLP and regional-level – RLP) participated in small-sided and conditioned games in which numerical relations between system agents were manipulated (5v5, 5v4 and 5v3). Typical grouping tendencies in sports teams (major ranges, stretch indices, distances of team centers to goals and distances between the teams' opposing line-forces in specific team sectors) were recorded by plotting positional coordinates of individual agents through continuous GPS tracking. Results showed that creation of numerical asymmetries during training constrained agents' individual dominant regions, the underloaded teams' compactness and each team's relative position on-field, as well as distances between specific team sectors. We also observed how skill level impacted individual and team coordination tendencies. Data revealed emergence of co-adaptive behaviors between interacting neurobiological social system agents in the context of sport performance. Such observations have broader implications for training design involving manipulations of numerical relations between interacting members of social collectives.

Editor: Ramesh Balasubramaniam, University of California, Merced, United States of America

Funding: This work was supported by the Foundation for Science and Technology (FCT, Portugal), through the grant SFRH/BD/73463/2010 awarded to the first author. The funder had no role in study design, data collection and analysis, decision to publish, or preparation of the manuscript.

Competing Interests: The authors have declared that no competing interests exist.

* Email: psilv@fade.up.pt

Introduction

Collective organizational principles underlying emergence of functional behaviors have been identified in many groups of biological organisms (e.g., flocks of birds, wolf packs, ant colonies) [1,2]. Observations of such superorganismic systems have revealed some advantages of swarming behaviors to achieve group goals, such as when feeding and maintaining member security. For instance, the labor of thousands of bees in a colony is collectively coordinated so that surrounding areas are surveyed most efficiently for food sources of nectar and pollen [3].

Human groups can also be considered as swarming superorganisms when individuals cooperate and coordinate their actions together to achieve common collective goals [4]. This sociobiological perspective can help explain various social-psychological phenomena such as the organization of labor by workers in a factory, how a traffic jam arises or the interpersonal rhythmic movements characterizing human activities like dancing or marching together.

Recently, this approach has been implemented to understand how interacting individuals coordinate their movements by detecting sensory information like the visual movement of others (see [5–8] as examples). Despite its obvious relevance, joint actions in the human performance domain of team sports has not received the same amount of empirical attention [9].

An *ecological dynamics* perspective to understand coordination in team sport social collectives views competing performers as biological agents functioning in integrated systems composed of many interacting subsystems (attackers and defenders) that can harness inherent self-organization tendencies to satisfy specific performance environment constraints [10,11]. From this theoretical rationale, sports teams have been modeled as social neurobiological systems whose agents co-adapt behaviors to changing ecological constraints of performance environments to achieve competitive goals [12,13].

These theoretical ideas have implications for current training methodologies in team sports systems seeking to promote activities of individual agents into functional coordinated performance modes needed to achieve effective competitive performance. A major principle that is paramount to achieve competitive performance goals in invasion games (like association football) is the coordinated effort to create numerical superiority in the vicinity of the ball (a type of swarming behavior) in attacking and defending sub-phases of play [14,15]. The relevance of this universal principle for successful performance in team sports was elucidated in studies of interpersonal coordination tendencies in competing agents by Vilar et al. [16]. They analyzed tendencies to maintain offensive and defensive numerical superiority in specific spatial sub regions of the performance environment by creating sudden defensive stabilities and offensive opportunities through collective behaviors during competitive football matches. More successful performance outcomes during attacking and defending sub-phases of play were directly related to the relative number of opposing players adopting a spatial location nearer to the ball (see [16]).

The creation of local numerical superiority through collective swarming behaviors when teams possess equal numbers of players is difficult to achieve without effective team coordination developed during training. To heighten awareness of such emergent interpersonal coordination tendencies during performance, coaches seek to simulate numerical asymmetries by designing training programs in which an attacking team is overloaded and a defending team is underloaded, respectively, containing more and fewer players. In such training practices, players learn to explore the interpersonal interactions that shape how different numerical relations can be suddenly created during attacking and defending sub-phases of play. In team sports training programs, small-sided and conditioned games (SSCGs) provide an important task vehicle used to constrain the emergence of interpersonal tactical behaviors in system agents through manipulations of numerical relations (in this paper such practice tasks are designated as small-sided "*and conditioned*" games because other constraints, besides field dimension, can be manipulated in order to shape specific behaviors; e.g., player numbers, rules, etc.).

The theoretical reasoning behind use of SSCGs is that they are simulations created during training to help team sports players to learn how to satisfy different constraints on their emergent collective behaviors. Indeed, they are important vehicles to aid sports teams, as complex neurobiological systems, to exploit inherent tendencies for co-adaptation and self-organization [1,17]. These properties of complexity have also been used to explain how agents in social neurobiological systems evolve and adapt their behaviors to satisfy evolutionary constraints [12]. Like such systems, players in sports teams use functional, context-dependent information to regulate their collective behaviors in dynamic performance environments. Previous research suggests that these emergent interpersonal coordination tendencies are predicated on perception of the action possibilities of nearby players [13,18] and the ball's displacement over space and time [19], which *afford* specific actions [20].

The concept of *affordances*, as originally postulated by Gibson [21], refers to the possibilities for action that emerge from the interactions of an organism with its environment. This concept is useful for explaining emergence of interpersonal interactions in team sports since the ability to perceive action possibilities for self in humans is complemented by their capacity to perceive another individual's *affordances* [22] and intentions [23]. As Gibson argued, the richest affordances are provided by interactions with others, since 'behavior affords behavior' (p135), signifying how the environment itself can also be perceived in relation to self and another person's abilities (see Witt et al. [24], [25]). Accordingly, an *ecological dynamics* approach advocates that the interpersonal synergies [26] established between system agents in sports teams can emerge through the perception of *shared affordances*. These are possibilities for action that players collectively perceive through their interacting behaviors with their colleagues and adversaries and that can be effectively designed into SSCGs [27,28]. For instance, a ball carrier in a SSCG can perceive a possibility for passing the ball to an unmarked teammate by also perceiving for him/her a possibility to receive the ball. In this example, both coordinating players perceive *affordances* for one another. The coordinated action of passing and receiving a ball composes a *shared affordance* that is specified to individuals forming a single synergy in different ways (see [17] for a detailed explanation on how shared affordances and synergies may form the basis of coordination of team tactical behaviors). Affordances are dynamic and coordination tendencies between interacting teammates, and between them and their opponents, can change due to the creation of overloads in attack and defense through swarming. In this sense, learning to suddenly outnumber the opposition by overloading in specific spatial areas of a SSCG training environment can help players to create numerical advantages by selectively picking up *shared affordances* that satisfy a team's momentary goals. This interactive process supports the emergence of swarming behaviors and the team's complex tactical performance [28]. However, the tactical behaviors exhibited by agents in team sports, like association football, that emerge at the group level (i.e., when swarming), due to the creation of unbalanced numerical relations, have seldom been investigated. In one exception, Travassos et al. [19] observed how, in the team sport of futsal, agents in a defending underloaded team, in a 5v4 + goalkeeper (gk) game context (a common situation where the goalkeeper of an attacking team plays as an outfield player to create a numerical advantage over a defending team), swarmed around the ball and protected their goal space. The players achieved this performance goal by synchronizing their own movements with the ball's lateral displacements in front of their own goal area. More information about team behaviors during asymmetrical game contexts is clearly needed. Such contexts emerge quite often in many team invasion games besides association football and futsal, such as waterpolo, rugby union, handball or hockey, when one player is 'sin-binned' or sent off temporarily or definitely. This information may be an asset for designers of team training programs to enhance understanding of emergent collective tactical behaviors, skill acquisition and decision-making as a consequence of the interplay of specific ecological constraints in a learning environment [29].

An important, related question concerns whether tactical behaviors emerging from manipulations of numerical relations between competing system agents might be influenced by performer skill level. Silva et al. [30] demonstrated that players of distinct competitive levels displayed different spatial distributions and movement oscillations on field during SSCGs, as a consequence of their skill level. Hence, it is important to understand how players' skill levels, within the ecological constraints of specific performance environments, can influence the interpersonal coordination tendencies afforded by differing numerical relations during training in SSCGs.

Previous investigations of coordination tendencies in team sport systems have revealed a number of reliable individual and compound performance variables [1] for assessing interpersonal coordination tendencies at different levels of system analysis (e.g. inter-individual, intra- and inter-team coordination levels).

Inter-individual coordination analyses have focused on cooperative tendencies amongst team members, providing information on the division of labor between agents [31]. For instance, recent work examined players' dominant regions in team sports of football and futsal by quantifying each individual's major ranges [32] and Voronoi cells [33], which depict the division of labor amongst team members. At a more macroscopic level of analysis, researchers have measured, for instance, teams' geometrical centers (or centroids) and stretch indices to assess intra-team coordination patterns [34,35]. These variables provide complementary information about emergent agent coordination tendencies, with the centroid highlighting the relative position of one team on field and the stretch index plotting the dispersion of players around the team center. *Intra-team analyses* also support identification of different characteristics of the coordination tendencies within each of the opposing teams.

At a larger scale of analysis, inter-team coordination focuses on the coordination patterns emerging *between* opposing teams and highlights the competitive interactions between players and teams to achieve specific performance goals. Knowledge about inter-team coordination has been obtained, for example, by quantifying distances between competing teams' centroids during performance [36]. An alternative to studying inter-team coordination tendencies involves analysis of specific sub-grouping alignments in sports teams, such as line-forces [37,38]. Line-forces provide (geometrically) an estimate of team cohesion (e.g., between players in a defensive line), representing the functional form in which players' attacking and defensive actions are co-aligned and co-organized according to specific team sectors (longitudinally, in attacking, midfield and defending team sectors or laterally, on the wings and middle axis of the field) [39]. Through this conception, inter-team coordination tendencies can be studied according to specific sub-grouping alignments, by measuring the distance between competing lines of players on field.

To summarize, due to the lack of empirical work addressing effects of different numerical relations on coordination tendencies in systems of interacting team sports players, we sought to analyze tactical behaviors emerging from swarming tendencies in SSCGs. To achieve this aim, we investigated whether different numerical relations between competing teams in association football impacted inter-individual, intra- and inter-team tactical behaviors (i.e., emerging in overloaded and underloaded teams), as well as the relative influence of player skill level, specifically on the: (i) players' division of labor, (ii) teams' relative positioning on field; (iii) teams' dispersion; and (iv), inter-team distances at specific locations.

Table 1. Number of shots and goals obtained by teams on each of the small-sided and conditioned games (SSCGs), according to skill.

SSCGs	National-level players				Regional-level players			
	Overloaded team		Underloaded team		Overloaded team		Underloaded team	
	Shots	Goals	Shots	Goals	Shots	Goals	Shots	Goals
5v5	6	1	4	4	3	2	4	4
5v4	8	2	2	2	8	3	2	2
5v3	11	5	4	4	12	5	5	5

The teams attacking the goal with a goalkeeper (overloaded teams) performed more shots in all treatments, with the exception of the regional-level players in the 5v5 treatment. The teams defending mini-goals (overloaded teams) always lost when playing under balanced numerical relations. This reflects the larger risks taken by this team defending goals without a goalkeeper. The underloaded teams performed fewer shots but the opportunities to shoot always ended in goals, depending only on the skill of the player to hit the target after a shooting opportunity was created.

Methods

Participants

Twenty male, youth football players (under-19 yrs) participated in this study, divided into two groups according to skill level (NLP, national-level of performance or RLP - regional-level of performance). Ten participants in the NLP group (mean age:

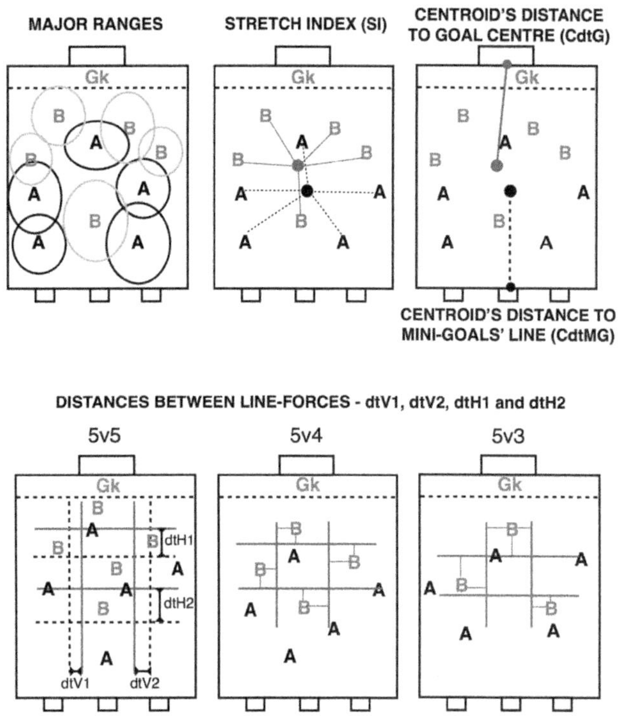

Figure 1. Illustration of inter-individual (major ranges), intra- (stretch index and centroids' distance to goals) and inter-team (distances between line-forces) variables used. The lower left panel illustrates the distances between opposing horizontal (dtH1 and dtH2) and vertical line-forces (dtV1 and dtV2) in the 5v5 condition. The lower middle and right panels illustrate the calculation of horizontal and vertical line-forces in the underloaded team with 4 and 3 players, respectively. All fields used were 47.3×30.6 m (length × width). The overloaded team attacked the goal with a goalkeeper and the underloaded team attacked the mini-goals.

17.64±0.67 yrs) played at a national-level in a top club from their country of origin (playing experience: 9.55±0.52 yrs). Two participants from this group played for their country's under-19 yrs national team. Participants in the RLP (age: 17.91±0.3 yrs) competed at a regional-level competition (playing experience: 9±1.9 yrs). All players or legal guardians (when under age) provided written informed consent to participate in the experiment. All procedures followed the guidelines stated in the Declaration of Helsinki and were approved by the Ethics Committee of the Faculty of Sports of Porto University.

Data collection

Within each group, participants were assigned to one of two technically-equivalent teams of five players by their coaches. Participants performed in three SSCGs in which the numerical relations of the two teams were manipulated. The first SSCG consisted of a 5-a-side plus goalkeeper (Gk) game (5v5+Gk). The goalkeepers played inside an area marked 5 m from the goal line and extending across the pitch width, while defending a 6×2 m (height × width) football goal. The team without a goalkeeper defended three mini-goals (1.2×0.8 m) located on the end line of the pitch. In the second and third SSCGs, the team playing with a goalkeeper was reduced to four (5v4+Gk) and three (5v3+Gk) outfield players, respectively. In accordance with pedagogical principles, this team was denominated the *underloaded* team, while the team with the same number of players was denominated the *overloaded* team. The objective of teams in all SSCGs was to score as many goals as possible and to prevent the opposing team from scoring goals (regardless of numerical overloaded or underloaded performance conditions and of the momentary score in the SSCG). The underloaded team attacked mini-goals without goalkeepers to maintain their chances of scoring when playing with a numerical disadvantage. Table 1 shows that both groups performed a similar number of shots and goals in all treatments. The effectiveness of the shots of both skill groups' underloaded teams confirms that, even when playing under a disadvantage of two fewer players, the chances of scoring were high (given that there was no GK). Effectively, there existed an attacking risk to the overloaded teams when possession was lost.

The length and width dimensions of the playing area were reduced, relative to official football field dimensions, to 47.3×30.6 m, given the number of players involved in the SSCG [40]. Each match lasted for 6 minutes interspersed with 6 minutes periods of rest to minimize the influence of fatigue on participants. During recovery periods, participants were allowed to recover actively at will and rehydrate. Time-motion analysis obtained through continuous GPS tracking showed similar physical profiles across treatments for the players of the overloaded teams. The players of the underloaded teams tended to augment the total distance covered and high intensity running activities when playing under a numerical disadvantage of two players (5v3 + Gk). These data signaled that accumulated fatigue of participants did not bias the results of the experiment.

Coaches were instructed not to provide any sort of encouragement or feedback to the players, before and during periods of data collection, as it could have distorted levels of practice intensity in individual participants [41].

All outfield players carried an unobtrusive global positioning tracking device (SPI Pro, GPSports, Canberra, Australia) to record their movement displacements with individual positional data (2D) at a sampling frequency rate of 15 Hz. The reliability of such devices has been previously well documented [42,43].

The performance area used in all treatments was calibrated with the coordinates of four GPS devices stationed in each corner of the pitch for approximately 2 minutes. The absolute coordinates of each corner were calculated as the median of the recorded time series, providing measurements that were robust to the typical fluctuations of the GPS signals. These absolute positions were used to set the Cartesian coordinate systems for each pitch, with the origin placed at the pitch center. Longitudinal and latitudinal (spherical) coordinates were converted to Euclidean (planar) coordinates using the Haversine formula [44]. Fluctuations in player positioning measures were reduced using a moving average filter with a time scale of 0.2 seconds and data resampling was employed to synchronize the time series of all players within each game.

Data analysis

Inter-individual coordination tendencies were analyzed measuring the dominant region of each player on field. To this effect, the major ranges of each player's displacement were calculated as the ellipse centered at the 2D mean location of each player (i.e., the locus), with semi-axes being the standard deviations in the longitudinal and lateral directions for each entire SSCG [32]. Analysis of ellipse shapes provides qualitative evaluation of the main directions of players' movements, their distribution and relative positioning on field. The areas of the ellipses were also calculated to furnish quantitative information of the amount of space that was under the dominant region of each player.

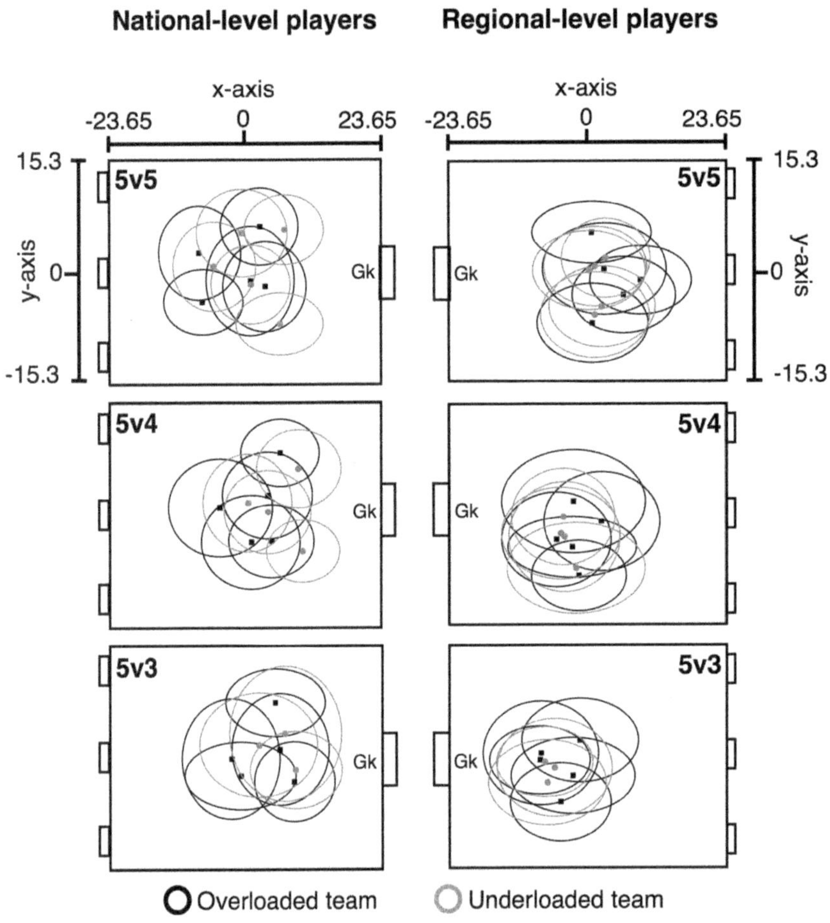

Figure 2. Major ranges of national- (NLP) and regional-level players (RLP) in each SSCG. Black and grey ellipses depict the major ranges of the overloaded and underloaded teams, respectively. Overloaded teams attack the goal defended by a goalkeeper. Lateral (y-axis) and longitudinal (x-axis) depict field coordinates.

To establish intra-team coordination we calculated the stretch index (SI) and the centroid's distance to the goal center (CdtG – in the case of the underloaded team) and to the end line where the mini-goals were placed (CdtMG – in the case of the overloaded team). The SI was calculated as the mean value of the distances of each player to their team's centroid, whereas the centroid was calculated as the average position of all outfield players of one team.

Inter-team coordination was examined through analysis of the distances separating the teams' horizontal and vertical opposing line-forces. We opted to record this variable instead of measurements of centroid distance values because the former does not capture the existence of eventual differences in the players' interactive behaviors at specific team locations (e.g., wings and sectors).

Each team's horizontal lines were calculated by averaging the longitudinal coordinate values of the two players furthest from, and nearest to their own goal line, which corresponded to the forward and back lines, respectively. Similarly, the vertical line-forces of each team were computed by averaging the mean lateral coordinates of the players furthest to the left and to the right on the pitch, corresponding to the left and right lines, respectively. Due to the small number of players participating in the SSCGs, only the wing lines and attacking and defending sectors were analyzed. Hence, the time series of the distances between forward-back and left-right lines of opposing teams were calculated according to team sectors, as follows: (i) dtH1 - distance between the back line of the underloaded team and the forward line of the overloaded team; (ii) dtH2 - distance between the forward line of the underloaded team and the back line of the overloaded team; (iii) dtV1 - distance between the left line of the overloaded team and the right line of the underloaded team; and (iv), dtV2 - distance between the right line of the overloaded team and the left line of the underloaded team.

All variables used in this study capture the interpersonal coordination tendencies at different levels of system analysis (inter-individual, intra- and inter-team coordination levels), as illustrated in Figure 1.

Statistical procedures

Mean ± standard deviations values of the ellipse areas were calculated for the numerically overloaded and underloaded teams according to skill level and different numerical relations. Given that the performance data of each team were analyzed separately and that there was a small number of participants per team (5 players in the overloaded team and 5, 4 and 3 players in the underloaded team), no inferential statistics were used to analyze major ranges areas.

The time series values of intra- (SI, CdtMG and CdtG) and inter-team (dtH1, dtH2, dtV1 and dtV2) variables were compared

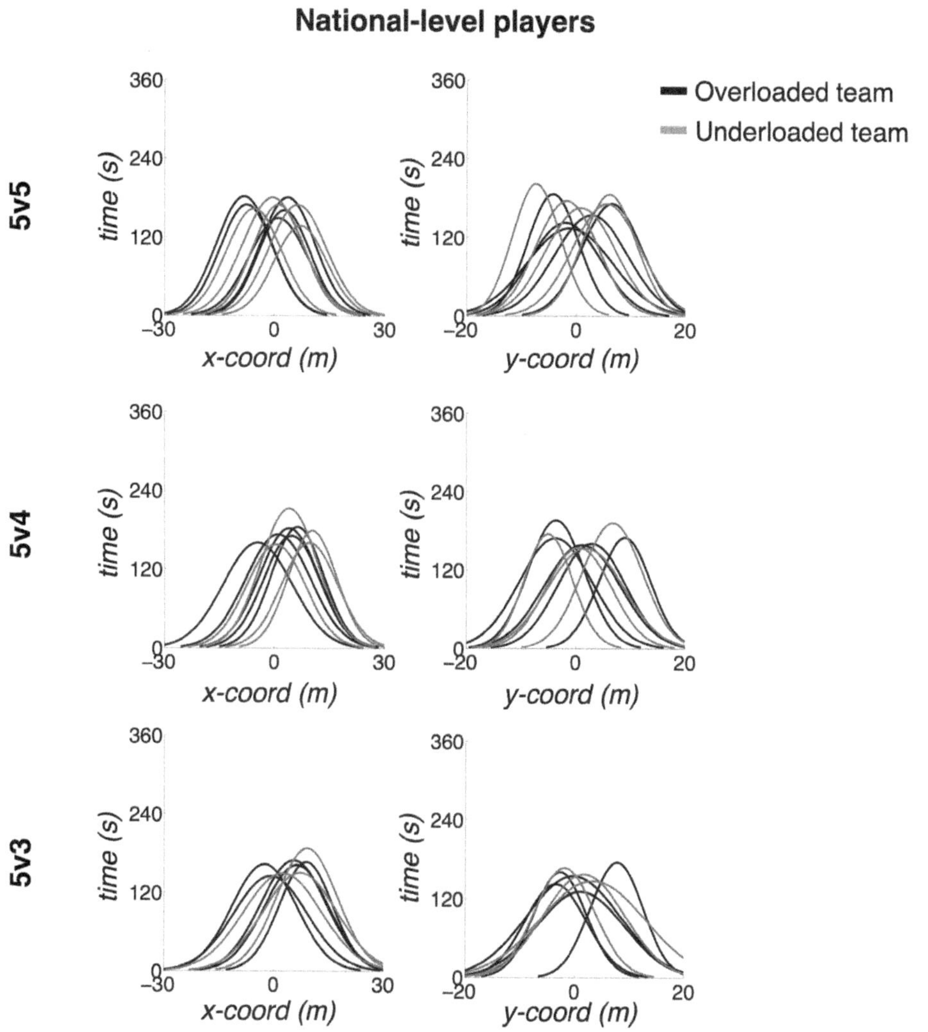

Figure 3. Normal density function of the players' distribution along the x- (longitudinal) and y-axes (lateral) – national-level players (NLP) distribution. Field coordinates vary between −23.65–23.65 and −15.3–15.3 for the x- and y-axes, respectively. The origin (0, 0) corresponds to the field center.

statistically through analysis of variance methods. Given that these time series are of a stochastic nature, the successive measures were only partly determined by previous values. Hence, the assumption of independence of the observations required to run the ANOVAs was overcome by sampling uncorrelated data points. To this effect, for each variable, time series values interspersed with a time interval (t) were selected to ensure that each observation recorded would be uncorrelated with previous selected values. Thus, the time series were fitted to autoregressive models (AR) of various orders (1 to 10) with the argument that, if the data came from an AR(p) process, then $t \geq p$. Thus, t can be estimated by solving the first p Yule-Walker equations with correlations estimated using the sample autocorrelation coefficients. The order of the process is, then, estimated to minimize the Schwarz's Bayesian criterion that represents a trade-off between the fit of the AR model and the number of parameters estimated [45]. Through the AR processes, 82% of the estimates were equal to $p = 4$ and lower. Based on this finding, measures of all intra- and inter-team variables were sampled at every 4 seconds of play (totaling 90 independent measures per variable). After this procedure, for each SSCG and group, we obtained a set of independent game situations containing identical variances, means and standard deviations of the original variables' time series.

Two-way ANOVAs were then conducted to examine the effect of skill (2 levels: NLP and RLP) and numerical relations (3 levels: 5v5, 5v4 and 5v3) on each intra- and inter-team variable. Statistical analysis of intra-team variables was run separately, according to the teams' numerical advantage – overloaded and underloaded teams. Given the large sample of data points analyzed (540 data points per variable), all statistical comparisons reported outcomes below the conventional statistical significance alpha value of $P = 0.05$. Thus, we focused on the magnitude of the effects (here reported as partial eta squared - η^2) obtained with the ANOVAs, following Cohen's guidelines [46]: (i) $0.01 \leq \eta^2 < 0.06$ – small effect; (ii) $0.06 \leq \eta^2 < 0.14$ – moderate effect; and (iii) $\eta^2 \geq 0.14$ – large effect. Bonferroni post-hoc pairwise comparisons and interaction effects were implemented when moderate or large effects of η^2 were identified.

For simplicity, when playing with equal number of players, the team attacking the goal with a goalkeeper and the team attacking the mini-goals were also denominated as overloaded and underloaded teams, respectively.

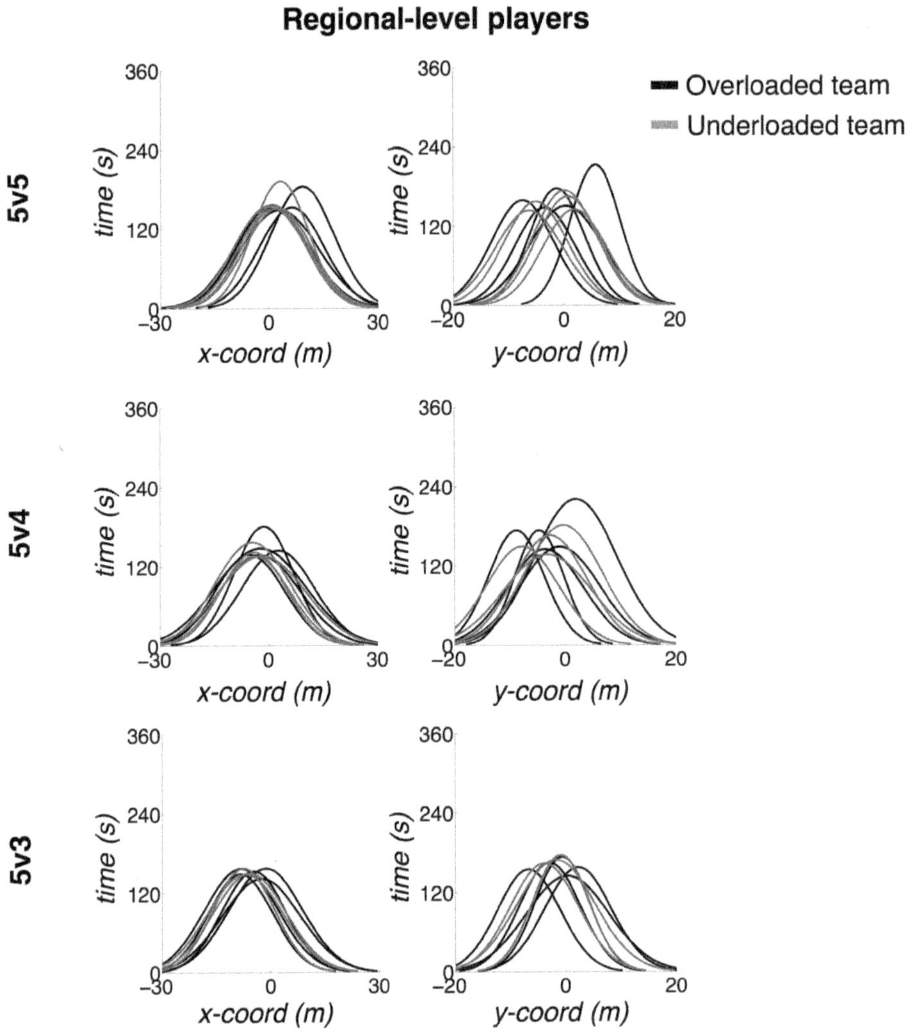

Figure 4. Normal density function of the players' distribution along the x- (longitudinal) and y-axes (lateral) – regional-level players (RLP) distribution. Field coordinates vary between −23.65–23.65 and −15.3–15.3 for the x- and y-axes, respectively. The origin (0, 0) corresponds to the field center.

Results

Inter-individual coordination (major ranges)

Figure 2 illustrates the major ranges and means ± standard deviations of the ellipse areas in each treatment for each group of players.

The ellipse areas of the RLP were more superimposed, displaying different shapes, compared to the NLP skill level. The latter displayed ellipses that were more rationally distributed according to corridors (left and right) and sectors (forward and back), presenting rounded shapes. Analysis of the distribution of players' movement coordinates in the x- (longitudinal) and y-axis (lateral) in Figures 3 and 4 confirm that NLP displayed differentiated distributions in the x-axis (Figure 3). In contrast, the RLP tended to play on very similar longitudinal coordinates of the field, only varying their positioning along the y-axis (Figure 4). The RLP also presented broader distributions along the x-axis, which caused their ellipses to be oval-shaped.

Additionally, the mean areas of ellipses in the NLP group presented a similar trend for both the overloaded and underloaded teams in the 5v5 and 5v4 condition (see Figure 5). In the 5v3 condition, both teams increased their mean areas but with the underloaded team displaying much larger mean ellipse areas than the overloaded team. This was evident in the ellipses of two out of the three players and also in the distribution of their coordinates in the y-axis (Figure 3) that was broader in the 5v3 treatment.

The RLP group displayed different mean areas across treatments for both teams, but identical mean areas for both underloaded and overloaded teams. The larger mean areas were registered in the 5v4 treatment.

Intra-team coordination (stretch index and centroids' distance to own goal and mini-goals' line)

Statistical analysis of SI showed a moderate effect of skill for the overloaded team, $F(1,534) = 71.759$, $P<0.001$, $\eta^2 = 0.12$. Higher mean values of SI were found for NLP ($M = 8.58$, $SE = 0.19$) than RLP ($M = 7$, $SE = 0.19$, see Figure 6, upper panel). No significant effects were observed for numerical relations, or the interactions (Table 2).

ANOVA of SI for the underloaded team presented a large effect of skill level, $F(1,534) = 101.23$, $P<0.001$, $\eta^2 = 0.16$, revealing higher mean values of SI for NLP ($M = 7.99$, $SE = 0.21$) than RLP

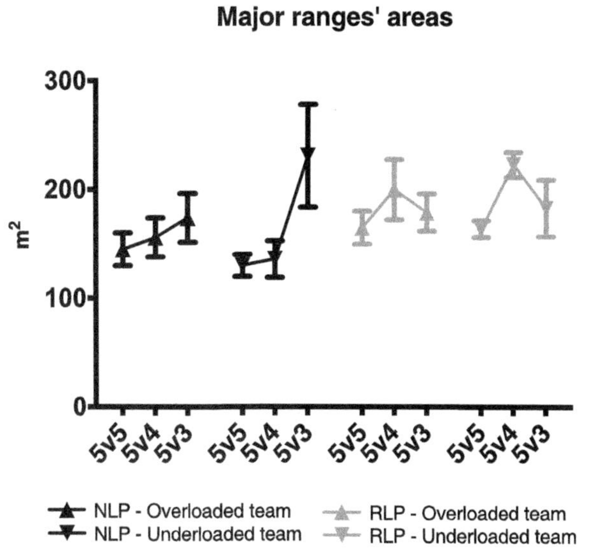

Figure 5. Major ranges areas of national- (NLP) and regional-level players (RLP) in each treatment. Error bars represent the standard error of the mean.

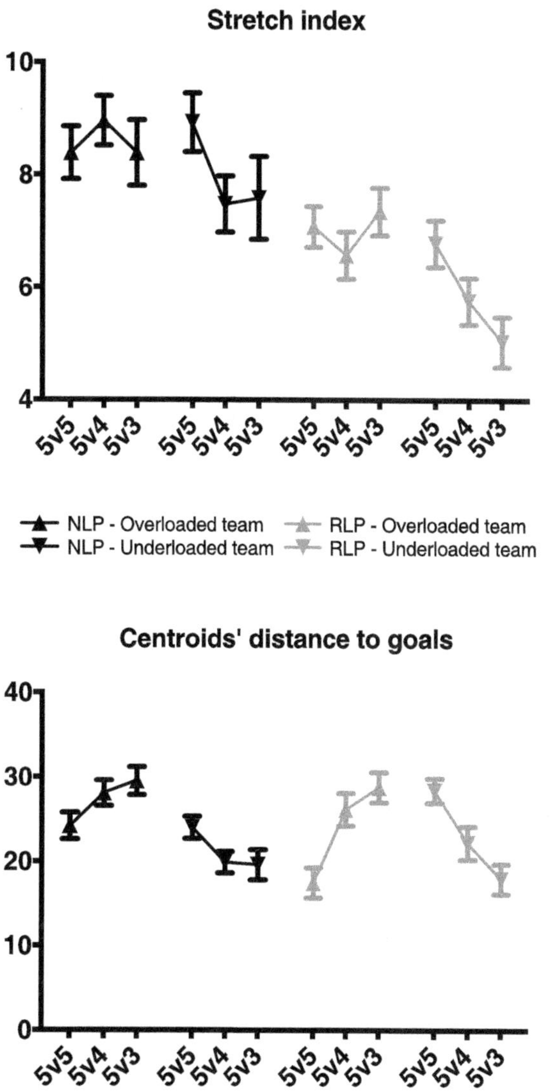

Figure 6. Mean stretch index (SI) and centroids' distance to goals' center (CdtG) and mini-goals line (CdtMG) of overloaded and underloaded teams across treatments and expertise groups. Error bars represent the standard error of the mean.

($M = 5.86$, $SE = 0.21$). Analysis of SI in the underloaded team also revealed a moderate effect of numerical relations, $F(2{,}534) = 19.66$, $P<0.001$, $\eta^2 = 0.07$. Bonferroni post hoc analyses showed higher mean values of SI for 5v5 ($M = 7.85$, $SE = 0.26$), than for 5v4 ($M = 6.62$, $SE = 0.26$, $P<0.001$) and 5v3 ($M = 6.31$, $SE = 0.26$, $P<0.001$). Interaction effects were negligible (see Table 2).

Concerning CdtMG, ANOVA revealed a large effect of numerical relations, $F(2{,}534) = 50.26$, $P<0.001$, $\eta^2 = 0.16$. Lower CdtMG mean values were found for 5v5 treatments ($M = 20.85$, $SE = 0.86$) than for 5v4 ($M = 27.13$, $SE = 0.86$, $P<0.001$) and 5v3 ($M = 29.15$, $SE = 0.86$, $P<0.001$, see Figure 6, lower panel). Skill level and interaction effects were not statistically significant (Table 2).

Concerning the CdtG of the underloaded team, a large effect was also obtained for numerical relations, $F(2{,}534) = 43.65$, $P< 0.001$, $\eta^2 = 0.14$, with larger mean values displayed for 5v5 ($M = 26.19$, $SE = 0.81$) than for 5v4 ($M = 21.05$, $SE = 0.81$, $P< 0.001$) and 5v3 ($M = 18.78$, $SE = 0.81$, $P<0.001$). Differences between 5v4 and 5v3 treatments were also observed ($P = 0.01$, $SE = 0.81$, see Figure 6, lower panel). No significant effects of skill level and interactions were observed.

Inter-team coordination (distances between opposing vertical and horizontal line-forces)

Despite not being sufficiently large to be conventionally considered a significant statistical effect, it is worth noting the interaction effect emerging for skill level and numerical relations, for confrontation of horizontal lines dtH1, $F(2{,}534) = 14.17$, $P< 0.001$, $\eta^2 = 0.05$, since it may have some practical significance (see discussion). Post-hoc analysis showed higher mean values of dtH1 for NLP ($M = 3.89$, $SE = 0.32$) than for RLP ($M = 2.82$, $SE = 0.32$, $P<0.001$) in the 5v5 treatment (Figure 7, upper panel). In contrast, in the 5v3, post hoc analysis reported lower mean values of dtH1 for NLP ($M = 2.05$, $SE = 0.32$) than RLP ($M = 3.3$, $SE = 0.32$, $P<0.001$). No differences were found between groups in the 5v4 treatment ($P = 0.07$).

Concerning dtH2, a moderate effect of numerical relation was observed, independent of skill level, $F(2{,}534) = 20.19$, $P<0.001$, $\eta^2 = 0.07$. Post-hoc analysis showed lower mean values of dtH2 in the 5v5 ($M = 4.02$, $SE = 0.34$) than in the 5v4 ($M = 5.02$, $SE = 0.39$, $P = 0.01$), and in the 5v3 ($M = 6.17$, $SE = 0.34$, $P< 0.001$). Significant differences were also found between the 5v4 and 5v3 treatments ($P = 0.002$).

Analysis of variance of dtV1 also registered a moderate effect for numerical relations, independent of skill level, $F(2{,}534) = 25.22$, $P<0.001$, $\eta^2 = 0.09$, but small effects for skill level and interactions (Table 2). Post-hoc tests revealed higher mean values of dtV1 for 5v3 ($M = 4.2$, $SE = 0.25$) than for 5v4 ($M = 2.97$, $SE = 0.25$, $P< 0.001$) and 5v5 ($M = 2.47$, $SE = 0.25$, $P<0.001$, see Figure 7, lower panel).

The ANOVA of dtV2 revealed a moderate effect for skill level, $F(1{,}534) = 33.4$, $P<0.001$, $\eta^2 = 0.06$, with larger mean values observed in the NLP ($M = 3.46$, $SE = 0.19$), compared to the RLP group ($M = 2.36$, $SE = 0.19$).

Table 2. ANOVA effect sizes.

Variables	Skill level (SL)	Numerical relation (NR)	SL × NR
SI	Overloaded: $\eta^2=0.12$*; Underloaded: $\eta^2=0.16$**	Overloaded: $\eta^2=0.001$; Underloaded: $\eta^2=0.07$*	Overloaded: $\eta^2=0.02$; Underloaded: $\eta^2=0.005$
CdtMG	$\eta^2=0.04$	$\eta^2=0.16$**	$\eta^2=0.02$
CdtG	$\eta^2=0.01$	$\eta^2=0.14$**	$\eta^2=0.02$
dtH1	$\eta^2=0.001$	$\eta^2=0.02$	$\eta^2=0.05$
dtH2	$\eta^2=0.01$	$\eta^2=0.07$*	$\eta^2=0.02$
dtV1	$\eta^2=0.004$	$\eta^2=0.09$*	$\eta^2<0.001$
dtV2	$\eta^2=0.06$*	$\eta^2=0.01$	$\eta^2=0.002$

Main effects of skill level and numerical relation and interaction effects of skill level x numerical relation on: (1) stretch index (SI); (2) centroid's distance to mini goals line (CdtMG); (3) centroid's distance to goal (CdtG); (4) horizontal lines' distances (dtH1 and dtH2) and (5) vertical lines' distances (dtV1 and dtV2).
*Moderate effect.
**Large effect.

Discussion

In this study we adopted an ecological dynamics perspective to investigate how players in football teams, here viewed as multi-agent neurobiological systems, co-adapted performance behaviors (by swarming) to the imposition of distinct numerical relations during SSCGs. Values of inter-individual (major ranges), intra- (stretch index and centroids' distance to goals) and inter-team (distance between horizontal and vertical line-forces) coordination patterns were analyzed during performance in SSCGs played under different numerical relations (5v5, 5v4 and 5v3). Additionally, differences in skill level were observed, between national- and regional-level players, to understand how skill level interacted with numerical relational constraints.

Inter-individual coordination within the team

The lower superimposition of the NLP ellipses (see Figures 2 and 3) reflected a more balanced occupation of different sections of the field, a basic principle required for successful performance in invasion team sports [15]. This process was not as clear in the RLP group whose major range tendencies reflected a poorer division of labor according to specific zones of the field [1].

Analysis of ellipse shapes also supported the assumption that the NLP participants were more tactically balanced. Their rounded shapes reflected the similarity of movement amplitudes in the longitudinal and lateral direction. In contrast, RLP participants tended to present larger movement amplitudes in the longitudinal direction, as specified by the oval-shaped ellipses displayed and also by the distribution of their movements in the longitudinal axis in all treatments (see Figure 4). Considering the fact that, in general, they also possessed wider major ranges areas, it seems that these players performed more runs in the longitudinal direction than in the lateral plane. Clearly, skill level constrained the perception of different action possibilities for each group and the distinct interaction possibilities captured by the division of positional roles on field (i.e., distinct shared affordances).

In the 5v3 treatment the NLP underloaded team presented a considerable larger mean area than the overloaded team. In fact, this was the largest mean ellipse area of all treatments and groups. This outcome can be interpreted as the capacity of NLP participants to cover a wider playing area when playing under a strong numerical disadvantage (with two players less than the opposition). Indeed, when playing against a numerical disadvantage of only one player (5v4), the areas covered were similar to when they played in a numerical balance. This finding implies that for the NLP group, a numerical difference of only one player was not enough to change the players' interpersonal coordination tendencies, probably due to their superior capacity of working together to compensate for the missing player. The larger mean ellipse areas observed in the NLP overloaded team during the 5v3 treatment might be related to the fact that more free space was available to be exploited since the opposing team had two fewer players.

Concerning the RLP group, it is not clear why these players displayed larger mean ellipses areas in the 5v4 and not in the 5v3 treatments and more research is needed to clarify understanding of this effect.

In general, results on inter-individual coordination tendencies suggested that skill level was determinant in the perception of different possibilities for action and in constraining decisions [30] emerging from each group of participants regarding their division of labor on field, here represented by distinct movement patterns and territorial occupation.

Intra-team coordination

The NLP group presented larger dispersion values than the RLP group in all treatments and teams (overloaded and underloaded team) and thus, a tendency to play in a more stretched way. However, playing against one or two fewer players did not provoke any significant changes in the dispersion values of both groups' overloaded teams.

The underloaded team of the NLP played in a more stretched way than the RLP team, perhaps reflecting their ability to spread out and cover the width of the field, when playing with a numerical disadvantage. In fact, during the defensive phase it is important that the defending team contracts to close down space near the ball but covering, at the same time, potential openings for the oppositions' passing lines. This observation signifies that players need to be spread out enough to be adjacent to different ball trajectories, according to the attackers' positions. Our findings concurred with data reported by Travassos et al. [47]. They showed that in non-intercepted passes in futsal, the distance of the second defender to the ball carrier decreased while the distance to the ball trajectory increased. In this sense, players can defend more efficiently if they are able to cover and press most of the possible passing lines available for an opponent, which implies that they should not be excessively contracted as a coordinating unit. By continually readjusting their positioning, based on defensive action

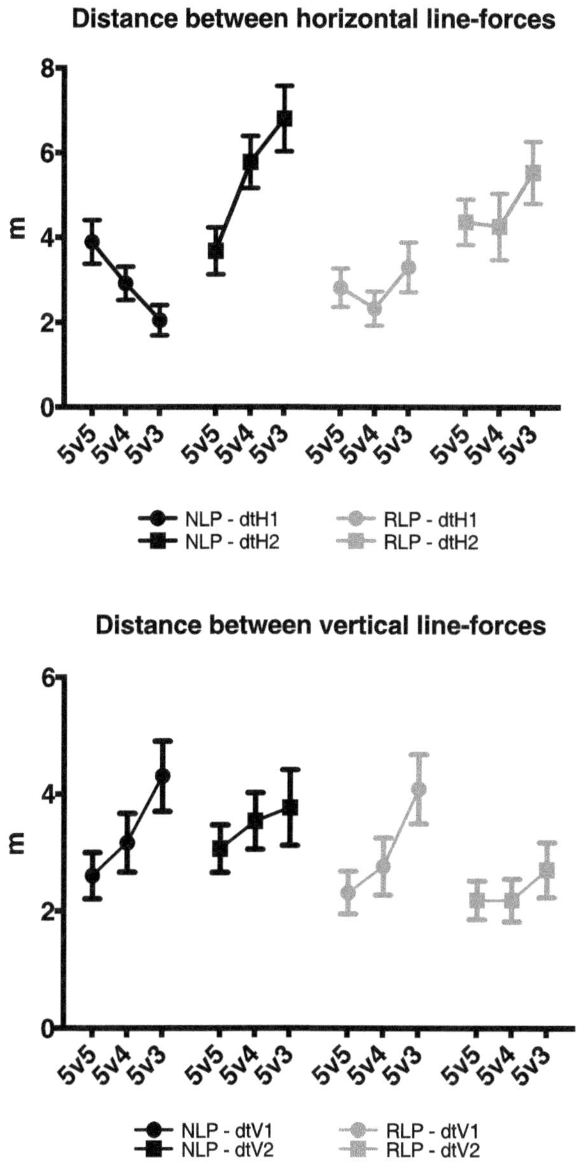

Figure 7. Mean distances between horizontal (upper panels - dtH1 and dtH2) and vertical lines (lower panels - dtV1 and dtV2) across treatments and expertise groups. Error bars represent the standard error of the mean.

possibilities for themselves and for teammates (e.g., covering space, closing passing lines, marking opponents, etc.), players can work to maintain the symmetry between competing teams in underloaded game contexts.

Nonetheless, in the underloaded teams, the values of SI decreased significantly across treatments, independent of skill level, signifying that the teams of both groups tended to contract when they were reduced in number. This finding was likely due to the fact that they spent more time performing defensive actions when underloaded. The NLP, however, presented similar dispersion values when playing with one and two players fewer, while the RLP group teams always tended to contract every time one player was omitted. Following the previous results of inter-individual coordination it seems plausible that this team maintained similar dispersion values through enlargement of their players' dominant regions. Thus, the same collective behavioral patterns were secured by distinct interpersonal coordination modes. This is another important characteristic of biological systems – the ability to degenerate behavior to satisfy different ecological constraints [48].

Concerning the teams' relative positioning on field (depicted by the centroid distance to the goal line), results showed that, as the numerical difference between teams increased, the overloaded team players moved further away from their mini-goals and approached the underloaded team's goal. This behavior was evident for both groups. In contrast, underloaded team players tended to be attracted backwards on field to defend their goal. Thus, the overloaded teams managed to acquire space near the opposing team's goal and forced them to move backwards. This result is in accordance with data reported in the study of Travassos et al. [49] in 5v4+Gk performance contexts in futsal. This coordination tendency was evident when underloaded teams were reduced by one player, while presenting similar CdtMG and CdtG values in the 5v4 and 5v3 treatments. These findings indicated the conditions that facilitated multi-agent collectives to act in a collectively coordinated manner, once players had become attuned to information from their opponents' actions.

Synthesizing these main findings, the manipulation of numerical asymmetries on field during training tasks influenced the dispersion values of the teams being underloaded and the relative positioning of both teams on field. Overloaded teams tended to advance on field when opponents lost players, but without impacting in their dispersion values. In contrast, underloaded teams tended to retreat nearer to their own goal and contract in order to protect it. In both situations, the data suggested that players were collectively attuned to shared affordances. Playing with fewer players might have offered fewer opportunities to keep possession of the ball and possibly constrained the emergence of a more compact defensive block. In contrast, playing with more players probably offered more possibilities for maintaining possession and attacking the opposition goal (which is typically the main performance behavior intended to be promoted through the creation of overloads). Skill level seemed most influential on the way each group of players spread out on field during play, although both groups presented similar trends in their emergent behaviors.

Inter-team coordination

With regards to the distances between horizontal line-forces, results showed that the NLP participants reduced the distance value dtH1 (i.e., distance between the back line of the underloaded team and the forward line of the overloaded team) as the numerical difference between both teams increased. The opposite effect emerged for the distance value of dtH2 (i.e., distance between the forward line of the underloaded team and the back line of the overloaded team).

By forcing an approach to the underloaded team's back line the NLP participants could have provoked the emergence of critical regions of performance [11] where the balance between the opposing line-forces could be perturbed leading the social neurobiological system to other performance outcomes like the creation of goal scoring opportunities. Critical regions of performance are characterized by low values of interpersonal distances between attackers and defenders that can lead to transitions in system organisational states, with eventual consequences for performance outcomes [11] as previously observed in studies of performance in several other team sports [10,50–52]. In our study, the proximity of the confronting line-forces could also

Table 3. Synthesis of inter-individual, intra- and inter-team behavioral trends across SSCGs.

Dominant regions	Teams' dispersion	Teams' relative positioning on field	Space between line-forces on wings	Space between line-forces on sectors
Overloaded team players: increased; Underloaded team players: increased;	Overloaded team: maintained; Underloaded team: decreased.	Overloaded team: approached the opponent's goal; Underloaded team: approached own goal.	dtV1: increased with numerical difference; dtV2: maintained across all numerical differences.	dtH1: decreased as the numerical difference increased for NLP; increased on 5v3 for RLP; dtH2: increased with the numerical difference.

Small-sided and conditioned games sequence: (i) 5v5 (ii) 5v4 and (iii) 5v3.
National- and regional-level players displayed the same behavioral trends, except for dtH1 (see table). Differences between groups were observed for the individual dominant regions, means of teams' dispersion and space between dtV2 line-forces.

have led to the emergence of critical states, an assumption that needs to be scrutinized in future studies.

On the other hand, the increase in the distance of dtH2 in both groups across SSCGs was attributed to the fact that the underloaded team, because of the numerical disadvantage, prioritized the closing of space near its goal by moving their lines backwards. This result corroborates previous findings regarding behaviors related to the CdtG, and is in accordance with data from previous work by Travassos et al. [49].

The same trend for dtH1 was not so clear in the RLP participants, since the mean distance values of both variables were roughly approximate in the 5v5 and 5v4 treatments, and increasing in the 5v3 treatment. Apparently, the players at that skill level did not press the underloaded team back line when they were in numerical disadvantage. In fact, the opposite occurred in the 5v3 treatment.

With respect to vertical lines, both groups displayed identical values for dtV1 (i.e., the distance between the left line of the overloaded team and the right line of the underloaded team), which increased with numerical differences between teams. On the opposite wing (i.e., dtV2 or the distance between the right line of the overloaded team and the left line of the underloaded team), the space between lines remained relatively constant across SSCGs conditions for both skill groups. This finding signifies that teams maintained relatively the same distances between vertical line-forces across treatments on only one of the two wings of the field. This outcome might have been constrained by other possible factors besides numerical relations, like the players' preferred foot and strategic options.

In sum, the most important effects were registered in the proximity between an overloaded team's attacking line and an underloaded team's defensive line, only in the NLP group. This outcome may have evidenced exploratory performance behaviors of an overloaded team when offensively pressing the reduced number of players in an underloaded team in order to disturb the equilibrium of opposing line-forces to create scoring opportunities. This type of exploratory activity may have emerged in the more skilled group perhaps due to their better technical skills and the capacity to dribble past opponents at critical values of interpersonal distances (see [53] for evidence on critical values of interpersonal distances between attacker-defender dyads in promoting dribbling actions).

Conclusions

Data from this study shed important insights on co-adaptive behaviors of agents in team sport systems performing under specific task constraints afforded by different numerical relations and skill levels in SSCGs (see Table 3 for a synthesis of main findings). Individual and team coordination tendencies were clearly constrained by the numerical relations between competing teams and the players' skill level. Skill levels provided different action possibilities available to synergistic groups of players, highlighting the importance of adapting training tasks to the players' individual characteristics in order to facilitate the emergence of required team behaviors. Accordingly, the findings of this study support the assumption that teams, here conceptualized as swarming neurobiological superorganisms, possess the ability to co-adapt to performance constraints that can be manipulated by practitioners during practice in SSCGs. Therefore, designing *shared affordances* for specific group tactics to emerge during practice through manipulations of numerical relations seems a feasible pedagogical methodology. In this study we identified the emergent behaviors constrained by different numerical relations in collective systems, which need to be considered when seeking to enhance the acquisition of specific skills and team tactical behaviors during training.

Future studies should identify the specific *affordances* supporting such tactical behaviors in order to provide deeper understanding of the players' actions and tactical relations during SSCGs. This information is deemed crucial for coaches to regulate their instructions and feedback provided to players.

Author Contributions

Conceived and designed the experiments: PS JG. Performed the experiments: PS. Analyzed the data: PS JG BT LV PA DA KD. Contributed reagents/materials/analysis tools: PS PA. Contributed to the writing of the manuscript: PS BT LV PA KD DA JG.

References

1. Duarte R, Araújo D, Correia V, Davids K (2012) Sport teams as superorganisms: implications of biological models for research and practice in team sports performance analysis. Sports Med 42: 633–642.
2. Sumpter DJT (2006) The principles of collective animal behaviour. Philosophical transactions of the Royal Society B: Biological Sciences 361: 5–22.
3. Kesebir S (2012) The Superorganism Account of Human Sociality: How and When Human Groups Are Like Beehives. Pers Soc Psychol Rev 16: 233–261.
4. Stearns S (2007) Are we stalled part way through a major evolutionary transition from individual to group? Evolution 61: 2275–2280.
5. Richardson MJ, Marsh KL, Isenhower RW, Goodman JRL, Schmidt RC (2007) Rocking together: dynamics of intentional and unintentional interpersonal coordination. Hum Mov Sci 26: 867–891.
6. Sebanz N, Bekkering H, Knoblich G (2006) Joint action: Bodies and minds moving together. Trends Cogn Sci 10: 70–76.
7. Schmidt R, Richardson M (2008) Dynamics of interpersonal coordination. In: Fuchs A, Jirsa VK, editors. Coordination: Neural, Behavioral and Social Dynamics. Verlag Berlin Heidelberg: Springer. pp. 281–308.
8. Marsh KL, Richardson MJ, Baron RM (2006) Contrasting approaches to perceiving and acting with others. Ecol Psychol 18: 1–38.

9. Hristovski R, Davids K, Araújo D, Passos P (2011) Constraints-induced emergence of functional novelty in complex neurobiological systems: a basis for creativity in sport. Nonlinear Dynamics Psychol Life Sci 15: 175–206.
10. Davids K, Button C, Araújo D, Renshaw I, Hristovski R (2006) Movement models from sports provide representative task constraints for studying adaptive behaviour in human movement studies. Adapt Behav 14: 73–94.
11. Passos P, Araújo D, Davids K (2013) Self-Organization Processes in Field-Invasion Team Sports. Sports Med 43: 1–7.
12. Passos P, Araújo D, Davids K, Gouveia L, Serpa S, et al. (2009) Interpersonal pattern dynamics and adaptative behavior in multiagent neurobiological systems: conceptual model and data. J Mot Behav 41: 445–459.
13. Button C, Chow J-Y, Travassos B, Vilar L, Duarte R, et al. (2012) A nonlinear pedagogy for sports teams as social neurobiological systems: how teams can harness self-organization tendencies. In: Ovens A, Hopper T, Butler J, editors. Complexity thinking in physical education. Oxon: Routledge. pp. 135–150.
14. Worthington E (1974) Learning and teaching soccer skills. Hollywood: Wilshire Book Company.
15. Teodorescu L (1977) Théorie et méthodologie des jeux sportifs; réunis Léf, editor: Les éditeurs français réunis.
16. Vilar L, Araújo D, Davids K, Bar-Yam Y (2013) Science of winning soccer: emergent pattern-forming dynamics in Association Football. Journal of Systems Science and Complexity 26: 73–84.
17. Silva P, Garganta J, Araújo D, Davids K, Aguiar P (2013) Shared knowledge or shared affordances? Insights from an ecological dynamics approach to team coordination in sports. Sports Med 43: 765–772.
18. Passos P, Milho J, Fonseca S, Borges J, Araujo D, et al. (2011) Interpersonal Distance Regulates Functional Grouping Tendencies of Agents in Team Sports. J Mot Behav 43: 155–163.
19. Travassos B, Araújo D, Vilar L, McGarry T (2011) Interpersonal coordination and ball dynamics in futsal (indoor football). Hum Mov Sci 30: 1245–1259.
20. Withagen R, Poel HJd, Araújo D, Pepping G-J (2012) Affordances can invite behaviour: Reconsidering the relationship between affordances and agency. New Ideas Psychol 30: 250–258.
21. Gibson J (1979) The ecological approach to visual perception. Hillsdale, NJ: Lawrence Erlbaum Associates.
22. Stoffregen T, Gorday K, Sheng Y-Y (1999) Perceiving affordances for another person's actions. J Exp Psychol Hum Percept Perform 25: 120–136.
23. Mark LS (2007) Perceiving the Actions of Other People. Ecol Psychol 19: 107–136.
24. Witt JK, Sugovic M, Taylor JET (2012) Action-specific effects in a social context: Others' abilities influence perceived speed. J Exp Psychol Hum Percept Perform 38: 715–725.
25. Witt JK, Sugovic M (2012) Does ease to block a ball affect perceived ball speed? Examination of alternative hypotheses. J Exp Psychol Hum Percept Perform 38: 1202–1214.
26. Riley M, Richardson M, Shockley K, Ramenzoni V (2011) Interpersonal synergies. Front Psychol 2: 1–7.
27. Davids K, Araújo D, Correia V, Vilar L (2013) How small-sided and conditioned games enhance acquisition of movement and decision-making skills. Exerc Sport Sci Rev 41: 154–161.
28. Araújo D, Silva P, Davids K (in press) Capturing group tactical behaviors in expert team players. In: Baker J, Farrow D, editors. Rotledge Handbook of Sport Expertise: Routledge.
29. Chow JY, Davids K, hristovski R, Araújo D, Passos P (2011) Nonlinear pedagogy: learning design for self-organizing neurobiological systems. New Ideas Psychol 29: 189–200.
30. Silva P, Aguiar P, Duarte R, Davids K, Araújo D, et al. (in press) Effects of pitch size and skill level on tactical behaviours of Association Football players during small-sided and conditioned games. International Journal of Sports Science & Coaching.
31. Eccles D (2010) The coordination of labour in sports teams. Int Rev Sport Exerc Psychol 3: 154–170.
32. Yue Z, Broich H, Seifriz F, Mester J (2008) Mathematical analysis of a soccer game. Part I: individual and collective behaviours. Studies in Applied Mathematics 121: 223–243.
33. Fonseca S, Milho J, Travassos B, Araújo D (2012) Spatial dynamics of team sports exposed by Voronoi diagrams. Hum Mov Sci 31: 1652–1659.
34. Frencken W, Lemmink K, Delleman N, Visscher C (2011) Oscillations of centroid position and surface area of soccer teams in small-sided games. Eur J Sport Sci 11: 215–223.
35. Duarte R, Araújo D, Folgado H, Esteves P, Marques P, et al. (2013) Capturing complex, non-linear team behaviours during competitive football performance. Journal of Systems Science and Complexity 26: 62–72.
36. Duarte R, Fernandes O, Folgado H, Araújo D (2013) Single camera analysis in studying pattern forming dynamics of player interactions in team sports. In: Davids K, Araújo D, Balague N, Button C, Passos P, editors. Complex systems in sport: Routledge.
37. Gréhaigne J-F, Bouthier D, David B (1997) Dynamic-system analysis of opponent relationships in collective actions in soccer. J Sports Sci 15: 137–149.
38. Grehaigne J-F, Godbout P (1995) Tactical knowledge in team sports from a constructivist and cognitivist perspective. Quest 47: 490–505.
39. Gréhaigne J-F (1988) Game systems in soccer from the point of view of coverage of space. In: Reilly T, Lees A, Davids K, Murphy WJ, editors. Science and Football. London: E. & FN Spon. pp. 316–321.
40. Hughes C (1994) The football association coaching book of soccer tactics and skills. Harpenden: Queen Anne Press.
41. Rampinini E, Impellizzeri FM, Castagna C, Abt G, Chamari K, et al. (2007) Factors influencing physiological responses to small-sided soccer games. J Sports Sci 25: 659–666.
42. Johnston R, Watsford M, Pine M, Spurrs R, Sporri D (2013) Assessment of 5 Hz and 10 Hz GPS units for measuring athlete movement demands. International Journal of Performance Analysis in Sport 13: 262–274.
43. Coutts AJ, Duffield R (2010) Validity and reliability of GPS devices for measuring movement demands of team sports. J Sci Med Sport 13: 133–135.
44. Sinnott RW (1984) Virtues of the Haversine. Sky and Telescope 68: 159.
45. Chatfield C (2003) The analysis of time series: an introduction. New York: Chapman & Hall.
46. Cohen J (1988) Statistical power analysis for the behavioral sciences. Hillsdale, NJ: Lawrence Erlbaum Associates.
47. Travassos B, Araújo D, Davids K, Vilar L, Esteves P, et al. (2012) Informational constraints shape emergent functional behaviours during performance of interceptive actions in team sports. Psychol Sport Exerc 13: 216–223.
48. Edelman G, Gally J (2001) Degeneracy and complexity in biological systems. Proc Natl Acad Sci U S A 20: 13763-13713-13768.
49. Travassos B, Araújo D, Duarte R, McGarry T (2012) Spatiotemporal coordination behaviors in futsal (indoor football) are guided by informational game constraints. Hum Mov Sci 31: 932–945.
50. Passos P, Araújo D, Davids K, Gouveia L, Milho J, et al. (2008) Information-governing dynamics of attacker-defender interactions in youth Rugby Union. J Sports Sci 26: 1421–1429.
51. Passos P, Araujo D, Davids K, Gouveia L, Serpa S, et al. (2009) Interpersonal Pattern Dynamics and Adaptive Behavior in Multiagent Neurobiological Systems: Conceptual Model and Data. J Mot Behav 41: 445–459.
52. Araújo D, Davids K, Bennett S, Button C, Chapman G (2004) Emergence of sport skills under constraints. In: Williams M, Hodges N, editors. Skill Acquisition in Sport Research, Theory and Practice. UK: Routledge. pp. 409–433.
53. Duarte R, Araújo D, Gazimba V, Fernandes O, Folgado H, et al. (2010) The ecological dynamics of 1v1 sub-phases in association football. Open Sports Sci J 3: 16–18.

4

Lower Body Symmetry and Running Performance in Elite Jamaican Track and Field Athletes

Robert Trivers[1]*, Bernhard Fink[2], Mark Russell[3], Kristofor McCarty[4], Bruce James[5], Brian G. Palestis[6]

1 Graduate Program in Ecology and Evolution, Rutgers University, New Brunswick, New Jersey, United States of America, **2** Courant Research Centre, Evolution of Social Behavior & Institute of Psychology, University of Göttingen, Göttingen, Germany, **3** Faculty of Health and Life Sciences, Northumbria University, Newcastle-upon-Tyne, United Kingdom, **4** Department of Psychology, Faculty of Health and Life Sciences, Northumbria University, Newcastle-upon-Tyne, United Kingdom, **5** MVP Track and Field Club, University of Technology, Kingston, Jamaica, **6** Department of Biological Sciences, Wagner College, Staten Island, New York, United States of America

Abstract

In a study of degree of lower body symmetry in 73 elite Jamaican track and field athletes we show that both their knees and ankles (but not their feet) are–on average–significantly more symmetrical than those of 116 similarly aged controls from the rural Jamaican countryside. Within the elite athletes, events ranged from the 100 to the 800 m, and knee and ankle asymmetry was lower for those running the 100 m dashes than those running the longer events with turns. Nevertheless, across all events those with more symmetrical knees and ankles (but not feet) had better results compared to international standards. Regression models considering lower body symmetry combined with gender, age and weight explain 27 to 28% of the variation in performance among athletes, with symmetry related to about 5% of this variation. Within 100 m sprinters, the results suggest that those with more symmetrical knees and ankles ran faster. Altogether, our work confirms earlier findings that knee and probably ankle symmetry are positively associated with sprinting performance, while extending these findings to elite athletes.

Editor: Patrizia d'Ettorre, University of Paris 13, France

Funding: The authors thank the Enhanced Education Foundation, the Ann and Gordon Getty Foundation, the Biosocial Research Foundation, the Center for Human Evolutionary Studies (CHES), and the German Science Foundation (DFG) for financial support. The funders had no role in study design, data collection and analysis, decision to publish, or preparation of the manuscript.

Competing Interests: With regard to the affiliation of coauthor Bruce James: Mr. James has provided the authors with access to the sample of elite athletes of this present study; he has also been involved in the on-site measurement logistics and activities in Kingston. Aside from this, Mr. James had neither a financial interest nor an influence on the outcome of the study results.

* Email: trivers@rci.rutgers.edu

Introduction

Trivers et al. [1] showed that Jamaican eight year olds of both sexes with more symmetrical knees were better sprinters 14 years later in both the 100 and the 200 m dashes, while symmetry of the upper body and feet did not predict sprinting speed, and ankle symmetry sometimes seemed to have a minor positive effect on sprinting speed. There are two separate reasons why we might expect symmetry of lower body traits to be positively associated with sprinting speed. Symmetry is inherently more efficient in races–it is less physically demanding and thus saves energy. This is presumably why the lower body asymmetry of Jamaican children 8.2 years of age is 1/3rd that of upper body asymmetry [2]. Walking and running are inherently symmetrical and should favor symmetrical traits associated with them while upper body movements may or may not be symmetrical (vide, laterality) [3,4].

On the other hand, it has been known since the 1950's from experimental work on *Drosophila* that stress during early development is associated with greater adult bodily asymmetry, as is genetic inability to deal with the stress (e.g., inbred vs. outbred). This led to the notion that fluctuating asymmetry (FA) – deviations from bilateral symmetry in paired traits, randomly distributed to the left and right side – is a measure of developmental instability, i.e., the inability of an organism genetically to buffer the system against stressors to achieve the optimal state, namely symmetry itself [5]. The key is that if a population shows true FA then it can be presumed to be attempting to be symmetrical, so that failure to do so is a measure of failure to reach–in the face of developmental perturbations–the phenotype that the genotype is aiming for. Once it was discovered that females in a variety of birds, insects and mammals preferred symmetrical males as mating partners, even in species lacking male parental investment, it became obvious that body symmetry must be positively associated with genetic quality–a resistance from disease, for example [6], and many other advantageous traits [7].

To test for associations between symmetry and athletic performance, we compared lower body symmetry (knees, ankles and feet) in a control sample of Jamaicans measured in the countryside, carefully matched to a sample of elite Jamaican athletes measured in Kingston (all members of the MVP Track and Field Association). Among the elite athletes we also obtained performance–best times in preferred events against world records–to see if variation in peak sprinting times was in part predicted by variation in lower body symmetry.

In this paper we show that elite athletes have markedly more symmetrical knees than countryside controls and also more symmetrical ankles, while symmetry of feet does not differ between the two. We further demonstrate that within elite sprinters, performance shows striking and consistent positive associations with both knee and ankle symmetry. To wit, taking all athletes together, knee symmetry predicts sprinting ability while ankle symmetry almost does so. By adding covariates, such as weight and age, knee and ankle symmetry remain as marginally significant predictors of athletic success at the highest level of elite performance. Considering only the 100 m sprinters ($n = 32$) we find positive correlations between degree of knee and ankle symmetry and world performance. It also seems noteworthy that overall symmetry decreases among those who run 200 m, 400 m or 800 m races, as if adapted to or caused by frequent left-hand turns.

Methods

Subjects

We recruited two groups of subjects: elite Jamaican track and field athletes and controls from the Jamaican countryside. The elite athletes were all members of the MVP Track and Field Club working out of University of Technology in Kingston. We were able to get a nearly complete sample of club membership (73 of 77). There are exclusive criteria for being members of MVP and it is highly sought after by up and coming Jamaican athletes. International Association of Athletics Federations (IAAF) scores allow comparisons across disciplines and genders [8] (www.iaaf.org) and we used these scores, which we calculated based on personal bests, as our measure of performance. Approximately 90% of MVP club members have IAAF scores above 1000, and 6 of our subjects have remarkably high scores (≥1200). Although their training all included sprinting, the athletes' best events varied, and in addition to comparing athletes and controls, we also compared symmetry of athletes whose specialties differed.

Control subjects consisted of individuals recruited in the countryside through word of mouth by someone who knew the community very well and had worked with the Jamaican Symmetry Project [2] since its inception in 1996. This person was given an exact list of the ages and sexes of the elite athletes we would be measuring in Kingston, so she could recruit a matching sample, which she did exactly. We then invited additional subjects who were within the age range of the elite athletes to appear and be measured, except that we discouraged all overweight individuals (which were overwhelmingly women) since we doubted there were many overweight elite athletes. The final number of control subjects was 116.

Elite athletes and controls were of very similar age (athletes: mean+/−SD = 23.0+/−3.2; controls 23.0+/−3.6; $t_{187} = 0.14$, $p = 0.89$). There is also no difference in variance in age between groups (Levene's test, $F = 1.68$, $p = 0.20$) and the ranges are as follows: elite 17.13–31.95; control 17.21–32.46.

Measurement of traits

Before traveling to Jamaica the three measurers met, and each measurer was exclusively allocated one trait to eliminate between-measurer effects. There were two sessions, each of approximately 6 hours, in which the measurement points for knees, ankles and feet were agreed upon and preliminary repeatability for each trait was established. Measurement points were the same as adopted in the Jamaican Symmetry Project in 1996 [2] and thus match the landmarks used in Trivers et al. [1].

When conducting the study in Jamaica, we measured the traits twice per side for each individual (second foot measurements missing for one subject). Repeated measurement is standard in FA studies, because the differences between sides are often so small that they can be similar in magnitude to measurement error [9–11]. Only by measuring each side at least twice can one demonstrate that the differences between sides reflect actual asymmetry, rather than measurement error. The calculated average of the two measurements were used in the subsequent statistical analysis.

To preserve anonymity each participant received a unique ID at arrival, printed on A6 cards, and only this number was used to assign his/her measurements. Measurements of the three lower body traits were all performed using a digital Vernier caliper (Preisser products, Germany) to an accuracy of 0.01 mm. To eliminate potential measurement biases, the calipers were closed after each measurement. In addition to the three lower body traits, weight and height were measured and age was self-reported. Collecting all measurement took approximately 10 minutes per participant and there was a time span of some 3–5 minutes between first and second measurements of a trait, in which participants completed measurements at another station before they returned for the second measurement. Each measurement was called out to an assistant sitting next to the investigator to ensure that the investigator could not memorize them.

The size of the left and right knee of each participant was measured as defined by the largest breadth, measured between the medial and lateral epicondyles of the femur. The investigator measuring ankles first located the widest point of the ankle by hand before putting the caliper in place. For both knee and ankle measurements, participants were seated on a chair with legs bent by 90° and measurements were taken by an investigator sitting in front of the participant. Somatometric landmarks were palpated and measurements were taken with constant pressure of the caliper to minimize soft tissue related measurement error. Foot length was measured bilaterally using standardized A3 graphical paper (resolution of 1 mm) that was then measured with calipers. In a seated position, participants were instructed to place both feet on to the paper in a manner which aligned the pternion to the head of the 2nd metatarsal axes of each foot in parallel. Using a leveling device, markings were placed at the pternion and at the tip of toe one of each foot. To ensure consistency of measurement, markings were placed at the tip of toe one irrespective of whether toes two through five would have elicited a greater foot length. The perpendicular distance between two parallel lines extrapolated from the original foot markings was deemed foot length.

Statistical analysis

Most analyses were performed using IBM SPSS Statistics 21. The presence of fluctuating and directional asymmetry (FA and DA) were assessed using the Excel template at www.biology.ualberta.ca/palmer/asym/FA/FA-Refs.htm#tools. With this template, the presence of significant FA (FA > measurement error) is demonstrated by a significant F-test for a sides X individuals interaction in a mixed model ANOVA [9,10]. DA is indicated by a significant effect of sides in the ANOVA model.

Significant DA was present in feet and ankles (see Measurements in the main text). To ensure that statistical tests are comparing FA and are not biased by directional differences between sides, we used the index of FA developed by Graham et al. [11]. This index is based on unrotated factors extracted from the covariance matrix of a principal component analysis of the mean right side measurements on a trait and the mean left side measurements. This first factor represents the covariance between

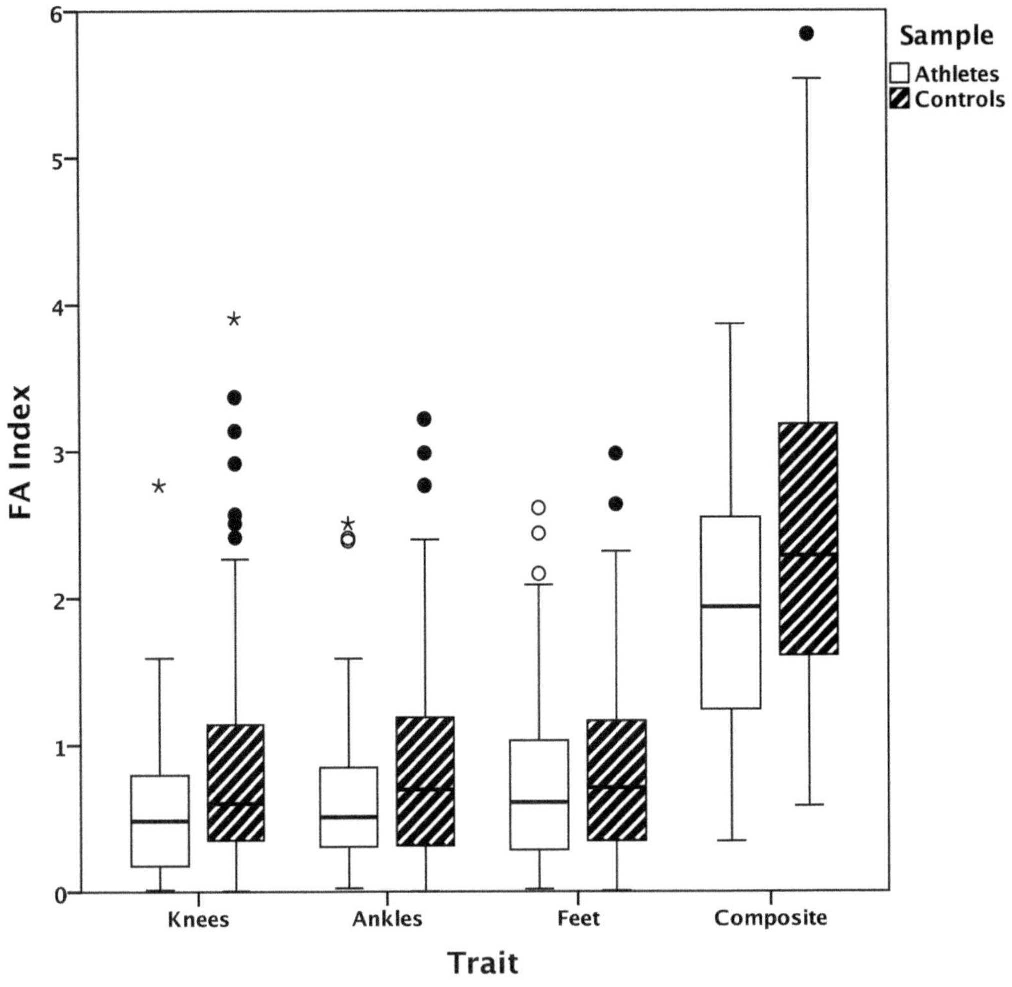

Figure 1. Boxplots for the three traits and their sum. FA is corrected for directional asymmetry using Graham et al.'s index (see Methods). Elite athletes (n = 73) are represented by open bars and controls (n = 116) by bars filled with diagonals. Circles represent outliers, with stars indicating extreme outliers; color of circles and stars corresponds to coloring in bars. Controls have significantly higher knee, ankle and composite FA than the athletes (see Tables 1–3).

sides, plus half the FA and half the remaining measurement error. The second factor represents half the FA and half the remaining measurement error. This second factor is therefore an index of FA and does not include DA, which would be extracted with the covariance between sides. When analyzing overall asymmetry, including DA, we use relative asymmetry (absolute asymmetry in a trait divided by trait size).

Unsigned FA (absolute value of right – left) has an asymmetrical frequency distribution with only half of a bell curve. However, FA should not then be transformed to achieve normality, because F-tests are robust and transformation may change the underlying relationships between FA and other variables [10,12]. Comparisons of FA are comparisons of variance in a trait, and comparisons of the means of two half-normal distributions gives an unbiased estimate of differences in variance [9,10]. Parametric correlation and regression analyses are also robust in this case [12]. To avoid inflating Type I error by conducting multiple tests, multivariate analyses were used whenever appropriate. When the dependent variables were FA in individual traits, the three traits were tested simultaneously using multivariate GLM in SPSS (MANOVA, MANCOVA). When testing dependent variable composite FA (sum of the FA index for the three traits) we used univariate GLMs (ANOVA, ANCOVA). When the FA values were the independent variables and athletic performance (indexed by IAAF scores) the dependent variable, we used multiple regression.

Significance tests were conducted with an alpha level of 0.05, and, whenever appropriate, effect sizes are given in addition to p-values. Tests are two-tailed except when testing for relationships between FA and racing performance. In these situations we use a directed test, a compromise between one and two-tailed testing for strongly directional hypotheses [13,14]. Our previous work [1] showed a positive relationship between symmetry (low FA) and sprinting and there is no reason to expect that greater symmetry would result in poorer performance, therefore we have a strong directional hypothesis. Our other comparisons are not as obviously directional: effects of weight, age, and gender on FA and on performance and effects of athletic training on FA.

The dataset is available in the Dryad repository (http://doi.org/10.5061/dryad.s3630).

Ethical statement

This research was approved by the Institutional Review Board of Rutgers University, protocol #14–425 M. All participants were

Table 1. Statistical comparisons of FA index between athletes and controls.

Treatment	Pillai's Trace	$F_{3,183}$	P	
Athlete vs. Control	0.083	5.55	0.001*	
Gender	0.013	0.83	0.48	
Gender X A v. C	0.041	2.59	0.055	
Factor	**Trait**	**$F_{1,185}$**	**P**	**Partial eta^2**
Athlete vs. Control	Knee	10.37	0.002*	0.053
Athlete vs. Control	Ankle	4.55	0.034*	0.024
Athlete vs. Control	Foot	0.62	0.43	0.003
Gender	Knee	2.24	0.13	0.012
Gender	Ankle	0.26	0.61	0.001
Gender	Foot	0.04	0.84	~0
Gender X A. v. C.	Knee	4.60	0.033*	0.024
Gender X A. v. C.	Ankle	0.001	0.97	~0
Gender X A. v. C.	Foot	3.13	0.079	0.017

Multivariate tests compare the three traits simultaneously (knee, ankle, foot). Statistically significant relationships (two-tailed tests, alpha = 0.05) are indicated with asterisks.

informed on the purpose of the study and gave written consent. Permission of legal guardians was also obtained for subjects below 18 years of age.

Results

Measurements

Mean values (+/−SD) for the three traits are as follows (all n = 189): right knee 96.80 mm+/−7.63; left knee 96.66+/−7.94; right ankle 67.99+/−5.40; left ankle 68.70+/−5.48; right foot 259.89+/−17.23; left foot 261.03+/−17.49. A Mixed Model Sides X Individuals ANOVA (see Methods) demonstrates significant FA in all 3 traits (FA > measurement error: knees $F_{188,378} = 1.96$; ankles $F_{188,378} = 2.91$; feet $F_{188.376} = 5.55$; all $p < 0.0001$) and significant directional asymmetry (DA) in ankles ($F_{1,188} = 34.76$, $p < 0.0001$) and feet ($F_{1,188} = 23.00$, $p < 0.0001$) but not knees ($F_{1,188} = 1.47$, $p = 0.23$). The left foot and ankle tended to be larger than the right: 64.0% of subjects had larger left ankles and 61.9% had larger left feet, with little variation among groups. The significant p-values are so low that they are still at the $p < 0.0001$ level even with any correction for multiple tests. Because of the presence of DA, we use FA values corrected for DA (see Methods).

Athletes vs. controls

Mean values of the FA index (corrected for DA) for athletes and controls are presented in Figure 1. The FA index was compared between elite athletes and controls in MANOVAs with dependent variables knee, ankle and foot asymmetry, and group (elite vs. control) and gender as the factors. There are significant differences between athletes and controls in knee and ankle asymmetry, but not in foot asymmetry (Table 1). There were no significant sex differences, but a significant gender x group interaction for knees because female controls had particularly high mean knee FA

Table 2. Statistical comparisons of composite FA index (knee, ankle, and foot FA combined) between athletes and controls.

Factor	$F_{1,185}$	P	Partial eta^2
Athlete vs. Control	13.24	<0.0001*	0.067
Gender	0.54	0.46	0.003
Gender X A. v. C.	0.07	0.80	~0
Factor	**$F_{1,183}$**	**P**	**Partial eta^2**
Athlete vs. Control	12.82	<0.001*	0.065
Gender	1.63	0.20	0.009
Gender X A. v. C.	0.002	0.96	~0
Age	0.33	0.56	0.002
Weight	1.99	0.16	0.011

Results are shown first with no covariates ($F_{3,185} = 4.86$, $p = 0.003$, adjusted $r^2 = 0.058$) and then with covariates age and weight added ($F_{5,183} = 3.46$, $p = 0.005$, adjusted $r^2 = 0.061$). Statistically significant relationships (two-tailed tests, alpha = 0.05) are indicated with asterisks.

(mean+/−SD = 1.04+/−0.82, n = 56; compare to Figure 1). Using composite asymmetry (sum of knee, foot, ankle) rather than individual traits again demonstrates significant differences between athletes and controls and no significant effect of gender, but also no significant gender x group interactions (Table 2).

Including weight and age as covariates does not change the key results Again significant differences between athletes and controls are present for composite FA (Table 2) and separately for knees and ankles, but not feet (Table 3). The gender x group interaction is now significant for both knees and feet, rather than just knees, but not when using composite FA. There is also a positive relationship between weight and foot FA, but the overall relationship with weight is marginal and there are no significant relationships between age and FA (Tables 2,3).

Within-athlete comparisons

Relationships between FA and performance of the athletes, measured by IAAF scores, were tested using multiple regression. For FA we used the residuals of a regression between FA corrected for DA and discipline, to control for effects of particular events on symmetry (see below). There is a significant negative relationship between composite FA and performance (i.e., more symmetrical athletes perform better; Table 4). Among individual traits, a significant relationship is present for knees, with ankles marginal (directional $p = 0.087$; Table 4). There is also a significant effect of gender. Even without considering covariates age and weight, the regression model explains 12 to 13% of the variance in performance (adjusted $r^2 = 0.12$ when using composite FA and 0.13 when using individual traits). Partial r^2 values indicate that knee or composite FA, depending on the model, are each related to approximately 5% of the variation in performance (Table 4).

When age and weight are added in as covariates, there is a strong positive relationship between age and performance, and the regression model explains 27 to 28% of the variance in performance (adjusted $r^2 = 0.27$ when using composite FA and 0.28 when using individual traits; Table 5). The relationship with composite FA remains significant and is related to 5% of the variation in performance, but relationships with weight and with individual traits are not significant (both knees and ankles are marginal; Table 5). The effect of gender is no longer significant, and likely resulted in part from a selection effect based on age: generally the most successful athletes are those most likely to continue competing as they age, and this may be especially true of women. Examination of the historical records of those six males and six females with the top ten finishes per sex (two of whom are in our sample) reveals that the age effect is probably not only due to selection–there is also typically a within-individual improvement with age for several years, but then a leveling off and a decline late in an athlete's career, circa 28 years (www.iaaf.org/athletes).

We also conducted analyses restricted to those whose best event is the 100 m sprint, because we predicted the relationship between FA and performance to be particularly important for sprinting events and our sample for sprinters, although small ($n = 32$), is larger than for any other events. Here we use the index of FA corrected for DA, but not the residuals with event, because we are testing within one event. A regression with dependent variable IAAF score and independent variables gender, knee, ankle, and foot FA is not significant ($F_{4,27} = 1.97$, $p = 0.13$, adjusted $r^2 = 0.11$) but suggests relationships with knee and ankle FA ($\beta = -0.33$, directional $p = 0.044$ and $\beta = -0.33$, $p = 0.045$, respectively), but not foot FA ($\beta = 0.18$, $p = 0.46$) or gender ($\beta = 0.10$, two-tailed $p = 0.56$). The overall regression model is significant when covariates age and weight are added ($F_{6,25} = 2.84$, $p = 0.030$, adjusted $r^2 = 0.26$), but the apparent relationships with knee and ankle FA are no longer significant (knees: $\beta = -0.11$, directional $p = 0.34$; ankles: $\beta = -0.24$, $p = 0.093$). For foot FA, $\beta = 0.13$, $p = 0.55$. Two-tailed p-values for the other variables are all greater than 0.05, but less than 0.10. Relationships with composite FA are not significant (directional $p = 0.31$ without covariates, 0.43 with covariates), because, within sprinters, foot FA trends opposite the predicted direction and therefore when knee and ankle FA are combined with foot FA the relationships become weaker. When using composite FA, significant effects of gender ($\beta = 0.62$, two-tailed $p = 0.017$), age ($\beta = 0.39$, $p = 0.024$), and weight ($\beta = 0.55$, $p = 0.034$) are all present and 25% of the variation in sprinting performance is explained ($F_{4,27} = 3.56$, $p = 0.019$, adjusted $r^2 = 0.25$). IAAF scores should not show significant differences between males and females, because they are calculated to allow comparison of relative performance regardless of gender. The significant relationship we find is likely a result of our sample happening to contain particularly successful female sprinters.

In addition to testing for relationships between FA and performance, we tested whether symmetry among athletes varied with their primary event, because events differ in the stresses they produce and may cause both fluctuating and directional asymmetry. Because of small sample sizes for several events, the events were combined into three categories: straight sprints (100 m, $n = 32$), longer races with turns (200 m, 400 m, 800 m; $n = 29$), and events with jumping or leaping (100 and 110 m hurdles, 400 m hurdles, long jump, high jump; $n = 11$) [the one shot-putter was excluded]. An ANOVA test revealed significant variation among these categories in relative composite FA (not corrected for DA): $F_{2,69} = 3.67$, $p = 0.031$. A Tukey's HSD post-hoc test revealed that longer distance runners were significantly more asymmetrical than sprinters. Means for sprinting and jumping events were similar. In a MANOVA, there were no significant differences among groups for the individual traits, but the trends for knees and especially ankles match the trend for composite FA (Fig. 2). If we use the FA index corrected for DA the patterns are similar, but are not significant (composite FA index, $F_{2,69} = 2.37$, $p = 0.10$). However, here we specifically want to test the effects of athletic stresses, which are often asymmetric, on overall symmetry and therefore DA should be included. Above we were interested instead in the relationships between developmental stability (indexed by FA) and performance, and thus needed to factor out DA.

Discussion

Jamaicans are the elite sprinters of the world. Why? If symmetry of knees and ankles is a factor, why should Jamaicans be especially symmetrical (there is no knowledge of whether they actually are)? One possibility is heterozygosity for genes important to sprinting. The slave trade greatly increased heterozygosity on the West African side by mixing genes up and down the West coast of Africa from Senegal to Nigeria [15,16]. Recently a mtDNA haplotype has been isolated that correlates with success in African American–but not Jamaican–sprinters [17]. Since there is a general (if often weak) positive relationship between heterozygosity and body symmetry [18] we are eager to do targeted studies of genomics on areas associated with sprinting, including energy substrate utilization, muscle fibre-type distribution and body composition analyses (with specific reference to the shape and size of the glutei maximi). Fast twitch (anaerobic) muscle fibres are characterized by specific adaptations which benefit the performances of explosive high-intensity actions such as those involved in sprinting. Notably, West Africans appear to have a higher fast twitch muscle fibre

Table 3. Statistical comparisons of FA index between athletes and controls, with age and weight added as covariates.

Treatment	Pillai's Trace	$F_{3,181}$	P	
Athlete vs. Control	0.083	5.43	0.001*	
Gender	0.023	1.43	0.24	
Gender X A v. C	0.046	2.94	0.035*	
Age	0.021	1.29	0.28	
Weight	0.036	2.23	0.087	
Factor	**Trait**	$F_{1,185}$	**P**	**Partial eta²**
Athlete vs. Control	Knee	10.21	0.002*	0.053
Athlete vs. Control	Ankle	4.52	0.035*	0.024
Athlete vs. Control	Foot	0.49	0.48	0.003
Gender	Knee	2.26	0.14	0.012
Gender	Ankle	0.38	0.54	0.002
Gender	Foot	1.74	0.19	0.009
Gender X A. v. C.	Knee	4.34	0.039*	0.023
Gender X A. v. C.	Ankle	0.002	0.96	~0
Gender X A. v. C.	Foot	4.50	0.035*	0.024
Age	Knee	0.13	0.72	0.001
Age	Ankle	0.88	0.35	0.005
Age	Foot	2.73	0.10	0.015
Weight	Knee	0.04	0.84	~0
Weight	Ankle	0.05	0.82	~0
Weight	Foot	6.57	0.011*	0.035

Multivariate tests compare the three traits simultaneously (knee, ankle, foot). Statistically significant relationships (two-tailed tests, alpha = 0.05) are indicated with asterisks.

content than do comparable Europeans (67.5% vs 59% in one sample [19], as cited in [20]).

An interesting problem arises. How much is genetic quality revealed by overall body symmetry and how much is it associated with symmetry of particular body parts? To give a (partly) counterintuitive example, over-all body symmetry, based on 10 measurements of race horses, is positively correlated with performance in competitive races, but both lower body asymmetry, especially of the knees, is a correlate and so also are features of the head [21], as if the symmetry of the apparatus controlling the running (brain, head, sensory organs) is as important as the parts doing the running (themselves already selected for symmetry as shown in the Jamaican children, see [1]). Møller and colleagues [22] also demonstrated a link between lower-body symmetry and locomotion (in chickens), but did not measure upper-body traits. Manning and Pickup [23] showed for humans that degree of nostril symmetry positively predicts running performance in middle-distance runners, which is plausible since middle distance

Table 4. Multiple regressions within athletes, testing for relationships with performance (IAAF scores).

Factor	Beta	Partial r^2	P
Individual Traits			
Resid. Knee FA	−0.22	0.05	0.040*
Resid. Ankle FA	−0.17	0.03	0.087
Resid. Foot FA	−0.09	0.01	0.20
Gender	0.31	0.10	0.007*
Composite FA			
Resid. Composite FA	−0.22	0.05	0.031*
Gender	0.33	0.11	0.004*

FA values are residuals of the FA index on the athletes' primary events. Results are shown first for individual traits ($F_{4,68} = 3.38$, $p = 0.014$, adjusted $r^2 = 0.12$) and then for composite FA ($F_{2,70} = 6.20$, $p = 0.003$, adjusted $r^2 = 0.13$). P-values for the predicted relationship between FA and performance are directional (see Methods), and statistical significance is indicated by asterisks.

Table 5. Multiple regressions within athletes, testing for relationships with performance (IAAF scores) with age and weight added as covariates.

Factor	Beta	Partial r^2	P
Individual Traits			
Resid. Knee FA	−0.16	0.03	0.084
Resid. Ankle FA	−0.16	0.03	0.081
Resid. Foot FA	−0.06	0.01	0.34
Gender	0.21	0.02	0.20
Age	0.41	0.19	<0.0001*
Weight	−0.15	0.01	0.35
Composite FA			
Resid. Composite FA	−0.18	0.05	0.046*
Gender	0.24	0.04	0.12
Age	0.42	0.20	<0.0001*
Weight	−0.12	0.01	0.44

FA values are residuals of the FA index on the athletes' primary events. Results are shown first for individual traits ($F_{6,66} = 5.43$, $p < 0.0001$, adjusted $r^2 = 0.27$) and then for composite FA ($F_{4,68} = 8.04$, $p < 0.0001$, adjusted $r^2 = 0.28$). P-values for the predicted relationship between FA and performance are directional (see Methods), and statistical significance is indicated by asterisks.

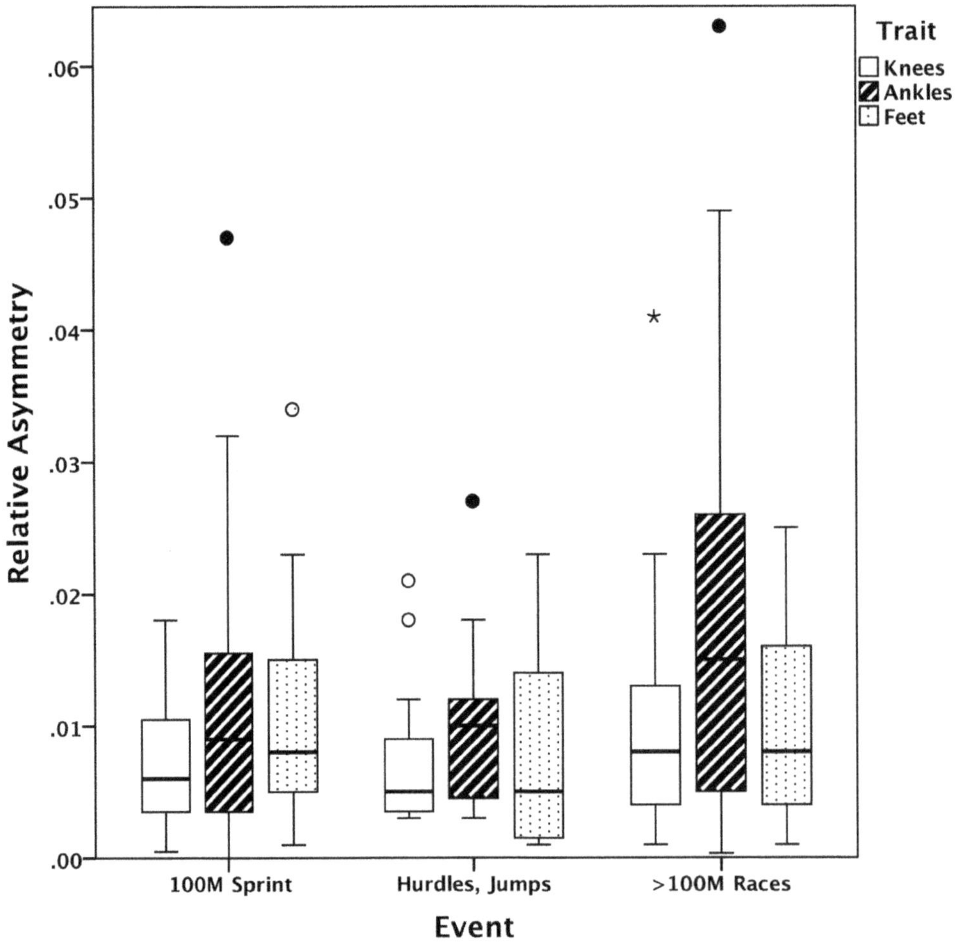

Figure 2. Boxplots for the three traits in athletes compared across events. These values reflect overall asymmetry, including FA and DA, divided by trait size. Knees are represented by open bars, ankles by bars filled with diagonals, and feet by bars filled with dots. Circles represent outliers, with stars indicating extreme outliers; color of circles and stars corresponds to coloring in bars.

running relies on oxygen much more than do sprints and symmetrical organs of air intake should maximize consumption. Foot asymmetry predicts physical aggressiveness in boys [24] and lower body symmetry predicts the same for college undergraduates [25], perhaps because stability is especially important in fights. Ear asymmetry, in turn, predicts tendency for women and girls to cradle a baby or doll, respectively, on the right side [3]. By contrast, Tomkinson, Popović and Martin [26] failed to find any significant differences between elite football (soccer) and basketball players, nor between elite (national league) and sub-elite (state leagues) categories of each. This is not surprising given their methodology. Numerous traits, soft body and hard, were measured for symmetry in each individual, and then averaged together so that a single average value was typically used. In our own work, symmetry of one part of the body (knees) suggests quality of associated parts as well, not just the bones of the knee but the attached cartilage, muscle, associated structures and developmental control. We know nothing about the details of this. The only part of the sprinting apparatus thought in advance to be important that we did not measure was the buttocks, hips, and glutei maximi (the largest and strongest muscles in the human body). Muscular strength measurements and imaging techniques such as dual-energy X-ray absorptiometry may allow a chance for progress on this (possibly key) variable.

A second problem has to do with cause and effect. If we find that those elite sprinters with the best times also have the most symmetrical knees, is it because those with symmetrical knees do well in advance or is it that intensive training leads to both success and more symmetrical knees? Of course it is likely that cause and effect go in both directions, and there is a weak trend toward decreased knee FA with age in the athletes ($r = -0.15$, $p = 0.22$). However, the fact that 8 year old knee FA predicts sprinting ability 14 years later [1] and that there are no statistically significant changes in symmetry with age in elite athletes, even though the older will have exposed themselves to symmetrical forces during training longer than the younger, suggests that knee symmetry is by no means a mere reflection of training.

In addition to the positive effects of symmetry on running performance that we demonstrate, we also find differences in symmetry between running events. Runners specializing in longer races are less symmetrical than sprinters, and this difference is particularly noticeable for the ankles. Why this is the case is unclear, but may relate to the asymmetrical stresses of events requiring turns and an increased prevalence of rearfoot striking in longer events, which would alter the distribution of stresses acting on the joints [27].

Acknowledgments

We are most grateful for the personal interest of Jeffrey Epstein and Gordon Getty. We thank Carla Hufschmidt and Tessa Cappelle for expert help in the field and John Graham for advice on analysis.

Author Contributions

Conceived and designed the experiments: RT. Performed the experiments: RT BF MR KM. Analyzed the data: BGP BF. Contributed reagents/materials/analysis tools: RT BF MR KM BJ. Contributed to the writing of the manuscript: RT BGP BF. Provided access to elite Jamaican athletes: BJ.

References

1. Trivers R, Palestis BG, Manning JT (2013) The symmetry of children's knees is linked to their adult sprinting speed and their willingness to sprint in a long-term Jamaican study. PLoS ONE 8: e72244.
2. Trivers R, Manning JT, Thornhill R, Singh D, McGuire M (1999) Jamaican symmetry project: long-term study of fluctuating asymmetry in rural Jamaican children. Hum Biol 71: 417–430.
3. Manning JT, Trivers RL, Thornhill R, Singh D, Denman J, et al. (1997) Ear asymmetry and left-side cradling. Evol Hum Behav 18: 1–14.
4. Manning JT, Trivers R, Thornhill R, Singh D (2000) The 2nd:4th digit ratio and hand preference in Jamaican children. Laterality 5: 121–132.
5. Van Valen L (1962) A study of fluctuating asymmetry. Evolution 16: 125–142.
6. Møller AP (2006) A review of developmental instability, parasitism and disease: infection, genetics and evolution. Infect Genet Evol 6: 133–140.
7. Møller AP, Swaddle JP (1997) Asymmetry, developmental stability and evolution. New York: Oxford University Press.
8. Spiriev B (2011) IAAF Scoring Tables of Athletics. Monaco: IAAF.
9. Palmer AR (1994) Fluctuating asymmetry analyses: a primer. In: Markow T, editor. Developmental Instability: Its Origins and Evolutionary Implications. Dordrecht: Kluwer. 335–364.
10. Palmer AR, Strobeck C (2003) Fluctuating asymmetry analyses revisited. In: Polak M, editor. Developmental Instability: Causes and Consequences. New York: Oxford University Press. 279–319.
11. Graham JH, Emlen JM, Freeman DC, Leamy LJ, Kieser JA (1998) Directional asymmetry and the measurement of developmental instability. Biol J Linn Soc 64: 1–16.
12. Gangestad SW, Thornhill R (1998) The analysis of fluctuating asymmetry redux: the robustness of parametric tests. Anim Behav 55: 497–501.
13. Rice WR, Gaines SD (1994) 'Heads I win, tails you lose': testing directional alternative hypotheses in ecological and evolutionary research. Trends Ecol Evol 9: 235–237.
14. Ruxton GD, Neuhäuser M (2010) When should we use one-tailed hypothesis testing? Methods Ecol Evol 1: 114–117.
15. Deason ML, Salas A, Newman SP, Macaulay V, Morrison EA, et al. (2012) Interdisciplinary approaches to the demography of Jamaica. BMC Evol Biol 12: 24.
16. Simms TM, Rodriguez CE, Rodriguez R, Herrera RJ (2010) The genetic structure of populations from Haiti and Jamaica reflect divergent demographic histories. Am J Phys Anthropol 142: 49–66.
17. Deason M, Scott R, Irwin L, Macaulay V, Fuku N, et al. (2012) Importance of mitochondrial haplotypes and maternal lineage in sprint performance among individuals of West African ancestry. Scand J Med Sci Sports 22: 217–223.
18. Vøllestad LA, Hindar K, Møller AP (1999) A meta-analysis of fluctuating asymmetry in relation to heterozygosity. Heredity 83: 206–218.
19. Bouchard C, Dionne FT, Simoneau JA, Boulay M (1992) Genetics of aerobic and anaerobic performances. Exerc Sport Sci Rev 20: 27–58.
20. Holden C (2004) Peering under the hood of Africa's runners. Science 305: 637–639.
21. Manning JT, Ockenden L (1994) Fluctuating asymmetry in race horses. Nature 370: 185–186.
22. Møller AP, Sanotra GS, Vestergaard KS (1999) Developmental instability and light regime in chickens (*Gallus gallus*). Appl Anim Behav Sci 62: 57–71.
23. Manning JT, Pickup LJ (1998) Symmetry and performance in middle distance runners. Int J Sports Med 19: 1–5.
24. Manning JT, Wood D (1998) Fluctuating asymmetry and aggression in boys. Hum Nat 9: 53–65.
25. Furlow B, Gangestad SW, Armijo-Prewitt T (1998) Developmental stability and human violence. Proc R Soc Lond B 265: 1–6.
26. Tomkinson GR, Popović N, Martin M (2003) Bilateral symmetry and the competitive standard attained in elite and sub-elite sport. J Sports Sci 21: 201–211.
27. Kulmala JP, Avela J, Pasanen K, Parkkari J (2013) Forefoot strikers exhibit lower running-induced knee loading than forefoot strikers. Med Sci Sports Exerc 45: 2306–2313.

5

Deceptive Body Movements Reverse Spatial Cueing in Soccer

Michael J. Wright[1]*, **Robin C. Jackson**[2]

1 Centre for Cognition and Neuroimaging, Department of Psychology, Brunel University London, Uxbridge, United Kingdom, **2** Centre for Sports Medicine and Human Performance, Department of Sport and Exercise Science, Brunel University London, Uxbridge, United Kingdom

Abstract

The purpose of the experiments was to analyse the spatial cueing effects of the movements of soccer players executing normal and deceptive (step-over) turns with the ball. Stimuli comprised normal resolution or point-light video clips of soccer players dribbling a football towards the observer then turning right or left with the ball. Clips were curtailed before or on the turn (−160, −80, 0 or +80 ms) to examine the time course of direction prediction and spatial cueing effects. Participants were divided into higher-skilled (HS) and lower-skilled (LS) groups according to soccer experience. In experiment 1, accuracy on full video clips was higher than on point-light but results followed the same overall pattern. Both HS and LS groups correctly identified direction on normal moves at all occlusion levels. For deceptive moves, LS participants were significantly worse than chance and HS participants were somewhat more accurate but nevertheless substantially impaired. In experiment 2, point-light clips were used to cue a lateral target. HS and LS groups showed faster reaction times to targets that were congruent with the direction of normal turns, and to targets incongruent with the direction of deceptive turns. The reversed cueing by deceptive moves coincided with earlier kinematic events than cueing by normal moves. It is concluded that the body kinematics of soccer players generate spatial cueing effects when viewed from an opponent's perspective. This could create a reaction time advantage when anticipating the direction of a normal move. A deceptive move is designed to turn this cueing advantage into a disadvantage. Acting on the basis of advance information, the presence of deceptive moves primes responses in the wrong direction, which may be only partly mitigated by delaying a response until veridical cues emerge.

Editor: Rouwen Canal-Bruland, VU University Amsterdam, Netherlands

Funding: The research was supported solely by Departmental research funds. The funders had no role in study design, data collection and analysis, decision to publish, or preparation of the manuscript.

Competing Interests: The authors have declared that no competing interests exist.

* Email: michael.wright@brunel.ac.uk

Introduction

A soccer player making a run with the ball will often execute a deceptive move known as a *step-over* in order to evade a defender. In recent decades, a number of international soccer players have become renowned for their skill in performing these moves, and awareness and appreciation of the step-over and its variants has increased amongst players, coaches and fans. This paper will examine how such deceptive moves produce their effects, and why even experienced players may be fooled by them.

Soccer is an example of an open-skill sport, that is, one where the environment and therefore the task at hand is constantly changing because of the actions of other players. Soccer players will benefit from being able to correctly predict the actions of their opponents because anticipation increases the time available for events such as intercepting a pass, blocking a shot at goal, or making a tackle. The importance, in interceptive sports, of body kinematics as a cue to future action, has been established in studies using point-light displays [1], [2]. Related studies have isolated which specific kinematic cues are predictive of the outcome of an action in sport, for example, the direction of a tennis serve [3], [4]. Furthermore, experiments within a range of interceptive sports, using video clips curtailed prior to critical events, consistently show better detection by experts of predictive information [2], [5], [6].

Competitive players also need to develop strategies to prevent their own actions from being anticipated. These strategies are broadly categorised as disguise or deception. Disguise strategies reduce the detectability of critical cues. For example, bowlers in cricket may minimize variations in different types of delivery such as topspinners and backspinners by keeping the movement pattern constant, except for the wrist action [7]. In the auditory modality, grunting by tennis players may be more than a vocal expression of effort, it may be an effective strategy in masking the sound of the racket-on-ball impact and thus degrading timing information [8].

Deception strategies introduce false or misleading cues that, if effective, result in the observer making an incorrect response [9]. Deceptive moves have been studied in rugby football [9–11], soccer [12–15] and tennis [16]. In these studies it was found that higher-skilled (HS) players are more accurate than lower-skilled (LS) players in predicting the outcome of deceptive moves, but that performance was nevertheless reduced by deception both for HS and LS players. This superior ability to anticipate both normal and deceptive action has been shown to depend on motor as well as sensory experience in the relevant sporting domain [17], [18].

When a visual cue directs attention to a visual location this has profound effects on the processing of information both at cued and uncued locations. The spatial cueing paradigm, whereby a visual cue stimulus can validly or invalidly indicate the location of a subsequent target, has given rise to many hundreds of experimental studies (see [19] for a review). A general finding is that reaction times (RTs) are faster for valid than for invalid cueing, so that the difference in RT provides an effective measure of spatial attention [20].

In a sport-related application of the spatial cueing paradigm [21], researchers studied directional judgements among novice basketball players. These experiments were based on the "head fake" in which a player attempts to deceive by gazing in one direction while passing or shooting the ball in another direction. Using stationary images of a basketball player about to pass the ball, the experiments demonstrated a spatial cueing effect of a player's head orientation, which produced a slowing of reaction times when incongruent with arm and body posture.

The use of stationary cues in spatial attention studies [14], [19] allows location and timing to be strictly controlled. On the other hand, Kibele [22] has proposed a cueing explanation for fast motor reactions in sports that is based on non-conscious analysis of perceived motion sequences of opponents. Could something as fluid and complex as a footballer's body movements act as an automatic spatial cue to the direction of play? A simpler case of cueing from biological motion is already known to occur: that is, the spatial cueing effect of point-light walker stimuli for left- or right- walking direction on detection of a brief visual target [23].

In the present study we investigate whether the kinematic body cues in typical one-on-one soccer play can produce a spatial cueing effect, and whether soccer expertise influences spatial cueing. The use of point-light stimuli allows the selective analysis of the effects of dynamical information, and we have tested the idea that the kinematics of a deceptive move reverses the spatial cueing effect.

Materials and Methods

Participants

Higher-skilled (HS) and lower-skilled (LS) male soccer players (age 18–33) were recruited by advertisement and personal contacts. HS players were defined as those currently belonging to a soccer club, training regularly, and competing in local or University leagues. LS participants comprised non-players or recreational players who did not train and did not play competitively. Demographic details and details of soccer experience were collected in a brief self-report questionnaire and are summarised in Table 1 for HS and LS participants; details of named clubs and leagues were checked online. Two different sets of participants undertook the two experiments.

Ethical Statement

The research was approved by the Psychology Research Ethics Committee of Brunel University before initiating the study. It followed British Psychological Society guidelines for research with human participants, in accordance with the Declaration of Helsinki. Written informed consent was obtained from all participants prior to taking part, and they were informed of the right to withdraw from the study.

Stimuli

Video clips (720×576 pixels, 24 bit colour) were made of three right-footed junior international level soccer players dribbling the ball towards a video camera (Panasonic NV GS400 recording at 25 frames/second) placed at a distance of 11.5 meters from the start of the player's run, in an indoor sports hall. The actors ran directly towards the camera, then on passing a floor marker, moved obliquely to the left or right as they would in evading a defending player's interception. The actors also performed a step-over in 50% of runs immediately prior to a direction change. The colour video was edited frame by frame to produce sparse binary (black/white) point-light representations consisting of 18 small disc markers on principal body joints and extremities (forehead, chin, L shoulder, R shoulder, L elbow, R. elbow, L wrist, R wrist, L pelvis, R pelvis, L knee, R knee, L ankle, R ankle, L toe, R toe, L heel, R heel). The ball was represented by a white disc matched to the silhouette of the ball in each frame, thus increasing in size as the player approached the camera. There was no representation of surface texture, depth, orientation or colour, either that of the player or that of the background in the point-light video. Occluded dots were masked. It is significant for the interpretation of results that the point-light player's head was represented by only two dots, one on the centre forehead and one on the chin. A sequence of stopped-motion frames from the point-light video of a step-over move is shown in Figure S1.

To generate the different levels of temporal occlusion, 6 normal and 6 deceptive source videos (two normal and two deceptive from each player) were cut off at various time points relative to the passing of the floor marker yielding 48 clips. Four occlusion levels were used relative to the final frame before the foot either made contact with (non-deceptive condition) or passed in front of (deceptive condition) the ball (−160, −80, 0 and +80 ms). In experiment 1, clips were presented in a pseudo-random order using Windows Media Player (Microsoft Inc.), with a 4 s blank interstimulus interval for responses. In experiment 2, stimuli were presented in random order and corresponding keyboard responses were recorded using e-prime2 (Psychology Software Tools, Inc.). They were viewed on a 43 cm computer screen at 120 cm viewing distance, and the players subtended approximately 7 deg vertically on closest approach. The point-light video was used in experiments 1 and 2, and the colour video was used for comparative purposes in experiment 1.

Design

The first experiment followed the design that is conventional for studying the effects of temporal occlusion on the ability to predict the outcome of an opponent's moves in a sport-related anticipation task. The purpose of this experiment was to compare the effects of low-resolution kinematic displays versus full video when HS and LS participants predict the direction of normal and deceptive soccer moves. The full video and point-light stimuli were presented in blocks, with order counterbalanced across participants; occlusion and deception variables were randomised within blocks, and the dependent measure was accuracy in predicting the final direction of the ball. The second experiment utilised the point-light video clips in the role of a spatial prime, and measured the reaction time (RT) to subsequent targets presented congruent or incongruent with the future trajectory of the ball. The purpose of this experiment was to establish whether body kinematic stimuli produce spatial cueing effects, whether deceptive primes produce reversed spatial cueing, and whether there are expertise differences in the normal and reversed cueing effects.

Procedures

Participants for experiment 1 were shown example clips of late-occluded video slides representing normal video with and without step-over, and point-light video with and without step-over, each with a brief identification from the experimenter. They were then instructed as follows: "Your task is to predict the direction that the player will take the ball, and you should respond as accurately as possible. To make the task more challenging, most of the clips are cut off before the ball changes direction. Please respond after every video clip, choosing the more likely alternative if you are unsure. If

Table 1. Soccer experience of the participant groups.

	Experiment 1		Experiment 2				
	Higher-skilled	Lower-skilled	Higher-skilled			Lower-skilled	
	Mean (*SD*)	Mean (*SD*)	Mean (*SD*)			Mean (*SD*)	
Age (years)	20.9 (2.9)	22.6 (4.6)	23.0 (3.7)			22.5 (3.3)	
Years playing	13.1 (3.9)	2.8 (4.1)	12.2 (6.1)			6.4 (6.2)	
Hours training/week	4.9 (2.8)	0.1 (0.45)	5.1 (3.6)			0.0 (0.0)	
				N	*N*	*N*	*N*
Amateur league (FA charter)				15	0	7	0
British Universities & Colleges Sport league				10	0	10	0
Other local league				2	0	2	0
Not competing in a league				0	20	0	19
Total *N*				27	20	19	19

you think he took the ball to your right, say "right". If you think he took the ball to your left, say "left"."

In experiment 2, the aim was to assess the effect of the video clips on a subsequent spatial target in the absence of any explicit interpretation or decision made on the video itself. Participants were shown example clips of the point-light player and the target stimuli. They were told that the soccer clips included both normal and deceptive (step-over) moves, but was not informative about the side of the target. For the experiment itself, on-screen instructions asked them to watch the video clips but respond only to the target. They were asked to press the "9" key with their right hand if the target was on the right and the "1 key with their left hand if the target was on the left. They were asked to respond as quickly and as accurately as possible.

Results

Experiment 1

Prediction of ball direction in normal and deceptive soccer moves using full video and point-light displays.

Twenty-seven higher-skilled (HS: $M=20.9$, $SD=2.9$ years of age) and 20 lower-skilled (LS: $M=22.6$, $SD=4.5$ years of age) soccer players viewed 48×2 s full video and 48×2 s point-light video clips and indicated the direction required for interception of a move (observer's left or right, forced choice). The dependent measure was percentage accuracy in judgment of direction. Expertise (HS, LS) was a between-participant variable, and stimulus format (full colour video, point-light), deception (normal, deceptive) and occlusion (−160 ms, −80 ms, 0 ms, +80 ms) were within-participant variables. Mauchly's test revealed a significant departure from sphericity for Occlusion ($W=.63$, $p<.005$) and Occlusion×Deception ($W=.60$, $p<.0005$), so a Greenhouse-Geisser correction was employed for these effects. Other data requirements for ANOVA were met. Partial eta squared (η^2_p) was taken as the measure of effect size appropriate for a mixed ANOVA [24]. Figures 1 and 2 summarise expertise effects, and the effects of temporal occlusion, video type, and deception. The corresponding statistical results from ANOVA are presented in Table 2.

Over all conditions, HS participants ($M=65.7\%$, $SD=8.82\%$) were more accurate than LS ($M=56.1\%$, $SD=6.2\%$). Differences were greater on deceptive moves (HS: $M=43.8\%$, $SD=15.5\%$; LS: $M=22.6\%$, $SD=13.8\%$) than on normal moves (HS: $M=87.6\%$, SD $=6.8\%$; LS: $M=89.6\%$, $SD=6.0\%$). Other significant effects of expertise such as a three-way interaction with occlusion and deception suggest that there are differences in the way that HS and LS participants processed cues. Significant within-group effects included a main effect of video type, with higher overall accuracy on full video ($M=62.9\%$, $SD=8.8\%$) than point-light ($M=58.8\%$, $SD=11.5\%$) stimuli. The largest effect size ($\eta^2_p=.92$) was found for the overall difference in accuracy between normal ($M=88.6\%$, SD $=6.5\%$) and deceptive ($M=32.2\%$, $SD=18.1\%$) moves. The variations in the shapes of the temporal occlusion curves in Figures 1 and 2 reflect significant interactions of temporal occlusion with video type and deception (Table 2) which would thus be consistent with variations in the pick-up of cues over time for the different video types and move types.

Planned comparisons were used to analyse the performance of HS and LS players on deceptive and normal moves, relative to a chance level of performance. As Table 3 shows, for normal moves, accuracy was better than chance at all occlusion levels for both higher-skilled and lower-skilled groups in both full video and point-light formats (one-sample t-tests). However, for deceptive moves, in both display conditions performance was below chance for early occlusion levels (LS: −160, −80, 0; HS: −160, −80 ms) and not significantly different from chance at late occlusion levels (LS: 80; HS: 0 ms). Performance at 80 ms for the higher-skilled group was also at chance in the point-light condition and was significantly above chance in the full video condition. Thus, the deceptive move successfully biased anticipation of ball direction in the wrong direction for both higher-skilled and lower-skilled groups, but higher-skilled players were able to show compensation particularly on late occluded clips (Figures 1, 2, Table 3).

The results showed a similar overall pattern of results for full video and point-light stimuli, but with superior performance on full video consistent with the reduction of spatial resolution and pictorial depth cues in the point-light kinematic representation. The performance of HS was superior to LS participants on deceptive trials, this corresponding to the significant interaction between expertise and deception in ANOVA. The fact that deceptive moves gave significant effects in the opposite direction to the veridical ball direction suggests that the deceptive move may cause a reversal of a spatial attention-biasing effect. This is tested in the next experiment.

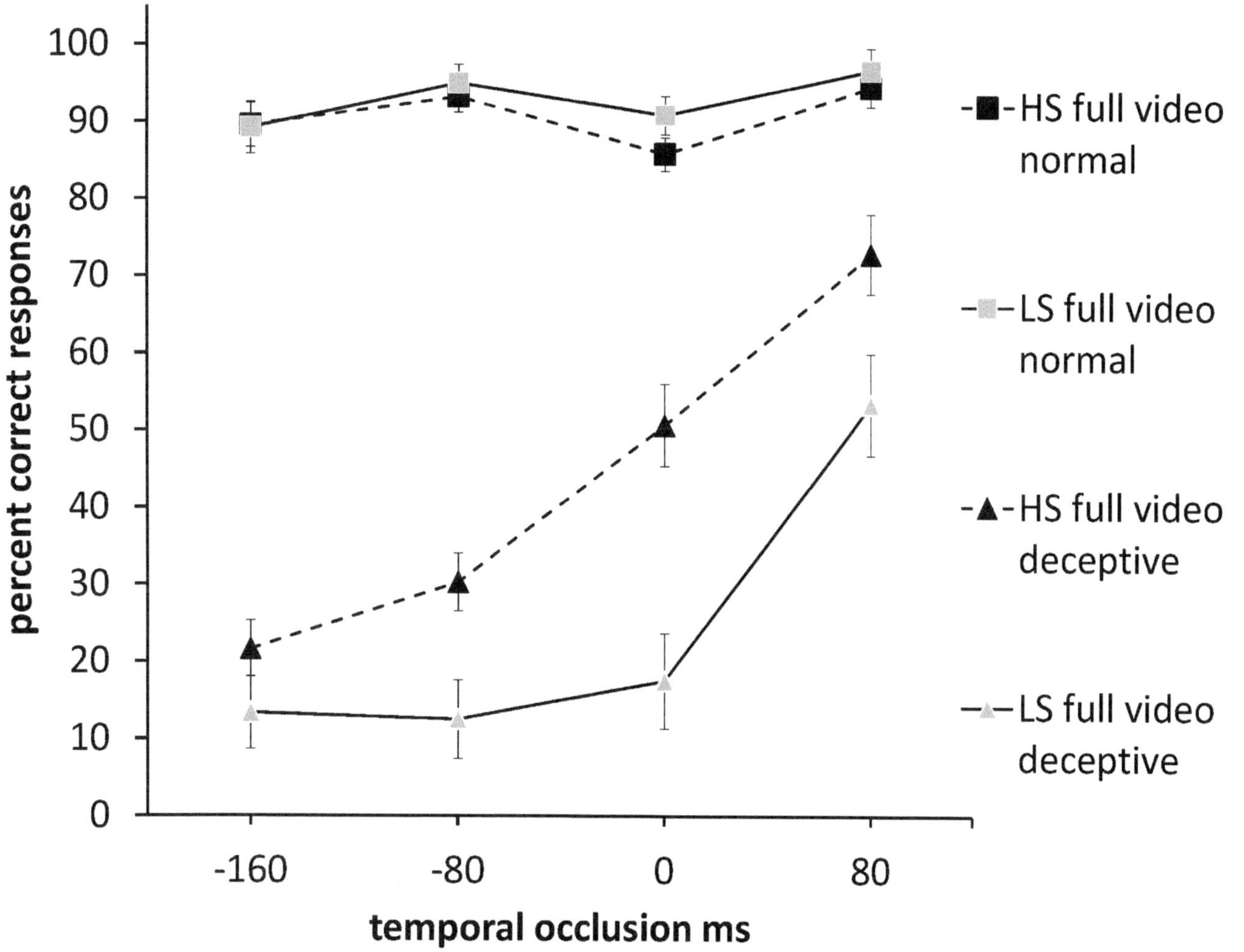

Figure 1. Accuracy in predicting the direction of the ball in normal and deceptive full colour soccer video clips in HS and LS players. Chance accuracy is 50%. The x-axis shows the temporal cut-off of the soccer video. Squares represent normal moves and triangles represent deceptive moves. Black symbols indicate HS players, and grey symbols LS players. Error bars are ± 1 SEM.

Experiment 2

Spatial cueing by normal and deceptive soccer moves in higher-skilled and lower-skilled groups.

In the second experiment, there were 19 higher-skilled males (HS: $M = 23.0$, $SD = 3.7$ years of age) and 19 lower-skilled males (LS: $M = 22.5$, $SD = 3.3$ years of age). The criteria for allocating participants to groups were the same as in Experiment 1, but no participants undertook both experiments. The cueing stimuli were identical with the point-light test set in Experiment 1, and each stimulus condition was presented twice, making 96 randomised trials. The stimulus sequence for a single trial is shown in Figure 3. The target stimulus was a small (0.5 deg) letter placed within a square box. The target letter could appear either in the left hand or in the right hand box on each trial. The onset of the target letter was 150 ms after the end of the video clip, and the duration was 150 ms. Instructions to participants indicated that they should watch the footballer but respond only to the target. The response required was a corresponding left-handed (key = 1) or right-handed (key = 9) keypress. Following the keypress there was a delay of 400 ms before the onset of the next video clip.

Mean errors (missed and incorrect responses to the target) ranged between 2.7%–3.7%, and were omitted from the analysis. All RT distributions departed significantly from normality (Kolmolgorov – Smirnov test, all $p<.05$). However, since the criterion for a cueing effect is a difference in RT between congruent and incongruent trials, the mean difference (RT incongruent – RT congruent) was computed for each within-participant variable (two levels of deception and four levels of occlusion). These cueing RT differences were consistent with a normal distribution for all eight variables (Kolmolgorov – Smirnov test, all n.s.) and Mauchly's test indicated no significant departures from sphericity. ANOVA was therefore conducted with the cueing RT differences as dependent variable, with all data requirements for ANOVA being met. The within subjects factors were deception (deceptive, normal) and occlusion (−160, −80, 0 and +80 ms temporal occlusion). The between-participant variable was expertise (lower-skilled, higher-skilled).

Normal soccer moves gave shorter reaction times (RTs) when congruent with the target, and deceptive soccer moves gave shorter RTs when incongruent with the target, that is the latter gave rise to a reversed cueing effect. The strongest effect observed on the incongruent – congruent RT difference was thus a significant main effect of deception, F (1, 36) = 19.22, $p<.0005$, $\eta_p^2 = .35$. As the graph in Figure 4 shows, cueing RT was

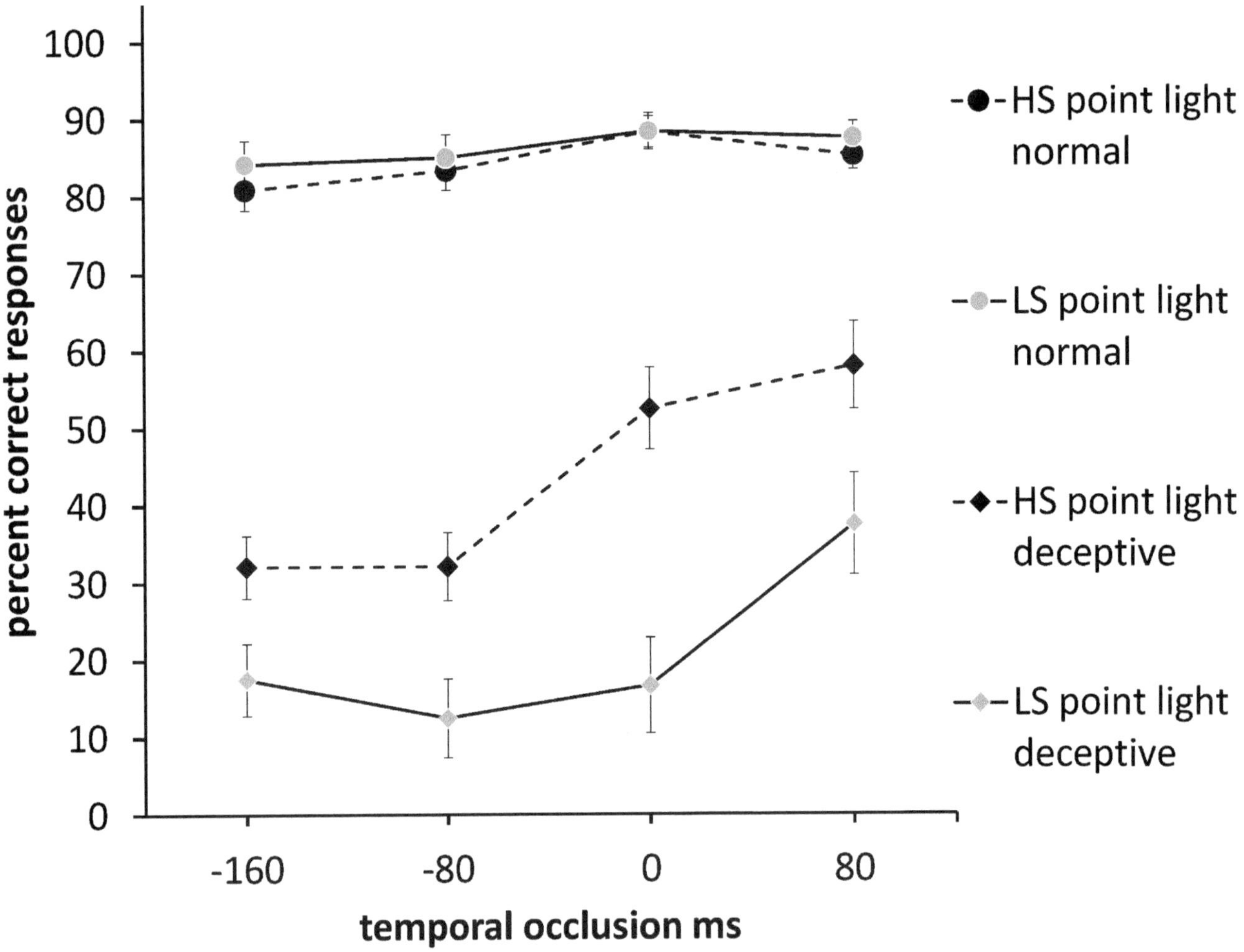

Figure 2. Accuracy in predicting the direction of the ball in normal and deceptive point-light soccer video clips in HS and LS players. Chance accuracy is 50%. The x-axis shows the temporal cut-off of the soccer video. Squares represent normal moves and triangles deceptive moves. Black symbols indicate HS players, and grey symbols LS players. Error bars are ± 1 SEM.

generally positive for normal moves and negative for deceptive moves. This means that for normal moves, when the target was congruent with the direction of play, RTs were shorter. Conversely, for deceptive moves, RTs were shorter when the target was incongruent with the direction of play, but congruent with the direction of the feint or bluff move. There was also a

Table 2. ANOVA results for experiment 1.

factor	*F*	*df*	*p*	η^2_p
Expertise	17.2	1,45	<.0005	.28
Video type	8.85	1,45	<.005	.16
Deception	506.1	1,45	<.0001	.92
Occlusion	42.5	2.3,102.6	<.0005	.49
Expertise × Deception	22.1	1,45	<.0005	.33
Video type × Occlusion	8.33	3,135	<.0005	.16
Deception × Occlusion	30.1	2.3,101.2	<.0005	.40
Expertise × Deception × Occlusion	3.66	2.3,101.2	<.05	.08
Video type × Deception × Occlusion	4.22	3,135	<.01	.09
All other interactions			n.s.	

Table 3. Accuracy of direction prediction compared with chance performance: entries in bold represent performance significantly below chance.

	lower-skilled			higher-skilled		
Full video	*t*	*df*	*p*	*t*	*df*	*p*
Normal −160 ms	10.1	19	<.0005	15.6	26	<.0005
Normal −80 ms	21.1	19	<.0005	19.4	26	<.0005
Normal 0 ms	15.9	19	<.0005	16.9	26	<.0005
Normal +80 ms	30.5	19	<.0005	14.4	26	<.0005
Deceptive −160 ms	**−8.5**	**19**	**<.005**	**−7.8**	**26**	**<.005**
Deceptive −80 ms	**−9.4**	**19**	**<.0005**	**−5.0**	**26**	**<.005**
Deceptive 0 ms	**−6.1**	**19**	**<.005**	.11	26	n.s.
Deceptive +80 ms	.56	19	n.s.	4.4	26	<.005
Point-light	*t*	*df*	*p*	*t*	*df*	*p*
Normal −160 ms	10.3	19	<.0005	12.5	26	<.0005
Normal −80 ms	13.1	19	<.0005	12.5	26	<.0005
Normal 0 ms	18.0	19	<.0005	17.8	26	<.0005
Normal +80 ms	22.6	19	<.0005	17.1	26	<.0005
Deceptive −160 ms	**−7.1**	**19**	**<.005**	**−4.4**	**26**	**<.005**
Deceptive −80 ms	**−11.8**	**19**	**<.0005**	**−3.4**	**26**	**<.05**
Deceptive 0 ms	**−6.5**	**19**	**<.005**	.69	26	n.s.
Deceptive +80 ms	−2.5	19	n.s.	.20	26	n.s.

Significance levels are based on planned comparisons against chance with one-sample t-tests, two-tailed, Bonferroni corrected.

significant main effect of occlusion, $F(3, 108) = 6.03$, $p<.005$, $\eta_p^2 = .14$. There were no significant differences due to expertise, and there were no other significant main effects or interactions. The direction of the occlusion effects was tested using polynomial contrasts, and these showed a linear relationship between cueing RT and occlusion level over the measured range, such that cueing RT becomes more positive with decreasing occlusion, $F(1,36) = 16.72$, $p<.0005$. $\eta_p^2 = .32$. Thus, for normal moves, increasing information from the video led to more normal cueing, that is, a bigger advantage for congruent moves. For deceptive moves, increasing information from the video led to a smaller disadvantage for congruent moves, that is a decreasing deceptive effect (Figure 4).

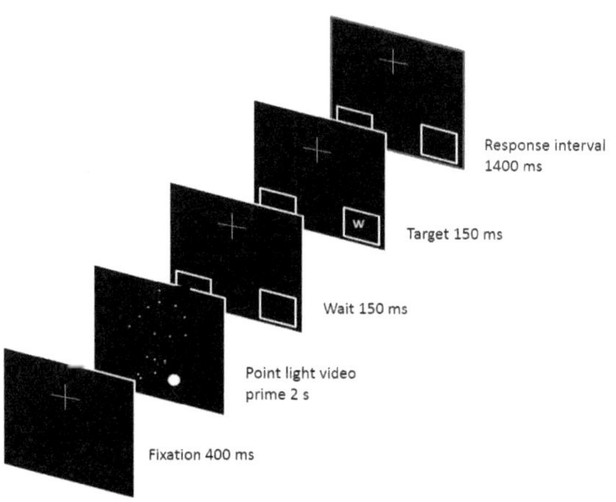

Figure 3. Stimulus sequence for a single trial of Experiment 2.

This implies that the critical cues that constitute the normal and deceptive moves had a different time-course, with the deceptive cues being earlier. Thus, rather than being identical up to the point the foot contacts or passes in front of the ball, the player's motion up to −160 ms is already generating a reverse cueing effect in the deceptive condition. Conversely, at this point there is no cueing effect for normal trials.

Discussion

The findings show that amateur soccer players in University and local league competitions are better than inexperienced or recreational players in predicting the direction of play. However both higher-skilled and lower-skilled players were adversely affected by deceptive moves, with LS significantly choosing the wrong direction at all levels of temporal occlusion, and HS significantly choosing the wrong direction for early-occluded sequences, and performing at or above chance level for late-occluded sequences. These results are broadly in line with previous findings in rugby football [9], [10] and tennis [16]. The first experiment showed that the effects of deception and expertise were similar in full video and point-light versions of the stimuli, although there was evidence of greater pickup of task-relevant cues from the full video stimuli. The expertise effects in Experiment 1 were not due to the verbal response mode because equivalent effects were found with manual response for full video [14] and point light [15] stimuli. The primary reason for conducting the first experiment was to establish expertise differences in an independent sample from the same recruitment pool and over the same range of temporal occlusion as the main (second) experiment and to establish the adequacy of the point-light stimuli for demonstrating effects of deceptive moves in comparison with full video stimuli.

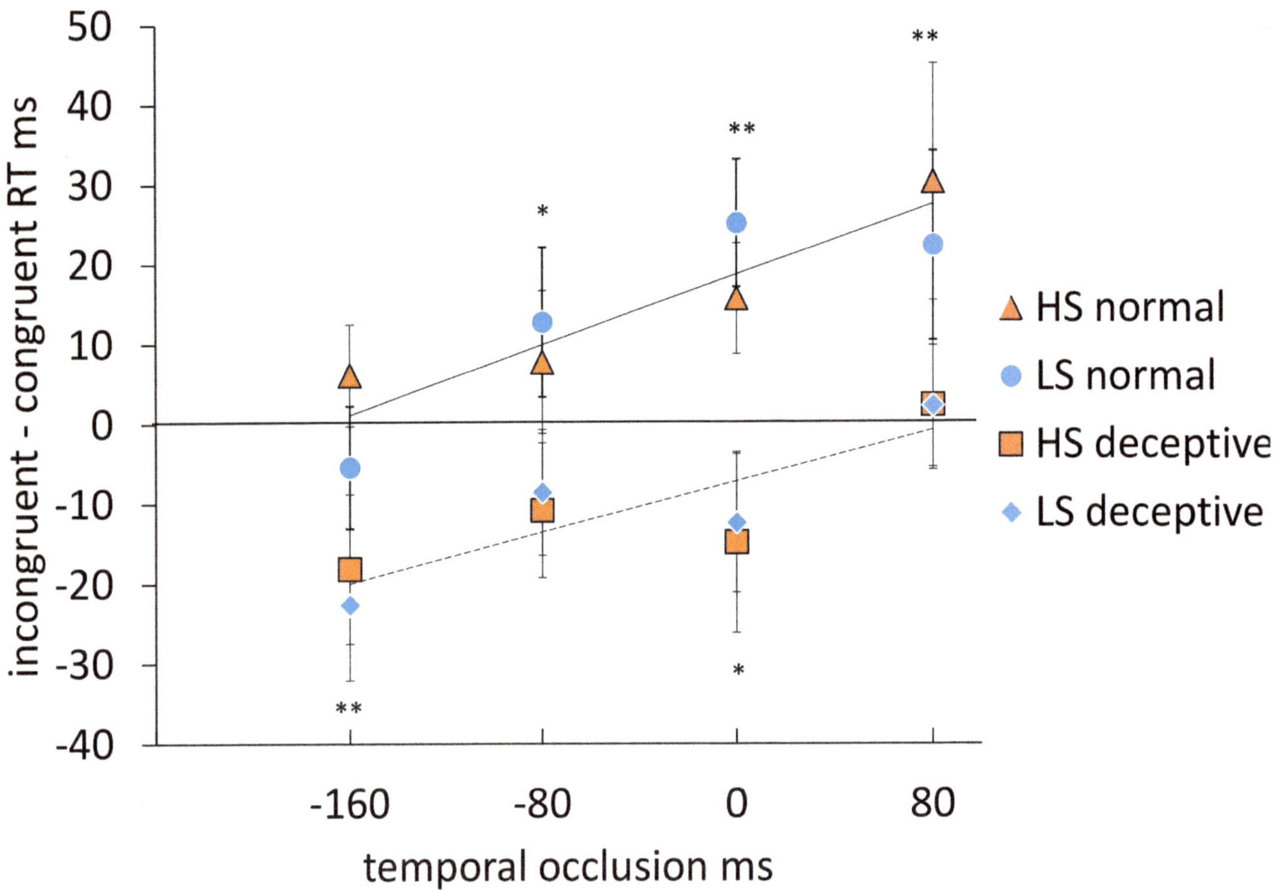

Figure 4. Cueing RT (incongruent minus congruent RT) is shown as a function of temporal occlusion for two types of cueing stimulus (normal and deceptive football moves) and two groups of participants (HS and LS). Regression lines were fitted to mean data by a least squares method (normal, solid line and deceptive, dashed line). One-sample t-tests show, for normal and deceptive moves, at which occlusion levels the mean cueing RT (across all participants) is significantly different from zero at $p<.05$ *, $p<.01$ **. Error bars are ± 1 SEM.

Caution must be exercised in extrapolating from these results to actual soccer play, because of concerns with ecological validity [25]. The angular size of the footballer stimuli on the computer screen was such that all the action was comfortably contained within the video frame, and was considerably smaller than would occur in a close interception on the pitch. The video stimuli were substantially impoverished compared with immersive 3D live action on the soccer field, and the element of sensory-motor interaction was absent. It is likely that higher-skilled players would be able to benefit from experience of these richer dynamic and contextual cues [26]. However the strengths of the reductive approach are that it allows isolation and analysis of specific cues, in particular, kinematic cues, and that it adds to a growing literature on biological stimuli as spatial cues.

An important development in understanding spatial attention is the evidence that a range of socially relevant stimuli can function as spatial cues. Both people within a scene and eyes within a face attract a strong fixation preference [27–29]. When we observe another person whose eyes are fixated on an object, our attention is directed towards that object. Direction of gaze acts as a spatial cue both in tightly-controlled laboratory experiments and in naturalistic scenarios [30], [31]. Social attention cues other than gaze have been less thoroughly studied but eye direction, head direction and hand gestures are all important components in directing social attention [32]. Gaze cues can also misdirect attention and this is one means whereby magicians create their tricks and illusions [33]. Although the walking direction of a point-light walker towards the left or right can produce a spatial cueing effect in the direction of motion [23], in the present experiment, cueing to a lateral target occurred when the net direction of locomotion of the point-light footballer was towards the observer. Kinematic cues can signal a future change of direction, and the step-over may resemble a mirror-image of the honest kinematic cues that are predictive of the direction of the turn. Thus in the present study, misdirection of spatial attention is proposed as the mechanism whereby deceptive soccer moves produce their effect.

Results indicated that the effects of normal and deceptive movements can be produced with purely kinematic, low-resolution, point-light information. Because the head was represented by only two vertical dots, these effects do not rely on direction of gaze. Furthermore, the cueing experiment indicated that in normal moves, spatial attention for targets in the future direction of ball play was cued by the player's body kinematics, whereas for deceptive moves, spatial attention was cued for targets on the opposite side to the future direction of ball play. It was shown that the time course of the reversed spatial priming in deceptive moves was earlier than the normal spatial priming in normal moves. This is consistent with the time-course and primary direction of the deceptive (step-over) and honest (outer foot pushing ball) movements.

Figure 4 showed that there was also a sustained cueing deficit for deceptive moves compared with normal moves across the whole −160 to +80 ms range. The dynamics of the deceptive move have a reversed spatial cueing effect like that of a normal move but in the wrong direction. The presence of deceptive moves thus opposes the overall attention cueing advantage that occurs with normal moves.

The present results exemplify the function of body kinematics as a cue for directing social attention; a function that is pre-eminent in dual interactions. One may suppose that the cueing of spatial attention by observed body kinematics is likely to be an evolutionary adaptation present in other mobile, visually proficient species. Cueing of spatial attention by body kinematics would help predators to anticipate the movements of prey, and equally it is advantageous for prey species to provide incongruent kinematic cues to evade predators. A good example of this is when wild mice execute sudden 90 degree turns [34]. Indeed spatial cueing by body kinematics may play a role in a wide range of within-species and inter-species behaviours that are reciprocal and time-critical.

In soccer, an advantage of acquiring deceptive skills such as the step-over is suggested by the current results. Not only can such moves frequently reverse the predictive decisions of opponents (Experiment 1), they can do so for HS as well as LS observers. On normal moves, HS and LS observers performed with similar levels of accuracy. On deceptive moves both showed high error rates relative to normal moves, but the HS observers were more accurate than LS, particularly on late-occluded stimuli. However, the spatial cueing effects on RT that occur in the absence of explicit identification of direction of play did not show any significant difference between HS and LS players. The different pattern of expertise effects in the two experiments could be explained by task differences, because the two tasks engage different attentional processes.

Evidently the spatial cueing effects of normal and deceptive movements in Experiment 2 are automatic, like those produced by arrow cues [19] gaze cues [31] or other biological motion cues [23] since they occur when the cue is not predictive of the target, and where instructions are given not to process the cue. The cueing effect on normal moves had the effect of speeding reaction times when the direction of the turn was congruent with the side of the target, and cue strength increased as more of the action was revealed with decreasing temporal occlusion. On deceptive moves, a reverse cueing effect occurred which had the effect of slowing reaction times to stimuli in the direction of the turn, relative to the incorrect direction. The reverse cueing effect decreased as more of the action was revealed with decreasing temporal occlusion, implying that the kinematics of the earlier parts of the deceptive move were more effective.

Thus correct prediction of the direction of a deceptive move requires a decision counter to an automatic adverse attention-biasing effect, and HS players achieved this more frequently than LS players in Experiment 1. This may require the move to be explicitly recognised as deceptive. In support of this view, HS players were found to be better than LS players at differentiating between normal and deceptive moves [15]. Secondly, it was found that the processing of deceptive moves recruited brain areas that are associated with error correction and inhibitory control, of which an example would be inhibiting an incorrect response tendency to a deceptive move [14]. Thirdly it would follow from this that for direction judgments in the presence of deception, accuracy should be increased by delaying a response, and that HS players should thus paradoxically have slower reaction times than LS, as has been found in the case of rugby sidesteps [10]. To the extent that HS players are able to correct, on some trials, an automatic response tendency based on spatial cueing by body kinematics, this could help account for the superior accuracy of HS players over LS players in direction prediction for deceptive moves.

Conclusions

Higher-skilled and lower-skilled soccer players were similar in accuracy of predicting the direction of play in normal and point-light soccer video clips, but both were inaccurate in direction prediction of deceptive moves. In relative terms, higher-skilled players were more accurate than lower-skilled players whose significantly below-chance accuracy, except at the latest occlusion level, implies a profound susceptibility to deception.

Occluded point-light video clips were shown to produce spatial cueing effects, thus body kinematics can direct attention in a predictive fashion. Reaction time to a small lateral letter target was faster when the side of the target corresponded with the occluded final direction of the soccer move, but only when it was a normal move. When it was a deceptive move, reaction time was faster when the target was incongruent with the (occluded) final direction of the move. Deceptive soccer moves produce reversed spatial cueing. The time course of normal and reverse cueing effects was consistent with the kinematics of the step-over (deceptive) and normal (honest) movements.

Supporting Information

Figure S1 Kinematics of a deceptive soccer move sampled at 80 ms intervals (left to right, top to bottom). The step-over begins in the top row. The player's right foot passes in front of the ball between the second and third frames of the middle row (marked with an x) then touches the ground and takes the player's weight. The bottom row shows the subsequent push with the player's left leg, and the left foot finally makes contact with the ball in the final frame, sending the ball to the player's left.

Data S1 Individual participants' data and results for Experiment 1.

Data S2 Individual participants' data and results for Experiment 2.

Author Contributions

Conceived and designed the experiments: MJW RCJ. Performed the experiments: MJW. Analyzed the data: MJW. Contributed reagents/materials/analysis tools: RCJ. Wrote the paper: MJW RCJ.

References

1. Abernethy B, Gill D, Parks SL, Packer ST (2001) Expertise and the perception of kinematic and situational probability information. Perception 30: 233–252.
2. Abernethy B, Zawi K, Jackson R (2008) Expertise and attunement to kinematic constraints. Perception 37: 931–948.
3. Williams AM, Huys R, Cañal-Bruland R, Hagemann N (2009) The dynamical information underpinning anticipation skill. Hum Mov Sci 28: 362–370. DOI: 10.1016/j.humov.2008.10.006
4. Cañal-Bruland R, Williams AM (2010) Recognizing and predicting movement effects identifying critical movement features. Exp Psychol 57: 320–326.

5. Abernethy B, Russell DG (1984) Advance cue utilisation by skilled cricket batsmen. Aust J Sci Med Sport 16: 2–10.
6. Abernethy B, Russell DG (1987) Expert-novice differences in an applied selective attention task. J Sport Psychol 9: 326–245.
7. Renshaw I, Fairweather MM (2000) Cricket bowling deliveries and the discrimination ability of professional and amateur batters. J Sports Sci 18: 951–957. DOI:10.1080/026404100446757
8. Sinnett S, Kingstone A (2010) A preliminary investigation regarding the effect of tennis grunting: Does white noise during a tennis shot have a negative impact on shot perception? PLOS ONE 5: e13148. DOI: 10.1371/journal.pone.0013148
9. Jackson R, Warren S, Abernethy B (2006) Anticipation skill and susceptibility to deceptive movement. Acta Psychol 123: 355–371.
10. Brault S, Bideau B, Kulpa R, Craig CM (2012) Detecting deception in movement: the case of the side-step in rugby. PLOS ONE 7: e37494.
11. Mori S, Shimada T (2013) Expert anticipation from deceptive action. Atten Percept Psychophys 75: 751–770. DOI: 10.3758/s13414-013-0435-z
12. Dicks M, Uehara L, Lima C (2011) Deception, individual differences and penalty kicks: implications for goalkeeping in Association football. Int J Sport Sci Coach 6: 515–521.
13. Savelsbergh GJP, Van der Kamp J, Williams AM, Ward P (2005) Anticipation and visual search behaviour in expert soccer goalkeepers. Ergonomics 48: 1686–1697. PubMed doi:10.1080/00140130500101346
14. Bishop DT, Wright MJ, Jackson RC, Abernethy B (2013) Neural basis of anticipation skill in soccer: an fMRI study. J Sport Exerc Psychol 35: 98–109. PubMed ID: 23404883
15. Wright MJ, Bishop DT, Jackson RC, Abernethy B (2013) Brain regions concerned with the identification of deceptive soccer moves by higher-skilled and lower-skilled players. Front Hum Neurosci 7: Art 851 1–15. Doi: 10.3389/fnhum.2013.00851.
16. Rowe R, Poulter DM, McKenna FP (2009) The effect of disguise on novice and expert tennis players' anticipation ability. J Appl Sport Psychol 21: 178–185.
17. Aglioti SM, Cesari P, Romani M, Urgesi C (2008) Action anticipation and motor resonance in elite basketball players. Nat Neurosci 11: 1109–1116. doi: 10.1038/nn.2182
18. Tomeo E, Cesari P, Aglioti SM, Urgesi C (2013) Fooling the kickers but not the goalkeepers: Behavioral and neurophysiological correlates of fake action detection in soccer. Cereb Cortex 23: 2765–2778. Doi: 10.1093/cercor/bhs279
19. Chica AB, Martín-Arévalo E, Botta F, Lupiáñez J (2014) The Spatial Orienting paradigm: How to design and interpret spatial attention experiments. Neurosci Biobehav Rev 40: 35–51.
20. Posner MI, Snyder CR, Davidson BJ (1980) Attention and the detection of signals. J Exp Psychol Gen 109: 160–174.
21. Kunde W, Skirde S, Weigelt M (2011) Trust my face: cognitive factors of head fakes in sports. J Exp Psychol Appl 17: 110–127.
22. Kibele A (2006) Non-consciously controlled decision making for fast motor reactions in sports – a priming approach for motor responses to non-consciously perceived movement features. Psychol Sport Exerc 7: 591–610.
23. Shi J, Weng X, He S, Jiang Y (2010) Biological motion cues trigger reflexive attentional orienting. Cognition 117: 348–354.
24. Richardson JTE (2011) Eta squared and partial eta squared as measures of effect size in educational research. Educ Res Rev 6: 135–147. doi:10.1016/j.edurev.2010.12.001.
25. Mann DL, Dicks M, Cañal-Bruland R, Kamp J van der (2013) Neurophysiological studies may provide a misleading picture of how perceptual-motor interactions are coordinated. Iperception 4: 78–80.
26. Farrow D, Abernethy B, Jackson RC (2005) Probing expert anticipation with the temporal occlusion paradigm: Experimental investigations of some methodological issues. Motor Control 9: 330–349.
27. Itier RJ, Villate C, Ryan JD (2007) Eyes always attract attention but gaze orienting is task-dependent: Evidence from eye movement monitoring. Neuropsychologia 45: 1019–1028. DOI: 10.1016/j.neuropsychologia.2006.09.004
28. Birmingham E, Bischof WF, Kingstone A (2008) Social attention and real-world scenes: The roles of action, competition and social content. Q J Exp Psychol 61: 986–998. DOI: 10.1080/17470210701410375
29. Yarbus AL (1967) Eye movements and vision. B. Haigh (Trans.) New York: Plenum Press.
30. Friesen CK, Kingstone A (1998) The eyes have it! Reflexive orienting is triggered by nonpredictive gaze. Psychon Bull Rev 5: 490–495.
31. Driver J, Davis G, Ricciardelli P, Kidd P, Maxwell E, et al. (1999) Gaze perception triggers reflexive visuospatial orienting. Vis Cogn 6: 509–540.
32. Langton SRH, Bruce V (2000) You must see the point: Automatic processing of cues to the direction of social attention. J Exp Psychol Hum Percept Perform 26: 747–757.
33. Kuhn G, Tatler BW, Cole GG (2009) You look where I look! Effect of gaze cues on overt and covert attention in misdirection. Vis Cogn 17: 925–944.
34. Walter RM (2003) Kinematics of 90° running turns in wild mice. J Exp Biol 206: 1739–1749.

6

PPARA Intron Polymorphism Associated with Power Performance in 30-s Anaerobic Wingate Test

Miroslav Petr[1]*, Petr Šťastný[2], Ondřej Pecha[3], Michal Šteffl[1], Ondřej Šeda[4], Eva Kohlíková[1]

1 Department of Physiology and Biochemistry, Faculty of Physical Education and Sport, Charles University in Prague, Prague, Czech Republic, 2 Department of Sport Games, Faculty of Physical Education and Sport, Charles University in Prague, Prague, Czech Republic, 3 Department of Kinanthropology and Humanities, Faculty of Physical Education and Sport, Charles University in Prague, Prague, Czech Republic, 4 Institute of Biology and Medical Genetics, the First Faculty of Medicine, Charles University and the General Teaching Hospital, Prague, Czech Republic

Abstract

To date, polymorphisms in several genes have been associated with a strength/power performance including alpha 3 actinin, ciliary neurotrophic factor, vitamin D receptor, or angiotensin I converting enzyme, underlining the importance of genetic component of the multifactorial strength/power-related phenotypes. The single nucleotide variation in peroxisome proliferator-activated receptor alpha gene (*PPARA*) intron 7 G/C (rs4253778; g.46630634G>C) has been repeatedly found to play a significant role in response to different types of physical activity. We investigated the effect of *PPARA* intron 7 G/C polymorphism specifically on anaerobic power output in a group of 77 elite male Czech ice hockey players (18–36 y). We determined the relative peak power per body weight ($P_{max}.kg^{-1}$) and relative peak power per fat free mass ($W.kg^{-1}{}_{FFM}$) during the 30-second Wingate Test (WT30) on bicycle ergometer (Monark 894E Peak bike, MONARK, Sweden). All WT30s were performed during the hockey season. Overall genotype frequencies were 50.6% GG homozygotes, 40.3% CG heterozygotes, and 9.1% CC homozygotes. We found statistically significant differences in $P_{max}.kg^{-1}$ and marginally significant differences in $P_{max}.kg^{-1}{}_{FFM}$ values in WT30 between carriers and non-carriers for C allele (14.6±0.2 vs. 13.9±0.3 $W.kg^{-1}$ and 15.8±0.2 vs. 15.2±0.3 $W.kg^{-1}{}_{FFM}$, $P = 0.036$ and 0.12, respectively). Furthermore, $P_{max}.kg^{-1}{}_{FFM}$ strongly positively correlated with the body weight only in individuals with GG genotypes ($R = 0.55$; $p < 0.001$). Our results indicate that *PPARA* 7C carriers exhibited higher speed strength measures in WT30. We hypothesize that C allele carriers within the cohort of trained individuals may possess a metabolic advantage towards anaerobic metabolism.

Editor: Balraj Mittal, Sanjay Gandhi Medical Institute, India

Funding: The authors report the following sources of funding: MSM 002160864 (Ministry of Education Youth and Sport), SVV 2012-265603 (Ministry of Education Youth and Sport), PRVOUK n. 38 (Ministry of Education Youth and Sport). The funders had no role in study design, data collection and analysis, decision to publish, or preparation of the manuscript.

Competing Interests: The authors have declared that no competing interests exist.

* Email: petr@ftvs.cuni.cz

Introduction

The study of genomic component of traits comprising athletic performance is at the center of the highly dynamic field of sports genomics. To date, polymorphisms in several genes have been associated with a strength/power performance including actinin, alpha 3 (*ACTN3*), ciliary neurotrophic factor (*CNTF*), vitamin D receptor (*VDR*), or info angiotensin I converting enzyme (*ACE*) [1–4]. The single nucleotide variation in peroxisome proliferator-activated receptor alpha gene (*PPARA*) intron 7 G/C (rs4253778; g.46630634G>C) has been repeatedly found to play a significant role in response to physical activity and other relevant gene-environment interactions [5]. Peroxisomes are organelles within the cell that play an important role in metabolism of fatty acids. They provide several essential metabolic functions such as shortening of very-long-chain fatty acids, later to be degraded in the mitochondria, and also help the cells to get rid of toxic peroxides. Peroxisomes proliferate and decrease in response to dietary lipids, hormones, hypolipidemic drugs, herbicides, and leukotriene antagonists, that bind to nuclear regulatory proteins called peroxisome proliferator-activated receptors (PPARs) proteins, which belong to the steroid hormone receptor superfamily. These receptors combine with the retinoid X receptors to form heterodimers that regulate genes involved in lipid and glucose metabolism, adipocyte differentiation, fatty acid transport, carcinogenesis, and inflammation [6–9]. PPARs exist in three different forms as PPAR-alpha (PPARα), PPAR-beta/delta (PPARβ/δ), and PPAR-gamma (PPARγ), which are encoded by similarly named genes – *PPARA*, *PPARD*, and *PPARG* [10]. PPARs act as ligand-activated transcription factors similar to other nuclear hormone receptors. Three variants of PPAR are distributed among various tissues. Unsaturated fatty acids bind to PPARα which is highly expressed in the heart, liver, kidney, and skeletal muscles [10], activating genes involved in fatty acid metabolism. During long-term fasting, the free fatty acids that are mobilized from adipose tissue bind to PPARα, enhancing hepatic fatty acid oxidation and production of ketone bodies, preventing hypoglycemia [11]. PPARα plays a role in the inflammatory response during atherosclerosis [12,13].

Several studies have associated *PPARA* gene variants with physical activity. For instance, it was associated with left ventricular growth in response to a ten-week exercise program with the largest increase found in 7C homozygotes [14]. Another study focusing on athletes in 13 different sport disciplines showed a linear trend of 7C allele with increasing anaerobic component of physical performance [15]. The analysis of muscle fiber composition in 40 young men revealed higher percentage of slow-twitch fibers in 7G homozygotes compared to 7C homozygotes [15], although a statistical significance could not be reached due to a low frequency of 7C/7C genotypes (n = 4). In another study *PPARA* intron 7 G/C variant along with *ACE* I/D variant were found to be the strongest predictors for muscle fiber type determination [16]. Group of Ahmetov et al. [17] included 7G allele of *PPARA* gene among ten "endurance alleles" whose number positively correlated with the proportion of slow-twitch muscle fibers, and with maximal oxygen consumption. According to Eynon et al. [18] endurance athletes showed a trend of a higher yet not significant proportion of the 7G/7G genotype compared with sprinters. Study of Lithuanian athletes had shown that male athletes with allele 7C had significantly higher muscle mass and better results in explosive strength of lower extremities than 7G/7G homozygotes [19]. On the other hand, 7C/7C genotype was more frequent among athletes in endurance and team sports than in speed/power and mix sports.

The objective of this study is to determine if previous findings of higher frequency of *PPARA* 7C allele in power/strength-oriented athletes would be supported by a positive trend to superior speed and power performance in a group of elite ice hockey players.

Materials and Methods

Subjects

All subjects (n = 77) were young, aged 18–36 y old, healthy, physically active Caucasian males – players of I. and II. National Czech ice hockey league. The detailed subject characteristics are shown in Table S1. The players were tested in the middle of the ice hockey season during the one-week competition break. None of our subjects followed low carbohydrate or energy restrictive diet before the tests. The Wingate test (WT30, described in detail below) results are referring to condition in season. Written informed consent was obtained from all subjects under protocols approved by the Institutional Ethics Committee of the Charles University of Faculty of Physical Education and Sport.

Anthropometric Measurement

Body weight (in kilograms) and height (in centimeters) were assessed prior to Wingate test to calculate an individual constant braking resistance. To estimate body fat percentage (BF) and fat free mass (FFM), the skinfold thickness was measured at seven sites (chest, midaxillary, triceps, subscapular, abdominal, suprailiac, front midthigh) by one trained technician using a Harpenden Skinfold Caliper (Baty International, Burgess Hill, UK) and formula by Jackson and Pollock was used [20].

Wingate Test

WT30 was used to diagnose an anaerobic power output of the tested group. Power output is calculated as a mean each 5 s. The best 5 s is called peak power, which is related to maximum and explosive strength abilities of individual [21]. The values can either be expressed in absolute values of peak power (P_{max}) expressed in Watt (W), relative peak power per body weight ($P_{max}.kg^{-1}$) expressed in Watt per body weight ($W.kg^{-1}$) or relative peak power per FFM expressed in Watt per FFM ($W.kg^{-1}{}_{FFM}$). P_{max} is regarded to mirror the alactate anaerobic processes, strength-speed abilities [22] and muscle rheological properties [23] of the tested subject. The WT30 test is a standard laboratory test for ice-hockey players and it is related to their skating performance [21,24]. The WT30 test was conducted on a calibrated friction loaded cycle ergometer (Monark 894E Peak bike, MONARK, Sweden) interfaced with a microcomputer. The cycle was equipped with toe-clips to prevent the subject's feet from slipping. The test consisted of a 30 s maximal sprint against a constant braking resistance dependent on the subjects' body mass (0.091 $kg.kg^{-1}$ body mass) according to the optimization tables of Bar-Or [22]. The test began from a rolling start, at maximal individual repetition against minimal resistance. When the maximum pedal rate was achieved, a countdown of "3-2-1-go!" was given before dropping the weight basket with a load. Prior to the test participants were instructed to pedal as fast as they could for 30 s.

DNA and Genotyping

Saliva samples were collected from individuals using FTA-cards (Whatman, USA). Samples (3 mm punch) were lysed and DNA was stabilized with DNA Extract All Reagents Kit (Applied Biosystems, USA) according to the manufacturers protocol. Selected loci were amplified in thermal cycler (Eppendorf, Germany), using TaqMan SNP Genotyping Assays (Assays IDs: C__2985251_10) and TaqMan Genotyping Master Mix (Applied Biosystems), in 20-µl reactions, each containing 10 µl of Master Mix, 1 µl of genotyping assay, 5 µl of DNase-free water and 4 µl of sample lysate. Cycling conditions were as follows: DNA polymerase activation at 95°C for 20 s, followed by 40 cycles of denaturation at 95°C for 3 s and Annealing/Extending step at 60°C for 20 s. PCR products were then subjected to Endpoint-genotyping analysis (program: post-genotyping, analysis mode: melting curves, detection format: dual color hydrolysis probe, color compensation: universal CC FAM(510) – VIC(580)) at LC 480 Light Cycler (Roche), in order to measure the relative amount of allele-specific fluorescence (FAM or VIC), which leads directly to the determination of individual genotypes.

Statistics

All the phenotype and genotype data are presented in the Supporting information file in form of Table S1. All variables were initially tested for normality using the Kolmogorov-Smirnov test. Since all the variables were normally distributed, the data are expressed as a mean ± SEM (Standard Error of the Mean). One-way analysis of variance (ANOVA) and independent samples t-test were used to evaluate differences between genotype groups. Pearson product-moment correlations and linear regression analyses specific for distinct genotype groups were performed to assess the relationships among continuous variables. Statistical significance was accepted at $P<0.05$ and p-values<0.1 were considered as marginally significant. All analyses were conducted using SPSS version 17.0 (SPSS, Inc., Chicago, IL).

Results and Discussion

As evident from the Table 1 listing the genotype and allelic frequencies of all 77 ice hockey players, the minor C allele was found at a frequency over 29%. Such frequency is substantially higher than those observed e.g. in reference Caucasian HapMap populations (19.6%), European healthy controls (Poles–21.3%, British–18.1%, Germans–17.9%) [14,25] and much higher than C allele frequencies detected in endurance-oriented cohorts [25,26]. The assumption of the Hardy-Weinberg equilibrium was tested

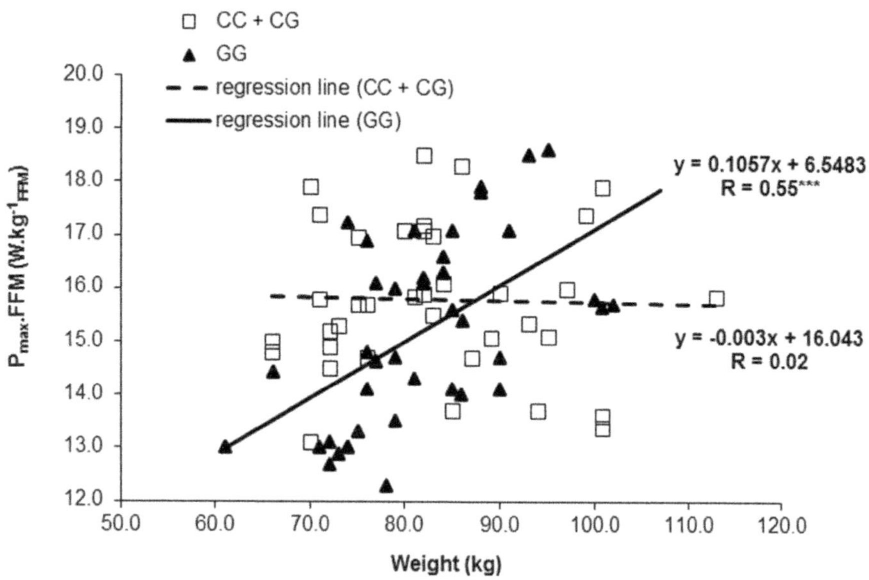

Figure 1. Effect of PPARA intron 7 G/C polymorphism on the relationship between body weight and P_{max}.FFM. ***$p<0.001$; R = Pearson product – moment correlation.

using Pearson χ^2 test. It was found that this test fails to reject the null hypothesis that the population is in Hardy-Weinberg equilibrium ($\chi^2 = 0.055$; df = 1; p = 0.97). There were no significant differences observed in age, anthropometric characteristics, or activity level across different *PPARA* genotypes (Table 2). We found statistically significant difference of $P_{max}.kg^{-1}$ and marginally significant difference of $P_{max}.kg^{-1}{}_{FFM}$ in WT30 between carriers and non-carriers for C allele (14.6±0.2 vs. 13.9±0.3 $W.kg^{-1}$ and 15.8±0.2 vs. 15.2±0.3 $W.kg^{-1}{}_{FFM}$, P = 0.036 and 0.12, respectively). The comparison among individual genotypes revealed no significant differences (P = 0.095 and 0.21 for $P_{max}.kg^{-1}$ and P_{max}.FFM, respectively) possibly reflecting relatively low number of CC homozygous in our group of athletes (N = 7). Furthermore, $P_{max}.kg^{-1}{}_{FFM}$ positive correlation with the body weight was significantly stronger in individuals with GG genotypes in comparison with carriers of the C allele (R = 0.55 [GG] vs. 0.02 [CG+CC], respectively; z-score = 2.538; p = 0.0055) as shown in Figure 1.

The present report is the first to demonstrate a higher relative peak power per body weight ($P_{max}.kg^{-1}$), and relative peak power per FFM ($P_{max}.kg^{-1}{}_{FFM}$) in WT30 in *PPARA* 7C allele carriers. Our results corroborate and extend the previous reports showing that 7C is a hot candidate of speed/power-related allele. Ice hockey is characterized by high intensity intermittent skating, rapid changes in velocity and duration, and frequent body contact. The intensity and duration of a particular shift determines the extent of the contribution from aerobic and anaerobic energy systems. Glycogen depletion studies show a preferential utilization of glycogen from the slow twitch fibers but also significant depletion from the fast twitch fibers. Although elite hockey players display a muscle fiber composition similar to untrained individuals [27], those with predominance of fast twitch fibers could have advantage in training of muscular strength and skating speed.

Better scores in WT30 in C allele carriers and positive peak power-increasing effect with body weight in GG genotypes do not have a clear explanation. Activation of PPARA favors lipid sparing [28], improves insulin sensitivity and affects some important cell functions [29]. Although 7 G/C polymorphism is located in noncoding region, it has been associated with a functional variant in a promoter or enhancer element of the *PPARA* gene that results in reduced *PPARA* gene expression [14]. It was shown that C allele carriers are possibly less responsive to β-adrenergic stimulation compared with GG homozygotes [30]. In fact, 7 C/C genotype and C allele containing haplotype significantly increased the risk for diabetes [31,32]. The consequences of these changes may have an important role in a muscle metabolism, such as inhibited glycogenolysis and partly limited glucose transport into a skeletal muscle. On the other hand, an increased expression of *PPARA* gene and the intermittent increase in fatty acid delivery to muscle during exercise training may both be important factors in enhancing muscle fatty acid oxidative capacity [33]. These processes are likely to be more active in 7G carriers. Under the circumstances it is possible that during intense exercise 7C carriers are more prone to rely on anaerobic processes what may be an adaptive stimulus leading to muscle fiber transformation. A muscle fiber composition have not been monitored in our study, but at least two studies associated *PPARA* 7 G/C genotypes with a muscle fiber specific composition in athletes [15,16]. Whilst initial composition is likely to be strongly influenced by genetic factors, training has significant effects on fiber shifts and related muscle

Table 1. PPARA 7 G/C genotype and allelic frequencies in 77 elite hockey players.

	GG	CG	CC	allele G	allele C
Frequencies (%)	0.51	0.40	0.09	0.71	0.29

Table 2. Basic descriptive statistics.

Variable	GG	CG	CC	CG + CC	p-value CC + CG vs. GG
N	39	31	7	38	
age	25.6±0.7	24.3±0.7	26.1±1.6	24.7±0.6	0.31
height (cm)	181.8±0.8	180.9±1.2	181.4±3.5	181.0±1.2	0.59
weight (kg)	81.9±1.5	82.2±2.0	86.5±4.9	83.0±1.8	0.63
FFM (kg)	75.0±1.2	76.2±1.7	76.9±3.9	76.3±1.5	0.49
$P_{max}.kg^{-1}$ ($W.kg^{-1}$)	13.9±0.3	14.7±0.2	14.3±0.6	14.6±0.2	0.036*
$P_{max}.FFM$ ($W.kg^{-1}{}_{FFM}$)	15.2±0.3	15.9±0.2	15.3±0.6	15.8±0.2	0.12

Data are expressed as mean ± SEM (Standard Error of the Mean); p-values are based on independent samples t-tests; *$p<0.05$.

metabolism changes. We propose an important role of *PPARA* 7 G/C polymorphism in these processes.

We are aware of several limitations of our study including relatively smaller sample size and potential effects of other environmental (e.g. dietary) or genetic factors. Validation in other cohorts and further studies are necessary to address the detailed role of the *PPARA* intron polymorphism within the complex phenotype of strength/power performance. All subjects included in our study were male elite ice hockey players, so whether the results are applicable to female population engaged in the same or similar sport discipline, is uncertain. Also, our findings most likely cannot be generalized to normal male population. Recent study in nonathletic population did not confirm any difference in strength parameters during static or dynamic conditions depending on 7 G/C polymorphism [34].

Our results regarding *PPARA* intron 7 G/C polymorphic site association with anaerobic power output may contribute to better understanding how genetics affects individual physiological variability resulting in different expression of muscle work. The C allele carriers might favor power/strength-oriented sport performance. Once the genetic variants related to athletes' performance are understood, it may be possible to develop genetic tests that may be used to identify sport talent. Furthermore, intervention genetic studies in the future may possibly uncover what training methods and approaches are potentially more beneficial for different genotypes.

Supporting Information

Table S1 Descriptive data of the 77 ice-hockey players. LBM - lean body mass; Pmax/kg - relative peak power per body weight.

Author Contributions

Conceived and designed the experiments: MP PŠ OP MŠ. Performed the experiments: MP PŠ MŠ EK. Analyzed the data: MP OP OŠ. Contributed reagents/materials/analysis tools: OŠ. Contributed to the writing of the manuscript: MP OŠ EK.

References

1. Windelinckx A, De Mars G, Beunen G, Aerssens J, Delecluse C, et al. (2007) Polymorphisms in the vitamin D receptor gene are associated with muscle strength in men and women. Osteoporos Int 18: 1235–1242.
2. De Mars G, Windelinckx A, Beunen G, Delecluse C, Lefevre J, et al. (2007) Polymorphisms in the CNTF and CNTF receptor genes are associated with muscle strength in men and women. J Appl Physiol 102: 1824–1831.
3. Druzhevskaya AM, Ahmetov II, Astratenkova IV, Rogozkin VA (2008) Association of the ACTN3 R577X polymorphism with power athlete status in Russians. Eur J Appl Physiol 103: 631–634.
4. Eynon N, Alves AJ, Yamin C, Sagiv M, Duarte JA, et al. (2009) Is there an ACE ID - ACTN3 R577X polymorphisms interaction that influences sprint performance? Int J Sports Med 30: 888–891.
5. Šeda O, Šedová L (2007) Peroxisome proliferator-activated receptors as molecular targets in relation to obesity and type 2 diabetes. Pharmacogenomics 8: 587–596.
6. Dubuquoy L, Dharancy S, Nutten S, Pettersson S, Auwerx J, et al. (2002) Role of peroxisome proliferator-activated receptor gamma and retinoid X receptor heterodimer in hepatogastroenterological diseases. Lancet 360: 1410–1418.
7. Spiegelman BM (1998) PPAR-gamma: adipogenic regulator and thiazolidinedione receptor. Diabetes 47: 507–514.
8. Mukherjee R, Jow L, Croston GE, Paterniti JR, Jr. (1997) Identification, characterization, and tissue distribution of human peroxisome proliferator-activated receptor (PPAR) isoforms PPARgamma2 versus PPARgamma1 and activation with retinoid X receptor agonists and antagonists. J Biol Chem 272: 8071–8076.
9. Cabrero A, Laguna JC, Vazquez M (2002) Peroxisome proliferator-activated receptors and the control of inflammation. Curr Drug Targets 1: 243–248.
10. Braissant O, Foufelle F, Scotto C, Dauca M, Wahli W (1996) Differential expression of peroxisome proliferator-activated receptors (PPARs): tissue distribution of PPAR-alpha, -beta, and -gamma in the adult rat. Endocrinology 137: 354–366.
11. Leone TC, Weinheimer CJ, Kelly DP (1999) A critical role for the peroxisome proliferator-activated receptor alpha (PPARalpha) in the cellular fasting response: the PPARalpha-null mouse as a model of fatty acid oxidation disorders. Proc Natl Acad Sci U S A 96: 7473–7478.
12. Staels B, Koenig W, Habib A, Merval R, Lebret M, et al. (1998) Activation of human aortic smooth-muscle cells is inhibited by PPARalpha but not by PPARgamma activators. Nature 393: 790–793.
13. Pyper SR, Viswakarma N, Yu S, Reddy JK (2010) PPARalpha: energy combustion, hypolipidemia, inflammation and cancer. Nucl Recept Signal 8: e002.
14. Jamshidi Y, Montgomery HE, Hense HW, Myerson SG, Torra IP, et al. (2002) Peroxisome proliferator-activated receptor alpha gene regulates left ventricular growth in response to exercise and hypertension. Circulation 105: 950–955.
15. Ahmetov II, Mozhayskaya IA, Flavell DM, Astratenkova IV, Komkova AI, et al. (2006) PPARalpha gene variation and physical performance in Russian athletes. Eur J Appl Physiol 97: 103–108.
16. Ahmetov II, Astratenkova IV, Druzhevskaia AM, Komkova AI, Liubaeva EV, et al. (2006) The association of gene polymorphisms with the muscle fiber type composition. Ross Fiziol Zh Im I M Sechenova 92: 883–888.
17. Ahmetov II, Williams AG, Popov DV, Lyubaeva EV, Hakimullina AM, et al. (2009) The combined impact of metabolic gene polymorphisms on elite endurance athlete status and related phenotypes. Hum Genet 126: 751–761.
18. Eynon N, Meckel Y, Sagiv M, Yamin C, Amir R, et al. (2010) Do PPARGC1A and PPARalpha polymorphisms influence sprint or endurance phenotypes? Scand J Med Sci Sports 20: e145–150.
19. Ginevičienė V, Pranckevičienė E, Milašius K, Kučinskas V (2010) Relating fi tness phenotypes to genotypes in Lithuanian elite athletes. Acta Medica Lituanica 17: 1–10.
20. Jackson AS, Pollock ML (1978) Generalized equations for predicting body density of men. Br J Nutr 40: 497–504.

21. Farlinger CM, Kruisselbrink LD, Fowles JR (2007) Relationships to skating performance in competitive hockey players. J Strength Cond Res 21: 915–922.
22. Bar-Or O (1987) The Wingate anaerobic test. An update on methodology, reliability and validity. Sports Med 4: 381–394.
23. Jelen K, Lopot F, Budka S, Novacek V, Sedlacek R (2008) Rheological properties of myometrium: experimental quantification and mathematical modeling. Neuro Endocrinol Lett 29: 454–460.
24. Cox MH, Miles DS, Verde TJ, Rhodes EC (1995) Applied physiology of ice hockey. Sports Med 19: 184–201.
25. Maciejewska A, Sawczuk M, Cieszczyk P (2011) Variation in the PPARalpha gene in Polish rowers. J Sci Med Sport 14: 58–64.
26. Ahmetov II, Popov DV, Mozhaiskaia IA, Missina SS, Astratenkova IV, et al. (2007) Association of regulatory genes polymorphisms with aerobic and anaerobic performance of athletes. Ross Fiziol Zh Im I M Sechenova 93: 837–843.
27. Montgomery DL (1988) Physiology of ice hockey. Sports Med 5: 99–126.
28. Lefebvre P, Chinetti G, Fruchart JC, Staels B (2006) Sorting out the roles of PPAR alpha in energy metabolism and vascular homeostasis. J Clin Invest 116: 571–580.
29. Guerre-Millo M, Gervois P, Raspe E, Madsen L, Poulain P, et al. (2000) Peroxisome proliferator-activated receptor alpha activators improve insulin sensitivity and reduce adiposity. J Biol Chem 275: 16638–16642.
30. Cresci S, Jones PG, Sucharov CC, Marsh S, Lanfear DE, et al. (2008) Interaction between PPARA genotype and beta-blocker treatment influences clinical outcomes following acute coronary syndromes. Pharmacogenomics 9: 1403–1417.
31. Cresci S (2008) PPAR Genomics and Pharmacogenomics: Implications for Cardiovascular Disease. PPAR Res 2008: 374549.
32. Flavell DM, Ireland H, Stephens JW, Hawe E, Acharya J, et al. (2005) Peroxisome proliferator-activated receptor alpha gene variation influences age of onset and progression of type 2 diabetes. Diabetes 54: 582–586.
33. Horowitz JF, Leone TC, Feng W, Kelly DP, Klein S (2000) Effect of endurance training on lipid metabolism in women: a potential role for PPARalpha in the metabolic response to training. Am J Physiol Endocrinol Metab 279: E348–355.
34. Broos S, Windelinckx A, De Mars G, Huygens W, Peeters MW, et al. (2011) Is PPARalpha intron 7 G/C polymorphism associated with muscle strength characteristics in nonathletic young men? Scand J Med Sci Sports.

Gender Differences in Emotional Responses to Cooperative and Competitive Game Play

J. Matias Kivikangas[1]*, Jari Kätsyri[2], Simo Järvelä[1], Niklas Ravaja[1,3]

1 Department of Information and Service Economy, Aalto University School of Business, Helsinki, Finland, **2** Department of Media Technology, Aalto University School of Science, Espoo, Finland, **3** Department of Social Research and Helsinki Institute for Information Technology, University of Helsinki, Helsinki, Finland

Abstract

Previous research indicates that males prefer competition over cooperation, and it is sometimes suggested that females show the opposite behavioral preference. In the present article, we investigate the emotions behind the preferences: Do males exhibit more positive emotions during competitive than cooperative activities, and do females show the opposite pattern? We conducted two experiments where we assessed the emotional responses of same-gender dyads (in total 130 participants, 50 female) during intrinsically motivating competitive and cooperative digital game play using facial electromyography (EMG), skin conductance, heart rate measures, and self-reported emotional experiences. We found higher positive emotional responses (as indexed by both physiological measures and self-reports) during competitive than cooperative play for males, but no differences for females. In addition, we found no differences in negative emotions, and heart rate, skin conductance, and self-reports yielded contradictory evidence for arousal. These results support the hypothesis that males not only prefer competitive over cooperative play, but they also exhibit more positive emotional responses during them. In contrast, the results suggest that the emotional experiences of females do not differ between cooperation and competition, which implies that less competitiveness does not mean more cooperativeness. Our results pertain to intrinsically motivated game play, but might be relevant also for other kinds of activities.

Editor: Marina Pavlova, University of Tuebingen Medical School, Germany

Funding: This study was partly supported by Finnish graduate school for User-Centered Technology. Experiment 1 of this research was funded by EU under the project "FUGA," Contract Number NEST-PATH-028765, and Experiment 2 was funded by Tekes, the Finnish Funding Agency for Technology and Innovation (www.tekes.fi/eng/), grant "Next Media", Decision Number 425/10. The funders had no role in study design, data collection and analysis, decision to publish, or preparation of the manuscript.

Competing Interests: The authors have declared that no competing interests exist.

* Email: matias.kivikangas@aalto.fi.

Introduction

Gender differences in competitiveness have been widely studied since after Darwin (see [1]), and males' greater tendency to compete has been reported in various contexts, such as career choices and labor market [2,3], negotiations and bargaining [4,5], economic experiments [6,7], and sports [8]. By contrast, females have been considered to be more cooperative (e.g., [9–12]). However, despite the difference in the behavioral preference, whether there is also a difference between genders in emotions behind the behavior has not been previously investigated.

When looking at the question regardless of gender, there is reason to expect that competition should be experienced more negatively than cooperation. According to appraisal theory, negative emotions are elicited by situations that are inconsistent with one's own goals [13]—and given that competitive situations include opposing goals between the participants, competition is by definition a threat of one's goals being blocked. Furthermore, evolutionary psychology suggests that in this regard, humans have evolved positive emotions to facilitate survival through cooperation, and negative emotions to defend against those who do not cooperate (e.g., [14]) and to help in competition for resources [15]. Consequently, competition should elicit more negative emotions than cooperation. Although there is no direct empirical evidence for differential emotional responses to competition and cooperation, for example students have been found to experience teaching more negatively when it is organized with competitive rather than cooperative goals [16]. Neuroscientific studies have indicated that in economic decision making games, cooperation is associated with reward system activations [17] and noncooperation is associated with neural activations suggestive of negative emotions [18].

Although theoretical considerations would suggest that competition is associated with negative emotions, during activities such as sports and games people in fact seem to derive great enjoyment from competition and actively seek it [19–21](cf. [22]). An explanation for this apparent discrepancy might be found in the motivational source for competition; that is, whether it is chosen voluntarily, constituting intrinsic motivation, or it is forced by external factors (extrinsic motivation). Self-determination theory [23] posits that voluntary participation in a challenging activity increases feelings of competence and autonomy as the goals are set by the person himself or herself, resulting in a high level of enjoyment. Although the motivation literature largely connects competition to extrinsic motivation and less positive emotions, competition can be subjectively viewed as intrinsically motivated as well [23,24]. In the terms of appraisal theory, if the person is motivated not by achieving victory and some extrinsic goals attached to it, but by playing itself, voluntary participation in competitive game play reinforces rather than blocks the player's goals.

Returning to gender differences, research evidence as described above suggests that males show a behavioral preference for competition over cooperation, whereas females prefer cooperation over competition—in fact, the (limited) evidence seems to suggest that these preferences hold regardless of whether the activity is extrinsically or intrinsically motivated (see [6,8,10,25–28]). Because preferences are based on emotions [29], this leads to the question whether males and females also show different emotional responses to competitive and cooperative activity modes; that is, whether males show more positive emotional responses during competition than females, and whether females show more positive responses during cooperation than males.

Present studies

We conducted two studies where we compared the emotional responses elicited by cooperative (participants have congruent goals – both win or lose together) and competitive (participants have mutually exclusive goals – if one wins, the other loses) game play. We used digital games for the research task because they provide an ecologically valid and culturally widespread intrinsically motivated activity in the modern Western world, and they also have the benefit of being relatively easily adaptable for experimental purposes—unlike, for example, sports, which have more physical and practical limitations. One previous study focusing on emotions elicited by competitive and cooperative games has already suggested that competition is more enjoyable (more positive emotion) than cooperation [30]; however, this study did not consider differences between males and females. As digital game playing is more popular among males than females [31] and females tend to dislike certain features of games (i.e., violence, negative gender stereotypes, and lack of social interaction; see [32]), we paid special attention to selecting games which would not be disproportionately more preferred by one gender.

In addition to self-report questionnaires, we used psychophysiological methods to study emotional experiences. There is compelling evidence that facial electromyography (EMG), electrodermal activity, and cardiac indices can be used to assess emotional valence, arousal, and attention, respectively [33,34]. Within the last decade these measurements have also been successfully applied to study emotions during digital game play ([35–38]; see also [39,40]). To summarize, facial EMG activity over zygomaticus major and orbicularis oculi (ZM and OO, activated when smiling) muscle areas are generally considered good indices for positive emotions, and activity over corrugator supercilii (CS) muscle area (activated when frowning) an index for negative emotions, while electrodermal activity (EDA) is a widely used measure for assessing arousal originating from physiological (i.e., sympathetic nervous system) activations [33,34]. In addition, heart rate (HR) is often used to assess arousal, although the dual innervation of heart by both the sympathetic and parasympathetic branches of the autonomous system makes the interpretation of HR changes difficult, particularly when using a more complex stimulus (see [39]).

Hypotheses

Based on the above considerations, we formulated the following hypotheses:

H1: Males will show higher positive emotion (as assessed by ZM and OO EMG activity and self-reports) in competitive than in cooperative game play.

H2: Females will show higher positive emotion (as assessed by ZM and OO EMG activity and self-reports) in cooperative than in competitive game play.

Given that there is evidence for both greater emotional expressiveness [41,42] and more intense emotional experiences [43] in females than males, greater overall facial EMG activation could be expected for females. However, this should not affect the differences between the competitive and cooperative modes.

Recent evidence indicates a degree of independence between positive and negative emotions (see [44]). Therefore it is possible that, as suggested by appraisal theory (negative emotions elicited by one's goals being blocked in competition) and some empirical findings [16], there would be more negative responses to competition (compared to cooperation) regardless of possible simultaneous positive responses. On the other hand, digital games are likely to enable intrinsic motivation when they are played by participants who voluntarily play games in their free time [45]. Consequently, given that the primary goal of intrinsically motivated participants is simply to enjoy playing the game rather than to win against the opponent, they might show no negative responses to competition. Considering these conflicting predictions, but seeing that there is no strong empirical evidence for either one, we present a research question:

RQ1: Is there a difference in negative emotion (as assessed by CS EMG activity and self-reports) between competition and cooperation, and is it associated with gender?

Finally, previous studies have reported that competition elicits higher self-reported arousal [30] and cardiovascular activity [46] than cooperation. Although males have been reported to be more responsive to changes in arousal [41], neither of these previous studies have given evidence that would support differences between the genders during competition and cooperation. This leads us to the following hypothesis:

H3: Both genders will show higher arousal (as assessed by EDA, HR and self-reports) in competitive than in cooperative game play.

Experiment 1

The first experiment was conducted using two activity modes, competitive and cooperative, during a digital game. In addition, we sought to demonstrate that our digital game playing results were not confounded by the unfamiliarity of the research laboratory environment (see [47]), as the ecological validity of the research environment may be of particular importance (cf. [25]). In order to address this issue, we repeated the experimental procedure both in laboratory and in a more familiar environment (participant's home).

Methods

Participants and ethics statement. Participants were 48 (18 female) volunteers, ranging from 18 to 34 years of age ($M = 24.0$, $SD = 4.09$), who played digital games on a regular basis (at least 4 hours per month). The number of female participants was smaller due to the difficulty of finding female volunteers with sufficient familiarity with digital games; however, we considered the ratio of females versus males to lie within acceptable limits. The participants were recruited in same-gender dyads by advertisements in gaming-related websites, student mailing lists, and student organizations. The dyads volunteered together, so they knew each other before the experiment. Although males and females were both considered regular players, when the previous experience of the particular game used in this experiment (Bomberman) was surveyed, males had more experience with it than females. This difference was taken into account in our statistical analyses.

We have complied with the APA's ethical standards and the Declaration of Helsinki in conducting the experiment. Participants were explicitly reminded that they could withdraw from the study at any time without negative consequences. Because the study did not concern medical research, the need for formal approval was, in accordance with Finnish law, waived by the ethics review board of our university. All participants received three movie tickets as compensation for their participation.

Materials. The game used was Bomberman (Hudson Entertainment, Redwood Shores, CA, 2006), played on PlayStation Portable handheld game console (Sony Computer Entertainment, Tokyo, Japan). Bomberman is a classic action game, in which two or more players are situated in a small maze and each player is using bombs to clear new routes and to attempt to eliminate the other players. The game was played in two two-player teams, with the two human participants assigned either to the same team (in cooperation) or different teams (in competition), while the remaining two characters were controlled by the computer. With the exception of team arrangements, the game was identical in both modes. Eliminating the opponent team was the only explicit goal in the game, and the success in this task (number of matches won) was displayed between the matches. For one match in the game, the last player in the maze was declared the winner (in the rare case of two players blasting each other at the same moment, a tie was declared). In our games, each match lasted between two and five minutes. Bomberman employs cartoonish graphics from isometric view and happy music and sounds. It does not contain realistic depictions of violence or negative gender stereotypes, and the nature of multiplayer game makes it inherently social.

Design and procedure. The experiment had a 2×2×2 mixed design, with gender (male, female) as the between-subjects factor, and activity mode (competition, cooperation) and environment (laboratory, home) as the two within-subjects factors. The experiment took place in two different locations: laboratory and the home of one of the two participants. In both locations, a practice session was followed by a rest period of 5 min (during which baseline physiological measurements were performed), and two 8-min play periods, one in competitive and one in cooperative mode. The participants played as many matches they could during the 8-min playing periods.

The order of environments was randomized, and the order of modes was counterbalanced across them (chosen randomly from two orders: BA AB or AB BA). When playing at a participant's home, the environment was ensured to be free of distractions (e.g., other people), and the illumination and immediate surroundings (such as chairs) were adjusted for comfortable play. In both locations the participants were seated next to each other, while the experimenter was located in an adjacent room during the actual measurements. The duration of the whole experiment was three to four hours, including the short trip between the locations, all conducted within a single day.

Physiological data acquisition. The physiological signals and environmental data were recorded from both players during all the play periods with two Varioport-B portable recorder systems (Becker Meditec, Karlsruhe, Germany), and preprocessed using Matlab software (version 2011a) and ANSlab (version 2.4, University of Basel, Germany) toolbox. All wirings were taped in place and attached to the recording device placed on a belt, not too tightly so that the participants' movements were not hindered. The electrodes were attached before the first practice session in the first location, and the recordings were run over the whole experiment, while baseline and play periods were marked with a hardware marker button. Baseline activity levels were recorded for all physiological signals, so that individual baseline differences could be partialled out in our analyses.

Facial EMG activity was recorded from the left CS (brow), ZM (cheek), and OO (near the corner of the eye) muscle regions. The electrodes were attached so that they would not enter the field of vision. Electrode wires were taped to the skin behind the ear and down to the back of the neck, so that they would not hinder any head movements. We used surface Ag/AgCl electrodes with a contact area of 4 mm diameter. Facial EMG signal was sampled at 1024 Hz at 57–390 Hz frequency range, rectified, and smoothed with a linear phase FIR filter using the Kaiser window method (101 coefficients, low-pass cutoff frequency 40 Hz). EDA signal was recorded using a constant 0.5 V voltage across Ag/AgCl electrodes with a contact area of 4 mm diameter, and sampled at 32 Hz. Electrodes were attached to the medial phalanges of the ring and little fingers of the participant's left hand using self-adhesive electrode collars and electrolyte gel. Ring and little fingers were used, instead of the more typically used index and middle fingers, because holding the game console left ring and little fingers free. Skin conductance level (SCL, an average over the whole period) was derived from the EDA signal. ECG was recorded with three electrodes in a modified Lead 2 placement, sampling at 512 Hz. Heart rates were extracted by identifying R-peaks from the signal in ANSlab software package (http://www.anslab.net).

In addition to the established physiological measurements, two accelerometers (sampling rate 32 Hz) were used to record body (sensor located on the participant's chest) and hand-held console (sensor located in the backside of the console) movements. Acceleration data were integrated over one second and 3-dimensional axes were added together and rectified. From earlier studies we had reason to suspect that player movements might be associated with emotions during digital game play [48].

Questionnaire data. All questionnaires were administered in Finnish and delivered on paper. For background variables, we asked the participants to assess their previous experience of the game and the game console device with 6-point scales, from "Never played before" to "Played more than 50 times". Given that the question related to the game device did not show any significant differences between genders when tested in the covariate analysis (see section Data analysis), it was discarded from our analyses. Trait questionnaire for Behavioral Inhibition and Activation System sensitivities (BIS and BAS) were used, as these are related to the propensity for negative and positive emotions due to punishment and reward [49].

Emotions were assessed by self-report measurements after both playing periods. Pleasure and Arousal scales from visual Self-Assessment Manikins (SAM; [50]), and shortened versions of Hostility (consisting of items "angry" and "hostile"), Fear ("frightened" and "nervous"), Joviality ("enthusiastic", "excited", and "delighted"), Serenity ("calm" and "relaxed"), and Sadness ("sad" and "downhearted") subscales from Positive and Negative Affect Scale (PANAS; [51]) were administered. The Hostility and Fear subscales represented high-arousal negative (high and low dominance), Joviality high-arousal positive, and Serenity and Sadness low-arousal positive and negative affect, respectively. We found that the variance for the negative affect scales was smaller, and that the distribution of Hostility skewed strongly towards minimum value.

In addition, the Social Presence module, an earlier version of Social Presence in Gaming Questionnaire or SPGQ [52], was used (17 items). This questionnaire evaluates the following aspects of inter-player involvement and awareness: Behavioral Involvement (e.g., "What the other did affected what I did" and "What I did affected what the other did"), Empathy (e.g., "When the other was happy, I was happy" and vice versa), and Negative Feelings (e.g., "I tended to ignore the other").

To examine potential confounds, Engagement and Spatial Presence subscales from the ITC-Sense of Presence Inventory with

27 items (ITC-SOPI; [53]) were administered, in addition to single items on 7-point scale to assess the anticipated threat, anticipated and experienced stressfulness and success ("How successful did you think you were in the previous game?"), and experienced performance ("How well did you perform, compared to your partner, in the previous game?"), mental struggling ("How much did you struggle to perform well in the previous game?") and interest in the game, both before (anticipated stress, threat, and success) and after the play period. The anticipated assessments were used as baseline scores for the experienced assessments, except for anticipated threat which was used as a threat appraisal assessment.

Discarded data. Following the recommendation of Simmons, Nelson, and Simonsohn [54], we report that other self-rating data (four trait questionnaires and one state questionnaire, and an experimental game experience questionnaire) and respiratory activity data were collected as a part of our routine experimental paradigm but were not included in the present report, because they were not relevant for the present hypotheses.

Data processing and analysis. Average physiological signals during the baseline and each of the playing periods were calculated for each participant. Logarithmic transformations were conducted for facial EMG, SCL, and acceleration data to normalize the distributions. The data were analyzed with Linear Mixed Models procedure with maximum likelihood estimation in SPSS 20, due to the requirements of dyadic and repeated structure of the data [55]. Playing period was specified as the repeated variable, and first-order autoregressive model was specified as the covariance structure for the residuals. The members of the dyad were not interchangeable (the condition conducted in home environment was one participant's home but not the other's), so statistical indistinguishability (see [55]) was tested to find out whether the model should take this into account by treating the members as different. Because no differences were found, the members could be treated as indistinguishable, and we defined Dyad×Participant as the subject for the repeated term. The nonindependence of participants within dyads was initially taken into account by including random intercepts with Dyad as subject variable into the model [55]; however, this random variable was dropped because its effect was not significant in any of our analyses and it prevented some models from converging.

We tested our hypotheses using a basic statistical model, which included mode (cooperation or competition), gender, and mode×gender interaction as independent variables. Unless mentioned otherwise, all of our reported are based on this basic model. In addition, we also ran expanded covariate models to check for the effects of potential confounds, as suggested by Simmons and others [54]. This model included the following variables as covariates: environment (home or laboratory), interaction for environment×host (which participant's home the home environment was), the order of modes (competition or cooperation first), the order of environments (home or laboratory first), baseline value of the dependent variable (when available), and previous experience with the game. The last item was included in the confound model because our preliminary analyses indicated that males had more experience with the game than females ($p<0.001$). Any other of the tested potential confounds (anticipated threat, or experienced engagement, spatial presence, interest, success, performance, or struggle) did not differ significantly between the genders, $ps>.1$, and were hence not included in the covariate model.

Given the large number of variables studied in the present investigation, we used False Discovery Rate correction [56] for the significance thresholds to control for the inflated possibility of false positives. FDR of 5% resulted in threshold of .025 (p-values larger than that were declared non-significant).

Results and Discussion

Results from the basic model analyses for all physiological variables are presented in Table 1, and for emotion self-report variables in Table 2. For the reader's convenience, we report the non-essential results, for body and console movement and social presence questionnaires, in Appendix S1 (Tables S1 and S2 in Appendix S1).

Hypothesis 1: higher positive emotion in competition for males. Hypothesis 1 was supported by the physiological measurements and self-reports: the significant interaction of mode and gender for both ZM and OO EMG activity (Figure 1, top panels) showed that males exhibited more positive emotion during competition than during cooperation (both $ps<.001$, see Table 1), and that they reported higher Joviality and SAM Valence in the competitive mode than in the cooperative mode, ($ps = .006$ and .005, Figure 1, bottom panels). See Table S1 in Appendix S1, for body and console movement results, and Table S2 in Appendix S1, for social presence results.

Hypothesis 2: higher positive emotion in cooperation for females. We found no support for Hypothesis 2, as there were no significant differences between cooperation and competition for females in ZM and OO EMG activity (Figure 1, top panels) or PANAS Joviality or SAM Valence (Figure 1, bottom panels).

Hypothesis 3: higher arousal in competition for both genders. HR was higher in the competitive versus cooperative mode ($p = .002$), but a significant interaction between mode and gender ($p = .004$) revealed that this effect was present only for males (Figure 2, top panel). SCL showed no significant main effect for mode, but instead an interaction similar to HR with a decrease for females and an increase for males from cooperative to competitive mode, although the interaction was not significant after FDR correction ($p = .030$). In self-reports, SAM Arousal showed the same interaction pattern where males reported higher and females (slightly) lower arousal during competition than during cooperation, ($p = .002$, Figure 2, bottom panel); but again the main effect for the mode was non-significant. In addition, self-reports related to low-arousal discrete emotions suggested that cooperation may have had a calming effect on both males and females: both genders reported feeling less Fear ($p = .012$), and more Serenity and Sadness ($p<.001$ and $p = .001$) during cooperation than competition.

Contrary to our Hypothesis 3, these results hence suggest that competition versus cooperation elicited opposite rather than similar effects between the genders (higher arousal in males and lower arousal in females).

Research question 1: is there more or less negative emotion in competition?. We found no association between mode and CS EMG activity or PANAS Hostility ($ps>.1$), and although participants reported experiencing more Fear and less Serenity and Sadness during competition (see above), this can be interpreted as an effect of arousal rather than negative emotion.

We conclude that competition does not seem to be experienced negatively as such (but see Table S2 in Appendix S1), at least in the intrinsically motivated competition used in this experiment.

Covariate models. The results for mode, gender, and their interaction did not notably change for any of the dependent variables for the covariate models that included environment, environment×host interaction, the order of modes and environments, and the baseline of the dependent. The only notable difference was that the weak interaction effect for SCL was even weaker ($p<.042$) when the covariates were included in the model.

Table 1. Experiment 1 Linear Mixed Models for Physiological Dependent Variables.

	Estimated Marginal Means (*SE*)				
Model Variables	**1**	**2**	*df*	*F*	*p*
Zygomaticus Major EMG activity (ln[μV])					
Mode	2.907 (0.088)	3.175 (0.087)	1,134.128	38.647	**<.001**
Gender	3.158 (0.104)	2.924 (0.134)	1,50.566	1.919	0.172
Mode×Gender	2.907 (0.107)	3.410 (0.107)	1,134.128	29.411	**<.001**
	2.907 (0.139)	2.941 (0.137)			
Corrugator Supercilii EMG activity (ln[μV])					
Mode	2.594 (0.101)	2.583 (0.101)	1,136.477	0.195	0.66
Gender	2.539 (0.121)	2.638 (0.160)	1,46.814	0.241	0.626
Mode×Gender	2.553 (0.122)	2.525 (0.122)	1,136.477	0.377	0.54
	2.635 (0.162)	2.640 (0.161)			
Orbicularis Oculi EMG activity (ln[μV])					
Mode	3.066 (0.073)	3.237 (0.073)	1,136.213	26.073	**<.001**
Gender	3.083 (0.087)	3.220 (0.113)	1,51.245	0.921	0.342
Mode×Gender	2.913 (0.090)	3.253 (0.089)	1,136.213	25.467	**<.001**
	3.219 (0.116)	3.221 (0.115)			
Skin conducance level (ln[μS])					
Mode	1.301 (0.088)	1.311 (0.088)	1,129.997	0.406	0.525
Gender	1.285 (0.099)	1.327 (0.145)	1,44.022	0.058	0.81
Mode×Gender	1.263 (0.100)	1.307 (0.100)	1,129.997	4.836	0.03
	1.340 (0.146)	1.315 (0.146)			
Heart rate (BPM)					
Mode	74.523 (1.561)	75.866 (1.552)	1,130.594	10.286	**0.002**
Gender	74.500 (1.925)	75.889 (2.410)	1,46.876	0.203	0.655
Mode×Gender	73.208 (1.945)	75.792 (1.940)	1,130.594	8.761	**0.004**
	75.838 (2.441)	75.941 (2.424)			

Note. Intercept is left out as uninformative from all models. Means 1 and 2 correspond to Cooperative and Competitive for Mode, and Male and Female for Gender, respectively. For Mode×Gender interactions, the rows denote Male and Female, and the columns denote Cooperative and Competitive, in that order. The *p*-values significant after controlling the false discovery rate are bolded.

Previous experience, despite of being reported significantly different for males and females, revealed no significant association with any of the dependent variables, in main effect nor in interaction between previous experience and gender.

Baseline was extremely significantly associated (all $ps<.001$, except $p = .003$ for Fear and .034 for Sadness) with almost all the variables (except for Serenity, n,s; for SAM there was no baseline), showing that there were significant individual differences between the participants. However, including these baseline values in our analyses did not change any of the above significant findings.

Order of mode and the environment did have a significant positive effect on the positive affect measures, i.e. ZM and OO EMG activity ($ps = .004$ and .008 for ZM, .006 and .016 for OO), and SAM Valence ($ps = .017$, and .018), as well as body and console movement ($p = .004$ and .025 for order of mode, but n.s. for environment). This shows that the later experimental periods elicited higher positive affect compared to earlier periods, and that home was experienced more positively than the laboratory, but that these effects did not affect the interactions between gender and mode (see above). Order of mode showed the same pattern as the positive emotions for HR ($p = .023$) but not for SCL ($ps > .1$). It seems plausible that the later experimental periods and periods at home have felt more comfortable and relaxed, allowing higher positive affect. This could also have lead to an effect for environment in Hostility, higher at the laboratory ($M = 1.936$, $SE = 0.099$) compared to home ($M = 1.499$, $SE = 0.100$, $t(166,172) = 2.844$, $p = .005$).

Experiment 2

In the second experiment we sought to test the findings from the first experiment with a different game, while addressing some concerns that might have affected its results. First, it is possible that the type of game (quick action) might have required a constant high level of arousal, effectively masking any arousal differences between the modes (Hypothesis 3), and possibly making the game more likable to males than females [57]. Consequently, we chose a new stimulus game that would not require constant quick action. A turn-based game would allow the participants to play the game on their own pace, which should allow for lower arousal levels and thereby provide better data on arousal differences in different conditions. This might also affect which processes are dominant on heart rate: if HR responded to arousal in a fast-paced game, it might be that during a less arousing game HR responds more to the attention component [58].

Table 2. Experiment 1 Linear Mixed Models for Self-Report Dependent Variables.

	Estimated Marginal Means (*SE*)				
Model Variables	**1**	**2**	*df*	*F*	*p*
PANAS-X Joviality					
Mode	4.795 (0.125)	5.004 (0.123)	1,129.863	3.033	0.084
Gender	4.885 (0.133)	4.914 (0.172)	1,59.348	0.019	0.892
Mode×Gender	4.612 (0.153)	5.158 (0.151)	1,129.863	7.946	**0.006**
	4.979 (0.198)	4.850 (0.195)			
PANAS-X Hostility					
Mode	1.752 (0.110)	1.765 (0.109)	1,123.946	0.016	0.899
Gender	1.695 (0.118)	1.822 (0.152)	1,53.679	0.435	0.512
Mode×Gender	1.678 (0.135)	1.711 (0.133)	1,123.946	0.034	0.853
	1.825 (0.174)	1.819 (0.172)			
PANAS-X Fear					
Mode	2.175 (0.100)	2.389 (0.099)	1,123.779	6.436	**0.012**
Gender	2.367 (0.110)	2.197 (0.142)	1,52.106	0.896	0.348
Mode×Gender	2.224 (0.123)	2.510 (0.121)	1,123.779	0.714	0.4
	2.125 (0.158)	2.268 (0.156)			
PANAS-X Serenity					
Mode	3.927 (0.129)	3.526 (0.127)	1,125.7	13.884	**<.001**
Gender	4.029 (0.143)	3.424 (0.184)	1,53.587	6.736	**0.012**
Mode×Gender	4.292 (0.158)	3.765 (0.156)	1,125.7	1.374	0.243
	3.561 (0.204)	3.286 (0.201)			
PANAS-X Sadness					
Mode	3.733 (0.071)	3.527 (0.070)	1,127.737	10.637	**0.001**
Gender	3.683 (0.078)	3.577 (0.100)	1,56.358	0.692	0.409
Mode×Gender	3.799 (0.087)	3.566 (0.086)	1,127.737	0.181	0.671
	3.666 (0.113)	3.488 (0.111)			
SAM Valence					
Mode	7.086 (0.147)	7.270 (0.145)	1,128.246	1.316	0.253
Gender	7.225 (0.153)	7.131 (0.190)	1,59.363	0.148	0.701
Mode×Gender	6.903 (0.184)	7.547 (0.181)	1,128.246	8.166	**0.005**
	7.269 (0.230)	6.994 (0.226)			
SAM Arousal					
Mode	6.188 (0.154)	6.366 (0.152)	1,124.389	1.282	0.26
Gender	6.386 (0.164)	6.168 (0.205)	1,55.956	0.69	0.41
Mode×Gender	6.050 (0.193)	6.722 (0.190)	1,124.389	9.798	**0.002**
	6.326 (0.241)	6.011 (0.237)			

Note. Intercept is left out as uninformative from all models. Means 1 and 2 correspond Cooperative and Competitive for Mode, and Male and Female for Gender, respectively. For Mode×Gender interactions, the rows denote Male and Female, and columns denote Cooperative and Competitive, in that order. The *p*-values significant after controlling the false discovery rate are bolded.

Second, it is possible that our dichotomy between competition and cooperation was too absolute, given that some activities may at the same time contain both coincidental and opposing goals between the participating individuals (cf. [59], pp. 254–256). For example, some sports activities combining both competition and cooperation have been reported to be more enjoyable than sports activities containing only either one of them [22]. Thus, we added a condition with both coincidental and opposing individual goals to the present study. Specifically, participants were assigned to the same team so that they scored wins or losses together against the computer-controlled team; however, at the same time they also competed individually for higher score within the team.

Third, we did not specifically (besides with subjective measures) control for the players' varying performance levels in the first experiment. In the second experiment, we recorded the personal and team victories and losses, and included them in our analyses.

Methods

Participants. The participants were 100 Finnish university students recruited in 50 same-gender dyads (21 female dyads). Due to technical difficulties, 9 of the dyads had to be removed from the

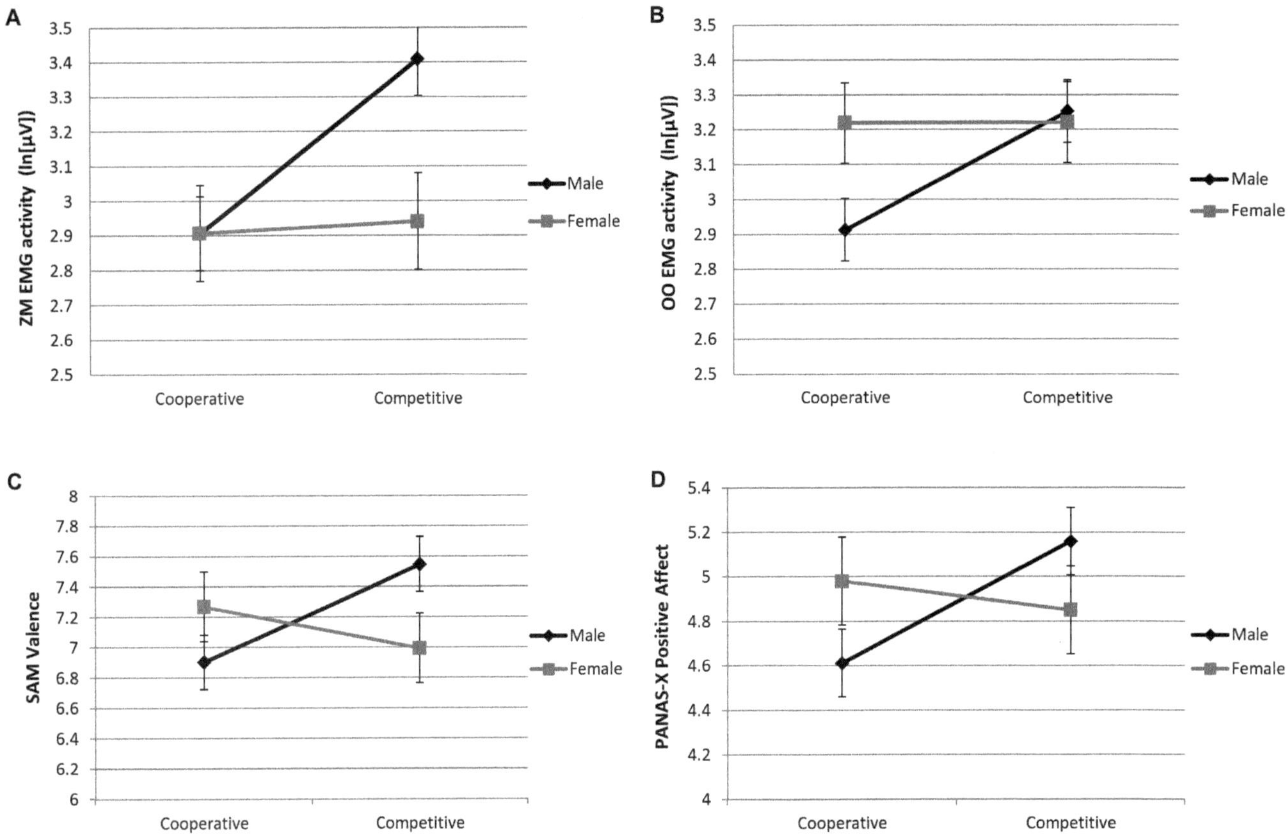

Figure 1. Gender differences in zygomaticus major (top left panel) and orbicularis oculi (top right) EMG activity, both associated with positive emotion, and self-reported pleasantness (bottom left) and positive affect (bottom right), across cooperative and competitive modes (Experiment 1). The error bars represent standard errors.

physiological dataset, which resulted in 82 participants in 41 dyads (16 female), with age ranging from 18 to 32 (M = 23.0, SD = 3.2 years). The participants received information and compensation and signed an informed consent form similarly as in Experiment 1.

Materials. The stimulus game was Hedgewars (http://hedgewars.org), an open-source clone of a popular commercial game Worms (Team 17). Hedgewars is a turn-based artillery game, which features two or more teams of cartoon-like characters on a two-dimensional map. The game's goal was to eliminate all other teams' characters by using various cartoonish weapons, either by reducing their health to zero or by managing to knock them into the water. Players had 45 seconds per turn to move a character (only one was moved at a time), choose a weapon, and shoot by adjusting the power and angle of the ballistic shot. Turn order was randomized. During the course of the game, players were able to gain new weapons by picking up boxes that landed on the map at constant intervals. Most of the game's weapons were turned off, however, so that the more experienced gamers would not have a significant edge over the less experienced ones, and to reduce the number of possible actions to a more manageable level.

Procedure. After the practice session and a 5-min baseline recording, the two players in each dyad sat next to each other in the laboratory and played the game on the same computer, sharing mouse and keyboard in turns to control the game. Separate computers on side desks were used for answering self-report questionnaires both before and after each experimental period.

Each dyad played the game in four different conditions, which were presented in a randomized order. The conditions were: (1) playing in the same team against a computer-controlled team (cooperation); (2) playing in the same team against a computer-controlled team with equal number of characters, while competing against each other for the higher score (cooperation-competition); (3) playing in different teams against each other, with equal number of computer-controlled characters in both teams (competition); and (4) playing in different teams against each other, without computer-controlled team members (competition without computer). Computer-controlled team characters were included in condition 3 in order to maintain both similar team sizes (six characters) and numbers of player-controlled characters (three characters) as in conditions 1 and 2. Computer-controlled team members were removed from condition 4 to control for the possible effects of computer-controlled within-team characters, keeping the player-controlled characters constant (resulting in three vs. three characters in condition 4, as opposed to six vs. six in other conditions). Of these, conditions 1 and 3 were equivalent to the cooperation and competition modes of Experiment 1, respectively.

When asked, 17 out of 82 participants (13.94%) reported erroneously after condition 2 that they had been playing condition 1, in contrast to only one or two mistakes in the other conditions. Apparently, the difference between conditions 1 and 2 was not as clear as differences between the other conditions, despite the fact that the playing condition was explicitly stated to the participants

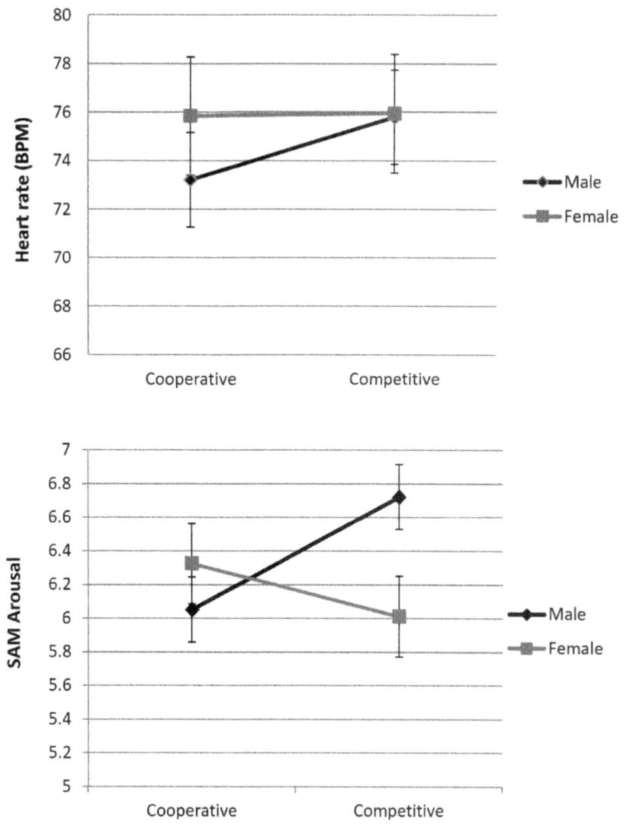

Figure 2. Gender differences in heart rate (left panel), associated with emotional arousal, and self-reported arousal (right panel), across cooperative and competitive modes (Experiment 1). The error bars represent standard errors.

before the beginning of each game. We removed these mistaken playing periods from our data.

Physiological data acquisition. Physiological data was acquired the same way as in Experiment 1, with the following exceptions to the processing of EDA and ECG signals. EDA signal was downsampled to 4 Hz and smoothed using Ledalab (V.3.2.5) toolbox for Matlab, and divided into phasic and tonic components using the non-negative deconvolution method [60]. The tonic component was averaged over each play period to skin conductance level (SCL). The advantage of this method is that because phasic variation is removed from the signal, it produces a less noisy measurement of the tonic component than direct averaging from the original signal. ECG signal was analyzed using the ECGLab toolbox for Matlab. R-peaks were identified from the original 512 Hz series and corrected for ectopic beats. Interbeat interval (IBI) time series was obtained, and HR was calculated as an inverse of IBI (i.e., 60000/IBI).

Questionnaires. All questionnaires were administered in Finnish on a computer. In pre-experimental questionnaires we asked the participants to evaluate their previous experience with Hedgewars game (the present game), Worms game (the game HW is a clone of), and artillery games in general. Because the previous experience with Worms differentiated the genders best, only this item was retained for further analyses. Similarly as in Experiment 1, pre- and post-condition questionnaires included PANAS-X Joviality, Fear, and Hostility scales (but not Serenity and Sadness); SAM Valence and Arousal scales, now added with Dominance scale; separate single items assessing anticipated threat, and anticipated and experienced struggle, success and stressfulness (anticipated assessments were again used as baseline scores, where applicable); and the Social Presence in Games Questionnaire; and BIS and BAS sensitivity scales as a trait questionnaire. In addition, we added the 5-point perceived comprehension scale from Social Presence Inventory (with items such as "My mood affected the mood of the other", both for me affecting the other and the other affecting me; [61]), shortened Attentiveness scale (2 items) from PANAS-X, and separate items for experienced frustration, being entertained, and intensity. We also had an open question to provide the participants a way to comment if something specific affected their answers.

Discarded data. In addition to the reported variables, we administered four state and eight trait questionnaires not relevant for the present study. Furthermore, we calculated various heart rate variability indices and compliance scores for all the physiological signals, which have been reported elsewhere [62,63]. We also measured body movement, but due to techical difficulties this data had to be discarded.

Data analysis. Data analysis was similar to Experiment 1, with minor modifications. In the basic model, instead of two-level mode, we used a four-level condition variable to test for differences between cooperation and competition, the final factors being gender, condition, and gender×condition interaction. The nonindependence of participants within dyads was taken into account by including random intercepts for dyads into the models of physiological (but not self-report) data. Unlike in the first experiment, variances for these intercepts were different from zero and were retained. The exception was the model with HR as dependent, for which the random effect was removed.

Similarly to the first experiment, we used a separate model to test for the effects of potential confounds. This model included the following covariate effects: order of conditions, baseline value of the dependent variable, previous experience with Worms game, game period length, and game scores. Game length was included because—unlike in Experiment 1—the playing time was not fixed. Game scores were included as a covariate because our preliminary analyses revealed that males were more successful against the computer opponents than females. Males also reported higher experienced performance than females ($M = 3.41$ for males and 2.98 for females, $t(81.301) = 2.612$, $p = .011$), but we discarded this variable from the covariate model as redundant after including game score. Other variables of interest were not significantly different between males and females in our preliminary analyses ($ps > .05$). Finally, FDR was calculated as in Experiment 1, resulting in threshold of 0.0178.

Results and Discussion

The results for all physiological variables are presented in Table 3, and for self-report variables in Table 4. Similarly as in Experiment 1, social presence results are available in Table S3 in Appendix S1.

Hypotheses 1 and 2: higher positive emotion in competition for males, and in cooperation for females; covariate models potentially explaining the differences to Experiment 1. Supporting Hypothesis 1, but not Hypothesis 2, significant interactions between condition and gender for ZM ($p = .002$) and OO EMG activities ($p = .009$; Figure 3, left and right panels, respectively) revealed that males, but to a lesser degree also females, had more positive emotional responses to competitive (conditions 3 and 4) than to cooperative (1 and 2) conditions (Table 3).

Self-reports, however, failed to support Hypotheses 1 and 2; that is, SAM Valence and PANAS Joviality showed no significant

Table 3. Linear Mixed Models for the Physiological Dependent Variables in Experiment 2.

	Estimated Marginal Means (*SE*)						
Model Variables	**1**	**2**	**3**	**4**	*df*	*F*	*p*
Zygomaticus Major EMG activity (ln[μV])							
Condition	1.46 (0.068)	1.491 (0.069)	1.699 (0.068)	1.721 (0.068)	3,206.116	29.538	**<.001**
Gender	1.769 (0.081)	1.417 (0.101)			1,40.898	7.364	**0.01**
Condition×Gender	1.56 (0.085)	1.668 (0.087)	1.928 (0.085)	1.918 (0.085)	3,206.116	5.26	**0.002**
	1.36 (0.106)	1.314 (0.107)	1.469 (0.106)	1.524 (0.106)			
Corrugator Supercilii EMG activity (ln[μV])							
Condition	1.063 (0.027)	1.074 (0.028)	1.021 (0.027)	0.991 (0.027)	3,211.781	13.552	**<.001**
Gender	0.984 (0.032)	1.091 (0.04)			1,41.149	4.303	0.044
Condition×Gender	1.008 (0.034)	1.007 (0.035)	0.959 (0.034)	0.962 (0.034)	3,211.781	2.619	0.052
	1.119 (0.042)	1.142 (0.043)	1.082 (0.042)	1.021 (0.042)			
Orbicularis Oculi EMG activity (ln[μV])							
Condition	1.606 (0.05)	1.626 (0.051)	1.817 (0.05)	1.828 (0.05)	3,208.14	34.546	**<.001**
Gender	1.854 (0.06)	1.585 (0.074)			1,40.977	7.952	**0.007**
Condition×Gender	1.69 (0.063)	1.75 (0.065)	1.989 (0.063)	1.985 (0.063)	3,208.14	3.994	**0.009**
	1.523 (0.078)	1.502 (0.08)	1.646 (0.078)	1.67 (0.078)			
Skin conductance level (ln[μS])							
Condition	2.204 (0.048)	2.205 (0.049)	2.227 (0.048)	2.231 (0.048)	3,222.169	3.317	0.021
Gender	2.244 (0.06)	2.19 (0.075)			1,41.061	0.318	0.576
Condition×Gender	2.24 (0.061)	2.243 (0.061)	2.243 (0.061)	2.251 (0.061)	3,222.169	1.96	0.121
	2.169 (0.076)	2.167 (0.076)	2.212 (0.076)	2.212 (0.076)			
Heart rate (BPM)[a]							
Condition	74.02 (0.96)	74.079 (0.969)	74.581 (0.958)	75.747 (0.957)	3,220.154	10.354	**<.001**
Gender	74.438 (1.174)	74.776 (1.464)			1,82.078	0.032	0.858
Condition×Gender	73.311 (1.203)	73.778 (1.216)	74.77 (1.198)	75.893 (1.197)	3,220.154	3.029	0.03
	74.729 (1.497)	74.381 (1.509)	74.392 (1.497)	75.601 (1.494)			

Note. Intercept is left out as uninformative from all models. Means 1 through 4 correspond to Cooperative, Cooperative and Competitive, Competitive, and Competitive Without Computer. Means 1 and 2 correspond to Male and Female for Gender. For Gender×Condition interactions, the rows denote Male and Female and the columns denote the Condition. The *p*-values significant after controlling the false discovery rate are bolded.
[a]Heart rate run with independent members.

Table 4. Linear Mixed Models for Self-Report Dependent Variables in Experiment 2.

	Estimated Marginal Means (*SE*)						
Model Variables	**1**	**2**	**3**	**4**	*df*	*F*	*p*
PANAS Joviality							
Condition	3.665 (0.089)	3.589 (0.094)	3.385 (0.089)	3.499 (0.089)	3,221.971	4.838	**0.003**
Gender	3.592 (0.096)	3.477 (0.117)			1,79.724	0.581	0.448
Condition × Gender	3.745 (0.113)	3.566 (0.121)	3.505 (0.112)	3.553 (0.113)	3,221.971	1.043	0.374
	3.586 (0.137)	3.612 (0.143)	3.266 (0.137)	3.445 (0.137)			
PANAS Hostility							
Condition	1.297 (0.073)	1.297 (0.08)	1.508 (0.072)	1.34 (0.073)	3,225.987	2.564	0.056
Gender	1.273 (0.063)	1.448 (0.077)			1,81.384	3.089	0.083
Condition × Gender	1.188 (0.092)	1.209 (0.104)	1.375 (0.092)	1.32 (0.092)	3,225.987	0.622	0.602
	1.406 (0.112)	1.385 (0.121)	1.641 (0.112)	1.359 (0.112)			
PANAS Fear							
Condition	1.451 (0.061)	1.445 (0.066)	1.422 (0.061)	1.48 (0.061)	3,221.643	0.283	0.837
Gender	1.391 (0.061)	1.508 (0.074)			1,78.575	1.469	0.229
Condition × Gender	1.339 (0.078)	1.406 (0.086)	1.375 (0.078)	1.444 (0.078)	3,221.643	0.629	0.597
	1.562 (0.095)	1.483 (0.101)	1.469 (0.095)	1.516 (0.095)			
SAM Valence							
Condition	6 982 (0.174)	7.03 (0.191)	6.417 (0.173)	6.709 (0.174)	3,224.437	3.364	0.019
Gender	7.034 (0.149)	6.535 (0.18)			1,79.531	4.543	0.036
Condition × Gender	7.526 (0.221)	7.077 (0.249)	6.646 (0.219)	6.886 (0.221)	3,224.437	1.836	0.141
	6.437 (0.268)	6.983 (0.289)	6.187 (0.268)	6.531 (0.268)			
SAM Arousal							
Condition	6.513 (0.16)	6.331 (0.171)	6.063 (0.159)	6.323 (0.16)	3,222.835	2.657	0.049
Gender	6.306 (0.161)	6.309 (0.196)			1,79.892	0	0.99
Condition × Gender	6.464 (0.203)	6.207 (0.222)	6.125 (0.202)	6.427 (0.203)	3,222.835	0.74	0.529
	6.563 (0.247)	6.454 (0.261)	6 (0.247)	6.219 (0.247)			
SAM Dominance							
Condition	6.546 (0.178)	6.573 (0.196)	5.177 (0.177)	6.443 (0.178)	3,224.032	17.802	**<.001**
Gender	6.398 (0.146)	5.972 (0.177)			1,78.522	3.434	0.068
Condition × Gender	7.092 (0.226)	6.882 (0.256)	5.167 (0.224)	6.449 (0.226)	3,224.032	2.809	0.04
	6 (0.274)	6.264 (0.296)	5.188 (0.274)	6.438 (0.274)			

Note. Intercept is left out as uninformative from all models. Means 1 through 4 correspond to Cooperative, Cooperative and Competitive, Competitive, and Competitive Without Computer. Means 1 and 2 correspond to Male and Female for Gender. For Gender × Condition interactions, the rows denote Male and Female and the columns denote the Condition. Note that the figures here are from the basic models without the confounding game result as covariate. The *p*-values significant after controlling the false discovery rate are bolded.

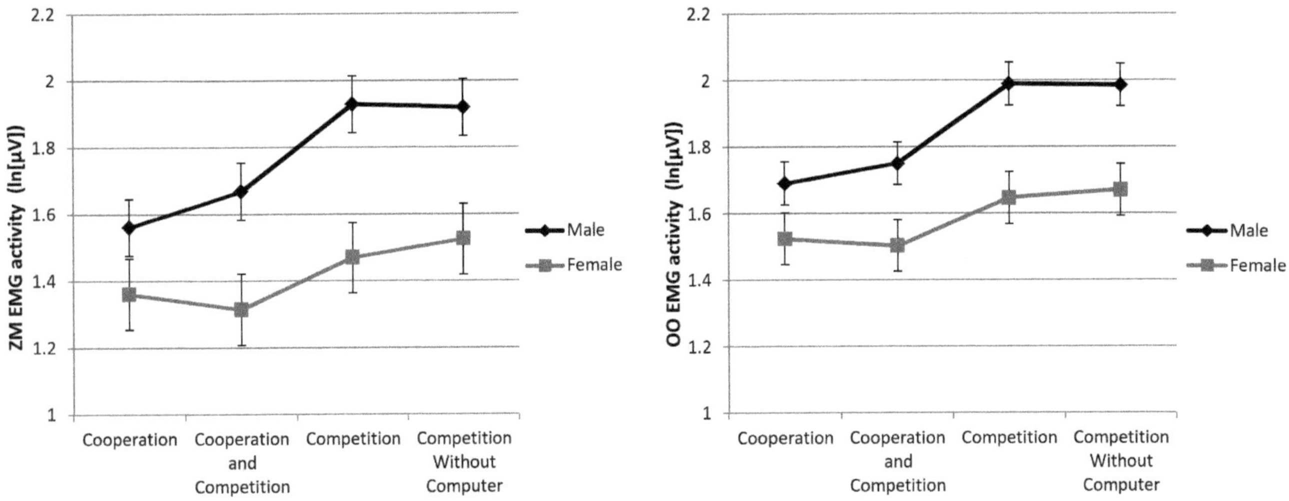

Figure 3. Gender differences in zygomaticus major (left panel) and orbicularis oculi (right panel) EMG activity, both associated with positive emotion, across the four conditions representing different modes of competitiveness (Experiment 2). The error bars represent standard errors.

interactions between gender and condition ($ps>.1$; see Table 4). The main effect for Joviality ($p=.003$, but for Valence, $p=.019$, n.s.) suggests that actually cooperative conditions were reported as more positive, both by males and females. However, the covariate models showed a strong positive effect for game result ($F(2, 223.861)=11.270$, $p<.001$ for Joviality, and $F(2, 244.533)=30.633$, $p<.001$ for Valence), indicating that winning the game resulted in higher self-reported positive emotions ($Ms=3.403$, 3.545, and 3.727 [Joviality], and 5.986, 6.737, and 7.350 [Valence] for game lost, game won by team member, and game won, respectively). It seems likely that emotional self-reports given after the game reflected emotional reactions to knowing the game's final score more than emotional reactions that were actually experienced during the game. Therefore, even if there were differences between genders across conditions, they would be confounded by the strong response to victory or defeat (cf. [64–66]). Unfortunately this limits the usefulness of these self-reports. It should be noted that in Experiment 1, although we did not control for victories and losses (and did not explicitly present the results to the participants as we did here), the participants played several matches during a fixed-length period and may have both won and lost during the game, thus on average probably reducing this effect. Physiological measurements, on the other hand, were collected during the game, while the winner was still unclear, and therefore reflected the emotions experienced *during* condition, instead of reflecting the response to game result afterwards.

In an attempt to control for the effect of game result, we ran post-hoc LMMs for Valence and Joviality separately for game won and lost. It was found that Joviality followed the pattern of physiological positive emotion measures when the game was won (but not when it was lost), although with power suffering from lower n the interaction was not significant ($p=.034$, main effect for condition at $p=.011$). Valence showed no significant associations ($p=.1$ for interaction, $p=.031$ for condition main effect when game was won). These might point to similar pattern to in the first experiment after victory but with no further means to distinguish the effect of the game result and the experience during play, this remains somewhat speculative.

Hypothesis 3: higher arousal in competition for both genders. As in Experiment 1, HR was strongly associated with conditions (main effect $p<.001$), and the increase in competitive conditions was somewhat stronger for males ($p=.030$ for the interaction), however the effect was nonsignificant when corrected for FDR. SCL showed no main effect for condition ($p=.021$, n.s.), and no interaction ($p>.1$). Although the game result did not have a significant effect on either physiological variable in the covariate model ($ps>.1$), the effects strengthened for HR ($p<.001$ for main effect and $p=.012$ for interaction), but weakened for SCL.

SAM Arousal showed a non-significant decrease (not increase) in competitive conditions in both basic ($p=.049$) and covariate ($p=.033$) models. (Game result was also only weakly associated with Arousal ($p=.023$) in the covariate model.)

The conclusion remains that there is no support for Hypothesis 3. Instead of an action game as in Experiment 1, we used a slower-paced turn-based game here. If the HR effect in Experiment 1 was simply a result of bodily activation and not the competition per se, it should have disappeared here. Instead, HR repeated the pattern resembling the one by positive affect measures, different from SCL that supposedly reflects the arousal closer, but also different from self-reported arousal (although the effect of game result might have affected this). The alternatives remain that HR responds successfully to arousal from the manipulation while SCL for some reason does not, or that while no differences can be found in arousal, HR might be associated specifically with high-arousal positive affect, seeing as how it follows the same pattern as ZM and OO EMG activity.

It has also been found that increasing tonic HR is related to decreasing attention (see [39]). For this, we ran a separate LMM with PANAS Attentiveness as dependent variable, but as the interaction was nonsignificant, it suggests that this explanation for HR was not valid here.

Research question 1: is there more or less negative emotion in competition?. Unlike in Experiment 1, the model for CS EMG activity revealed an effect for condition ($p<.001$), showing higher activity in cooperative – not competitive – conditions. This rather points to reciprocal activation of positive and negative emotions, not to uncoupled activation as did the results of Experiment 1, given that self-reported Hostility and Fear did not corroborate these results.

Post-hoc analyses of potential explanators for gender differences. To investigate the gender differences more in depth, some variables measured as potential confounds were examined separately in the analysis phase. Control questions included items about how stressed the participants were about the upcoming match and how threatening they considered it, both related to a potential explanation of risk-aversiveness [2,6], by which females tend to view a competition as a threat rather than a challenge and therefore react with more stress; and an item about how well they anticipated they would perform during the upcoming match, related to a potential explanatory variable of self-confidence (regardless of skills or performance, males tend to believe they will perform well; [3,6]). Furthermore, the trait Behavioral Inhibition System (BIS) and Behavioral Activation System (BAS) sensitivity between genders was also compared, because the former is associated with sensitivity to anticipated negative and the latter with anticipated positive emotions [49]. Post-hoc analyses were conducted for these variables from both experiments, with gender, mode/condition, and their interaction as predictors, and the repeated effect defined as described for the basic analyses (except for BIS and BAS sensitivity, which were single trait scores and therefore could not have a repeated effect).

The results can be found from Tables S4 and S5 in Appendix S1. In short, we found that females tended to negligibly anticipate more stress ($p = .139$ in Experiment 1, $p = .023$ in Experiment 2), possibly associated with the gender difference in BIS sensitivity ($p = .001$), but no difference in anticipated threat, playfulness, or BAS measures, and the higher self-confidence in males was explained by their previous experience with the game.

Covariate models. As explained above, game result did not had no significant effects on any of the physiological variables, but it exerted a strong effect on most self-reports (with the exception of Fear, $p > .2$). This supports the interpretation that self-reports reflected the game result more than actual affect during play, while physiological signals were unaffected by this.

Of the other covariates, period length was negatively associated with OO ($p < .001$; $p = .030$ for ZM) EMG activity, suggesting that the shorter (with more effective – and possibly more entertaining – single shots) games were experienced more positively than the lengthier ones. Order of period was positively associated with CS EMG activity ($p = .006$), and negatively with SCL and HR, ($p < .001$ and $p = .005$), but not to ZM or OO EMG activity as in Experiment 1. Baseline values were strongly associated with the physiological dependent variables (and self-reported Joviality and Fear) with all $ps \leq .003$, again illustrating that individual differences matter, but they did not change the general results.

Other findings. SAM Dominance showed a significant effect for condition interaction ($p < .001$), both genders reporting clearly lower ratings during the competitive condition where the participant was teamed with a computer player. This pattern looks similar to patterns in Joviality, Hostility (inversely), Valence, Arousal, and Behavioral Involvement and Perceived Comprehension (the social presence results in Table S3 in Appendix S1), which seems too regular to be coincidence. Because more than one participant commented for the open question that the computer team mate "made stupid choices that I felt I could not affect" (such as who to target and the weapon choices), this might have been seen as hindering the participants' own goals due to their different (and invisible) logic, possibly affecting emotion and social presence. This effect was probably not explained by the computer players' poorer performance; we tested this with a post-hoc analysis by using a basic LMM with the single item "I felt frustrated" as the dependent variable and by controlling the game result as a random variable, but found no main effect for condition ($p > .5$) and no interaction ($p = .092$). Apparently, these results may have been caused by the observation that the reasons for the computer players' choices were undecipherable, and this might lead to reduced positive emotions, dominance, and self-reported social presence. This interpretation is related to findings that computer player's presence adversely affects the physiological assessment of social presence (see [62,63]).

General Discussion

Earlier research suggests that males prefer competition and females prefer cooperation. For instance, in economic experiments [6] and cognitive tasks [2,3] males choose competition (over non-competitive scoring) more often than females; in sports and games male motivations are more oriented to competition than female motivations [8,28]; and it has been even suggested that females are biologically wired to be more cooperative [9] (see also [17]). Because preferences are based on emotions [29] it would be expected that these preferences are mirrored by similar differences in emotions. Our two studies examined the differences between male and female emotional responses to competition and cooperation during and after (intrinsically motivated) game play, controlling for various confounding factors. In both experiments, we found strong support for Hypothesis 1 that males would exhibit more positive emotions during competitive than cooperative game play, but no support for Hypothesis 2 that females would show more positive emotions during cooperative game play. The physiological evidence based on both zygomatic and orbicularis EMG responses (associated with positive emotions; see [34,67,68]; for studies in game context, see e.g., [65,69]) was strong, revealing the same positive association with competitive game play for males and a lack of difference between modes for females in both experiments. Self-reported positive emotions corroborated this evidence in Experiment 1. In Experiment 2 the self-reported positive emotions followed the same pattern for males only to a limited extent, but the explicit way of declaring the winner after the game may have affected these results. We also found that these results held regardless of skills and previous experience with the game, perceived performance, the initial interest in the activity, and whether the participants won or not.

Although cooperation and competition are often discussed as polar opposites to each other (e.g., [10,17,70]), which leads to the assumption that not preferring competition indicates preference for cooperation, it is important to note that the specific evidence on female tendency for cooperation is much weaker than the evidence on male preference for competition. Actually, it has been a long-standing issue that despite the idea of female cooperativeness present in the gender roles (e.g., [71]), female self-perceptions (e.g., [11,12]), and evolutionary psychological theories [7,10], the experimental evidence has been hard to find and conflicting [72–74]. Furthermore, both reviews on the subject [6,72] state that the occasional gender difference in cooperativeness seems to be very context sensitive. As the most research on the subject is from social dilemmas (such as dictator games) instead of real-life behavior, it is not clear whether any possible differences even could be generalized to another particular context—and the only previous study from gaming context [30] did not report gender effects for cooperation or competition. Our results support the view that, in addition to females not preferring cooperation over competition, females are not more cooperative than males. The between-subjects comparison of physiological responses is problematic because of large individual differences present in these measures [75], but the fact that zygomatic activity was overall higher in males while females are generally more prone to present that activity higher [41] suggests—along with self-reports—that this conclusion is not too far-fetched here. Whether this is generalizable to intrinsically motivated activities beyond simple digital games is a question left for future research.

The theoretical basis behind the gender difference in tendency to compete is, as stated, much better established than the evidence on differences in cooperation. Several mechanisms have been proposed in the literature, among others the females' higher risk-aversiveness and male overconfidence: the former refers to the female tendency to view a competition as a threat rather than a challenge, and the latter to results that, regardless of skills or performance, males tend to believe they will perform well [2,3,6]. We did not measure risk-aversiveness and self-confidence as such, but we did have control questions for potential confounds on how stressed the participants were about the upcoming match, how threatening they considered it, and how well they anticipated they would perform during the upcoming match. Our post-hoc investigation revealed that there was no difference in anticipated threat, nor in anticipated success between genders—although the males did anticipate better success than females before the match (indicating higher self-confidence), this difference was explained by the difference in previous experience with the game. However, anticipated stress was a bit higher for females (in Experiment 2), and we also found higher Behavioral Inhibition System sensitivity in females—a measure that indexes the biological system behind responding to anxiety-relevant cues in environment [49]. While connection of stress and BIS sensitivity and the female tendency to higher BIS sensitivity scores have been reported earlier [76,77], the evidence suggests that higher BIS sensitivity should be associated with more negative emotions (rather than less positive; see [44], for evidence for separability of positive and negative), yet our analyses of the physiological or self-reported negative emotions did not show a gender difference (RQ1). Hence, at least with our limited measures, gender differences in self-confidence did not receive support as an explanation for the gender differences in emotions, and similar threat appraisal results for males and females failed to support the other viable explanation based on risk-aversiveness in females. Although females reported more stress, which would be consistent with the risk-aversiveness explanation, there was no interaction effect on stress between gender and mode. While it is conceivable that a lower level of stress would make it easier to experience positive emotions, it is unlikely to be the sole source of the difference in positive emotions between genders.

Another possibility to explain the difference in responses to competition is provided by the framework of the self-determination theory [23], and the findings that positive and negative affect has a somewhat direct association with intrinsic and extrinsic motivation, respectively (in the context of sports, see [78]; for digital games, see [79]). It might be that—instead of e.g., higher reward-seeking behavior in males—the mechanism for both competitive preferences and consequent positive affect stems from the cultural gender expectations that perpetuate the higher male need for competence (e.g., [80]) and the needs satisfaction fulfilled by competition. For example, Gneezy, Leonard, and List [81] report how a matrilineal society in India with different gender roles shows the pattern of higher female preference for competition, and this would be also in line with the findings that masculine gender roles are associated with increasing intrinsic motivation in competition [25]. Further, the findings about male overconfidence (e.g., [3]) might be related to high perceived competence that comes with the gender expectations. While we assumed a game being played by people who like to play games an intrinsically motivated activity, the motivation is not a binary state, but a continuum, allowing differences in the level of intrinsic motivation (cf. [78]). Our results could therefore reflect the culturally higher male need for competence and fulfillment of that need by competition. Without explicit measurements, however, we do not know how the participants would have reported their needs or motivation, so this explanation remains conjectural.

Our Hypothesis 3 concerned higher arousal in competition, compared to cooperation, regardless of gender. The findings were conflicting. Heart rate, a signal often associated with arousal [33], was higher in competition for males but not for females in both experiments, an effect closely resembling to the one of positive affect measures. On the other hand, skin conductance level, the most widely used measure of physiological arousal [33,39,82], did not show a significant difference between the modes, and the self-reports supported HR in Experiment 1, but lacked any effect in Experiment 2. Given that the neural control of electrodermal activity is exclusively under sympathetic nervous system while the heart rate is innervated by both sympathetic and parasympathetic pathways, the skin conductance could be considered a more reliable index of arousal during complex stimuli [39]. On the other hand, electrodermal responses habituate quickly [82], which might lead to weakened differences in measures of tonic skin conductance level during longer experimental periods, though we have not found this to be a problem in our previous experiments. Another possibility comes from following the line of explanations about gender role expectations presented above. Given that the cardiovascular activity respond to gender-roles—whether the participants consider the task something their gender should be capable at [83,84]—HR might show a sensitivity to specifically high-arousal positive affect in the context of competitive digital game (cf. [39]). HR results could therefore indicate that the participants considered winning in a digital game more relevant to males. Again, as we did not assess gender-role orientation and perceived ability, this remains speculative.

Other Findings. Social presence was found to be linked to positive affect at least to some extent, which is not surprising per se [85,86]. However, we also found that certain emotional states normally labeled as negative (such as schadenfreude and revengefulness) might be associated with positive affect. As they were experienced as part of the (playful) competitive setup, this might be a sign of so-called meta-emotions (cf. [21,87]). Social presence also responded to the presence of computer-controlled characters, showing that the social presence might be reduced because of them (cf. [62,63], for assessment of social presence with so-called physiological linkage),

There have been only preliminary indications what would be the association between body or hand movement and emotions [88], but according to our results they seem to be closely related with the cooperative-competitive manipulation. This might suggest that movement is related to positive emotions during competition, presumably as the participants move more when they are having fun with a friend, or perhaps to arousal, if results with heart rate can be interpreted as such. As the acceleration sensors are becoming more commonplace within consumer electronics, they might become an easy way to assess at least some aspects of emotions, if the association can be ascertained and replicated in the vastly different situations those devices are used.

Limitations and Future Directions. Due to difficulty of recruiting female digital game players in both experiments the number of participants was unequal, and specifically the number of females was not as high as we hoped. The lack of statistical power is an undeniable limitation of this study, but the convergence in the results gives us confidence in them. However, as the participants were self-selected volunteers, it is possible that, for example, the female sample reflects the general population poorer than the male sample, given that playing digital games is more common in males [31].

We used digital games to set up competitive and cooperative situations and assumed that they constitute an intrinsically motivated activity for participants who (according to their own statement) like to play digital games. Further studies should take into account the explicitly stated motivation (cf. [22]). It has been also shown that competitive orientation affects the intrinsic motivation and the emotional response to competition [8,19]. For example, it is conceivable that the participants with a high desire to win [19] would have had more positive responses to a more competitive game and to actually winning, whereas the participants with low desire to win could have less positive responses to a more competitive game and perhaps less responsivity in general to winning or losing. Future studies should include a competitiveness measure to control this.

It is possible that the comparisons of EMG activity levels are affected by mostly social smiles instead of smiles resulting from emotions [89]. However, our results indicated that almost actually always males almost always actually smiled more (see Figures 1 and 3), and as female smiles are especially prominent for social situations [42], this speaks against the behavioral ecology interpretation, as that should have led to more smiles in females.

A separate potential limitation related to the tasks and competition rules is the fact that when manipulating cooperative and competitive game conditions, we necessarily also vary the opposition: i.e., as the conflict structure in the game is 2 vs. 2, in cooperative mode the participants are in the same two-character team against two computer-controlled characters, and in competitive mode they are in the opposing teams (with a computer-controlled character). Because of the interconnected structure of the 2 vs. 2 set-up, a purely symmetrical cooperation-competition (where the teammates and the opposition would not also change) was not possible. According to Ravaja and others [86], the (controller of the) opponent has effect on the emotional experience at least in competitive game play. In their study, the human opponent elicited more positive emotions than computer-controlled opponent, and a friend as an opponent elicited also more positive emotions than a stranger and this might have affected our main effects (difference between cooperation and competition) as well. The fact that many emotion and social presence self-reports showed clearly lower ratings when the computer-controlled characters were present (compared to otherwise identical competitive condition where they were not) might suggest that the interconnectedness has had an effect—while on the other hand, the lack of difference in physiological responses implies that this has not affected the general emotional states. With other types of tasks where the interconnectedness between mode and opponent is not an issue (see [22]), there would be no need for computer-controlled team members—although this would also severely limit the types of competition.

It has been shown that personal relationship and mediation may affect emotional reactions to digital games [64,85,86,90,91]. As in our experiment the participants were friends and they sat side by side in the same room, it is possible that the emotional responses were more positive due to the closeness of the participants, perhaps in interaction with the cooperation/competition manipulation. In future studies it could be tested if there is interaction between mediation, relationship, and competitiveness, although it should be noted that the relationship also may affect the social reasons to smile [42].

Conclusions. Our study is the first to examine the gender differences in emotional responses to cooperation and competition. We found that males experience the competition more positively than cooperation, that females do not have different emotional reactions to competition and cooperation, and that the males' probably experienced the competition as more positive than the females experienced either mode. These results suggest that while we consider the activity in our study, playing digital games, intrinsically motivated, the males have higher enjoyment than females, which might lead to the higher preference to competition that has been established in the research literature. The results also do not support the view that females are more cooperative than males, even if they are less competitive, implying that—contrary how they are sometimes discussed—cooperation and competition are not polar opposites.

Supporting Information

Appendix S1 Results for body and console movement and social presence evaluations for Experiment 1, social presence evaluations for Experiment 2, and post-hoc analyses for potential explanators for gender differences in both experiments.

Appendix S2 In accordance with the guidelines of PLOS ONE concerning data availability, Appendix S2 contains the final SPSS files for Experiments 1 and 2. The raw data can be made available by request.

Acknowledgments

The authors wish to thank the reviewers and associate professor Jeff Larsen of Texas Tech University for helpful comments that improved this article significantly.

Author Contributions

Conceived and designed the experiments: JMK NR JK SJ. Performed the experiments: SJ JMK. Analyzed the data: JMK JK NR. Contributed reagents/materials/analysis tools: JMK. Wrote the paper: JMK JK NR SJ.

References

1. Knight J (2002) Sexual stereotypes. Nature 415: 254–256. Available: http://dx.doi.org/10.1038/415254a. Accessed 28 August 2010.
2. Gupta ND, Poulsen A, Villeval MMC (2005) Male and Female Competitive Behavior - Experimental Evidence. Available: http://ssrn.com/abstract=906766. Accessed 18 February 2011.
3. Niederle M, Vesterlund L (2007) Do women shy away from competition? Do men compete too much? Q J Econ 122: 1067–1101.
4. Small D, Gelfand M, Babcock L, Gettman H (2007) Who goes to the bargaining table? The influence of gender and framing on the initiation of negotiation. J Pers Soc Psychol 93: 600–613. doi:10.1037/0022-3514.93.4.600.
5. Walters AE, Stuhlmacher AF, Meyer LL (1998) Gender and negotiator competitiveness: A meta-analysis. Organ Behav Hum Decis Process 76: 1–29. doi:10.1006/obhd.1998.2797.
6. Croson R, Gneezy U (2009) Gender differences in preferences. J Econ Lit 47: 448–474.
7. Van Vugt M, De Cremer D, Janssen DP (2007) Gender differences in cooperation and competition: the male-warrior hypothesis. Psychol Sci 18: 19–23.
8. Gill D, Dowd DA, Williams L, Beaudoin CM, Martin J. (1996) Competitive orientations and motives of adult sport and exercise participants. J Sport Behav 19.

9. Yamasue H, Abe O, Suga M, Yamada H, Rogers M a, et al. (2008) Sex-linked neuroanatomical basis of human altruistic cooperativeness. Cereb cortex 18: 2331–2340.
10. Taylor SE, Klein LC, Lewis BP, Gruenewald TL, Gurung RAR, et al. (2000) Biobehavioral responses to stress in females: Tend-and-befriend, not fight-or-flight. Psychol Rev 107: 411–429. doi:10.1037/0033-295X.107.3.411.
11. Cloninger CR, Svrakic DM, Przybeck TR (1993) A psychobiological model of temperament and character. Arch Gen Psychiatry 50: 975–990.
12. Ahlgren A, Johnson DW (1979) Sex Differences in Cooperative and Competitive Attitudes From the 2nd Through the 12th Grades. Dev Psychol 15: 45–49. doi:10.1037/h0078076.
13. Scherer K, Schorr A, Johnstone T (2001) Appraisal Processes in Emotion: Theory, Methods, Research. Scherer K, Schorr A, Johnstone T, editors Canary, NC: Oxford University Press.
14. Petersen MB, Sznycer D, Cosmides L, Tooby J (2012) Who Deserves Help? Evolutionary Psychology, Social Emotions, and Public Opinion about Welfare. Polit Psychol 33: 395–418.
15. Campbell A (2005) Aggression. In: Buss D, editor. The Handbook of Evolutionary Psychology. New York, NY: John Wiley. pp. 628–652.
16. Sherman LW (1986) Cooperative versus competitive educational psychology classrooms: A comparative study. Teach Teach Educ 2: 283–295. Available: http://dx.doi.org/10.1016/S0742-051X(86)80008-7. Accessed 17 April 2012.
17. Decety J, Jackson PL, Sommerville J a, Chaminade T, Meltzoff AN (2004) The neural bases of cooperation and competition: an fMRI investigation. Neuroimage 23: 744–751.
18. Sanfey AG, Rilling JK, Aronson JA, Nystrom LE, Cohen JD (2003) The neural basis of economic decision-making in the Ultimatum Game. Science (80-) 300: 1755–1758. Available: http://www.sciencemag.org/content/300/5626/1755.abstract. Accessed 18 July 2011.
19. Franken RE, Brown DJ (1995) Why do people like competition? The motivation for winning, putting forth effort, improving one's performance, performing well, being instrumental, and expressing forceful/aggressive behavior. Pers Individ Dif 19: 175–184. doi:10.1016/0191-8869(95)00035-5.
20. Scanlan TK, Lewthwaite R (1986) Social Psychological Aspects of Competition for Male Youth Sport Participants: IV. Predictors of Enjoyment. J Sport Psychol 8: 25–36.
21. Vorderer P, Hartmann T, Klimmt C (2003) Explaining the enjoyment of playing video games: the role of competition. In: Marinelli D, editor. ICEC '03 Proceedings of the second international conference on Entertainment computing. ICEC '03. Pittsburgh, PA: Carnegie Mellon University. pp. 1–9. Available: http://dl.acm.org/citation.cfm?id=958735. Accessed 24 October 2011.
22. Tauer JM, Harackiewicz JM (2004) The effects of cooperation and competition on intrinsic motivation and performance. J Pers Soc Psychol 86: 849–861.
23. Deci EL, Ryan RM (1985) Intrinsic motivation and self-determination in human behavior. New York, NY: Plenum.
24. McAuley E, Tammen V (1989) The effects of subjective and objective competitive outcomes on intrinsic motivation. J Sport Exerc Psychol 11: 84–93. Available: http://selfdeterminationtheory.org/SDT/documents/1989_McAuleyTammen_JESP.pdf. Accessed 18 December 2013.
25. Conti R, Ann M, Picariello ML (2001) The impact of competition on intrinsic motivation and creativity: considering gender, gender segregation and gender role orientation. Pers Individ Dif 30: 1273–1289. doi:10.1016/S0191-8869(00)00217-8.
26. Crocker PRE, Graham TR (1995) Coping by competitive athletes with performance stress: Gender differences and relationships with affect. Sport Psychol 9: 325–338.
27. Gill D, Dzewaltowski D (1988) Competitive Orientations Among Intercollegiate Athletes: Is Winning The Only Thing. Sport Psychol 2: 212–221.
28. Greenberg BS, Sherry JL, Lachlan K, Lucas K, Holmstrom A (2010) Orientations to Video Games Among Gender and Age Groups. Simul Gaming 41: 238–259. Available: http://sag.sagepub.com/cgi/doi/10.1177/1046878108319930. Accessed 13 March 2013.
29. Scherer KR (2005) What are emotions? And how can they be measured? Soc Sci Inf 44: 695–729. Available: http://ssi.sagepub.com/cgi/doi/10.1177/0539018405058216. Accessed 18 September 2013.
30. Schmierbach M (2010) "Killing Spree": Exploring the Connection Between Competitive Game Play and Aggressive Cognition. Communic Res 37: 256–274. Available: http://crx.sagepub.com/cgi/content/abstract/37/2/256. Accessed 31 March 2012.
31. Williams D (2006) A Brief Social History of Game Play. In: Vorderer P, Bryant J, editors. Playing video games: Motives, responses, and consequences. Mahwah, NJ: Lawrence Erlbaum Associates. pp. 197–212.
32. Hartmann T, Klimmt C (2006) Gender and Computer Games: Exploring Females' Dislikes. J Comput Commun 11: 910–931.
33. Bradley MM (2000) Emotion and motivation. In: Cacioppo JT, Tassinary LG, Berntson GG, editors. Handbook of Psychophysiology. New York, NY: Cambridge University Press. pp. 602–642.
34. Lang PJ (1995) The emotion probe. Studies of motivation and attention. Am Psychol 50: 372–385. doi:10.1037/0003-066X.50.5.372.
35. Kivikangas JM, Chanel G, Cowley B, Ekman I, Salminen M, et al. (2011) A review of the use of psychophysiological methods in game research. J Gaming Virtual Worlds 3: 181–199. doi:10.1386/jgvw.3.3.181_1.
36. Mandryk RL (2008) A physiological approach for continuously modeling user emotion in interactive play environments. Meas Behav 2008: 93–94. Available: http://www.hci.usask.ca/uploads/153-Symposium_vandenHoogen_Mandryk.pdf. Accessed 17 December 2012.
37. Mandryk RL, Atkins M (2007) A fuzzy physiological approach for continuously modeling emotion during interaction with play technologies. Int J Hum Comput Stud 65: 329–347.
38. Nacke LE, Stellmach S, Lindley CA (2010) Electroencephalographic Assessment of Player Experience: A Pilot Study in Affective Ludology. Simul Gaming. Available: http://sag.sagepub.com/cgi/doi/10.1177/1046878110378140. Accessed 3 February 2011.
39. Ravaja N (2004) Contributions of psychophysiology to media research: review and recommendations. Media Psychol 6: 193–235.
40. Simons RF, Detenber BH, Roedema TM, Reiss JE (1999) Emotion processing in three systems: the medium and the message. Psychophysiology 36: 619–627.
41. Lang PJ, Greenwald MK, Bradley MM, Hamm AO (1993) Looking at pictures: affective, facial, visceral, and behavioral reactions. Psychophysiology 30: 261–273. doi:10.1111/j.1469-8986.1993.tb03352.x.
42. LaFrance M, Hecht M a., Paluck EL (2003) The contingent smile: A meta-analysis of sex differences in smiling. Psychol Bull 129: 305–334.
43. Fujita F, Diener E, Sandvik E (1991) Gender differences in negative affect and well-being: the case for emotional intensity. J Pers Soc Psychol 61: 427–434.
44. Larsen JT, McGraw AP (2011) Further Evidence for Mixed Emotions. J Pers Soc Psychol 100: 1095–1110. doi:10.1037/a0021846.
45. Ryan RM, Rigby CS, Przybylski AK (2006) The Motivational Pull of Video Games: A Self-Determination Theory Approach. Motiv Emot 30: 344–360.
46. Harrison LK, Denning S, Easton HL, Hall JC, Burns VE, et al. (2001) The effects of competition and competitiveness on cardiovascular activity. Psychophysiology 38: 601–606. doi:10.1111/1469-8986.3840601.
47. Takatalo J, Häkkinen J, Kaistinen J, Nyman G (2011) User Experience in Digital Games: Differences Between Laboratory and Home. Simul Gaming 42: 656–673. Available: http://sag.sagepub.com/cgi/doi/10.1177/1046878110378353. Accessed 28 September 2010.
48. Poels K, de Kort YAW, Ijsselsteijn WA (2008) Observational Coding of Players' Behavior as a Continuous Measure of Digital Game Experience. Paper presented at the annual meeting of the International Communication Association, TBA, Montreal, Quebec, Canada. Available: http://www.allacademic.com/meta/p232172_index.html. Accessed 7 December 2012.
49. Carver CS, White TL (1994) Behavioral inhibition, behavioral activation, and affective responses to impending reward and punishment: The BIS/BAS Scales. J Pers Soc Psychol 67: 319–333.
50. Lang PJ (1980) Behavioral Treatment and Bio-Behavioral Assessment: Computer Applications. In: Sidowski JB, Johnson JH, Williams TA, editors. Technology in mental health care delivery systems. Norwood, NJ: Ablex Publishing. pp. 119–137.
51. Watson D, Clark LA, Tellegen A (1988) Development and validation of brief measures of positive and negative affect: The PANAS scales. J Pers Soc Psychol 54: 209–238. doi:10.1037/0022-3514.54.6.1063.
52. De Kort YAW, IJsselsteijn W, Poels K (2007) Digital games as social presence technology: Development of the Social Presence in Gaming Questionnaire (SPGQ). Proc PRESENCE: 195–203. Available: http://home.ieis.tue.nl/ydkort/de kort et al Digital games as social presence technology PRESENCE 2007.pdf. Accessed 25 February 2014.
53. Lessiter J, Freeman J, Keogh E, Davidoff J (2001) A Cross-Media Presence Questionnaire: The ITC-Sense of Presence Inventory. Presence Teleoperators Virtual Environ 10: 282–297.
54. Simmons JP, Nelson LD, Simonsohn U (2011) False-positive psychology: undisclosed flexibility in data collection and analysis allows presenting anything as significant. Psychol Sci 22: 1359–1366.
55. Kenny DA, Kashy D, Cook W (2006) Dyadic data analysis. New York: Guilford Press.
56. Benjamini Y, Hochberg Y (1995) Controlling the false discovery rate: A practical and powerful approach to multiple testing. J R Stat Soc Ser B 57: 289–300.
57. Weaver AJ, Jensen JD, Martins N, Hurley RJ, Wilson BJ (2011) Liking violence and action: An examination of gender differences in children's processing of animated content. Media Psychol 14: 49–70.
58. Lee S, Lang A (2009) Discrete Emotion and Motivation: Relative Activation in the Appetitive and Aversive Motivational Systems as a Function of Anger, Sadness, Fear, and Joy During Televised Information Campaigns. Media Psychol 12: 148–170.
59. Salen K, Zimmerman E (2004) Rules of Play. Game design fundamentals. Cambridge, MA: MIT Press.
60. Benedek M, Kaernbach C (2010) Decomposition of skin conductance data by means of nonnegative deconvolution. Psychophysiology 47: 647–658. doi:10.1111/j.1469-8986.2009.00972.x.
61. Biocca F, Harms C (2003) Guide to the Networked Minds Social Presence Inventory v. 1.2: Measures of co-presence, social presence, subjective symmetry, and intersubjective symmetry. Available: http://cogprints.org/6743/.
62. Järvelä S, Kivikangas JM, Kätsyri J, Ravaja N (2013) Physiological linkage of dyadic gaming experience. Simul Gaming 45: 24–40. doi:10.1177/1046878113513080.
63. Spapé MM, Kivikangas JM, Järvelä S, Ravaja N (2013) Keep your opponents close: social context affects EEG and fEMG linkage in a turn-based computer game. PLoS One 8. doi:e78795. doi:10.1371/journal.pone.0078795.
64. Kivikangas JM, Ravaja N (2013) Emotional responses to victory and defeat as a function of opponent. IEEE Trans Affect Comput 4: 173–182.

65. Ravaja N, Turpeinen M, Saari T, Puttonen S, Keltikangas-Järvinen L (2008) The psychophysiology of James Bond: phasic emotional responses to violent video game events. Emotion 8: 114–120.
66. Van den Hoogen W, Poels K, IJsselsteijn WA, de Kort YAW (2012) Between Challenge and Defeat: Repeated Player-Death and Game Enjoyment. Media Psychol 15: 443–459.
67. Bolls PD, Lang A, Potter RF (2001) The effects of message valence and listener arousal on attention, memory, and facial muscular responses to radio advertisements. Communic Res 28: 627–651. doi:10.1177/009365001028005003.
68. Larsen JT, Norris CJ, Cacioppo JT (2003) Effects of positive and negative affect on electromyographic activity over zygomaticus major and corrugator supercilii. Psychophysiology 40: 776–785. doi:10.1111/1469-8986.00078.
69. Hazlett RL (2006) Measuring Emotional Valence during Interactive Experiences: Boys at Video Game Play. Proceedings of SIGCHI '06 conference on Human Factors in computing systems. pp. 1023–1026. doi:10.1145/1124772.1124925.
70. Loch CH, Galunic DC, Schneider S (2006) Balancing cooperation and competition in human groups: the role of emotional algorithms and evolution. Manag Decis Econ 27: 217–233.
71. Gladstone EC, O'Connor K (2013) At First Sight: How Facial Femininity Signals Cooperativeness and Undermines Negotiators. Acad Manag Proc 2013: 17524. Available: http://proceedings.aom.org/content/2013/1/17524.abstract. Accessed 17 March 2014.
72. Balliet D, Li NP, Macfarlan SJ, Van Vugt M (2011) Sex differences in cooperation: a meta-analytic review of social dilemmas. Psychol Bull 137: 881–909. Available: http://www.apa.org/pubs/journals/releases/bul-137-6-881.pdf.
73. Anthony D, Horne C (2003) Gender and cooperation: explaining loan repayment in micro-credit groups. Soc Psychol Q 66: 293–302. Available: http://www.jstor.org/stable/1519827. Accessed 18 March 2014.
74. Simpson B (2003) Sex, Fear, and Greed: A Social Dilemma Analysis of Gender and Cooperation. Soc Forces 82: 35–52.
75. Reeves B, Geiger S (1994) Designing experiments that assess psychological responses to media messages. In: Lang A, editor. Measuring psychological responses to media messages. Hillsdale, NJ: Lawrence Erlbaum Associates Inc. pp. 165–180.
76. Heponiemi T, Keltikangas-Järvinen L, Puttonen S, Ravaja N (2003) BIS/BAS sensitivity and self-rated affects during experimentally induced stress. Pers Individ Dif 34: 943–957.
77. Jorm A, Christensen H (1999) Using the BIS/BAS scales to measure behavioural inhibition and behavioural activation: Factor structure, validity and norms in a large community sample. Pers Individ Dif 26: 49–58.
78. Vallerand RJ, Losier GF (1999) An integrative analysis of intrinsic and extrinsic motivation in sport. J Appl Sport Psychol 11: 142–169.
79. Przybylski AK, Weinstein N, Ryan RM, Rigby CS (2009) Having to versus wanting to play: background and consequences of harmonious versus obsessive engagement in video games. Cyberpsychology Behav 12: 485–492.
80. Fredricks JA, Eccles JS (2002) Children's Competence and Value Beliefs From Childhood Through Adolescence: Growth Trajectories in Two Male-Sex-Typed Domains. Dev Psychol 38: 519–533. doi:10.1037/0012-1649.38.4.519.
81. Gneezy U, Leonard KL, List JA (2008) Gender Differences in Competition: Evidence from a Matrilineal and a Patriarchal Society. Econometrica 77: 1637–1664. Available: http://www.nber.org/papers/w13727. Accessed 28 May 2012.
82. Dawson ME, Schell AM, Filion DL (2000) The electrodermal system. In: Cacioppo JT, Tassinary LG, Berntson GG, editors. Handbook of Psychophysiology. New York, NY: Cambridge University Press. pp. 200–223.
83. Weidner G, Messina CR (1995) Effects of gender-typed tasks and gender roles on cardiovascular reactivity. Int J Behav Med 2: 66–83. doi:10.1207/s15327558ijbm0201_6.
84. Wright RA, Murray JB, Storey PL, Williams BJ (1997) Ability analysis of gender relevance and sex differences in cardiovascular response to behavioral challenge. J Pers Soc Psychol 73: 405–417. doi:10.1037/0022-3514.73.2.405.
85. Gajadhar BJ, de Kort YAW, IJsselsteijn WA (2008) Shared fun is doubled fun: player enjoyment as a function of social setting. In: Markopoulos P, Ruyter B, IJsselsteijn W, Rowland D, editors. Fun and Games 2008, LNCS. Lecture Notes in Computer Science. Berlin, Heidelberg: Springer Berlin Heidelberg, Vol. 5294. pp. 106–117. doi:10.1007/978-3-540-88322-7.
86. Ravaja N, Saari T, Turpeinen M, Laarni J, Salminen M, et al. (2006) Spatial presence and emotions during video game playing: Does it matter with whom you play? Presence Teleoperators Virtual Environ 15: 381–392.
87. Bartsch A, Vorderer P, Mangold R, Viehoff R (2008) Appraisal of Emotions in Media Use: Toward a Process Model of Meta-Emotion and Emotion Regulation. Media Psychol 11: 7–27.
88. De Kort YAW, Van Den Hoogen W, IJsselsteijn WA (2009) Effects of sensory immersion on behavioural indicators of player experience: movement synchrony and controller pressure. Proceedings of DiGRA 2009.
89. Fridlund AJ (1994) Human facial expression: An evolutionary view. San Diego, CA: Academic Press.
90. Gajadhar BJ, de Kort YAW, IJsselsteijn WA (2009) Rules of Engagement: Influence of co-player presence on player involvement in digital games. Int J Gaming Comput Simulations 1: 14–27. doi:10.4018/jgcms.2009070102.
91. Ravaja N (2009) The Psychophysiology of Digital Gaming: The Effect of a Non Co-Located Opponent. Media Psychol 12: 268–294.

8

Row for Your Life: A Century of Mortality Follow-Up of French Olympic Rowers

Juliana Antero-Jacquemin[1,2]*, François Deni Desgorces[1,2], Frédéric Dor[1], Adrien Sedeaud[1], Amal Haïda[1], Philippe LeVan[3,4], Jean-François Toussaint[1,2,5]

1 Institut de Recherche bioMédicale et d'Epidemiologie du Sport (IRMES), Institut National du Sport de l'Expertise et de la Performance (INSEP), Paris, France, **2** Université Paris Descartes, EA 7329, Sorbonne Paris Cité, Paris, France, **3** Comité National Olympique et Sportif Français (CNOSF), Medical Commission, Paris, France, **4** Institut National du Sport de l'Expertise et de la Performance (INSEP), Medical Department, Paris, France, **5** Centre d'Investigations en Médecine du Sport, Hôpital Hôtel-Dieu, Assistance Publique-Hôpitaux de Paris, Paris, France

Abstract

Background/Aim: Strenuous endurance training required to participate in the highest sports level has been associated with deleterious effects on elite athletes' health and cardiac abnormalities. We aimed to describe overall mortality and main causes of deaths of male French rowers participating in at least one Olympic Game (OG) from 1912 to 2012 in comparison with the French general population.

Methods: Identity information and vital status of French Olympic rowers were validated by National sources from 1912 to 2013 (study's endpoint) among 203 rowers; 52 out of 255 (20.3%) were excluded because their vital statuses could not be confirmed. Main causes of deaths were obtained from the National registry from 1968 up to 2012. Overall and disease-specific mortalities were calculated through standardised mortality ratios (SMRs) with its 95% confidence intervals (CIs). The overall mortality was calculated for the whole rowers' cohort (PT) and for two periods apart: (P1) including rowers from 1912 to 1936 OG, a cohort in which all rowers have deceased and (P2) considering rowers from 1948 to 2012 OG.

Results: Among the 203 rowers analysed, 46 died before the study's endpoint, mainly from neoplasms (33%), cardiovascular diseases (21%) and external causes (18%). PT demonstrates a significant 42% lower overall mortality (SMR: 0.58, 95% CI: 0.43–0.78, $p<0.001$), P1 a 37% reduction (SMR: 0.63, 95% CI: 0.43–0.89, $p=0.009$) and P2 a 60% reduction (SMR: 0.40, 95% CI: 0.23–0.65, $p<0.001$) compared with their compatriots. Mortality due to cardiovascular diseases is significantly reduced (SMR: 0.41, 95% CI: 0.16–0.84, $p=0.01$) among rowers.

Conclusions: French Olympic rowers benefit of lower overall mortality compared with the French general population. Among rowers' main causes of death, cardiovascular diseases are reduced in relation to their compatriots. Analytical studies with larger samples are needed to understand the reasons for such reductions.

Editor: Alejandro Lucia, Universidad Europea de Madrid, Spain

Funding: This work was supported by a grant from the Ministry of Sports, Youth, Popular Education and Community life of France [Project n°12-R-10]. The funders had no role in study design, data collection and analysis, decision to publish, or preparation of the manuscript.

Competing Interests: The authors have declared that no competing interests exist.

* Email: juliana.antero@insep.fr

Introduction

Rowing has been reported as a safe contactless sport with low injury rate, providing health benefits to its practitioners [1,2]. Although high occurrence of cardiac diseases, and alterations on cardiovascular morphology has been previously reported in university rowers [3,4], epidemiological studies have described higher life expectancy in Harvard and Yale university rowers as in Oxford-Cambridge boat racers compared with their non-athletic referents [5,6].

If regular physical activity has been demonstrated to provide large health benefits [7–9] studies have reported that strenuous exercises and training of elite athletes could be associated with deleterious effects [10]: cardiac abnormalities [11,12] more likely triggering a sudden death during high demanding effort [13,14], with higher incidence rate among men varying according sports practice [15] and deregulated inflammatory responses [16]. In addition, training cessation after international career has showed to be deleterious in retired athletes [17–20]. Conversely, a recent meta-analysis of epidemiological studies has concluded that top-level athletes live longer than the general population [21].

Olympic Games (OG) are the highest competition level for rowing athletes; thus Olympians are exposed to the most extraneous training program and performance exigencies. This study aims to assess the overall mortality and main causes of deaths of male French Olympic rowers competing from 1912 up to 2012 compared with their referents in the French population.

Methods

Design and participants

Retrospective cohort study of French Olympic rowers. The cohort was composed of all male rowers who represented France in at least one OG, from 1912 up to 2012, and had their vital status validated by the National registry of Identification of Physical Persons (RNIPP). Coxswains were not accounted as rowers.

Three periods were taken into account to analyse rowers' overall mortality. The first (P1) included only rowers that participated in the OG from 1912 up to 1936. This period was chosen for a separated analysis because all rowers, who participated in those games, had already deceased, allowing for a complete follow-up until the entire cohort's extinction. The second period (P2) is an uninterrupted period of OG after World War II, from 1948 to 2012. Finally, we considered the total period (PT), analysing the totality of rowers participating in the OG from 1912 up to 2012 (Figure 1). The discontinuity at the rowers' entry in the cohort between 1912–1920 and 1936–1948 is related to the Games interruption due both World Wars.

Data collection

Data concerning rowers' biography came from historians' sources as previously reported [22]. These records were confirmed by data of the International Olympic Committee (olympic.org) and the French Federation of Rowing (http://www.avironfrance.asso.fr/). Rowers' identity information and vital statuses were collected since their first Olympic participation up to January 1st 2013 (study's endpoint) from the RNIPP via INSEE (National Institute of Statistics and Economical Studies), which registers vital status of all French people since 1891. Hence, rowers born before 1891 were not included in the study.

The causes of death of each deceased subject were obtained from the CépiDc (Epidemiologic Centre on Medical Causes of Death). Currently, causes of deaths occurring on French territory are available via National registry from 1968 up to January 1st, 2012. Thus, only deaths occurring during this period were submitted to investigation of its causes.

This study was approved by the Advisory Committee on Information Processing in Research in the Field of Health (CCTIRS) and the French National Commission for Data Protection and Liberties (CNIL).

Statistical Analysis

We compared the mortality of French rowers with the French general population by calculating overall and disease-specific Standard Mortality Ratio (SMR) and its 95% confidence intervals (CI). SMR is the ratio between the number of deaths observed in the rowers' cohort and the number of expected deaths if the athletes had the same death rates of the French population with age and period adjustment [23]. The source for general population death rates was the French life tables available at the Human Mortality Database (http://www.mortality.org/) via CépiDc.

The number of expected deaths was therefore calculated by multiplying male French death rates by the rowers' person-years at the corresponding age and period. Person-years were computed so that each rower contributes for one record of each year during his follow-up.

The rowers' follow-up starts with their date of first OG participation and finishes with their date of death (if concerned) or

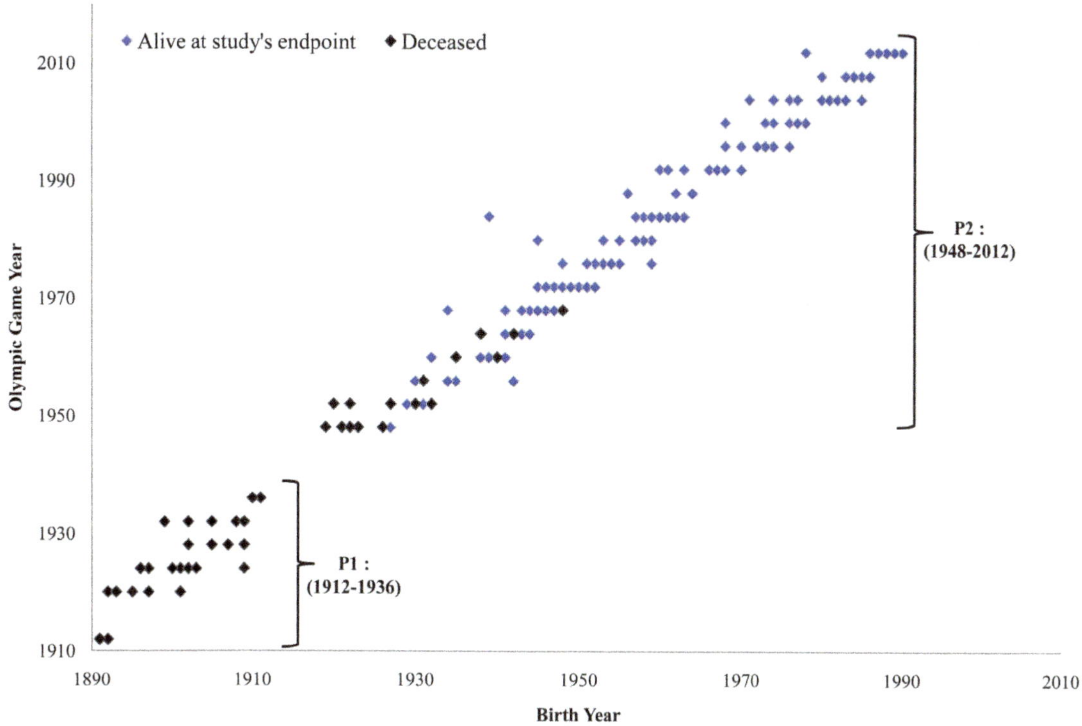

Figure 1. French Olympic rowers by Olympic Games and birth year. Black diamond represents deceased subjects and blue diamond represents the subjects alive at the study's endpoint. The two periods studied apart are schematically indicated.

with the study's endpoint. The rowers' entries in the cohort are represented in Figure 1.

The observed and expected survival estimations were illustrated by Kaplan-Meier curves [24] and were compared with use of the log-rank test.

For the disease-specific mortality we compared each cause of death found among rowers with the specific rate in the general population by calculating SMR's for the available identification period, 1968 to 2012. Causes of death were classified according to the International Classification of Diseases - ICD (8th revision before 1978, 9th revision between 1979 and 1999, 10th Revision after 2000).

The 95% confidence intervals were calculated using the exact method [25]. R software v2.14.0 was used for the analysis.

Results

Overall mortality

A total of 255 male rowers represented France in the Olympics from 1912 up to 2012. All rowers verified by the RNIPP had their vital status validated, except for fifty-two (20.3%) who were not included in the study since they were born prior to 1891 (n = 10) or their date or place of birth were not properly validated (n = 42). Therefore, the analyses were performed on 203 French rowers.

Among rowers' cohort, 46 deaths occurred before the study's endpoint; 30 within P1 (Table 1). The age of death ranged from 35 to 100 years old. The mean age of death was 72.5 (±15.6) in P1 and 74.0 (±9.1) in P2. The PT overall mortality is significantly reduced by 42% compared with the French general population. Significant overall mortality reduction is also observed among rowers for both cohort periods considered apart (Table 1).

The rowers observed and expected survival curves are illustrated in Figure 2. The rowers observed curve is significantly different from the expected curve derived from the matched general French population ($p = 0.008$). The observed rowers' curve diverges and shifts to the right early in the follow-up period. The gap widens until 45 years of follow-up, and narrows afterwards until the end of follow-up. With increasing time, progressively fewer rowers contribute to the survival estimate.

Main causes of death

Among the 46 deaths observed, 36 occurred during the available period of death's cause identification (1968–2012). From those, 3 died abroad and their cause of death were not available. Therefore, 33 rowers had their underlying cause of death identified. The main causes of death (Table 2) observed were neoplasms, n = 11(33%), followed by cardiovascular diseases n = 7 (21%) and external causes n = 6 (18%). The ICD chapter of external cause comprises deaths related to accidents, homicides, suicides and falls. The remaining causes observed (nervous system diseases, genitourinary diseases, respiratory diseases, skin diseases and ill-defined conditions) together account for 27% of all causes of death identified. Concerning the three main causes observed among French Olympic rowers, cardiovascular diseases are 59% significantly lower than found in the general population. Neoplasms and external causes are not significantly different from the general population (Table 2).

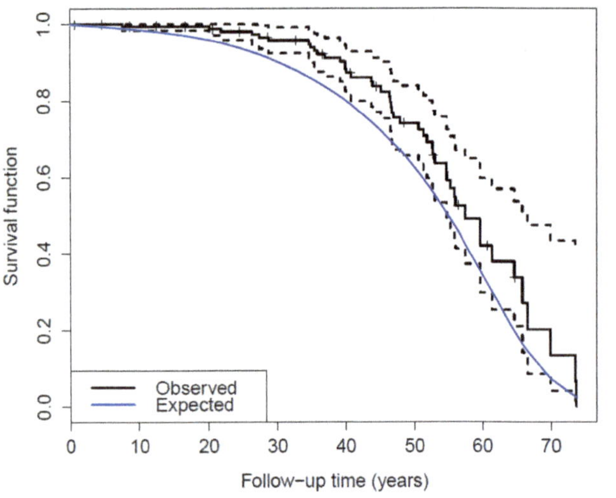

Figure 2. French Olympic rowers' observed and expected survival curves. Rowers' observed survival is represented by the solid black curve and its dashed confidence interval. The blue curve refers to the expected survival derived from the matched general French population.

Discussion

To our knowledge the present study is the first to describe a survival advantage of elite rowers compared with their referents in the general population. The follow-up over the last century shows a 42% reduction of the overall mortality of French Olympic rowers. The early cohort of rowers (P1) followed until its complete extinction as well rowers competing post Wars up to 2012 (P2) showed a consistent mortality reduction.

The difference between observed and expected survival curves since the beginning of the follow-up illustrates the rowers' survival advantage over the general population. This advantage, visible since the beginning of the follow-up, increases with time and rowers deviate most from the expected when they are 50 to 70

Table 1. French Olympic rowers' cohort description and their overall mortality compared with the French general population.

Cohort	PT (n = 203)	P1 (n = 30)	P2 (n = 173)
Cohort's entry period	1912–2012	1912–1936	1948–2012
Nb. of person-years	6724.2	1528.4	5195.8
Mean age at cohort's entry in years (SD)	24.1 (±3.6)	24.1 (±3.7)	24.1 (±3.6)
Mean follow-up time in years (SD)	33.8 (±18.5)	48.4 (±15.7)	31.0 (±17.7)
SMR (95% CI)*	0.58 (0.43–0.78)	0.63 (0.43–0.89)	0.40 (0.23–0.65)
p-value	<0.001	0.009	<0.001

*SMR lower than 1.0, indicates a reduced mortality of rowers compared with the reference population.

Table 2. French Olympic rowers' main disease-specific mortality compared with the French general population.

Main causes of death (n)	Observed/Expected deaths	SMR (95% CI)	p-value
Neoplasms (11)	11/18.4	0.59 (0.29–1.07)	0.09
Cardiovascular diseases (7)	7/17.0	0.41 (0.16–0.84)	0.01
External causes (6)	6/5.7	1.0 (0.38–2.29)	0.99

years old. At older ages the rowers' survival approaches the curve of their compatriots.

The increased selectivity of the Olympics in the modern era may require increased training intensity and may further develop the use of enhancing performance techniques, with potential adverse effects on athletes' health [26]. The consequence of such period changes on elite rowers' mortality will only be fully acknowledged after the entire extinction of the current young rowers, as it will allow a complete retrospective analysis. Up to now, our results suggest that recent rowers' longevity (P2) follows the survival advantage trend observed among P1 rowers; the mortality difference with the general population even seems to widen. However our results should be cautiously interpreted as we compare healthy individuals at cohort's entry with the general population, including ill and handicapped individuals. This "healthy worker effect" [27] probably overestimates the mortality reduction found among rowers.

French rowers' survival advantage appears associated with a reduced mortality from cardiovascular diseases. The benefits of leisure endurance sports on the cardiovascular health are well known in the general population [28,29] but some studies have underlined possible risks to the cardiovascular system due to excess training [13,30,31]. The preparation to OG includes important training volumes with rowers reaching more than 1000 h of training per year [32]. Such training loads undertaken during years of practicing produces major adaptations of the athletes' cardiovascular system [4,33] a phenomenon probably enhanced by a previously selection process [34,35]. Among French Olympic rowers, rather than a risk, the cardiovascular adaptation to training requirements to access the OG seems to be protective in light of the 59% mortality reduction found among them. Previous studies assessing cardiovascular diseases of endurance elite athletes as defined by the ICD show: a 51% reduction among Finish long distance running and cross country skiing [36] and a 37% reduction among French cyclists [37]. Finally, our findings among Olympic rowers are also in line with longevity studies assessing rowers from lower competitive level [5,6].

Similar reduced overall mortality have been reported among other elite athletes cohorts [21,36,38,39], including recent findings considering endurance athletes [40]. A study of French cyclists in the *Tour de France* with comparable methods - although the number of subjects and follow-up period are different - has shown a 41% reduction of cyclists overall mortality [37]. Although road cycling risks are greater than rowing [2], French rowers and cyclists presents similar mortality advantage over their compatriots. Yet, the lower injury incidence among rowers might be behind the contrast with American football players' mortality [41]. Despite an overall mortality reduction of 47% the players presented an increased mortality due to neurodegenerative diseases claimed to be related with concussive blows to the head.

We limited our cohort to Olympic athletes in order to focus on the highest sports level for which health consequences of intense training remains debatable [10]. Nevertheless, our results are based on a small absolute number of subjects, especially those concerning causes of death; hence they should be interpreted with caution. In addition, we are not able to determine how the excluded athletes might alter the magnitude of our findings. Finally, except for age and period, we could not adjust for potential confounding factors. Our methods advantage, however, relies on an extensive follow-up of French Olympic rowers followed during a century of OG, allowing for a complete follow-up of the rowers competing in the first Games. In addition, the vital status and causes of deaths assessed and validated by National sources reduces uncertainty.

Further investigations based on larger cohorts and in a large variety of countries are now needed to better apprehend elite athletes' reduced mortality. As it is out of an observational study's scope to determine causality, analytical studies are necessary to explain elite athletes' survival advantage. The assessment of lifestyle or physical activity post-career of elite athletes may provide better understanding of their mortality determinants.

Conclusions

French elite rowers followed-up during a century of Olympic Games benefit of lower overall mortality compared with the French general population. The cohort composed only of deceased rowers from the early Olympic Games analyzed apart and followed until its complete extinction shows also an important mortality reduction. Among elite rowers' main causes of death, cardiovascular diseases are reduced in relation to their compatriots. Analytical studies with larger samples controlling for confounders such as elite athletes' training-load and lifestyle after career are needed to understand the reasons behind elite athletes' survival advantage.

Acknowledgments

The authors thank the Institut National du Sport de l'Expertise et de la Performance (INSEP) for their full support.

All authors had full access to the data and were fully involved in the data analysis.

Author Contributions

Conceived and designed the experiments: JAJ FDD FD PLV JFT. Performed the experiments: JAJ AS AH. Analyzed the data: JAJ FDD FD JFT. Contributed reagents/materials/analysis tools: JAJ AS AH. Wrote the paper: JAJ FDD FD.

References

1. Brosh S, Jenner JR (1988) Injuries to rowers. Br J Sports Med 22: 169–169. doi:10.1136/bjsm.22.4.169.
2. Shephard RJ (1998) Science and medicine of rowing: A review. J Sports Sci 16: 603–620. doi:10.1080/026404198366416.
3. Moorstein B (1968) Life expectancy of Ivy League rowing crews. JAMA 205: 106.
4. duManoir GR, Haykowsky MJ, Syrotuik DG, Taylor DA, Bell GJ (2007) The effect of high-intensity rowing and combined strength and endurance training on left ventricular systolic function and morphology. Int J Sports Med 28: 488–494. doi:10.1055/s-2006-955897.
5. Hartley PHS, Llewellyn GF (1939) The longevity of oarsmen: A study of those who rowed in the Oxford and Cambridge boat race from 1829–1928. Br J Sports Med 1: 657–662.
6. Prout C (1972) Life expectancy of college oarsmen. JAMA 220: 1709–1711. doi:10.1001/jama.1972.03200130039008.
7. Warburton DER, Nicol CW, Bredin SSD (2006) Health benefits of physical activity: the evidence. CMAJ Can Med Assoc J J Assoc Medicale Can 174: 801–809. doi:10.1503/cmaj.051351.
8. Bize R, Johnson JA, Plotnikoff RC (2007) Physical activity level and health-related quality of life in the general adult population: a systematic review. Prev Med 45: 401–415. doi:10.1016/j.ypmed.2007.07.017.
9. Sallis RE (2009) Exercise is medicine and physicians need to prescribe it! Br J Sports Med 43: 3–4. doi:10.1136/bjsm.2008.054825.
10. Predel H-G (2014) Marathon run: cardiovascular adaptation and cardiovascular risk. Eur Heart J: eht502. doi:10.1093/eurheartj/eht502.
11. Gerche AL, Burns AT, Mooney DJ, Inder WJ, Taylor AJ, et al. (2011) Exercise-induced right ventricular dysfunction and structural remodeling in endurance athletes. Eur Heart J: ehr397. doi:10.1093/eurheartj/ehr397.
12. Ector J, Ganame J, Merwe N van der, Adriaenssens B, Pison L, et al. (2007) Reduced right ventricular ejection fraction in endurance athletes presenting with ventricular arrhythmias: a quantitative angiographic assessment. Eur Heart J 28: 345–353. doi:10.1093/eurheartj/ehl468.
13. Drezner JA (2008) Contemporary approaches to the identification of athletes at risk for sudden cardiac death. Curr Opin Cardiol 23: 494–501. doi:10.1097/HCO.0b013e32830b3624.
14. Marijon E, Tafflet M, Celermajer DS, Dumas F, Perier M-C, et al. (2011) Sports-related sudden death in the general population. Circulation 124: 672–681. doi:10.1161/CIRCULATIONAHA.110.008979.
15. Marijon E, Bougouin W, Périer M, Celermajer DS, Jouven X (2013) Incidence of sports-related sudden death in France by specific sports and sex. JAMA 310: 642–643. doi:10.1001/jama.2013.8711.
16. Cooper DM, Radom-Aizik S, Schwindt C, Zaldivar F Jr (2007) Dangerous exercise: lessons learned from dysregulated inflammatory responses to physical activity. J Appl Physiol Bethesda Md 1985 103: 700–709. doi:10.1152/japplphysiol.00225.2007.
17. Yoshiga CC, Higuchi M, Oka J (2002) Serum lipoprotein cholesterols in older oarsmen. Eur J Appl Physiol 87: 228–232. doi:10.1007/s00421-002-0627-z.
18. Petibois C, Cassaigne A, Gin H, Déléris G (2004) Lipid profile disorders induced by long-term cessation of physical activity in previously highly endurance-trained subjects. J Clin Endocrinol Metab 89: 3377–3384. doi:10.1210/jc.2003-031311.
19. Witkowski S, Spangenburg EE (2008) Reduced physical activity and the retired athlete: a dangerous combination? Br J Sports Med 42: 952–953. doi:10.1136/bjsm.2008.054353.
20. Marquet L, Brown M, Tafflet M, Nassif H, Mouraby R, et al. (2013) No effect of weight cycling on the post-career BMI of weight class elite athletes. BMC Public Health 13: 510. doi:10.1186/1471-2458-13-510.
21. Garatachea N, Santos-Lozano A, Sanchis-Gomar F, Fiuza-Luces C, Pareja-Galeano H, et al. (2014) Elite Athletes Live Longer Than the General Population: A Meta-Analysis. Mayo Clin Proc 89: 1195–1200. doi:10.1016/j.mayocp.2014.06.004.
22. Clarke PM, Walter SJ, Hayen A, Mallon WJ, Heijmans J, et al. (2012) Survival of the fittest: retrospective cohort study of the longevity of Olympic medallists in the modern era. BMJ 345: e8308.
23. Bernard P-M, Lapointe C (1987) Mesures Statistiques en Épidémiologie. PUQ. 329 p.
24. Pohar M, Stare J (2006) Relative survival analysis in R. Comput Methods Programs Biomed 81: 272–278. doi:10.1016/j.cmpb.2006.01.004.
25. Liddell FD (1984) Simple exact analysis of the standardised mortality ratio. J Epidemiol Community Health 38: 85–88.
26. Deligiannis A, Björnstad H, Carre F, Heidbüchel H, Kouidi E, et al. (2006) ESC study group of sports cardiology position paper on adverse cardiovascular effects of doping in athletes. Eur J Cardiovasc Prev Rehabil Off J Eur Soc Cardiol Work Groups Epidemiol Prev Card Rehabil Exerc Physiol 13: 687–694. doi:10.1097/01.hjr.0000224482.95597.7a.
27. Last JM (1995) A Dictionary of Epidemiology. 3rd ed. Oxford, UK: Oxford University Press.
28. Schnohr P, Marott JL, Lange P, Jensen GB (2013) Longevity in male and female joggers: the Copenhagen City Heart Study. Am J Epidemiol 177: 683–689. doi:10.1093/aje/kws301.
29. Wang H, Dwyer-Lindgren L, Lofgren KT, Rajaratnam JK, Marcus JR, et al. (2012) Age-specific and sex-specific mortality in 187 countries, 1970–2010: a systematic analysis for the Global Burden of Disease Study 2010. Lancet 380: 2071–2094. doi:10.1016/S0140-6736(12)61719-X.
30. Möhlenkamp S, Lehmann N, Breuckmann F, Bröcker-Preuss M, Nassenstein K, et al. (2008) Running: the risk of coronary events. Prevalence and prognostic relevance of coronary atherosclerosis in marathon runners. Eur Heart J 29: 1903–1910. doi:10.1093/eurheartj/ehn163.
31. Mont L, Elosua R, Brugada J (2009) Endurance sport practice as a risk factor for atrial fibrillation and atrial flutter. Europace 11: 11–17. doi:10.1093/europace/eun289.
32. Fiskerstrand A, Seiler KS (2004) Training and performance characteristics among Norwegian international rowers 1970–2001. Scand J Med Sci Sports 14: 303–310. doi:10.1046/j.1600-0838.2003.370.x.
33. Pelliccia A, Kinoshita N, Pisicchio C, Quattrini F, Dipaolo FM, et al. (2010) Long-term clinical consequences of intense, uninterrupted endurance training in olympic athletes. J Am Coll Cardiol 55: 1619–1625. doi:10.1016/j.jacc.2009.10.068.
34. Kujala UM, Sarna S, Kaprio J, Tikkanen HO, Koskenvuo M (2000) Natural selection to sports, later physical activity habits, and coronary heart disease. Br J Sports Med 34: 445–449. doi:10.1136/bjsm.34.6.445.
35. Ruiz JR, Gómez-Gallego F, Santiago C, González-Freire M, Verde Z, et al. (2009) Is there an optimum endurance polygenic profile? J Physiol 587: 1527–1534. doi:10.1113/jphysiol.2008.166645.
36. Sarna S, Sahi T, Koskenvuo M, Kaprio J (1993) Increased life expectancy of world class male athletes. Med Sci Sports Exerc 25: 237–244.
37. Marijon E, Tafflet M, Antero-Jacquemin J, Helou NE, Berthelot G, et al. (2013) Mortality of French participants in the Tour de France (1947–2012). Eur Heart J: eht347. doi:10.1093/eurheartj/eht347.
38. Gajewski AK, Poznańska A (2008) Mortality of top athletes, actors and clergy in Poland: 1924–2000 follow-up study of the long term effect of physical activity. Eur J Epidemiol 23: 335–340. doi:10.1007/s10654-008-9237-3.
39. Juliana Antero-Jacquemin, Aurélien Latouche, Jean-François Toussaint (2014) French Olympic Athletes Show a 50% Reduced Mortality Rate. Abstract: Volume 46:5.
40. Ruiz JR, Fiuza-Luces C, Garatachea N, Lucia A (2014) Reduced Mortality in Former Elite Endurance Athletes. Int J Sports Physiol Perform. doi:10.1123/ijspp.2013-0492.
41. Lehman EJ, Hein MJ, Baron SL, Gersic CM (2012) Neurodegenerative causes of death among retired National Football League players. Neurology. Available: http://www.ncbi.nlm.nih.gov/pubmed/22955124. Accessed 14 September 2014.

9

The Very High Premature Mortality Rate among Active Professional Wrestlers Is Primarily Due to Cardiovascular Disease

Christopher W. Herman[1]*, Anna S. C. Conlon[2], Melvyn Rubenfire[2], Andrew R. Burghardt[1], Stephen J. McGregor[1]

1 Eastern Michigan University, Ypsilanti, Michigan, United States of America, 2 University of Michigan, Ann Arbor, Michigan, United States of America

Abstract

Purpose: Recently, much media attention has been given to the premature deaths in professional wrestlers. Since no formal studies exist that have statistically examined the probability of premature mortality in professional wrestlers, we determined survival estimates for active wresters over the past quarter century to establish the factors contributing to the premature mortality of these individuals.

Methods: Data including cause of death was obtained from public records and wrestling publications in wrestlers who were active between January 1, 1985 and December 31, 2011. 557 males were considered consistently active wrestlers during this time period. 2007 published mortality rates from the Center for Disease Control were used to compare the general population to the wrestlers by age, BMI, time period, and cause of death. Survival estimates and Cox hazard regression models were fit to determine incident premature deaths and factors associated with lower survival. Cumulative incidence function (CIF) estimates given years wrestled was obtained using a competing risks model for cause of death.

Results: The mortality for all wrestlers over the 26-year study period was.007 deaths/total person-years or 708 per 100,000 per year, and 16% of deaths occurred below age 50 years. Among wrestlers, the leading cause of deaths based on CIF was cardiovascular-related (38%). For cardiovascular-related deaths, drug overdose-related deaths and cancer deaths, wrestler mortality rates were respectively 15.1, 122.7 and 6.4 times greater than those of males in the general population. Survival estimates from hazard models indicated that BMI is significantly associated with the hazard of death from total time wrestling ($p<0.0001$).

Conclusion: Professional wrestlers are more likely to die prematurely from cardiovascular disease compared to the general population and morbidly obese wrestlers are especially at risk. Results from this study may be useful for professional wrestlers, as well as wellness policy and medical care implementation.

Editor: Carmine Pizzi, University of Bologna, Italy

Funding: The authors have no funding or support to report.

Competing Interests: The authors have declared that no competing interests exist.

* Email: cherman2@emich.edu

Introduction

Much attention has been given in the popular media to the occurrence of premature deaths associated with professional wrestling, a choreographed form of high-impact athletic entertainment. Over the past twenty-five years, professional wrestling has become increasingly popular within the United States and numerous national wrestling organizations were in existence throughout the 1980s, 1990s, and early 2000s. World Wrestling Entertainment Inc. (WWE) is currently the largest professional wrestling organization in the world, generating nearly $500 million annually in revenues [1].

The potential for both acute and chronic injury exists among professional wrestlers, especially when considering the intensity of their efforts and their year-round competition. Abuse of androgenic anabolic steroids (AAS) was especially prevalent in professional wrestling throughout the 1980s and early 1990s until a widely publicized federal trial regarding AAS abuse in 1992 [2]. Both AAS and analgesic abuse have been linked to cardiovascular disease [3,4]. The abuse of these drugs may play a role in the premature cardiac-related deaths of professional wrestlers that receive media attention.

While most professional wrestlers have an exaggerated muscular physique, many are visibly obese with truncal obesity suggesting the presence of the metabolic syndrome (pre-diabetes) and some are morbidly obese [5,6]. There is a consistent relationship between obesity defined by the body mass index (BMI), visceral fat represented by waist, diabetes, hypertension, coronary disease, stroke, as well as premature death [7–9]. While it is understood that BMI is not the most effective measurement of body fatness among a highly muscular athletic population such as professional wrestlers, BMI values may be more representative of the actual body compositions of the wrestlers in the higher BMI ranges. In a recent study of NFL players, increased size measured by BMI was associated with increased blood pressure (BP), as well as increased triglycerides, LDL cholesterol, and fasting glucose levels, as well as lower HDL cholesterol levels [10].

The media has closely examined professional wrestler deaths that may be associated with some of the aforementioned occupational and lifestyle factors, but no epidemiological research has formally analyzed the mortality rates and survivability of the wrestlers over a long period of time. Therefore, the purpose of this study was to determine the survival estimates for professional wrestlers active between 1985 and 2011. Mortality of professional wrestlers was compared to that of the general population.

Methods

Ethics Statement

All data were de-identified for the purposes of this analysis.

A comprehensive review was conducted of the 557 regularly employed male professional wrestlers who were consistently active between January 1, 1985 and December 31, 2011. All subjects were employed by various national professional wrestling organizations during this time period [11–14]. Data was collected between January 2009 and December 2011. No permits were required for the described study, which complied with all relevant regulations. Active wrestlers who made their professional debut after June 30, 2011 were excluded. Regular employment was defined as performers featured on pay-per-view television broadcasts, live television programming, television tapings, or those who traveled as a featured performer on untelevised arena tours (also known as house shows) for at least six months or longer. Wrestler birth name, stage name, billed height, billed weight, BMI, date of birth, sex, race, age, and when applicable, cause of death, date of death, and age at death were collected from various public sources including The Wrestling Observer Newsletter [11], other wrestling-related internet sites [13,15–17], and the WWE's officially licensed published Encyclopedia [14]. Complete information was available for 536 of the 557 wrestlers who were entered into survival analyses and hazard models described below.

The effects of age, BMI, height, weight, and the amount of time wrestled on five year and ten year survival were assessed using logistic regression models. Definitions for body mass index (kg/m^2) were as follows: optimal 20–24.9; overweight 25–29.9; stage 1 obesity 30–34.9; stage 2 obesity 35–39.9; and stage 3 or morbid obesity equal to or greater than 40 kg/m^2.

Calculations of Mortality Rates

Mortality rates in the professional wrestlers were calculated and expressed as a percentage over time in years and as deaths per 100,000 per year and determined by age and cause of death. The rates were compared to the most recently available published population rates from the Centers for Disease Control (CDC) in 2007 [18]. The total number of person-years for each age cohort was calculated, and the expected number of deaths for each age group was obtained based on the 2007 CDC reported mortality rates for each group. The standardized mortality ratio (SMR) was calculated as the observed number of deaths divided by the expected number of deaths for each age group. Finally, P-values were calculated using a chi-square test to determine whether the observed number of deaths in each age group was significantly different from the expected number of deaths, with the null hypothesis being that the death rate of wrestlers within each age group is equal to the United States population death rate for that group.

Survival Analysis

Kaplan-Meier survival estimates were obtained and Cox proportional hazards models were fit to determine incident professional wrestlers' premature death and factors associated with lower survival rates. Logistic regression models were used to determine factors related to the odds of five year and ten year survival after start of career. The Kaplan-Meier plot for years wrestled at time of death does not take into account years wrestled prior to 1985. In a separate Cox regression analysis we found the time wrestled prior to 1985 was not significantly associated with the hazard of death for years wrestled after 1985. Therefore, Kaplan-Meier analyses and hazard models only consider survival probability from the start of a wrestler's career (or 1985, whichever was later). Product-limit survival estimates were also determined for wrestlers by cause of death.

Statistical analysis was performed using the R statistical software package version 2.13.1 and SAS statistical software, version 9.2 [19,20].

Results

557 males (495 survivors and 62 deceased) were included in this study. All survivor ages were calculated as of December 31, 2011. The average age when subjects started their professional wrestling career was 29.0±6.4 years. Approximately 78% of the wrestlers in this study were Caucasian, while Hispanic, Black, Asian/Pacific Islander and wrestlers of other races consisted of approximately 9%, 6%, 6%, and 1% of the sample, respectively. Demographic data for survivors and wrestlers who died within five years and ten years from the start of their career are displayed in Table 1 and Table 2, respectively.

All wrestler mortality rates were compared to those of 2007 CDC published mortality rates [18]. The total mortality over the 26-year study period was 0.007 per person-year, or 708 deaths per 100,000 per year. Specific mortality rates by BMI category for wrestlers are illustrated in Table 3. A comparison between wrestler age-adjusted mortality rates and CDC mortality rates for the general population are detailed in Table 4.

Overall, wrestler mortality rates for age groups 25–34, 35–44, and 45–54 were 1.3, 2.9, and 2.9 times greater than the 2007 CDC mortality rates for males of the same age groups. Mortality rates were also compared between the wrestlers and general population for a variety of causes of death. Among the wrestler deaths, the percentages of wrestler deaths attributed to cardiovascular disease, acute drug intoxications, and cancer were 35.5%, 17.8%, and 8.8% of total deaths, respectively. For cardiovascular-related deaths, drug overdose-related deaths and cancer deaths, the wrestler mortality rates were respectively 15.1, 122.7 and 6.4 times greater than those of males in the general population [18].

Survival Estimates

Because the CDC does not publish age-adjusted mortality rates by cause of death, a series of survival analyses were completed to develop a more formal understanding of the survivability of professional wrestlers. Survival estimates and 95% confidence intervals (CI) are presented in Figure 1. Approximately 16% of wrestlers died by the time they were 50 years of age. Additionally, survival estimates and 95% CI from the start of the wrestler's career or 1985 (whichever is later) were calculated. A professional wrestler who has been active for 10 years has a 5% mortality (survival =0.95 (95% CI: 0.93, 0.97)), compared with an 18% mortality (survival =0.82 (95% CI: 0.77, 0.87)) 25 years after the start of their career. The wrestler's starting age was not significantly associated with the hazard of mortality over time

Table 1. Five-Year Survival for Professional Wrestlers.

Variable	Total (n = 557) Mean (SD)	Alive 5 years after start (n = 503 out of 515 with at least 5 years of follow-up) Mean (SD)	Dead by 5 years after start (n = 12 out of 515 with at least 5 years of follow-up) Mean (SD)	P-value for odds of death by 5 years, given start age
Starting Age (yrs)	29.3 (6.4)	29.3 (6.6)	32.0 (6.6)	0.17
BMI (kg/m^2)	33.3 (5.1)	33.4 (4.9)	37.7 (10.7)	0.01*
Height (m)	1.87 (0.13)	1.87 (0.09)	1.87 (0.13)	0.90
Weight (kg)	116.8 (24.9)	117.1 (24.1)	135.5 (58.5)	0.03*

* Statistical significance between survivors and deceased at the 0.05 level

after starting their wrestling career (HR 1.03 (95% CI: 0.99, 1.06); p = 0.13) with every increase in starting age category.

Figure 2 displays survival probability by BMI category by age for the wrestlers. In a univariate Cox proportional hazards model for survival, BMI was significantly associated with overall survival, with the hazard ratio for death increasing by a factor of 1.86 (95% CI: 1.40, 2.48; p<0.0001) for each increase in BMI category. Figure 3 reports survival probability for BMI by years since the start of a wrestling career. A separate Cox proportional hazards model for survival found that BMI was significantly associated with the hazard of death after controlling for age. The hazard ratio (HR) for death increased by a factor of 2.12 (95% CI: 1.50, 2.81; p<0.0001) for each increase in BMI category. Figure 4 demonstrates the probability of death by causes (e.g. cardiovascular disease, drug-related death) given the number of years wrestled.

Discussion

Our study of active professional wrestlers over the past quarter of a century confirms there is an alarmingly high premature mortality rate. Wrestlers between the ages of 25 and 49 were 4.5 times more likely to die than the general population as reported by the CDC in 2007. Leading causes of mortality among wrestlers, as calculated using cumulative incidence functions, were cardiovascular-related (22 out of 62 deaths; 38%), drug-related (including overdoses of prescription drugs; 14.8%), and cancer (11.5%) throughout a 26-year wrestling career. Professional wrestlers who survived to their mid-fifties had a subsequent mortality rate comparable to the general population, as reported in Table 3.

Ninety-eight percent of wrestlers had a BMI ranging from overweight to morbidly obese, and approximately 21% were classified as stage 2 or morbidly obese. The overall mean [SD] BMI for the surviving wrestlers in this study was 32.7 kg/m2 [±4.4] and mean BMI for deceased wrestlers was 37.1 [±8.1] by last available weight. A similar association between obesity in professional athletes and mortality has been demonstrated in retired National Football League (NFL) Players. In a report from 1994, retired NFL players experienced an overall 46% lower mortality rate compared with the general population, but retired offensive and defensive linemen with a higher BMI had a 52% greater risk of dying from heart disease [21].

In the current study, obesity as defined by categories of BMI was associated with total mortality for wrestlers. Morbidly obese wrestlers had a 14% chance of mortality after only seven years of competition, and this increased to 23% after twenty years of wrestling. Duration of active wrestling has a strong relationship with mortality. Those who debuted prior to age 25 years had a 16% chance of mortality after twenty years of competition. Specifically, the aforementioned cumulative incidence function estimates indicated that there was a higher incidence of death among wrestlers from drug-related and cardiovascular causes over the 26-year study period.

Our findings suggest many of the premature deaths in active professional wrestlers result from adverse health behaviors including the abuse of performance enhancing drugs, the abuse of prescription and non-prescription drugs, and obesity that may be related to the duties performed and injuries sustained [3,4,6,22–24]. It is reasonable to assume chronic musculoskeletal injuries resulting in abuse of pain-relieving prescription drugs play a role in the premature drug-related deaths and possibly suicide among some wrestlers. It is also plausible that the painful injuries are self-treated with high doses of non-steroidal anti-inflammatory drugs (NSAIDs), which can cause or worsen hypertension and increase the risk of heart and kidney failure [25–27].

Considering the increasing popularity of professional wrestling as a form of entertainment, it would seem prudent for the wrestlers and their employers to further establish health screening efforts and treatments designed to prevent premature deaths related to performance enhancing drugs, prescription drugs, NSAIDs, eating disorders, and metabolic (diabetes) and cardiovascular diseases.

Table 2. Ten-Year Survival for Professional Wrestlers.

Variable	Total (n = 557) Mean (SD)	Alive 10 years after start (n = 419 out of 445 with at least 10 years of follow-up) Mean (SD)	Dead by 10 years after start (n = 26 out of 445 with at least 10 years of follow-up) Mean (SD)	P-value for odds of death by 10 years, given start age
Starting Age (yrs)	29.3 (6.4)	29.7 (6.7)	31.2 (7.1)	0.28
BMI (kg/m^2)	33.3 (5.1)	33.5 (5.0)	37.0 (8.2)	0.004*
Height (m)	1.9 (0.1)	1.86 (0.09)	1.90 (0.14)	0.07
Weight (kg)	116.8 (24.9)	117.2 (23.6)	136.2 (48.8)	0.001*

* Statistical significance between survivors and deceased at the 0.05 level

Table 3. Comparison of Mortality rates by BMI Categories for Wrestlers by Gender.

BMI Category by # of males	Mortality rate Per 100,000 (Males)	Hazard Ratio (Vs. Optimal Group)
Optimal (n = 5)	0	1.00
Overweight (n = 106)	36	1.98
Obese 1 (n = 326)	5197	3.91
Obese 2 (n = 81)	3047	7.73
Morbidly Obese (n = 37)	6810	15.29

Based upon our findings and the known association between obesity and hypertension, professional wrestlers should be regularly advised regarding their blood pressure and risk factors for hypertension, and treated appropriately. Even mild increases in blood pressure are associated with an increase in cardiovascular event (CVE) rate. There is a direct, linear relationship between BP and risk of stroke and other cardiovascular events with a systolic BP of greater than 115 mmHg; a 20 mmHg increment of systolic BP doubles the risk of CVE across a range from 115/75 to 185/115 mmHg [28]. Subjects with high normal BP are at twice the risk of developing hypertension than those with lower values and therefore over time are at greater risk of events and may require antihypertensive medication in the future.

To our knowledge, there is no published reference regarding blood pressure and prevalence of hypertension in professional wrestlers. However, there have been studies of active professional football players including offensive and defensive linemen who have a similar body habitus, similar training, potential for anabolic steroid abuse, and performance associated injuries requiring pain relief. Compared to over 1900 healthy matched controls, among 504 NFL professional football players with an average age of 26 years, there was a nearly 3 fold (13.8%% vs. 5.5%) incidence of hypertension (BP>140/90 mmHg) and prehypertension (120–139 mmHg systolic or 80–89 mmHg diastolic) (64.5% vs. 24.2%), $p<0.001$ for both. The mean BMI of offensive and defensive lineman was 37.8 kg/m^2 and 35.7 kg/m^2 respectively. The combined prevalence of hypertension and prehypertension was 91% in the largest players. Higher BMI was associated with each of the measurable coronary risk factors including higher BP, LDL cholesterol, triglycerides, and fasting glucose, and decrease in HDL cholesterol [10]. The NFL has plans to investigate the mechanisms of hypertension including the use of NSAIDs, strength and resistance training, salt intake, and sleep disordered breathing.

It is well known that diabetes mellitus (DM) is a metabolic disorder characterized by increased mortality rates and importantly implicated in the atherogenic process [29]. Further, in addition to vascular disease, diabetes is associated with substantial premature death from several cancers, infectious diseases, external causes, intentional self-harm, and degenerative disorders, independent of several major risk factors [30]. While we don't have data on the prevalence of diabetes in our wrestler cohort, considering their BMI [10] and use of steroids, and androgens, it is highly likely there is an increase incidence of both diabetes and the metabolic syndrome whose components are each risk factors or markers for coronary disease. Moderate to severe obesity, both central and abdominal, which is very prevalent in the wrestlers, is associated with an abnormal fasting blood sugar, hypertension, low HDL cholesterol, and elevated triglycerides, each of which increases the risk of diabetes and coronary atherosclerosis, coronary events, and cardiovascular mortality [31].

It is important to note that many of the professional wrestlers analyzed in the present study did not directly compete for WWE, which is currently the world's largest professional wrestling

Table 4. Comparison of Total Wrestler and CDC Mortality rates by Age Group.

Age Group (years)	Person- years in group	# Dead in Age Group	CDC Mortality Rate (Per 100,000)	Expected deaths (person-years *CDC rate/10000)	SMR (observed deaths/ expected)	Chi-square p-value
20–24	252	0	145	0.37	0	0.82
25–29	1118	2	140	1.57	1.28	0.96
30–34	1697	13	148	2.51	5.18	<0.0001*
35–39	1698	9	185	3.14	2.87	0.002*
40–44	1395	12	277	3.86	3.11	0.0001*
45–49	1077	13	424	4.57	2.85	0.0002*
50–54	713	3	647	4.61	0.65	0.60
55–59	421	2	922	3.88	0.52	0.48
60–64	236	4	1328	3.13	1.28	0.84
65–69	109	3	2002	2.18	1.37	0.83
70–74	23	0	3047	0.70	0	0.81
75–79	8	1	4817	0.39	2.59	0.85

*Statistical significance between wrestler and 2007 CDC rates at the 0.05 level.

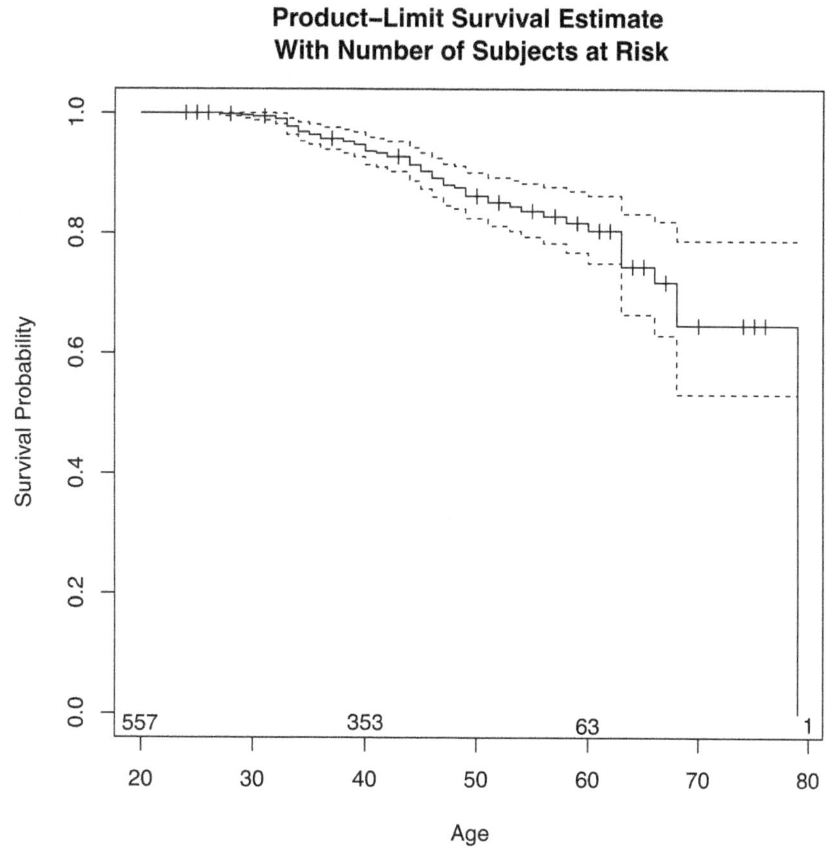

Figure 1. Survival probability by age.

organization that instituted a Talent Wellness Program in 2006 to address some of the health concerns among their performers [32,33]. The program components include 'an aggressive substance abuse and drug testing policy' and 'a cardiovascular testing and monitoring program' [32]. Currently, there is one other national professional wrestling organization and information on any associated corporate wellness policy is not publicly available. Results from this study are associated with professional

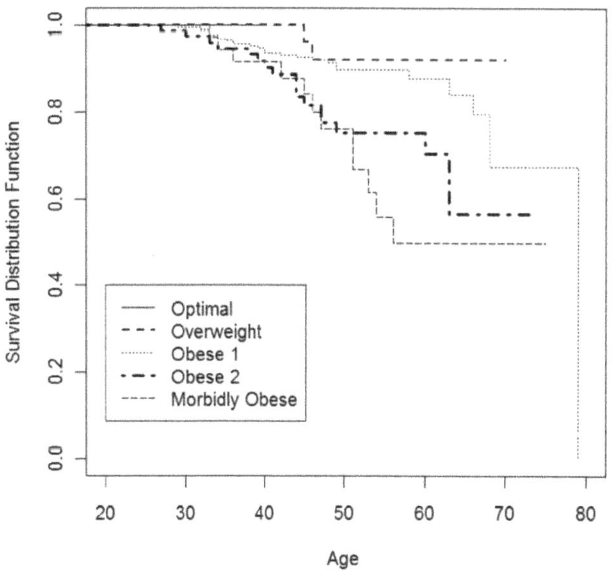

Figure 2. Survival probability for BMI by age for wrestlers.

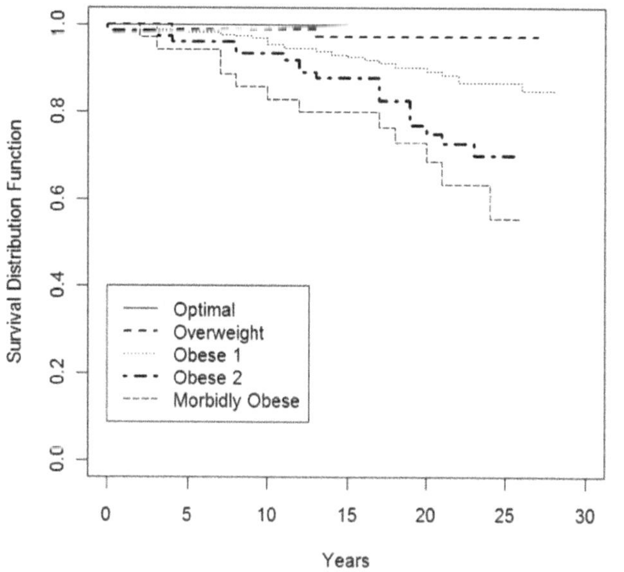

Figure 3. Wrestler survival probability for BMI by years from start of career.

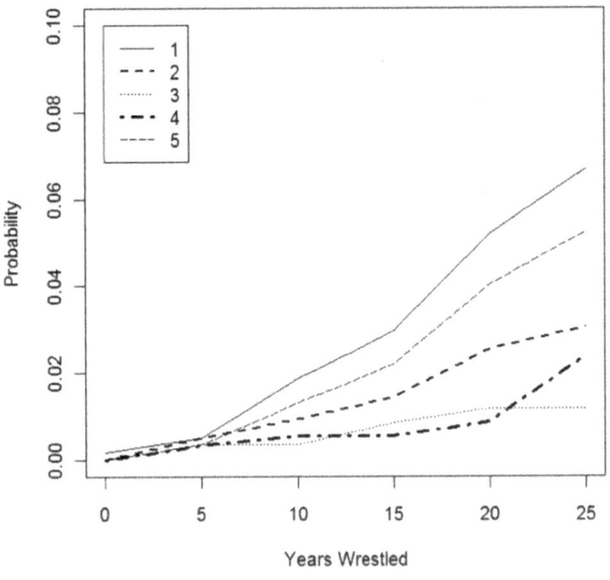

Figure 4. Cumulative incidence function estimates given years wrestled for cause of death. Figure 4 Note: 1 = Cardiovascular-Related Death; 2 = Drug-Related Death; 3 = Non-Drug Suicide and Homicide; 4 = Cancer Death; 5 = Other Cause of Death.

wrestlers in the industry as a whole and not with any specific professional wrestling organization.

There are several limitations to our study, the primary being the reliability of data collection. Rather than the standard of medical record review for each participant, we used non-scientific websites and other public data sources such as publications and websites. These sources of information are similar in nature to those employed by a recent study of professional cyclists [34]. We also used cause-of-death information from these sources to compare mortality rates with the CDC, which more formally confirms causes of death. The veracity of information in the present study is supported by the fact that premature wrestler deaths have been publicized and extensively scrutinized. In conjunction with the publicly acknowledged wellness violations among some of these individuals, the circumstances of these deaths are publicly accepted. We concluded the information obtained is reasonable and can be used to support more accurate studies using standard methods with medical records. Additionally, in this observational study, it is not appropriate to state that a causal relationship exists between participation in a professional wrestling organization and survivability. With the exception of age, height, weight, BMI, and time-period wrestled, we were not able to adjust for any other potential confounding factors. This is somewhat similar to the aforementioned cycling study [34]. Furthermore, while we defined obesity by BMI, which has not been validated in wrestlers with scientific methods of measuring body fatness, it is reasonably assumed that any potential exaggeration in weight per unit height among the wrestlers was likely consistent across all BMI categories for all of the performers. In the present study, while there was no loss to follow-up for overall mortality, the cause and/or date of mortality were not found for a few of the deceased wrestlers and it is possible that a wrestler may have met the requirements for dataset inclusion but was accidentally omitted. Finally, small sample sizes for the wrestlers <25 years and >56 years of age limited the analysis in these groups.

Conclusion

Considering the very high rate of premature mortality from cardiovascular disease, cancer, and substance abuse, the health and wellbeing of professional wrestlers who are part of the entertainment industry need an intense prevention strategy with aggressive treatment of each of the risk factors. Results from this study may be useful for professional wrestlers, and may be useful for the development of future wellness policy and medical care implementation among professional wrestling organizations.

Author Contributions

Conceived and designed the experiments: CH AC MR AB SM. Performed the experiments: CH AC. Analyzed the data: CH AC MR AB SM. Wrote the paper: CH AC MR SM.

References

1. (30 Sept 2011) WWE Income Statement. Available: Rehttp://ir.corporate.wwe.com/asreported.aspx?keyreport = 592&keytable = 1&iid = 4121687. Accessed 2011 December 15.
2. (13 April 2009) WWE and Steroids: Still A Tough Target. Available: http://sports.espn.go.com/espn/e60/columns/story?columnist=assael_shaun&id=4055522. Accessed 2011 December 15.
3. Nascimento JH, Medei E (2011) Cardiac Effects of Anabolic Steroids: Hypertrophy, Ischemia, and Electrical Remodeling as Potential Triggers of Sudden Mortality. Mini Review of Medicinal Chemistry 11: 425–429.
4. Carman WJ, Su S, Cook SF, Wurzelmann JI, McAffe A (2011) Coronary Heart Disease Outcomes among Chronic Opioid and Cyclooxygenase-2 Users Compared With A General Population. Pharmacoepidemiology and Drug Safety 20: 754–762.
5. Park YW, Zhu S, Palaniappan L, Heshka S, Carnethon MR, et al. (2003) The metabolic syndrome: Prevalence and associated risk factor findings in the US population from the third national health and nutrition examination survey, 1988–1994. Archives of Internal Medicine 163: 427–436.
6. Hu G, Qiao Q, Tuomilehto J, Balkau B, Borch-Johnsen K, et al. (2004) Prevalence of the metabolic syndrome and its relation to all-cause and cardiovascular mortality in non-diabetic European men and women. Archives of Internal Medicine 164: 1066–1076.
7. Stein CJ, Colditz GA (2004) The Epidemic of Obesity. The Journal of Clinical Endocrinology & Metabolism 89: 2522–2525.
8. Manson JE, Bassuk SS (2003) Obesity in the United States: A Fresh Look At Its High Toll. The Journal of the American Medical Association 289: 229–230.
9. Wolin KY, Carson K, Colditz GA. (2010) Obesity and Cancer. The Oncologist 15: 556–565.
10. Tucker AM, Vogel RA, Lincoln AE, Dunn RE, Ahrensfield DC, et al. (2009) Prevalence of Cardiovascular Disease Risk Factors Among National Football League Players. Journal of the American Medical Association 301: 2111–2119.
11. (n.d.) The Wrestling Observer Newsletter Online. Available: http://www.f4wonline.com. Accessed 2010 October 2.
12. (n.d.) The Internet Wrestling Database. Available: http://www.profightdb.com. (n.d.)
13. (n.d.) World Wrestling Entertainment, Inc. Available: http://www.wwe.com. Accessed 2011 December 31.
14. Shields B, Sullivan K (2009) WWE Encyclopedia: The Definitive Guide to World Wrestling Entertainment. Indianapolis, IN: DK Publishing - Brady Games, a division of Penguin Group (USA), Inc.
15. (n.d.) Wrestlers That Have Passed Away (In chronological order). Available: http://www.pwwew.net/people/dead.htm. Accessed 2011 December 31.
16. (n.d.) Wrestler Deaths & Obituaries. Available: http://wrestlingtruth.com/news/category/wrestling-deaths/. Accessed 2010 December 1.
17. Cohen E (n.d.) Wrestling's Dirty Secret. Available: http://prowrestling.about.com/od/whatsrealwhatsfake/a/wrestlersdeaths.htm. Accessed 2010 November 1.
18. Xu J, Kochanek KD, Murphy SL, Tejada-Vera B (2010) Deaths: Final Data for 2007. National Vital Statistics Reports 58: 22.
19. (2011) R: A language and environment for statistical computing. Vienna, Austria: R Foundation for Statistical Computing.
20. (2011) SAS Version 9.2. Cary, NC: SAS Institute, Inc.
21. Barson S, Rinsky R (1994) Health Hazard Evaluation Report, National Football League Players Mortality Study. Atlanta, GA: National Institute for Occupational Safety and Health.
22. Michaels S (2006) Heartbreak and Triumph: The Shawn Michaels Story. Stamford, CT: World Wrestling Entertainment. 352 p.

23. Hart B (2008) Hitman: My Real Life in the Cartoon World of Wrestling. New York: Grand Central Publishing. 592 p.
24. Foley M (2010) Countdown to Lockdown: A Hardcore Journal. New York: Grand Central Publishing. 400p.
25. Knauf H, Bailey MA, Hasenfuss G, Mutschler E (2006) The influence of cardiovascular and anti-inflammatory drugs on thiazide-induced hemodynamic and saluretic effects. European Journal of Clinical Pharmacology 62: 885–892.
26. Lapi F, Azoulay L, Yin H, Nessim SJ, Suissa S (2013) Concurrent Use of Diuretics, Angiotensin Converting Enzyme Inhibitors, and Angiotensin receptor Blockers with Non-Steroidal Anti-Inflammatory Drugs and Risk of Acute Kidney Injury: Nested Case-Control Study. BMJ 346.
27. Trelle S, Reichenbach S, Wandel S, Hildebrand P, Tschannen B, et al. (2011) Cardiovascular safety of non-steroidal anti-inflammatory druges: network meta-analysis. BMJ 342.
28. Lewington S, Clark R, Qizilbash N, Peto R, Collins R (2002) Age-specific relevance of usual blood pressure to vascular mortality. Lancet 360: 1903–1913.
29. Berry C, Tardif J-C, Bourassa MG (2007) Coronary Heart Disease in Patients with Diabetes: Part I: Recent Advances in Prevention and Noninvasive Management. Journal of the American College of Cardiology 49: 632–642.
30. Emerging Risk Factors Collaboration S, Kaptoge SR, Thompson S, Di Angelantonio A, Gao E, et al. (2011) Diabetes Mellitus, Fasting Glucose, and Risk of Cause-Specific Death. New England Journal of Medicine 364: 829–841.
31. Malik S, Wong ND, Franklin SS, Kamath TV, L'Italien GJ, et al. (2004) Impact of the metabolic syndrome on mortality from coronary heart disease, cardiovascular disease, and all causes in United States adults. Circulation 110: 1245–1250.
32. (27 Feb 2006) WWE Talent Wellness Program. World Wrestling Entertainment, Inc. Available: http://corporate.wwe.com/documents/TalentWellnessProgramOutline2-27-06CORPweb.pdf. Accessed 2010 December 18.
33. Deitch C (2 Dec 2010) Heavyweight Champions. Pittsburgh City Paper. Available: http://www.pittsburghcitypaper.ws/gyrobase/Content?oid=oid%3A88609. Accessed 2010 December 9.
34. Marijon E, Tafflet M, Antero-Jacquemin J, El Helou N, Berthelot G, et al. (2013). Mortality of French participants in the Tour de France (1947–2012). European Heart Journal. doi: 10.1093/eurheartj/eht347.

10

Do Coaches Perceive Themselves as Influential on Physical Activity for Girls in Organised Youth Sport?

Justin M. Guagliano[1]*, Chris Lonsdale[2], Richard R. Rosenkranz[1,3], Gregory S. Kolt[1], Emma S. George[1]

1 School of Science and Health, University of Western Sydney, Sydney, Australia, **2** Institute for Positive Psychology and Education, Australian Catholic University, Sydney, Australia, **3** Department of Human Nutrition, Kansas State University, Manhattan, Kansas, United States of America

Abstract

Participation in organised youth sports (OYS) has been recommended as an opportunity to increase young peoples' physical activity (PA) levels. While coaches can potentially influence athletes' PA levels, what has not been explored is the question; do coaches perceive themselves as influential on PA for girls in OYS? Participants were 30 coaches of girls OYS teams aged 9–17 years in the Greater Sydney Metropolitan Area, Australia. Participants took part in a semi-structured interview that lasted approximately 30 minutes. They responded to questions regarding their perceived role as coaches, their perceptions of themselves as role models for PA, their views on their athletes' current PA levels, their opinions on improving their athletes' PA levels, and their perceived challenges as coaches in OYS. Many coaches considered themselves role models for PA due to their own involvement in organised sports. Coaches felt that they were conscious of girls' PA levels during training and could accurately gauge how active girls were. Coaches perceived their training sessions to provide sufficient PA and thus, did not feel the need to try to increase PA during training. Many coaches were cautious about conducting training sessions where the PA intensity was high for prolonged periods because they believed that it could potentially result in dropout from OYS. Coaches' perceived time commitment to OYS, variability of skill/experience amongst girls, and poor parental support as major challenges they experienced in OYS. This study provided a unique insight from the perspective of coaches in OYS. Most coaches felt that they had the potential to influence PA for girls in OYS; however, coaches may underestimate or not fully realise the impact they can have on the girls they coach. Future research should focus on educating coaches to capitalise on the opportunity they have to promote PA through OYS.

Editor: Naoyuki Hayashi, Tokyo Institute of Technology, Japan

Funding: This study was funded by the School of Science and Health at the University of Western Sydney. The funders had no role in study design, data collection and analysis, decision to publish, or preparation of the manuscript.

Competing Interests: The authors have declared that no competing interests exist.

* Email: j.guagliano@uws.edu.au

Introduction

Organised youth sports (OYS) is a structured physical activity (PA) setting for children and adolescents that is governed by the rules of the sport being played [1]. In OYS, athletes attend training sessions and games under supervision of one or more adults, who most often assume the role of team coach [1,2]. Coaches in OYS are in an ideal position to impact the health and well-being of children and adolescents. Due to their role in OYS, coaches can carry considerable influence, as they are viewed as experts by their athletes [3]. Similarly, Smith and Smoll [4] have suggested that coaches can have a strong impact on children and adolescents within an OYS context due to the amount of direct involvement they have with their athletes on a weekly basis. Coaches also have considerable reach, as high proportions of children and adolescents participate in OYS around the world [5]. The most recent prevalence data indicate that, approximately 66% of all Australian children (67% of all boys and 65% of all girls) participate in at least one OYS (including dance) outside of school hours [6,7]. Through their participation in OYS, children and adolescents have the potential to be exposed to an array of physical and psychosocial health and developmental benefits [8–11].

Arguably, one of the most pertinent attributes of OYS is its potential to contribute significantly to moderate-to-vigorous physical activity (MVPA) levels of participating children [12,13]. Children and adolescents should engage in at least 60 minutes of MVPA daily and vigorous PA, including activity that strengthens muscle and bone, should be incorporated at least three times per week [14–16]. However, since a sizeable proportion of children and adolescents around the world do not meet the recommended levels of daily MVPA [5]. In Australia, a recent report found that less than one-fifth of Australian children and adolescents, aged 5–17, met recommended physical activity guidelines every day of the week [6]. This issue is even more concerning when examining youth PA levels separately, by gender. Girls are less physically active than boys throughout childhood [17,18] and their participation in PA declines more sharply than in boys as they transition into adolescence [17,19]. As such, girls have been identified as a high priority group for PA promotion [20], therefore participating in OYS can have major public health implications. Although participation in OYS provides an ideal opportunity for children and adolescents to accumulate substantial amounts of MVPA, participation in OYS does not guarantee MVPA. Studies have found that children and adolescents spend large proportions of time during OYS inactive or in light PA [12,21,22]. Furthermore, coaches spent a considerable proportion of training time in management and knowledge delivery contexts [12], where it is likely that children and adolescents would be relatively inactive [23].

Coaches, therefore, have the opportunity to influence their athletes' PA levels, particularly during training where coaches are better able to dictate the intensity of PA, compared to a game. However, the way coaches perceive themselves with regards to influencing girls' PA is not clear and further exploration is warranted due to the high proportion of children who participate in OYS and the myriad of health and developmental benefits children and adolescents stand to gain through the setting. OYS presents a good opportunity to participate in PA and has the potential to be a powerful health-promoting environment for children and adolescents, where coaches are at the helm.

To our knowledge, no study has explored whether coaches perceive themselves as influential on PA for girls participating in OYS. Further, only a few cross-sectional studies have examined children and adolescents' PA levels in OYS [12,21,22], finding that children and adolescents spent large proportions of time during OYS inactive or in light PA. Coaches' views on their athletes' current PA levels and their opinions on improving their athletes' PA levels, however, have not been investigated. Lastly, coaches' perceived challenges in OYS have also not previously been considered, and as such, this information could provide valuable insight on aspects of the coaching experience that could inform future studies aiming to increase PA in OYS. Accordingly, this study aimed to explore OYS coaches': (1) perceived role as a coach; (2) perception of themselves as role models for PA; (3) views on their athletes' current PA levels; (4) opinions on improving their athletes' PA levels; and (5) their perceived challenges as coaches in OYS.

Methods

Study design and procedures

This study conforms to the consolidated criteria for reporting qualitative research (COREQ) developed by Tong, Sainsbury, and Craig [24]. Between July and August 2012, each of the 30 coaches recruited took part in one in-depth semi-structured interview with the primary author (JMG). Interviewing is one of the most commonly used methods in qualitative research [25] and is a method capable of providing rich and comprehensive data [26]. Semi-structured interviews also provide the interviewer with the flexibility to further explore participants' responses [27].

The interview questions, prompts, and probes used in this study are outlined in Table 1. The development of the interview questions was guided by the aforementioned study aims. Most interview questions were open-ended to elicit a wide range of responses and prompts and probes were used to encourage further discussion, when required. To ensure content validity, the interview guide was iteratively developed by all members of the research team; reviewing content, structure, and wording of the questions. The research team also assessed the ordering of the interview questions and length of the interview. The questions were pilot tested on three adults who had coaching experience in a range of sports to ensure appropriate face validity.

Each participant was informed that the current study would be disseminated as part of JMG's doctoral thesis and associated publications, and all participants provided verbal and written informed consent prior to participating in their interview. All interviews were conducted face-to-face, and the majority of the interviews took place at a training ground prior to one of the participants' regular scheduled training sessions (23/30 interviews). Interviews were also conducted at participants' homes (5/30) or at a local café (2/30 interviews), as these locations were most convenient for the coaches. Each interview was conducted in a private or semi-private location and only the participant and the primary author were present during the interviews. The interviews lasted approximately 30 minutes, ranging from 28–40 minutes. At the conclusion of each interview, the participant received a $50 gift card as compensation for their time. Following each interview, field notes were made by JMG reflecting any key moments or quotes that occurred.

All interviews were conducted by JMG, who has conducted prior research on the chosen organised sports [12]. He has four years of personal experience coaching childrens' organised sport teams, and has played soccer for over 20 years. JMG is also working towards a doctoral degree in the area of PA promotion in children and youth, and currently holds an honours bachelor's degree in community health sciences. This knowledge and experience of sports and coaching was useful, because it helped build rapport with participants, and ensured jargon used by the coaches was understood. Most participants did not have any prior relationship with the research team; however, five coaches were involved in a previous study [12].

Participants

A convenience sample of OYS coaches who coached club and representative level teams of girls aged 9 to 17 years participated in this study. In this study, a club-level coach coaches athletes that have registered with an OYS club and have been assigned to a team. Representative athletes are also registered with an OYS club; however, these athletes were selected members of a team. Representative athletes represent their district and compete in a higher level of competition than club athletes. The representative-level is not the highest level of competition in OYS; however, higher levels of competition were not discussed in this study.

Participants were recruited from OYS clubs playing netball, basketball, and outdoor soccer (football) in the Greater Sydney Metropolitan Area, Australia. These organised sports were chosen because of their popularity amongst girls (in terms of participation rates) in Australia [28]. Initially, a member of each of the organised sport club's executive committee was contacted by the primary author (JMG), to provide information about the study. Clubs then provided contact details (a phone number and/or an email address) of interested participants who were coaching girls' teams in the appropriate age range. Detailed study information was then sent via email to each potential participant and coaches were included based on their willingness to participate in the study. The Human Research Ethics Committee of the University of Western Sydney approved this study.

Participant characteristics are detailed in Table 2. In total, 30 coaches (10 coaches from each of the three organised sports) participated. Coaches were aged 18–69 years (mean age $= 42.2 \pm 13.2$ years) and had an average of 13.3 ± 11.8 years of coaching experience. The majority of the coaches were male (63%), married (57%), educated at a tertiary level (57%), held a form of coaching credential related to their sport (90%), and were overweight (43% with ≥ 25 BMI<30) or obese (30% with BMI≥ 30), based on participants' self-reported height and weight.

Data analysis

Interviews were audio-recorded and transcribed verbatim by JMG. During transcription, further notes were added to the

Table 1. Interview questions, prompts, and probes.

• How do you describe your role as a coach?
• In terms of physical active, do you see yourself as a role model for your athletes?
○ In relation to having a healthy/active lifestyle?
• In what ways do you think you can influence the health behaviours of your athletes?
• How active do you think the athletes are during training?
• Can you tell me about the major demands or challenges you face as a coach?
○ Personal (e.g., lack of time, work or family commitments)
○ Athletes (e.g., lack of motivation, interest, or discipline)
○ Parents
○ Facilities/equipment
• If you were asked to make changes to your team with regard to promotion of greater physical activity levels during training time, what factors would influence your ability to do that?
• How important is it to you that your athletes are physically active during training?
• Can you identify ways you could increase children's physical activity levels during organised sport training?
• How do you plan what you're going to do for a training session? Take me through your process.
• How important is it to you that your athletes are physically active outside of organised sport?
• To what degree do you think you are responsible for influencing the physical activity behaviours of your athletes outside of organised sport?

original field notes made during post-interview reflection. After transcription, 20% of transcripts were returned to corresponding participants for verification. To ensure equal representation, two participants (a male and a female) were selected from each sport for verification. Participants made no changes to their transcripts.

Using a long table approach, content analysis was conducted using guidelines established by Côté, Salmela, Baria, and Russell [29]. Due to the exploratory nature of this study, an interpretational approach to analysis was used [30]. Côté et al. [29], described two separate phases for interpretational qualitative analysis: (1) data organisation (or creating tags) and (2) data interpretation (or creating categories). The process used to analyse the data is illustrated in Figure 1. A decision-making heuristic for the analysis of unstructured qualitative data by Côté and Salmela [31] was also used.

During the data organisation phase, text from each transcript (and corresponding field notes) were divided into segments called meaning units to produce a set of concepts that reflected meaningful pieces of information [29]. Text was divided into meaning units directly on each transcript, where tags were assigned to each meaning unit. Tagging was performed by JMG. A separate document was kept as an inventory of all the accumulated tags for the second phase of the analysis. For the data interpretation phase, the inventory of tags from all transcripts was examined by JMG and ESG. For our purposes, a deductive process was used to underpin the coding framework and help organise tags; where tags fell within five overarching categories (the aims of this study). An inductive process, however, was used to group tags with similar meaning together, which led to the emergence of themes and sub-themes within each overarching category. Disagreements while categorising were discussed with two members of the research team (CL and GSK) until a consensus was reached.

Sample size was determined *a priori* to ensure equal representation of the three organised sports. Transcripts were analysed after all interviews were conducted, in the order in which the interviews were conducted to determine theoretical saturation. Côté et al. [29] stated that theoretical saturation is reached when new data fits adequately into the existing framework. Theoretical saturation was determined to have occurred following the 23rd interview.

In order to assess classification consistency, a random sample of 25% of tags was selected for independent classification under mutually exclusive categories and themes by a member of the research team familiar with the study aims but removed from data analysis until this point (RRR). Agreement was determined by comparing RRR's independent classification of a random sample of tags with the classification of tags conducted by the rest of the research team. Seventy percent agreement was set as the minimum acceptable level of agreement. Agreement was also assessed using Cohen's kappa coefficient. RRR's independent classification of a random sample of tags showed a high level agreement with the rest of the research team (88.6% agreement, kappa coefficient = 0.88).

Results

A summary of the main themes, sub-themes, and example quotes that emerged from the 30 in-depth semi-structured interviews with OYS coaches are presented by category in Tables 3 to 7. The five categories are presented in the following order: (1) participants' perceived role as coaches (five themes, three sub-themes); (2) their perception of themselves as role models for PA (two themes, no sub-themes); (3) their views on their athletes' current PA levels (five themes, no sub-themes); (4) their opinions on improving their athletes' PA levels (five themes, two sub-themes); and (5) their perceived challenges as coaches in OYS (four themes, nine sub-themes).

Perceived role as coaches

Coaches described roles in which they could be influential to their athletes, such as being a mentor or role model. The most common influential perceived role that coaches cited, though, was as a teacher:

Table 2. Characteristics of Participating Coaches.

Variable	Netball (n = 10)	Basketball (n = 10)	Soccer (n = 10)
Mean age (±SD)	41.8(18.8)	38.8(12.3)	45.8(5.4)
Sex, n			
Male	2	8	9
Female	8	2	1
Mean height (cm) (±SD)	165.7(9.4)	179.3(11.4)	176.2(10.8)
Mean weight (kg) (±SD)	74.6(13.1)	83.3(20.2)	94.4(15.2)
Mean body mass index (±SD)	27.2(4.2)	25.6(4.3)	30.3(5.3)
Marital Status, n			
Married	4	5	8
Divorced	1	1	0
Not married	5	4	2
Level of education, n			
University or higher	2	3	1
Certificate/diploma	3	3	5
Trade/apprenticeship	1	0	1
Secondary school	3	2	2
Less than secondary school	1	2	1
Annual income, n			
$100,000+	3	2	7
$80,000–$99,999	1	5	1
$60,000– $79,999	1	0	1
$40,000–$59,999	2	0	1
$20,000–$39,999	0	2	0
<$20,000	3	1	0
Mean years coaching (±SD)	18.5(16.3)	12.8(8.7)	8.5(7.2)
Mean number of sports coaching (±SD)	1(0)	1.1(0.3)	1.5(0.9)
Mean number of age groups coaching (±SD)	1.8(0.6)	2.8(0.8)	1.7(1.0)
Coaches with coaching credentials, n	10	10	7

Note: n = number of coaches.

"Mainly I'm like a teacher and that's what I want to be seen as because that's what I'm doing - teaching the girls about netball... skills, strategy and so on." [Netball coach 13].

Within this theme, coaches described the need to foster sports-related development, promote the development of life skills, and to create a positive environment for their athletes. Sport-specific development was the focal point for many coaches, with a particular focus on teaching athletes skills, tactical/strategic awareness, and preparedness relevant to their sport. Another predominant topic discussed by coaches was their efforts to try to teach life skills through sport. The most frequently discussed life skills were accountability, confidence, respect, and social skills. Many considered generating a positive team environment to be an important aspect of their role as a coach. In particular, coaches identified the need to create an environment that was fun, friendly, and supportive.

Other coaches perceived their role to be that of a facilitator, which was described by coaches as someone who organises aspects of OYS (e.g., plan training sessions, set line ups, ensure equal playing time), or as a disciplinarian, which was described as someone who is strict and resolves conflicts amongst athletes. Perceived roles as a facilitator or disciplinarian, however, were not as common as the previously mentioned perceived roles.

Coaches' perceptions of themselves as role models for PA

When asked, most coaches thought of themselves as a role model for PA, but many had not considered it before.

"I suppose I haven't thought about it before now... But, I think it's [being a role model] a given, you know, it's just an understanding you have, that if you're coaching and you're still playing they'll look up to you." [Soccer coach 5].

Other coaches cited their participation at training, their current involvement in the sport (as an athlete in a team), a physically active lifestyle, and their age and longevity in the sport as reasons for perceiving themselves as role models for PA for their athletes.

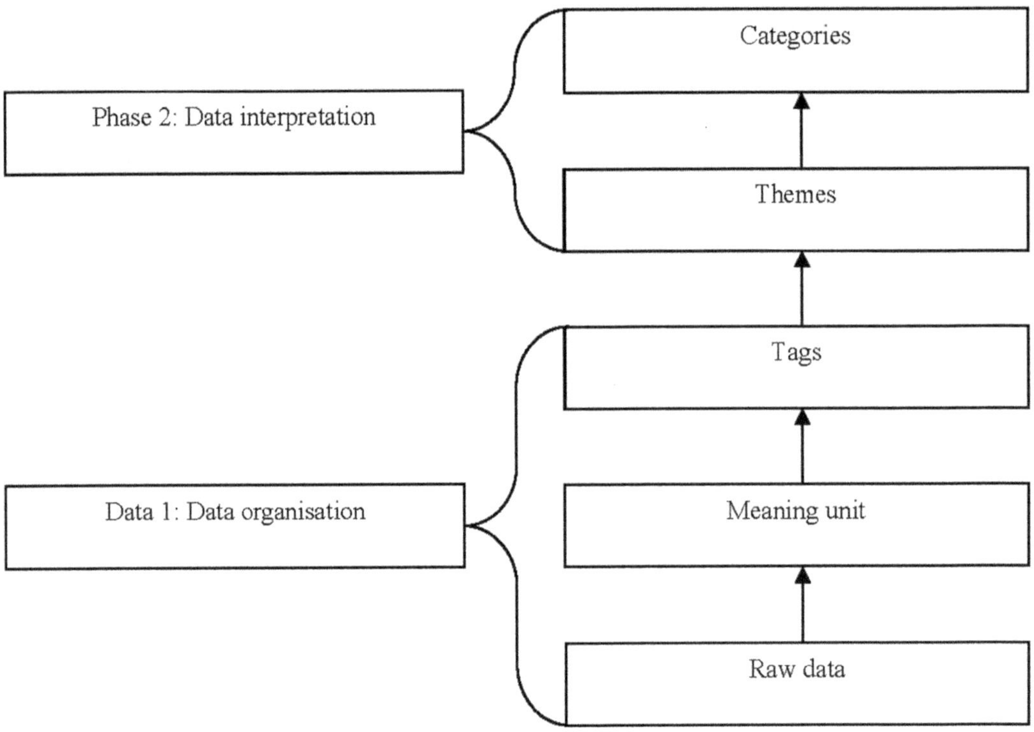

Figure 1. Data analysis process.

While most coaches considered themselves role models for PA, the view was not shared by all coaches. Poor fitness levels, old age, injury or health problems, and retirement from organised sports were the most common reasons for coaches not perceiving themselves as role models. Although some coaches did not perceive themselves as particularly good role models for the

Table 3. Perceived role as coaches: summary of categories, themes, sub-themes, and example quotes.

Category	Themes	Sub-themes	Example quotes
Perceived role as a coach	Teacher	To foster sports-related development	"My main role is to teach them how to be better soccer players. I focus on developing their soccer skills, preparing them for games and keeping them focused" [SC 6].
		To foster the development of other life skills	"For the girls, I would hope I'm seen as kind of like a life coach. I try focus on teaching them things they can learn through sport that can be used later in life like I tell them if you lose a ball, you have to make sure you get back and try to win it back because you are not helping the team if you don't – that's being accountable" [SC 3].
		To create positive environment	"…I'm a bit of a joker at times and I try to keep the atmosphere as light, fun, and friendly as possible and I think I have a pretty good rapport with the kids" [NC 15].
	Role Model		"I see myself as a role model for the girls… I'm only a little bit older than the girls on my team and I want them to know that I don't care if other people judge me because I play sport and if they say things like 'oh it's not girly to be running around playing sport getting sweaty'. I want to show them that it's just sports, I do it, and everyone should be doing it, really. [NC 17].
	Mentor		"I'm more of a mentor, someone who's guiding them to achieve the goals that they want and helping them develop the skills that they need to achieve those goals" [SC 10].
	Facilitator		"I organise their training sessions once a week, prepare them for the game… make sure they are ready to go, that they know what we're doing, adjusting positions, making sure everyone has equal court time… and I take care of all the paperwork."[NC 16].
	Disciplinarian		"A lot of people will tell you I'm a meanie (laughs). So, I suppose I'm a disciplinarian because I'm strict." [BC 20].

SC = soccer coach; NC = netball coach; BC = basketball coach.

Table 4. Coaches' perceptions of themselves as role models for physical activity: summary of categories, themes, sub-themes, and example quotes.

Category	Themes	Sub-themes	Example quotes
Coaches' self-perceptions as role models for athletes	Positive self-perception as a role model for physical activity		"They see me play on Monday nights in the men's comp and I train with them all the time, running around; so hopefully they see me as a role model both for basketball skills as well as the fitness aspect of it." [BC 25].
			"I've never really thought about it, but yeah, I haven't not played sport (laughs)... and most of the kids that I coach know that I've played at a pretty high level too. So I'd consider myself a pretty good role model." [BC 20].
			"I do because this is my lifestyle. I find it odd that people aren't physically active, you know (laughs). I'm a PE teacher, I coach, play, umpire, I'm in an old ladies representative team as well, so you know, it's just what I am about and hopefully some of that rubs off." [NC 13].
			"...not only in the teams that I'm coaching but also in my general life with people around the netball courts. I'm definitely a role model to people around the netball courts in terms of longevity, how long can you do this sport? And people just sort of respect that I think." [NC 8].
	Negative self-perception as a role model for physical activity		"...probably not in the physical activity sense – I'm a bit passed that... I'm not the fittest 50-year old I know." [NC 15].
			"Probably not, you're talking to an old bugger here." [SC 6].
			"Not since my knees have gone on me." [BC 11].
			"Oh look, probably not. I don't actually play netball anymore, I did for 15 years previously, but my physical activity has sort of taken a dip." [NC 16].

SC = soccer coach; NC = netball coach; BC = basketball coach.

reasons listed above, some recognised the importance and the opportunity they had to be role models.

> *"I see the importance of people like me being a role model for our players... the truth is you don't have to be a physically fit person to inspire others to be fit. But, role modelling is always important and there is an opportunity as coaches to be a fantastic role model." [Basketball coach 29].*

Perceived levels and importance of PA

Coaches' perceived importance related to athletes' PA during training. Coaches' perceptions relating to the importance of athlete PA during training were not universal. The majority of coaches, however, perceived PA to be important during training, with some stating that being physically active is more important to them than winning.

> *"...keeping the girls active at training is very important, it's one things I really try to do. I love seeing the girls improve their fitness, their skills... and hey, if we get some wins along the way, that's great too (laughs)." [Basketball coach 11].*

Some coaches mentioned that a physically active training session was needed to keep girls motivated and engaged. Other coaches stated that the athletes would benefit by being physically active during training because their fitness levels will allow them to outperform their opposition late in games.

Also, a few coaches discussed how they front-loaded their training sessions to include higher intensity PA at the beginning of the season and purposefully dropped the PA intensity at training as the season went on. The reason that coaches did this was because they felt girls' fitness levels were not maintained over the off-season, so the focus of training sessions at the beginning of the season was to regain girls' fitness. Once coaches felt the girls' fitness was regained, the focus of their training sessions shifted to skill development, where coaches perceived PA intensity to drop.

> *"Early in the year, fitness training was huge because the girls were pretty low in fitness, you know, they had the summer holidays and they hadn't done much. But, as we move on during the season, ball skills and controlling the ball become paramount... then it's lots of drills and getting their positions right. So the intensity at training drops a bit because we do more drills and focus less on the fitness aspect." [Soccer coach 9].*

Coaches who felt that their athletes' PA level during training was not important tended to believe that it was more important to focus on teaching sport-related skills and skill development. These coaches were willing to sacrifice PA intensity to achieve this.

Perceived levels of PA. Most coaches felt that they were conscious of their athletes' PA levels and that they were able to gauge how active the girls were at training. Furthermore, the majority of coaches considered high intensity PA to be inherent in OYS.

> *"I'm always on them about different things, trying to keep the intensity up... and as a coach you can gauge how the team is training ... so, if the group is down then I can quickly gauge that the intensity is down and I'll try to pick it up." [Basketball coach 20].*
> *"...I try to keep the girls moving and high intensity activity is natural in soccer." [Soccer coach 1].*

Training session preparation. Coaches' training preparation responses were highly variable, ranging from developing a meticulously written training plan to no planning at all. In this sample of coaches, very few coaches actually wrote down their

Table 5. Coaches' perceived levels and importance of physical activity: summary of categories, themes, sub-themes, and example quotes.

Category	Themes	Sub-themes	Example quotes
Coaches' perceived levels and importance of physical activity	Athlete physical activity during training is important		"Yeah because if they get too many drink breaks they shut off, they're not motivated, they're not active, and they talk. Then the training session just drags out and doesn't become a good training session." [SC 24].
			"The more you keep them active at training the easier it'll be coping in game situations when they're under pressure in the final quarter because they'll have that fitness. So, you know, it's really really important for them, far more than the club player who may only play a quarter or two." [NC 23].
			"…at the beginning of the season they're a lot more active and we do a lot more running than they would later in the season later." [SC 6].
	Athlete physical activity during training is not important		"I'd rather they be focused and lazy than running around not listening at all. I think that's more important… I've got to get across what we're trying to do – the skills and how we'll implement that in a game." [NC 16].
	Training planning		"I wing it. I've been coaching for so many years I just make it up as I go." [NC 14].
			"I write down what I want at the beginning of the year, but no, I don't write a formalised plan for each session it's more of a general idea." [BC 11].
			"….the less committed the team is the less time I put into making a training session." [BC 27].
	Athlete physical activity outside of orgnanised youth sport is important		"…anything they can do outside netball is only going to improve performance and make things easier during netball. So, that is important to me but I can't demand it and I don't initiate conversations about be active outside netball." [NC 23].
			"Nowadays what we do as coaches is not enough because the kids aren't doing anything outside of the sports they play." [BC 21].
			"For rep players it's important." [BC 22].
			"If you want to play at an elite level, one 2-hour training session a week is not going to get you there." [BC 19].
	Athlete physical activity outside of orgnanised youth sport is not important		"I believe that people should be active, especially kids, during and outside of sports. But, with the team that I'm coaching now, if I could get them all to training and get them to come to the game, that's two activity sessions a week and I'd be satisfied with that. If I was coaching a rep team, I'd expect them to do more than that." [NC 8].

SC = soccer coach; NC = netball coach; BC = basketball coach.

plan for training, with many claiming that they just mentally prepare for their training sessions.

> *"I usually just plan in my head on my way to training, so it's mentally written down… so, there is the warm up that I want to do, there are certain drills I want to do and there is a cool down…." [Netball coach 12].*

Some coaches discussed having general or thematic (e.g., shooting drills, passing drills) training session plans in mind rather

Table 6. Coaches' perceptions on improving athlete physical activity: summary of categories, themes, sub-themes, and example quotes.

Category	Themes	Sub-themes	Example quotes
Coaches' perceptions on improving athlete physical activity	Perceives a need to increase athlete physical activity during training		"…there probably is a need to increase activity, but it might be hard to convince the girls." [NC 17]
	Does not perceive a need to increase athlete physical activity during training		"No there's no need, I'm fairly happy with where we're at. I've been doing this for a while." [BC 19].
	Methods to increase physical activity during training	Coach-specific methods	"Make sure that you're prepared and organised and that you set out a specific training schedule so that there isn't any down time." [BC 21].
			"focus more on constant running or movement and less standing time, less watching, less waiting, and less listening to instructions from myself…." [BC 30].
		Drill modification	"…using modified drills. So, smaller groups and lots of equipment so they're really just keep chugging through." [NC 13].
	Perceived responsibility to influence physical activity outside of organised youth sports		"No, I don't think I'm responsible for the girls outside of the sport… I don't have that much of an influence outside of soccer." [SC 4].
			"With the rep players we encourage them to do things outside of netball but not with the club players." [NC 23].
			"I don't feel a responsibility, but I'll use the word opportunity again, I think there's a huge opportunity as a coach." [BC 29].
	Coach has the ability to impact health behaviours		"…I think I can because coaches I've had have had an impact on me and my sisters as well, I think I can…." [NC 7].
	Coach does not have the ability to impact health behaviours		"We [as coaches] only see the kids twice a week, once at training and once at the game, so I think parental influence is far outweighing anything I can do as a coach." [NC 15].
			"…because I only see them for probably 2 hours a week I think other influences like parents, schools, and even friends would play a much larger role in influencing their physical activity." [NC 16].

SC = soccer coach; NC = netball coach; BC = basketball coach.

than including specific drills, claiming that they are experienced enough to come up with specific drills on-the-spot. Some even claimed that they would just "wing it" during their training sessions, relying on their coaching experience to develop a session as-they-go. Some coaches with multiple teams admitted that they spent less time preparing training sessions for their less competitive teams. The majority of coaches said that their focus at training was based on observed weaknesses from the previous game.

Coaches' perceived importance related to athletes' PA outside of OYS. Athletes' PA outside of OYS was perceived as being important by most coaches. This was due to the perceived positive effect it would have on performance in OYS. Also, being physically active outside of OYS was perceived as being more important for representative athletes compared to club athletes by coaches; especially if there was a desire to play at an elite level. It appeared that coaches were content if club athletes attended their weekly training session and game, but for representative athletes the expectation to be physically active went beyond weekly training and games; these athletes were expected to be physically active in some way outside of OYS.

Some coaches reflected on changes in norms from their childhood where playing outside was regarded as a norm, compared to now where coaches perceive children to be doing very little outside of OYS.

> *"I remember when I was a kid, you get home from school, you go down to your mate's place and play basketball, footy, soccer, whatever, or you're on your push bike… now you don't see any push bikes or anything like that. It's a completely different lifestyle than when I was a kid. [Basketball coach 21].*
>
> *"It's not like it used to be back when I was a kid, we used to play outside until it got dark every night after school. Things have changed and I think that the kids have got to do something outside of your training session to get better, I think a lot of kids today come to training and that's it for the week." [Basketball coach 29].*

Coaches' perceptions on improving athlete PA

Perceived need to increase athlete PA during training. Few coaches perceived the need to increase PA because they were content with the level of PA during their training

Table 7. Coaches' perceived challenges: summary of categories, themes, sub-themes, and example quotes.

Category	Themes	Sub-themes	Example quotes
Coaches' perceived challenges	Coaches' perceived personal challenges	Time commitment to coaching	"There's a high level of commitment required in coaching you have the campaign, training, match day, phone calls and emails to organise everyone, etcetera, etcetera. It can be pretty time consuming." [SC 4].
			"After having a whole shift at work all day and then having to organise the drills and getting them down-pat that's one barrier for me because this is my first year coaching." [SC 9].
		Weak in some coaching aspect	"I'm good at the coaching and the motivating and leadership skills; but the technical skills is not my expertise, you know, I haven't really played a lot of soccer." [SC 5].
			" One of my weaknesses is getting kids focused when they need to be focused. When I was a younger coach, kids were having fun but they weren't actually getting better because there would be no focus at training." [BC 27].
			"I'm coaching the kids based on my own experiences, you know, I haven't had any formal training so, that's a big barrier for me." [SC 28].
		Work commitments	"I'm really really busy with work and I really try hard just to find the time to put the effort into being with the girls but often I have to get someone else to run training because I can't make it." [SC 10].
	Coaches' perceived challenges relating to their athletes	Athletes' variability in skill/experience	"I suppose one of the big barriers I have with the 11's is that there is such a wide array of skill and experience. So, I have some girls that are really, really advanced and you have some that aren't, like I've got two girls playing their first year of netball. So, it's hard trying to catch them up as well as making the ones who want to advance not bored." [NC 12].
		Athletes' lack of interest/focus	"…they do chatter a lot and that can be a problem sometimes, to keep them interested and keep them focused on what they're meant to doing." [SC 10].
		Athletes' lack of motivation/commitment	"…lack of motivation is a barrier sometimes. Sometimes the girls probably don't take it as seriously as they should and some girls just see training as a social thing; which it definitely can be. But, it's important that they make an effort to train hard otherwise why bother coming?" [BC 30].
		Athlete management	"Sometimes the girls don't listen to what I tell them to do, like if I tell them to do warm up laps they'll complain and it becomes a negotiation, which wastes time." [NC 17].
			"There's always one or two in most teams where you'll find a personality where you've got to work really hard to work out where they're coming from or what their problem is without having them blow up or getting upset or whatever. It's definitely an obstacle – one that you don't need." [NC 23].
			"I've got one girl who hasn't spoken all year and one who is deaf so, she can't get instructions from me. With those girls in particular, it's been very difficult for me." [SC 5].
	Coaches' perceived challenges relating to their athletes' parents	Managing parental expectations/perceptions	"…dealing with the parents is a big one… playing time; expectations on the teams' performance; their opinions on where I should be playing their daughter; parents who are yelling at refs, opposing parents, players… you name it." [SC 3].
		Parental commitment	"The main barrier is getting the children to training. That's the main barrier. All the children like to play and as a general rule you'll get the children there on a Saturday to play, but the lack of commitment by the parents to get their kids to training is huge" [NC 8].
	Coaches' perceived challenges relating to promoting physical activity.		"There's just not enough time to do anything besides basketball. We only have two sessions a week for two hours." [BC 21].

SC = soccer coach; NC = netball coach; BC = basketball coach.

sessions. Some coaches, however, reported having to reduce the intensity of their training sessions because of the girls' disinclination to train at a high intensity.

> *"...the girls were just not keen to put the effort into the training sessions that I was running.... I've had to re-adjust my focus and my expectations for the girls and I'm happy where we sit now with the level of activity" [Soccer coach 2].*

A major concern raised by coaches was a fear of athlete dropout if the PA intensity during training in OYS was too high.

> *"You can't push some of these girls too much, because they'll quit. You can try to be motivational to get them to be more active, but you can't force them, you know." [Basketball coach 22].*
>
> *"...there's a lack of fitness in probably two-thirds of the side and there's a reluctance to put the effort in.... So, if I were to step up the intensity, there would be more of a dropout rate. A lot of the girls fake injury to sit out as it is." [Soccer coach 4].*
>
> *"...they would revolt [if the coach tried to increase PA]. They would just go 'no, I'm not doing it' or they wouldn't come to training. So, you've really got to gauge how far you can push them. [Netball coach 15].*

One coach, however, emphasised the need to take advantage of the time spent in OYS because she has noticed that the girls who she coaches are less active and has noticed changes in body shape and their physical ability.

> *"...compared to 10 years ago, the girls I coach are generally less active, and I've noticed that they don't have the same gross motor skills as they would've had 10 years ago. I definitely see a change in body shape and physical ability. So, I think we need to take advantage of the time kids are at basketball because for some, this is all the activity they get in a week." [Basketball coach 21].*

Methods to increase PA during training. Although most coaches did not feel the need to increase PA during their training sessions, they were, however, able to identify ways to increase training session PA if they needed to. Coaches suggested improving their organisation, increasing preparation for training, developing more specific training plans, and reducing waiting (i.e., in lines during drills or during drill tranisition) and instruction time. They also suggested modifying drills to include smaller groups and having more equipment available.

Perceived responsibility to influence PA outside of OYS. Although most coaches felt that their athletes should be physically active outside of OYS, very few felt it was their responsibility to influence PA outside of OYS. Coaches felt that they had very little influence over their athletes' PA behaviours outside of OYS, most commonly citing parents as more influential in this respect. Peers were also considered by coaches to have a greater influence on PA levels outside of OYS than they did.

The comparison between representative athletes and club athletes emerged once again while discussing coaches' perceived responsibility to influence PA outside of OYS. Some coaches thought it was more likely that they could encourage representative athletes to train in their free time outside of OYS as opposed to club athletes; however, this was seldomly discussed.

Although not feeling a responsibility to influence PA outside of OYS, some acknowledged that coaches in OYS have a substantial opportunity to do so. See Table 6 for supporting quotes.

Coaches' perceived ability to impact health behaviours. When coaches were asked if they felt they had the ability to impact girls' health behaviours, coaches took a very pragmatic approach. Some coaches stated they have had coaches that have had a lasting impact on them, so it was plausible that they could have a lasting impact on their athletes. There were no identifible charateristics that were apparent among coaches with differing opinions of their perceived ability to impact girls' health behaviours (i.e., sport coached, coach's gender, coaching experience).

Interestingly, PA was rarely discussed as a health behaviour when identifying whether coaches thought they could impact their athletes' health behaviours or not. Often the conversation shifted from the designed focus on PA to coaches discussing their attempts to inform their athletes about healthy eating.

> *"I try to encourage healthier eating, like I had one girl that used to eat a meat pie before a game, so I tried to get her in the habit of eating the correct foods before games. That's one area where I think I can leave an impression.... what they eat and how they prepare is important and I think I can help with that." [Netball coach 18].*

Most coaches, though, perceived their ability to impact girls' health behaviours was limited. Insufficient exposure and influence were the main reasons that coaches could not impact girls' health behaviours. Again, parents, teachers, and peers were considered to have a greater influence on girls' health behaviours.

Coaches' challenges in OYS

Coaches' perceived personal challenges relating to OYS. Few coaches felt they had any personal challenges while coaching in OYS. The perceived time needed to commit to OYS was, however, the main issue identified by coaches who did report having personal challenges. The time needed for administrative tasks as well as preparing for training were the two biggest time consumers, with the latter particularly affecting less experienced coaches. Some coaches discussed an over-commitment to their sport; this included coaching and refereeing multiple teams and games, respectively.

> *"Maybe an over-commitment to basketball... I can only be in one place at one time and sometimes it clashes with training. It takes a toll on you, some nights I'm coaching non-stop." [Basketball coach 20].*
>
> *"...Friday nights I'm here coaching three teams and reffing two, so it's just bang-bang-bang five games in a row." [Basketball coach 25].*

Some coaches felt that they were weak in some aspects of coaching, which they perceived as a limitation in their coaching ability. Perceived coaching weaknesses included poor sport-specific technical skills, difficulty keeping athletes focused on the task at hand, and lack of formal training. Work commitments also emerged as an issue faced by coaches occasionally, but were not commonly discussed.

Coaches' perceived challenges relating to their athletes. A predominant challenge coaches discussed was the wide variation in athletes' skill levels and experience within a team.

Some coaches described the dilemma of trying to find the right balance at training, where the skilled/experienced athletes feel engaged without leaving the less skilled/experienced athletes to fall further behind.

Girls' focus and interest levels posed problems for coaches as well, with the main reported obstacle being that girls talk too much during training. Some coaches described training as a "social gathering" and felt that girls' motivation and commitment was lacking. As a negotiation with the girls, some coaches have implemented "talk time" where they are allowed to talk at certain points of the training session, in an effort to minimise conversations that are not sports-related.

> *"I've had to implement, what I call, 'talk time' to keep the conversations to a minimum during training... see a lot of them went to primary school together and they're at different high schools. So, it's like a reunion every Wednesday night." [Soccer coach 9].*

Athlete management was another theme that emerged as an athlete-related challenge, which related to non-compliance with coach instructions, difficult athletes, and athletes with disabilities. See Table 7. for supporting quotes.

Coaches' perceived challenges relating to their athletes' parents. All coaches, at one point or another, experienced some sort of issue relating to their athletes' parents during their years coaching OYS. Athletes' playing time was one of the most common complaints from parents. Parental commitment to OYS was cited as a major issue for coaches as well, with the main perceived issue being parents' unreliability when it came to getting their daughters to training.

Also, one coach was frustrated with some parents' lack of interest in the sport that their daughter was playing and felt that the lack of parental support could impact on further participation in OYS.

> *"It annoys me when the parents aren't quite on the same wavelength as you because I love this stuff [netball], okay, and I think most of the girls do too. So, it bothers me when parents don't take any interest in it and I'd bet there are probably kids who stop playing netball because they don't have any support from their mum or dad." [Netball coach 13].*

Another coach noticed that, as the girls on his team got older, fewer parents were attending their daughters' training and game sessions.

> *"When I started coaching them at 12... all the parents were there and now, no parents are there." [Soccer coach 1].*

Coaches' perceived challenges relating to promoting PA. Frequency and duration of training sessions were the most commonly cited challenges with regard to promoting PA. Coaches felt they had too little time at training to discuss anything outside of the sport they were coaching.

Discussion

To our knowledge, this is the first study to explore whether coaches perceive themselves as influential on PA for girls participating in OYS. More specifically, we explored coaches' perceived role as coaches, their perception of themselves as role models for PA, their views on their athletes' current PA levels, their opinions on improving their athletes' PA levels, and their perceived challenges during OYS. Our analysis of 30 in-depth semi-structured interviews suggests that most coaches feel that they have the potential to influence PA for girls in OYS. It is possible, though, that coaches may underestimate or not fully realise the impact they can have on the girls they coach in OYS.

When asked about their perceived role as a coach, a range of influential roles were discussed. The perception of being a teacher, role model, or mentor resonated with many of the coaches in this study. The fact that several influential roles resonated with coaches is a positive finding from a PA promotion standpoint, as Smith and Smoll [4] have suggested that coaches can have a strong impact on children and adolescents due to consistent direct involvement with them. Not surprisingly, coaches primarily reported that it was their responsibility to provide sport-specific development (e.g., technical skills, tactical awareness, preparedness). Coaches also reported, however, that it was part of their role to create a positive environment (e.g., fun, friendly, supportive) and to foster the development of life skills, which was also found in recent study by Vella et al. [32]. Those authors also noted that the responsibility coaches felt to develop athletes' life skills was an important extension to existing literature and our study lends support to that finding.

While some coaches had never considered it before the interview, the majority perceived themselves to be role models for PA, particularly if they were still currently involved in organised sports in some capacity (i.e., active participants during training or currently playing in a team). Although no direct comparisons are available, Drummond et al. examined student and health educators' perceptions in relation to role modelling exercise [29]. The authors found that 90% (18 out of 20) of health educators perceived themselves as role models for exercise for their students, citing their participation level as the main reason for this perception [33]. In contrast to our findings, however, nonparticipation in sports was not cited as a reason for health educators not perceiving themselves as role models for exercise in the study by Drummond et al. [33].

Most coaches stated that being physically active during OYS was important. Coaches reported that they were conscious of their athletes' PA levels and had the ability to gauge their athletes' PA levels. The presumption by many, however, was that high-intensity PA was inherent to OYS. So, it is not surprising that most coaches felt it was unnecessary for them to try to increase girls' PA levels and reduce their inactivity during training. Smith and Smoll's [4] research, however, indicates that coaches have limited awareness of their actions during OYS and state that increasing awareness is essential for change to occur. Therefore, low-cost methods, such as pedometers or direct observation systems (e.g., the System for Observing Fitness Instruction Time [34]), could be used to provide coaches with objectively measured feedback on girls' PA levels, and self-monitoring could be introduced to coaches in an effort to assist in optimising time spent in training during OYS.

An interesting theme that emerged was the concern held by coaches that girls might drop out of OYS if, for a prolonged period training, PA intensity was too high. Coaches' recognition that they could be responsible for prompting athletes' withdrawal is a positive finding. Youth athletes in other studies have ranked their coach as the most influential person in making the decision to withdraw from OYS [35], where one study found that coaches influenced nearly one-third of athletes to withdraw from OYS [36]. Of the extensive literature that exists relating to athlete dropout from OYS [37–39], as far as we are aware, high-intensity

PA is not commonly reported as a reason for withdrawal from OYS among athletes. One study sampled nearly 400 athletes and reported over 30 reasons for athlete withdrawal from OYS and none of the athlete-reported reasons related specifically to PA intensity. This is not to say that high-intensity PA cannot influence girls' decision to withdraw from OYS. Though, as far as we are aware, coaches' perception that girls may withdraw from OYS due to high intensity PA does not appear to be in line with athlete-reported reasons for dropping out of OYS. Further exploration on this topic is warranted and should be taken into consideration in any PA promotion interventions in OYS involving girls.

Generally, coaches in this study reported spending little time preparing for training sessions. The majority of coaches said that they relied on their experience to create impromptu training sessions. Mandic and colleagues have suggested that coaches should ensure that training session drills are structured to maximise PA intensity [40]. Further supporting a structured training session, a recent study conducted in a physical education setting found a negative correlation between time spent in management (i.e., drill transition, instruction) and student MVPA [23]. Without prior preparation, there is a greater likelihood that time at training is not being used as efficiently as it can be, and PA intensity could potentially drop.

Coaches reported that they were capable of altering their training sessions to increase girls' PA, if they felt they needed to. Coaches were able to identify numerous strategies that could be employed in their training sessions to increase opportunities to be active, reduce inactivity, and improve their efficiency and management of training. Many of the strategies that coaches identified have also been recommended within a physical education setting; and included: using smaller groups, providing more equipment, reducing waiting, and reducing instruction time to increase girls' opportunities to be physically active [41,42]. However, coaches' awareness of these strategies may not necessarily mean they will employ them because knowledge can be a poor predictor of behaviour [43]; especially if coaches' perception of girls' PA during training is already considered adequate. Approaches are needed, then, to ensure that coaches are not only aware of strategies to increase opportunities to be active (and reduce inactivity), but also have the belief that as a result of implementing these strategies it can lead to positive outcomes (e.g., health benefits) [43].

Most coaches stated that being physically active during OYS was important, however, rarely discussed the health benefits associated with being physically active. Coaches in this study felt confident discussing the sport they coached, but may lack confidence discussing the more general health benefits associated with PA. Coaches' perceived ability to impact girls' health behaviours was also discussed, and few coaches felt that they could have an impact on the health behaviours of the girls they coached. This belief may represent a missed opportunity for coaches to make a meaningful impact on girls' health behaviours as girls can learn behaviours from their coaches, particularly if the girls admire their coach [44]. Coaches did not feel that they were able to impact their girls' health behaviours, and two of the main reasons for this were a perceived lack of influence and limited exposure to their athletes. However, Smith and Smoll [4] suggest the contrary, coaches can greatly impact their athletes. Interestingly, PA was rarely mentioned as a health behaviour that coaches felt they could impact, rather healthy eating was commonly discussed instead. This may be due to coaches' perception that PA is inherent to OYS.

Outside of OYS, coaches discussed changes in norms from their childhood where unstructured leisure-time PA was regarded as a norm. They also perceived there to be a decline in PA amongst children and adolescents, however, very few coaches felt responsible for influencing girls to be physically active outside of OYS. Even though most coaches perceived their role to be one that could be influential to their athletes in OYS, it appears many of them do not perceive their influence to extend outside of OYS. Coaches suggested that parents and peers had a greater influence on PA outside of OYS than coaches did. There is ample evidence to support coaches' claims that parents and peers are influential in supporting children to be physically active [45–47]; however, one study found that physical education teachers were as influential as parents in supporting adolescents' PA outside of school [48]. While this is not a direct comparison, it is possible that OYS coaches can also greatly influence girls' PA outside of OYS and coaches are underestimating the impact they can have.

The most commonly perceived personal challenge experienced by coaches was the amount of time they felt they needed to commit to OYS. Administrative tasks and preparing for training were considered the two biggest perceived consumers of coaches' time. Many coaches, however, stated that they relied on their experience to plan training sessions somewhat spontaneously. Coaches also identified a number of challenges relating to coaching their athletes. The predominant issue was the amount of variation in skill level and experience within their teams. Some coaches found it difficult to keep the skilled/experienced girls engaged during training without having the less skilled/experienced girls falling further behind, likely increasing the amount of instruction needed. These findings could potentially result in training sessions that do not maximise athletes' opportunities to be physically active. These are important findings as previous literature has shown that for the majority of time during OYS athletes are inactive or in light PA [12,13,21,22]. Furthermore, Dudley et al. [23] found negative correlations between instruction/management and MVPA. This valuable insight could inform future studies aiming to increase PA in OYS.

Coaches also reported girls' focus/interest levels, motivation/commitment, and athlete management as challenges. Although coaches identified these as challenges, they seemed confident in their ability to deal with them, often detailing how they overcome them.

When coaches discussed their perceived challenges in relation to parents, an interesting finding from a PA promotion perspective was that some coaches believed that they were able to identify girls on their teams who had low parental support. Coaches reported being frustrated with some parents' lack of commitment and support for their daughters. A coach commented on how annoyed she was with parents who did not take any interest in the sport their daughter played, and suggested that girls with a lack of parental support are likely to stop playing OYS. This is an encouraging finding as there is strong evidence to suggest that parental support is linked with children's PA behaviours [49–52] and children's participation in OYS [53,54]. Furthermore, Lubans, Sylva, and Morgan [55] found that in older adolescents, parental support was significantly correlated with MVPA; however, one coach commented on his observation that parents' presence during OYS has decreased as the girls he coached got older. Given that girls' PA levels tend to decrease sharply in adolescence [17,19], maintaining parental support may be an important factor to consider in efforts to increase and maintain PA levels in girls as they transition into adolescence and adulthood. As coaches in this study were able to identify athletes lacking this much-needed parental support, coaches may be able to play an important role maintaining parental support and should be examined further.

Some potential limitations should be considered when interpreting these findings. Firstly, it is possible that coaches offered socially desirable viewpoints during their interview. Secondly, a convenience sample was used, possibly introducing an element of selection bias. That said, a wide array of responses from a diverse sample of coaches was collected. Lastly, female-coaching perspectives may be underrepresented as our sample contained more men than women; however, male coaches are more prevalent than female coaches in OYS [56]. Despite these limitations, the present study provides unique insight into coaches' perceptions of themselves as being influential on PA for girls in OYS. Also, rigorous research methodology was employed to ensure the trustworthiness of the data. We used several strategies [57] to strengthen the credibility of our data, for example, investigator triangulation during the interpretation phase, individual classification during data analysis, reflexivity, and member checking. Along with aiding in the credibility of the data, the above-mentioned strategies also protected against individual perceptual biases [58]. According to Lincoln and Guba [59], demonstrating credibility may be considered sufficient to support the notion of dependability. Further, we have established acceptable confirmability by using published guidelines to analyse our data [29,31] and, as mentioned above, employed strategies to reduce individual perceptual biases. Lastly, concerning transferability, Lincoln and Guba [59] suggested that transferability is primarily the responsibility of the researcher interested in transferring the findings to another context or population than that of the original study. Lincoln and Guba [59] also state that so long as the original study presents sufficient descriptive data to allow comparisons the issue of transferability has been adequately addressed. The current study provided a thorough description of the research context and adequate descriptive data allowing other researchers to make judgement on how practical a transfer of the results are to a different context or population.

Considering the high proportion of children that participate in OYS, and the myriad of health and developmental benefits associated with the setting, OYS has the potential to be a powerful health-promoting environment for children and adolescents. Recently a number of studies have examined OYS clubs as a setting to promote health [9,10,60]. These studies illustrate a wide range of health-promoting capabilities OYS can provide and the importance of OYS clubs. However, only one study recognised that OYS clubs can play a role in promoting PA [60]. Our study provides a unique perspective on OYS coaches' perceptions of themselves as being influential on PA for girls in OYS. Further, coaches in this study (whilst not the primary focus) indicated that they were confident discussing healthy eating with the girls on their team. They may, however, underestimate or not fully realise the impact they can have. To further enhance the health-promoting capabilities of OYS, there should also be an emphasis placed on educating coaches to capitalise on the opportunity they have to promote PA to the girls they coach. This information on OYS can be used as a platform on which to inform policies, programs, and interventions to develop strategies to increase girls' PA levels through OYS.

Acknowledgments

We would like to thank the coaches for their participation in this study and Dr. Rebecca Olson for her constructive criticism of our research methodology.

Author Contributions

Conceived and designed the experiments: JMG RRR GSK CL. Performed the experiments: JMG. Analyzed the data: JMG CL RRR GSK ESG. Contributed to the writing of the manuscript: JMG CL RRR GSK ESG.

References

1. Janssen I (2014) Active play: An important physical activity strategy in the fight against childhood obesity. Canadian Journal of Public Health 105: e22–e27.
2. Smoll FL, Smith RE (2002) Children and youth in sport: A biopsychosocial perspective (2nd ed.). Dubuque, IA: Kendall-Hunt.
3. Conroy DE, Coatsworth JD (2006) Coach training as a strategy for promoting youth social development. The Sport Psychologist 20: 128–144.
4. Smith RE, Smoll FL (1997) Coaching the coaches: Youth sports as a scientific and applied behavioral setting. Current Directions in Psychological Science 6: 16–21.
5. Tremblay MS, Gray CE, Akinroye K, Harrington DM, Katzmarzyk PT, et al. (2014) Physical activity of children: A global matrix of grades comparing 15 countries. Journal of Physical Activity and Health 11: S113–S125.
6. Active Healthy Kids Australia (2014) Is sport enough? The 2014 Australian report card on physical activity for children and young people. Adelaide, South Australia: Active Healthy Kids Australia. 1–49 p.
7. Australian Bureau of Statistics (2012) Children's participation in sport and leisure time activities, 2003 to 2012. Catalogue No. 4901.0. Canberra: Australian Bureau of Statistics; 2012.
8. Fraser-Thomas J, Côté J, Deakin J (2005) Youth sport programs: An avenue to foster positive youth development. Physical Education & Sport Pedagogy 10: 19–40.
9. Geidne S, Quennerstedt M, Eriksson C (2013) The youth sports club as a health-promoting setting: An integrative review of research. Scandinavian Journal of Public Health 41: 269–283.
10. Kokko S, Kannas L, Villberg J (2009) Health promotion profile of youth sports clubs in Finland: club officials' and coaches' perceptions. Health Promotion International 24: 26–35.
11. Strong WB, Malina RM, Blimkie CJ, Daniels SR, Dishman RK, et al. (2005) Evidence based physical activity for school-age youth. The Journal of Pediatrics 146: 732–737.
12. Guagliano JM, Rosenkranz RR, Kolt GS (2013) Girls' physical activity levels during organized sports in Australia. Medicine & Science in Sports & Exercise 45: 116–122.
13. Wickel EE, Eisenmann JC (2007) Contribution of youth sport to total daily physical activity among 6-to 12-yr-old boys. Medicine & Science in Sports & Exercise 39: 1493–1500.
14. World Health Organization (2010) Global recommendations on physical activity for health.
15. Department of Health and Aging (2014) Australia's physical activity & sedentary behaviour guidelines for children (18–64 years). Canberra: Commonwealth of Australia.
16. Department of Health and Aging (2014) Australia's physical activity & sedentary behaviour guidelines for young people (13–17 years). Canberra: Commonwealth of Australia.
17. Troiano RP, Berrigan D, Dodd KW, Mâsse LC, Tilert T, et al. (2008) Physical activity in the United States measured by accelerometer. Medicine and Science in Sports and Exercise 40: 181–188.
18. Hardy LL, Okely AD, Dobbins TA, Booth ML (2008) Physical activity among adolescents in New South Wales (Australia): 1997 and 2004. Medicine & Science in Sports & Exercise 40: 835–841.
19. Kimm SY, Glynn NW, Kriska AM, Barton BA, Kronsberg SS, et al. (2002) Decline in physical activity in black girls and white girls during adolescence. New England Journal of Medicine 347: 709–715.
20. Camacho-Miñano MJ, LaVoi NM, Barr-Anderson DJ (2011) Interventions to promote physical activity among young and adolescent girls: A systematic review. Health Education Research 26: 1025–1049.
21. Leek D, Carlson JA, Cain KL, Henrichon S, Rosenberg D, et al. (2011) Physical activity during youth sports practices. Archives of Pediatrics & Adolescent Medicine 165: 294–299.
22. Sacheck JM, Nelson T, Ficker L, Kafka T, Kuder J, et al. (2011) Physical activity during soccer and its contribution to physical activity recommendations in normal weight and overweight children. Pediatric Exercise Science 23: 281–292.
23. Dudley DA, Okely AD, Cotton WG, Pearson P, Caputi P (2012) Physical activity levels and movement skill instruction in secondary school physical education. Journal of Science and Medicine in Sport 15: 231–237.
24. Tong A, Sainsbury P, Craig J (2007) Consolidated criteria for reporting qualitative research (COREQ): A 32-item checklist for interviews and focus groups. International Journal for Quality in Health Care 19: 349–357.
25. Bryman A (2012) Social research methods. New York, NY: OUP Oxford.
26. Creswell JW (2012) Qualitative inquiry and research design: Choosing among five approaches. Thousand Oaks, CA: Sage Publications, Inc.

27. Boeije HR (2009) Analysis in qualitative research. Thousand Oaks, CA: Sage Publications Limited.
28. Australian Bureau of Statistics (2009) Children's participation in organised sport and dancing.
29. Côté J, Salmela JH, Baria A, Russell SJ (1993) Organizing and interpreting unstructured qualitative data. The Sport Psychologist 7: 127–137.
30. Tesch R (1990) Qualitative research: Analysis types and software tools. Philadelphia, PA: RoutledgeFlamer, Taylor & Francis Inc.
31. Côté J, Salmela JH (1994) A decision-making heuristic for the analysis of unstructured qualitative data. Perceptual and Motor Skills 78: 465–466.
32. Vella SA, Oades L, Crowe T (2011) The role of the coach in facilitating positive youth development: Moving from theory to practice. Journal of Applied Sport Psychology 23: 33–48.
33. Drummond JL, McGuire JG, Bennett G (2002) Student perceptions of exercise role modelling by secondary health educators. Health Education Journal 61: 78–86.
34. McKenzie TL, Sallis JF, Nader PR (1991) SOFIT: System for observing fitness instruction time. Journal of Teaching in Physical Education 11: 195–205.
35. Rottensteiner C, Laakso L, Pihlaja T, Konttinen N (2013) Personal Reasons for Withdrawal from Team Sports and the Influence of Significant Others among Youth Athletes. International Journal of Sports Science and Coaching 8: 19–32.
36. Armentrout S, Kamphoff C (2011) Organizational barriers and factors that contribute to youth hockey attrition. Journal of Sport Behavior 34: 121–136.
37. Hedstrom R, Gould D (2004) Research in youth sports: Critical issues status. White Paper Summaries of Existing Literature.
38. Fraser-Thomas J, Côté J, Deakin J (2008) Understanding dropout and prolonged engagement in adolescent competitive sport. Psychology of Sport and Exercise 9: 645–662.
39. Fraser-Thomas J, Côté J (2006) Youth sports: Implementing findings and moving forward with research. Athletic Insight 8: 12–27.
40. Mandic S, Bengoechea EG, Stevens E, de la Barra SL, Skidmore P (2012) Getting kids active by participating in sport and doing It more often: focusing on what matters. International Journal of Behavioral Nutrition and Physical Activity 9: 86.
41. Rink J, Hall TJ, Williams LH (2010) Schoolwide physical activity: A comprehensive guide to designing and conducting programs. Champaign, IL: Human Kinetics.
42. Kelder SH, Mitchell PD, McKenzie TL, Derby C, Strikmiller PK, et al. (2003) Long-term implementation of the CATCH physical education program. Health Education & Behavior 30: 463–475.
43. Ajzen I, Joyce N, Sheikh S, Cote NG (2011) Knowledge and the prediction of behavior: The role of information accuracy in the theory of planned behavior. Basic and Applied Social Psychology 33: 101–117.
44. Blomquist KB (1986) Modeling and health behavior: Strategies for prevention in the schools. Health Education 17: 8–11.
45. Fitzgerald A, Fitzgerald N, Aherne C (2012) Do peers matter? A review of peer and/or friends' influence on physical activity among American adolescents. Journal of Adolescence 35: 941–958.
46. Trost SG, Sallis JF, Pate RR, Freedson PS, Taylor WC, et al. (2003) Evaluating a model of parental influence on youth physical activity. American Journal of Preventive Medicine 25: 277–282.
47. Cox M, Schofield G, Kolt GS (2010) Responsibility for children's physical activity: Parental, child, and teacher perspectives. Journal of Science and Medicine in Sport 13: 46–52.
48. McDavid L, Cox AE, Amorose AJ (2012) The relative roles of physical education teachers and parents in adolescents' leisure-time physical activity motivation and behavior. Psychology of Sport and Exercise 13: 99–107.
49. Bélanger M, Casey M, Cormier M, Filion AL, Martin G, et al. (2011) Maintenance and decline of physical activity during adolescence: Insights from a qualitative study. International Journal of Behavioral Nutrition and Physical Activity 8: 117.
50. Bradley R, McRitchie S, Houts R, Nader P, O'Brien M (2011) Parenting and the decline of physical activity from age 9 to 15. International Journal of Behavioral Nutrition and Physical Activity 8: 33.
51. Sallis JF, Prochaska JJ, Taylor WC (2000) A review of correlates of physical activity of children and adolescents. Medicine and science in sports and exercise 32: 963–975.
52. Bauer KW, Nelson MC, Boutelle KN, Neumark-Sztainer D (2008) Parental influences on adolescents' physical activity and sedentary behavior: longitudinal findings from Project EAT-II. International Journal of Behavioral Nutrition and Physical Activity 5: 12.
53. Eime RM, Harvey JT, Craike MJ, Symons CM, Payne WR (2013) Family support and ease of access link socio-economic status and sports club membership in adolescent girls: a mediation study. International Journal of Behavioral Nutrition & Physical Activity 10: 50.
54. Timperio A, van Stralen M, Brug J, Bere E, Chinapaw M, et al. (2013) Direct and indirect associations between the family physical activity environment and sports participation among 10–12 year-old European children: testing the EnRG framework in the ENERGY project. Int J Behav Nutr Phys Act 10: 15.
55. Lubans DR, Sylva K, Morgan PJ (2007) Factors associated with physical activity in a sample of British secondary school students. Australian Journal of Educational & Developmental Psychology 7: 22–30.
56. Leberman S, LaVoi N (2011) Juggling balls and roles, working mother-coaches in youth sport: Beyond the dualistic worker-mother identity. Journal of Sport Management 25: 474–488.
57. Krefting L (1991) Rigor in qualitative research: The assessment of trustworthiness. The American Journal of Occupational Therapy 45: 214–222.
58. Patton MQ (2001) Qualitative research & evaluation methods. Thousand Oaks, CA: Sage Publications Inc.
59. Lincoln YS, Guba EA (1985) Naturalistic inquiry. Beverly Hills, CA: Sage.
60. Kelly B, King L, Bauman AE, Baur LA, Macniven R, et al. (2014) Identifying important and feasible policies and actions for health at community sports clubs: A consensus-generating approach. Journal of Science and Medicine in Sport 17: 61–68.

11

Effects of 12 Weeks High-Intensity & Reduced-Volume Training in Elite Athletes

Anders Kilen[1], Tanja Hultengren Larsson[1], Majke Jørgensen[1], Lars Johansen[2], Susanne Jørgensen[2], Nikolai B. Nordsborg[1]*

1 Department of Nutrition, Exercise and Sport, University of Copenhagen, Copenhagen, Denmark, **2** Team Denmark, Copenhagen, Denmark

Abstract

It was investigated if high-intensity interval training (HIT) at the expense of total training volume improves performance, maximal oxygen uptake and swimming economy. 41 elite swimmers were randomly allocated to a control (CON) or HIT group. For 12 weeks both groups trained ~12 h per week. HIT comprised ~5 h vs. 1 h and total distance was ~17 km vs. 35 km per week for HIT and CON, respectively. HIT was performed as 6-10×10-30 s maximal effort interspersed by 2–4 minutes of rest. Performance of 100 m all-out freestyle and 200 m freestyle was similar before and after the intervention in both HIT (60.4±4.0 vs. 60.3±4.0 s; n = 13 and 133.2±6.4 vs. 132.6±7.7 s; n = 14) and CON (60.2±3.7 vs. 60.6±3.8 s; n = 15 and 133.5±7.0 vs. 133.3±7.6 s; n = 15). Maximal oxygen uptake during swimming was similar before and after the intervention in both the HIT (4.0±0.9 vs. 3.8±1.0 l $O_2 \times min^{-1}$; n = 14) and CON (3.8±0.7 vs. 3.8±0.7 l $O_2 \times min^{-1}$; n = 11) group. Oxygen uptake determined at fixed submaximal speed was not significantly affected in either group by the intervention. Body fat % tended to increase ($P = 0.09$) in the HIT group (15.4±1.6% vs. 16.3±1.6%; $P = 0.09$; n = 16) and increased ($P < 0.05$) in the CON group (13.9±1.5% vs. 14.9±1.5%; n = 17). A distance reduction of 50% and a more than doubled HIT amount for 12 weeks did neither improve nor compromise performance or physiological capacity in elite swimmers.

Editor: Jeffrey M. Haddad, Purdue University, United States of America

Funding: This work was funded by Team Danmark. The funders had no role in study design, data collection and analysis, decision to publish, or preparation of the manuscript.

Competing Interests: The authors have declared that no competing interests exist.

* E-mail: nnordsborg@nexs.ku.dk

Introduction

High-intensity interval training (HIT), such as 4-6×30 s all-out exercise bouts interspersed by 3–5 minutes of rest, has proved to be a potent stimulus for muscular and cardiovascular adaptation in untrained persons [1] and athletes [2]. In untrained participants, as little as three sessions of HIT per week for 6 weeks causes a ~7% increase of maximal oxygen uptake ($VO_{2\ max}$) and reduces the respiratory exchange ratio ~0.01 at 65% of $VO_{2\ max}$ [3]. Thus, adaptations after HIT are comparable to adaptations after 40–60 minutes of cycling at 65% of VO_{2max} [3]. In highly trained cyclists, VO_{2max} has been found to improve ~6–8% after HIT [4] but also to be unaffected in other athletic populations such as recreational runners [5]. In addition, HIT can improve work efficiency ~3–6% in recreational runners and soccer players [5–7] which is of importance for performance [8]. With regards to performance, brief intense exercise capacity can be improved ~7% and time to exhaustion in a prolonged endurance exercise test can be more than doubled in untrained individuals following HIT [3,9]. In trained individuals performance of brief intense exercise, intermittent running and endurance exercise, such as a 40 km cycling time trial improves ~5–6% after HIT [2,4].

At the muscular level in untrained subjects HIT induces mitochondrial biogenesis [9], reduces lactate production [10] and increases capacity for lipid oxidation [3]. In trained subjects, skeletal muscle oxidative enzymatic potential is not always improved [5,6] but has been observed to increase after one week of HIT in elite distance runners [11]. Thus, the mechanisms responsible for performance improvements with HIT may be different in untrained and trained subjects. There is evidence that HIT leads to a reduction in plasma K^+ concentration and increased ability to work at high intensities. Reduced plasma K^+ appears to result from increased skeletal muscle Na^+, K^+ pump [5]. However, the role of K^+ in muscle fatigue is unclear [12]. If HIT improves performance either by inducing mitochondrial biogenesis or by increasing Na^+, K^+ pump expression or both, an associated physiological response can be expected. For example, reduced blood lactate concentration, reduced blood acidity and/or reduced blood K^+ concentrations during standardized exercise could be expected. However, only a very limited number of studies have investigated changes in metabolic markers in response to HIT in elite athletes [11,13] and no studies have done so when HIT has been performed for more than four weeks. Thus, it is unclear if an added amount of HIT in elite athletes at the expense of total training volume for a prolonged period causes changes in blood markers of metabolism such as pH, lactate and K^+.

Most HIT studies have investigated interventions lasting from two weeks [3] to ten weeks [2,14,15] and it is unknown if HIT at the expense of training volume continues to induce physiological and performance beneficial adaptations if the intervention period is prolonged. In addition, studied populations are either untrained [3] or elite trained without prior systematic engagement in HIT, such as recreational runners [5,6,16] or highly trained cyclists [4,13]. Thus, it also remains unanswered if a substantial increase in the amount of HIT training in an elite population that regularly perform HIT is of similar benefit as populations not previously engaged in HIT. Finally, most studies have included less than ten athletes. Thus, there is a need for studies to include a larger number of subjects in order to detect possibly small differences in outcome measures.

In the present study, performance and physiological adaptations to HIT was investigated in competitive swimmers. Swimmers were selected because HIT training has been a part of competitive swim training for decades [17], however swim training often focuses on a high distance at medium to low intensity [18]. This appears contradictory to the high anaerobic energy demand that exists during competition, where 13 of the 16 Olympic events have race times less than 130 seconds. Thus, competitive swimmers appear to be a good model to investigate if more HIT training at the expense of low intensity high-volume training induces further physiological adaptations and improves performance. A few studies have addressed the impact of HIT in swimming, but these were either performed on children [19], after a 4 months break [20] or without physiological measurements, except from blood lactate [21].

When training volume is drastically reduced in endurance athletes, total caloric intake is not necessarily adjusted accordingly [22]. Additionally, the low total exercise time spent on HIT does not allow the higher intensity to compensate for the reduced total volume in terms of total energy expenditure. Thus, added HIT at the expense of total training distance for a prolonged period of time may increase body weight and/or body fat percentage. This possibility is of obvious importance for elite athletes but has never been addressed in an elite population subjected to HIT at the expense of total training volume. In swimming, added body weight may both be detrimental to performance due to increased frontal area but could also be of benefit due to increased buoyancy.

The purpose of the present study was to investigate if an increased amount of HIT at the expense of a reduced training volume would 1) improve swimming performance; 2) improve swimming specific VO_{2max}; 3) improve swimming economy; 4) alter the metabolic response to swimming at a fixed speed and 5) induce increased body fat.

It was hypothesized that the intervention would improve performance, which could be explained by improved swimming economy and increased swimming maximal oxygen uptake and possibly be associated with reduced disturbances of lactate, pH and K^+ levels at submaximal swimming speeds. Further, it was hypothesized that the reduced training volume would result in elevated body weight due to increased body fat.

Methods

Participants

Forty-one healthy Danish national level senior elite swimmers (30 males and 11 females) were recruited for the study. Age: 20.0±2.7 years, height 179.9±6.5 cm and body mass 72.0±10.6 kg. The athletes had been training and competing on a regular basis for a minimum of 5 years, and they were swimming 8–16 hours per week with an average weekly distance of 20.000 m–60.000 m. The enrolled swimmers primarily competed in 50 m–200 m events. Two swimmers were specialized in 400 m and 800 m events. All participants were fully informed of possible risks and discomforts associated with the experimental procedures before they gave their written informed consent to participate. Written informed consent was obtained from one parent if participants were under 18 years. This study conformed to the code of Ethics of the World Medical Association (Declaration of Helsinki) and all procedures were approved by the Ethics Committee of Copenhagen and Frederiksberg communities.

Intervention Period and Training

An intervention period lasting 12 weeks was carried out in the competitive mid-season from February to May. A two-group parallel longitudinal study design was used. Subjects from four different teams were randomly assigned to either an intervention group (HIT group; n = 20, 14 males and 6 females) or control group (CON group; n = 21, 16 males and 5 females). From each team, swimmers were assigned to both HIT and CON groups. In the HIT group, regular training volume was reduced by 50% and the amount of high intensity training was more than doubled. In table 1, a simplified summary of training data is provided based on team coaches' registration and training reports from participating swimmers. In the CON group, training was continued as usual. All training sessions were supervised and logged by team coaches who had received detailed instructions by the research team. Additional dry-land training with focus on core-stability was performed for approximately 20 minutes per day and strength training with focus on upper body strength was performed for up to 2 hours per week. Participating swimmers were instructed to maintain their regular eating habits but this was not controlled.

Experimental protocols

Before (PRE) and after (POST) the HIT intervention period, participants underwent a series of physiological evaluations: body composition analyses; determination of swimming economy and swimming peak oxygen uptake in a custom built swim flume; a pool based 5×200 m freestyle swim test with increasing speeds and blood analyses. Additionally, performance was evaluated by analyses of 100 m freestyle all-out and 200 m freestyle completed in competition. Details for each procedure are given below. All subjects completed familiarization to all physiological tests six weeks before PRE-testing. The familiarization trial; PRE-trial and POST-trials followed the same time schedule so that an individual underwent testing at the same time of day on all occasions. First experimental day was always a Friday and the second experimental day was either the following Saturday or Sunday. Swimmers were instructed not to do any training on the experimental days prior to testing. Swimmers were also instructed to eat at least two hours before the first test and to keep a record of food intake. Participants received written and verbal instructions to repeat the food consumption schedule on the three test occasions. For logistic reasons, several of the enrolled swimmers did not complete the evaluations. Thus, the number of evaluated swimmers is given for each reported variable.

Laboratory analyses

On the first experimental day, body composition was determined by Dual x-ray absorptiometry (DEXA) scanning (Lunar Prodigy, GE Healthcare, UK). Subsequently, swimming economy and maximal oxygen uptake during freestyle swimming was measured in a custom built swimming flume. Pulmonary oxygen uptake and ventilation were measured breath-by-breath (Cosmed Quark b2, Milan, Italy). Swimmers completed a five minutes warm-up at submaximal speed chosen so that the swimmers reported the swim to be "easy". Subsequently, swimming economy was analyzed by completion of a six minutes continuous swim at the same speed as during warm-up. Based on the pre-test results, the speed was selected to represent ~60% of $VO_{2\ max}$. After three minutes of rest, a progressive test to exhaustion was

Table 1. Training intensity and volume.

	Total volume and hours		Li -Aerobic		Hi - Aerobic		HIT	
Week	**CON**	**HIT**	**CON**	**HIT**	**CON**	**HIT**	**CON**	**HIT**
PRE	13 h	13 h	10.7 h	10.7 h	1.3 h	1.3 h	1.0 h	1.0 h
	34 km	34 km	31.7 km	31.7 km	1.5 km	1.5 km	0.8 km	0.8 km
1–2	13 h	13 h	10.7 h	6.7 h	1.3 h	1.3 h	1.0 h	5.0 h
	34 km	17 km	31.7 km	12.0 km	1.5 km	1.0 km	0.8 km	4.0 km
3–4	20 h	20 h	16.4 h	10.4 h	2.0 h	2.0 h	1.6 h	7.6 h
	52 km	26 km	48.4 km	17.6 km	2.3 km	2.3 km	1.3 km	6.1 km
5–6	13 h	13 h	10.7 h	6.7 h	1.3 h	1.3 h	1.0 h	5.0 h
	34 km	17 km	31.7 km	12.0 km	1.5 km	1.0 km	0.8 km	4.0 km
7–8	13 h	13 h	10.7 h	6.7 h	1.3 h	1.3 h	1.0 h	5.0 h
	34 km	17 km	31.7 km	12.0 km	1.5 km	1.0 km	0.8 km	4.0 km
9–10	11 h	11 h	8.5 h	5.0 h	1.0 h	1.0 h	1.5 h	5.0 h
	24 km	12 km	22.0 km	7.2 km	0.8 km	0.8 km	1.2 km	4.0 km
11–12	13 h	13 h	10.7 h	6.7 h	1.3 h	1.3 h	1.0 h	5.0 h
	34 km	17 km	31.7 km	12.0 km	1.5 km	1.0 km	0.8 km	4.0 km

Training time and milage averaged for every 2nd week and split into three major training categories. CON: Control groups; INT: intervention group. Li-Aerobic: Technical training, Recovery and low to moderate aerobic training with % of maximal heart rate < 70%. Hi-Aerobic: Intense aerobic training aiming at eliciting close to maximal heart rate and >90% of VO_{2max}. HIT: "High-Intensity Training" with maximal effort for 20–90 s and a rest: work ratio > 4.

completed with speed increasing ~0.1 $m \times s^{-1}$ every minute. The duration of the incremental test varied between four and eight minutes. The incremental test design was based on pilot studies, where it was found that longer test durations caused premature fatigue.

Pool testing

On the second experimental day, pool tests were completed in a 25 m six lane pool. All testing was performed using freestyle technique. First, the swimmer completed a warm-up of ten minutes followed by 5×200 m at increasing pace. The pace was determined so that the first three 200 m were submaximal (subjectively rated as "very easy" to "somewhat hard"). For the first three 200 m, two groups were designed based on individual level in the initial testing. One group paced at 160.2±1.7 s; 155.5±1.9 s and 150.6±1.9 s. The other group paced at 170.0±1.0 s; 165.3±1.9 s and 160.8±1.0 s. The final two 200 m were paced individually (subjective rating "hard, but not maximal" and "maximal") with average pacing of all trials being 138.0±5.6 s and 130.0±5.9 s in the first group and 149.2±5 s and 142.6±7.3 s in the second group. The same pace scheme was used on all test occasions. Pacing was controlled by the scientific staff with audio signals given every 25 m. Each 200 m was started in the water from the wall and swimmers used tumble turns. One minute after each swim, a finger capillary blood sample was obtained and used for analyses of blood lactate concentration (YSI 1500 Sport, Yellow Springs Instruments, USA). Additionally, after the first, third and fifth 200 m and three minutes after the fifth 200 m an additional capillary sample was obtained and analyzed for blood pH and $[K^+]$ (GEM premier 4000). Arm stroke frequency and swim time was registered for each 200 m using a stop watch with frequency count function (Seiko S141, Tokyo, Japan).

After 4½ hours of recovery, swimmers did a 15-minute warm-up followed by an all-out 100 m freestyle. Subjects started with a standardized push off from the wall. To avoid pacing and racing strategies, the 100 m was completed by one swimmer at a time. After 20 minutes of recovery (range from 15–25 minute), the swimmers completed a 200 m freestyle at competition like conditions with heats of three swimmers and start from the block. In this analysis, subjects were matched according to expected best time.

Statistics and calculations

Statistical analyses were performed using SPSS, Statistics 20.0. Data distribution and variance was visually inspected and found to be normally distributed with homogeneous variance between groups. Differences between groups were analyzed using a mixed model [23] with fixed factors: "Group" (Control, Intervention); "Trial" (PRE, POST) and subject specified to identify repeated observations. If significant main effects or interactions were present post hoc test were applied by use of t-tests with Bonferroni adjustment. The level of significance was set to $p<0.05$. Results are reported as means ± standard deviations (SD). The number of participants varies between analyses due to either logistic or technical difficulties. The number of participants is reported for each analysis. An inference about population effects approach was applied to the primary outcome variables of the present study [24]. The change from pre to post was calculated and evaluated relative to 0 by a one-sample t-test. A 90% confidence interval was calculated and the probability of a beneficial or harmful effect was inferred by defining threshold values and using a t-distribution.

Results

Performance

Performance of 100 m all-out freestyle (Fig. 1A) was similar before and after the intervention (Trial: $p=0.34$; Group: $p=0.97$; Trial×Group: $p=0.16$) in both the HIT (60.4±4.0 s vs. 60.3±4.0 s; n = 13; $p=0.75$) and CON (60.2±3.7 s vs. 60.6±3.8 s; n = 15; $p=0.09$) group. Likewise, performance of 200 m freestyle (Fig. 1B) in simulated competition was similar

(Trial: $p=0.65$; Group: $p=0.97$; Trial×Group: $p=0.99$) before and after the intervention in both the HIT (133.2±6.4 s vs. 132.6±7.7 s; $n=14$; $p=0.75$) and CON (133.5±7.0 s vs 133.3±7.6 s; $n=15$; $p=0.75$) group. Also, average speed of a 200 m freestyle performed after four preceding 200 m swims with increasing speed was similar (Trial: $p=0.36$; Group: $p=0.32$; Trial×Group: $p=0.48$) before and after the intervention in both the HIT and CON group ($1.48\pm0.10\ m\times s^{-1}$ vs. $1.50\pm0.08\ m\times s^{-1}$; $n=15$; $p=0.26$ and $1.52\pm0.09\ m\times s^{-1}$ vs. $1.52\pm0.09\ m\times s^{-1}$; $n=16$;$p=0.88$). Stroke- rate and length was similar (Trial: $p=0.39$; Group: $p=0.52$; Trial×Group: $p=0.65$) during the paced 200 m before and after the invention in both the HIT (29.9 ± 2.3 strokes×min^{-1} vs. 29.8 ± 2.3 strokes x min^{-1}; $n=15$; $p=0.70$) and CON (29.4 ± 3.3 strokes×min^{-1} vs. 29.0 ± 3.6 strokes×min^{-1}; $n=16$; $p=0.43$) group.

Maximal oxygen consumption during flume swimming

$VO_{2\ max}$ determined during freestyle swimming with increasing speed in a flume (Fig. 2) was similar (Trial: $p=0.08$; Group: $p=0.76$; Trial×Group: $p=0.35$) before and after the intervention in both the HIT ($4.0\pm0.9\ lO_2\times min^{-1}$ vs. $3.8\pm1.0\ lO_2\times min^{-1}$; $n=14$; $p=0.09$) and CON group ($3.8\pm0.7\ lO_2\times min^{-1}$ vs. $3.8\pm0.7\ lO_2\times min^{-1}$; $n=11$; $p=0.56$). In contrast, $VO_{2\ max}$ expressed relative to body weight was affected by the intervention (Trial: $p=0.01$; Group: $p=0.95$; Trial×Group: $p=0.26$) with a decrease in HIT ($55.7\pm7.2\ mlO_2\times min^{-1}\times kg^{-1}$ vs. $52.7\pm7.0\ mlO_2\times min^{-1}\times kg^{-1}$; $n=14$; $p=0.02$) and no significant difference in CON ($55.0\pm5.9\ mlO_2\times min^{-1}\times kg^{-1}$ vs. $53.8\pm6.4\ mlO_2\times min^{-1}\times kg^{-1}$; $n=13$; $p=0.31$).

Swimming economy

VO_2 determined at a fixed submaximal speed before and after the intervention was similar (Trial: $p=0.37$; Group: $p=0.37$; Trial×Group: $p=0.74$) in both the HIT ($2.4\pm0.7\ lO_2\times min^{-1}$ vs. $2.4\pm0.7\ lO_2\times min^{-1}$; $n=13$; $p=0.39$) and CON ($2.6\pm0.6\ lO_2\times min^{-1}$ vs. $2.6\pm0.6\ lO_2\times min^{-1}$ $n=14$; $p=0.68$) groups.

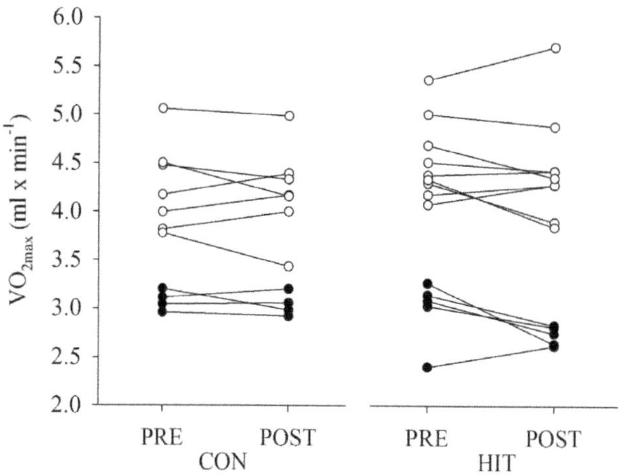

Figure 2. Oxygen uptake. Maximal oxygen uptake (VO_{2max}) determined during freestyle swimming in a swimming flume with increasing water speed until exhaustion in two groups of swimmers before (PRE) and after (POST) a training intervention. One group performed usual swim-training (CON) and another group reduced their training volume by 50% and more than doubled the amount of high-intensity training (HIT). On average, VO_{2max} was similar before and after the 12 week intervention period in both groups. Individual data is presented. Open circles: male; Closed circles: female.

Ventilation

V_E determined at a fixed submaximal speed before and after the intervention was similar (Trial: $p=0.17$; Group: $p=0.58$; Trial×Group: $p=0.92$) in both the HIT ($63.0\pm26.9\ l\times min^{-1}$ vs. $61.4\pm27.1\ l\times min^{-1}$; $n=15$; $p=0.40$) and CON ($58.9\pm13.5\ l\times min^{-1}$ vs. $57.0\pm11.1\ l\times min^{-1}$; $n=15$; $p=0.26$) groups. $V_E\times VO_2^{-1}$ determined at a fixed submaximal speed before and after the intervention was similar (Trial: $p=0.59$; Group: $p=0.29$; Trial×Group: $p=0.95$) in both the HIT ($24\pm4\ l\times min^{-1}$ vs. $23\pm4\ l\times min^{-1}$; $n=15$; $p=0.67$) and CON ($24\pm4\ l\times min^{-1}$ vs. $22\pm4\ l\times min^{-1}$; $n=15$; $p=0.73$) groups.

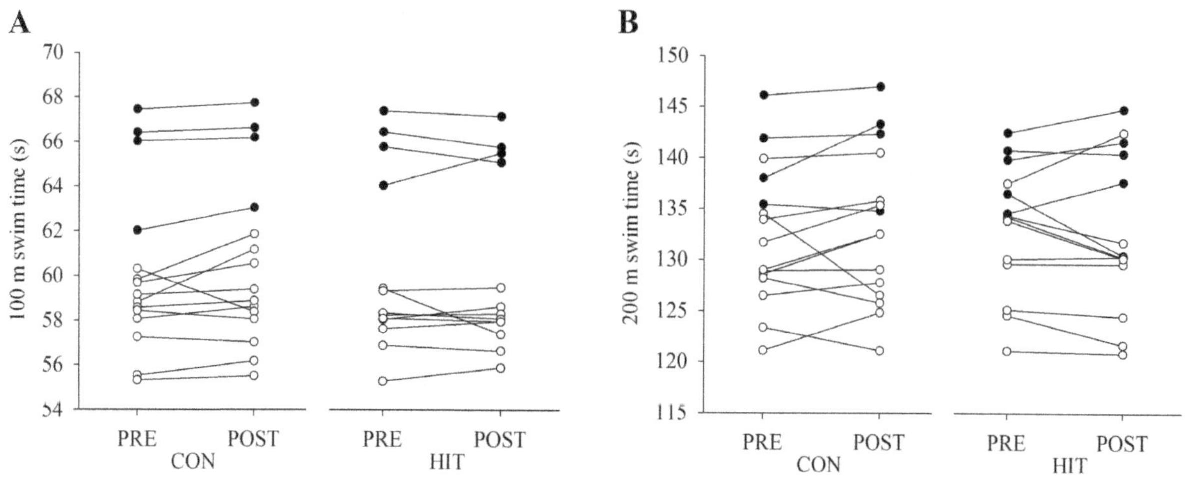

Figure 1. Swimming performance. Performance of 100 m freestyle all-out, starting with wall push-off and one swimmer in the pool at a time (A) and 200 m freestyle in a competition setting, starting from blocks in heats of 3–4 swimmers (B) as determined before (PRE) and after (POST) a training intervention. One group performed usual swim-training (CON) and another group reduced their training volume by 50% and more than doubled the amount of high-intensity training (HIT). On average, both the 100 m and 200 m performance was similar before and after the 12 week intervention period in both groups. Individual data is presented. Open circles: male; Closed circles: female.

Respiratory exchange ratio

The respiratory exchange ratio determined at a fixed submaximal speeds before and after the intervention was similar (Trial: $p=0.47$; Group: $p=0.37$; Trial×Group: $p=0.61$) in both the HIT (0.87 ± 0.04 vs. 0.87 ± 0.04; $n=13$; $p=0.88$) and CON (0.88 ± 0.02 vs. 0.88 ± 0.04; $n=13$; $p=0.38$) groups.

Blood lactate, pH and K^+ response to increasing swimming speed

Blood lactate response to increasing swimming speeds during five times 200 m freestyle was similar (Trial: $p=0.60$; Group: $p=0.90$; Sample: $p<0.001$; Trial×Group×Sample: $p=0.31$) before and after the intervention in both the HIT and CON group (Fig. 3). Furthermore, the change in blood lactate concentration from the 3rd 200 m to the sample obtained after the 5th 200 m (Table 2) was similar (Trial: $p=0.66$; Group: $p=0.32$; Trial×Group: $p=0.55$). Blood pH response to the third and fifth swim interval was similar (Trial: $p=0.81$; Group: $p=0.74$; Trial×Group: $p=0.82$ and Trial: $p=0.62$; Group: $p=0.25$; Trial×Group: $p=0.77$, respectively) before and after the intervention in both groups (Table 2). Likewise, blood K^+ response to the third and fifth swim interval was similar (Trial: $p=0.89$; Group: $p=0.57$; Trial×Group: $p=0.74$ and Trial: $p=0.36$; Group: $p=0.74$; Trial×Group: $p=0.99$, respectively) before and after the intervention in both groups (Table 2).

Body composition

Body fat percent as determined by DEXA scanning was affected by the intervention (Trial: $p=0.01$; Group: $p=0.51$; Trial×Group: $p=0.99$). For the HIT group ($n=16$) the increase did not reach statistical significance ($15.4\pm1.6\%$ vs. $16.3\pm1.6\%$; $p=0.09$). In the CON group ($n=17$) body fat percent increased from $13.9\pm1.5\%$ to $14.9\pm1.5\%$ ($p=0.04$).

Results from the inference about population effects approach is presented in Table 3.

Discussion

The major findings were that more than a doubling of high-intensity training (HIT) in combination with a 50% reduction of training volume for 12 weeks did not change swimming performance, swimming specific VO_{2max}, swimming economy, blood metabolic markers or body composition as compared to a control group. However, VO_{2max} normalized to body weight was reduced in the HIT group only.

The current observation that added HIT and reduced training volume for 12 weeks does not improve performance as compared to high volume training is in agreement with a previous study of ten elite swimmers, where 6.5 weeks of HIT after a four months break yielded similar performance improvements as in a control group [20]. The result is also consistent with unaltered performance after 5 weeks in-season HIT training in younger (~16-17 years) swimmers [21]. However, in children (~10 years) 5 weeks of HIT improved swimming performance in competition [19] indicating that the investigated age group may be of importance. The unaltered performance after HIT in adult swimmers is in contrast to recreational runners who improved time to exhaustion in tests lasting 1–3 minutes [5,16,25] and ~5–6 minutes [15]. Furthermore, in athletes that have not previously engaged in HIT performance can also be improved by added HIT and reduced volume [26,27]. Because the swimmers investigated in the present study had performed HIT for a number of years as a part of their regular training, an upper limit may exist to the amount of HIT that can be applied and still yield physiological adaptation and performance enhancement. In this context it may be of importance to consider that technique in swimming is a major determinant of performance [28] and thus HIT induced physiological adaptations may be less important in swimming as compared to for example running or cycling. Notably, the reduction of training volume in the CON group did not compromise performance. Thus, the increased amount of HIT allowed a drastic distance reduction without compromising performance. The reduced distance and increased recovery time is important for yearly training planning because periodic HIT may allow time to other important training focuses such as technical and/or tactical skills.

The present observation of unaltered swimming specific VO_{2max} after a prolonged period of HIT training is in accordance with observations from moderately trained runners [5,6] but in contrast to the increase observed in well-trained cyclists after 4

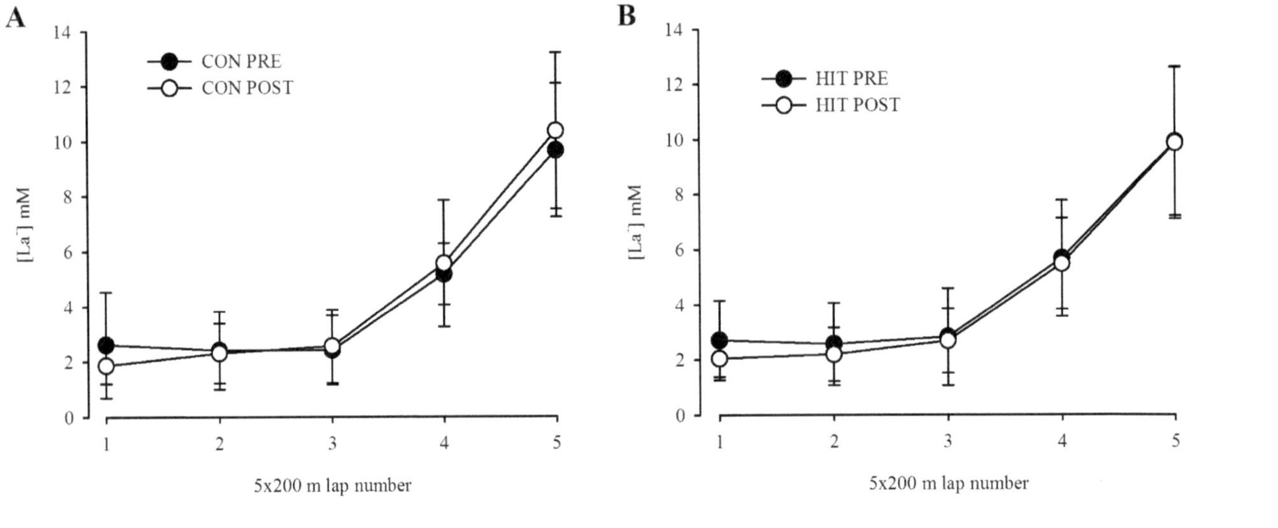

Figure 3. Blood lactate. Blood lactate determined from a finger capillary sample obtained 1 minute after each of five 200 m freestyle completed at increasing speeds (see methods) in two groups of swimmers before (PRE) and after (POST) a training intervention. One group performed usual swim-training (CON) and another group reduced their training volume by 50% and more than doubled the amount of high-intensity training (HIT).

Table 2. Blood metabolites.

Blood variable	Test	Intervention group Pre	Post	n	Control group Pre	Post	n
pH	3rd 200 m	7.39±0.04	7.40±0.04	15	7.39±0.04	7.39±0.03	16
pH	5th 200 m	7.23±0.06	7.22±0.07	15	7.20±0.09	7.20±0.07	17
ΔpH	3rd → 5th	0.17±0.05	0.18±0.06	15	0.19±0.07	0.19±0.06	16
ΔLactate	3rd → 5th	7.8±2.7 mM	7.2±2.6 mM	15	8.2±2.6 mM	8.3±2.6 mM	17
K^+	3rd 200 m	4.78±0.35 mM	4.74±0.44 mM	15	4.69±0.23 mM	4.66±0.36 mM	16
K^+	5th 200 m	5.15±0.53 mM	5.01±0.61 mM	15	5.09±0.88 mM	4.95±0.56 mM	17
ΔK^+	3rd → 5th	0.43±0.54 mM	0.27±0.67 mM	15	0.38±0.85 mM	0.34±0.56 mM	16

Blood variables obtained from a fingertip sample after the 3rd and 5th of five 200 m swims performed at increasing speeds before and after a 12 week intervention period. The third 200 meter was swum on a identical speed before and after the intervention whereas the fifth 200 meter was swum with maximal effort.

weeks of added HIT [13] and in moderately trained cyclist after 6 weeks of HIT [29] as well as findings from untrained subjects [3]. There are several possible explanations for the observed unaltered VO_{2max}. Importantly, the current population had a much higher training volume and longer history than previously studied populations. Thus, a natural plateau in VO_{2max} may have been reached prior to the initiation of the study. This suggestion is somewhat supported by the observation that HIT induces similar increases in VO_{2max} as low-intensity high-volume training in young swimmers aged ~10 years [19] as well as in adult swimmers when preceded by a four months break [20]. It may also be considered that swimming VO_{2max} may not have been limited by the central cardiovascular capacity as expected during running or cycling [30] but more so by the upper body capacity to extract oxygen. This suggestion is substantiated by the finding that seasonal fluctuations in a Olympic level swimmers VO_{2peak} appears unrelated to running VO_{2peak} [31]. As such, the current finding of unaltered VO_{2max} may indicate unaltered muscular respiratory capacity and this suggestion is in agreement with a previous study that found unaltered muscular oxidative capacity in trained populations after a period of HIT [2]. It is of interest to note that the previously reported improvement of running economy, which was associated with reduced VO_2 but unchanged RER at submaximal speeds [6] could not be verified in the present study of elite athletes. Importantly, a reduced VO_{2max} relative to body weight was apparent in the HIT group but not the CON group. However, it could not be demonstrated that the change in normalized VO_{2max} differed between groups. Further, both groups experienced a gain of body weight of ~1 kg which was not significantly different between groups (data not shown).

The present investigation of blood metabolic markers in response to increasing swimming speed demonstrated the expected increases of blood lactate, K^+ and H^+ concentrations. However, the hypothesis of reduced extracellular accumulation of blood lactate, K^+ and H^+ in the HIT group after the intervention period could not be verified. This is in apparent contrast to the observation that HIT can increase muscle Na^+, K^+ ATPase expression and reduce plasma K^+ concentration at the end of 1–2 minutes exhaustive runs in recreational runners [5,32]. After HIT plasma K^+ may also be reduced during the recovery from exercise [32,33], but this is not always the case [5]. In the present study, samples were obtained one minutes after an exhaustive 200 m swim that lasted ~2 minutes, which corresponds well to the samples obtained during early recovery in previous studies [16,33].

The present observations are in accordance with unaltered plasma K^+ concentrations after HIT during submaximal workloads and after an incremental test [5]. It can be speculated that reduced plasma K^+ concentrations may have existed in the present study if the swimmers had been evaluated after a constant speed swim to exhaustion [5]. However, this type of test does not correspond to the competition performed by swimmers and most other athletes.

During the 5×200 m pool test with gradually increasing swimming speed, blood lactate concentration was unaltered. Additionally, the change in blood lactate concentration from the 3rd to the 5th 200 m was unaltered by the intervention, indicating that the muscular lactate production and release was similar before and after HIT. This is supported by the unaltered changes in plasma pH observed during the 5×200 m steptest before and after the HIT period. The current observations are in agreement with the finding that blood and muscle lactate as well as muscle H^+ accumulation and muscular expression of monocarboxylate transporters (MCT) 1 and 4 is unaltered after HIT in recreational runners [5,16]. However, muscular MCT1 expression has also been observed to increase after HIT in recreational runners [25] and the reason for this discrepancy between previous studies is unclear but may be related to differences in the applied HIT protocols.

Metabolites were measured in plasma during recovery in the present study and it cannot be excluded that undetected changes in other compartments and at other time-points existed. Previous studies have demonstrated that HIT reduces K^+ accumulation in the interstitial space in untrained subjects [34] and that changes in K^+ plasma concentrations occurs within 10–30 s after onset and termination of exercise [35,36] and that plasma K^+ concentration is sensitive to training [37]. Additionally, muscle lactate and H^+ accumulation can be reduced by HIT [38] and with respect to sample timing, exercise induced changes in lactate and H^+ homeostasis persist for several minutes into recovery in both intramuscular [39] and in the plasma compartment [38]. Thus, training induced changes in muscular capacity for handling K^+, H^+ and lactate usually translates into altered plasma accumulation [34] and is detectable during recovery, which suggests that the present observations of unaltered plasma metabolite response is representative for the events at the muscular level.

Only the CON group showed an increase of body fat during the intervention period, but a similar and close to significant increase was apparent in the HIT group. This finding demonstrates that a drastic shift in training volume does not necessarily translate into

Table 3. Inference of effects.

	100 m	200 m	$VO_{2\,max}$	$VO_{2\,sub}$	RER_{sub}	$[La^-]_{max}$	pH_{max}	$[K^+]_{max}$
HIT								
90% C.I.	[−0.3;0.5]	[−0.9;2.0]	[−280;−5]	[−110;33]	[−0.02;0.02]	[−0.66;1.3]	[−0.03;0.01]	[−0.5;0.22]
P	0.72	0.48	0.09	0.44	0.90	0.59	0.49	0.51
Threshold	0.2 s	0.2 s	150 ml	−100 ml	−0.02	0.5 mM	0.02	0.2 mM
Inference								
- Beneficial	31%	68%	0%	9%	5%	36%	22%	6%
- Trivial	57%	15%	53%	91%	88%	56%	76%	55%
- Harmful	12%	17%	47%	0%	7%	8%	2%	39%
CON								
C.I.	[−0.9;0.0]	[−2.3;0.7]	[−150;67]	[−110; 68]	[−0.02;0.01]	[−0.39;1.9]	[−0.04;0.03]	[−0.52;0.24]
P	0.12	0.375	0.49	0.707	0.285	0.267	0.901	0.525
Threshold	0.2 s	0.2 s	150 ml	−100 ml	−0.02	0.5	0.02	0.2 mM
Inference								
- Beneficial	1%	13%	0%	6%	9%	65%	18%	7%
- Trivial	19%	12%	94%	92%	91%	32%	70%	54%
- Harmful	80%	75%	6%	2%	0%	3%	12%	39%

The 90% confidence interval (90% C.I.) for the observed change in primary outcome variables within each group and the P-value (P) for a one-sample t-test with the null-hypothesis $\mu = 0$. A subjectively chosen threshold for the minimal change that could be considered beneficial (Threshold) was used to calculate the chance that the observed changes would be beneficial, trivial or harmful (Inference). One group performed usual swim-training (CON) and another group reduced their training volume by 50% and more than doubled the amount of high-intensity training (HIT).

to altered body composition. This observation is in agreement with unaltered body composition, despite a one week change in total daily energy expenditure in trained athletes [22].

The present study is the longest running HIT intervention in an elite-population and at the same time includes more subjects than most previous studies [2,18]. Despite the long intervention period, relatively large group of subjects and carefully controlled training and testing, some concerns need attention. It may be speculated that some, but not all, swimmers can benefit from HIT and if there is any chance that HIT can improve performance of some but not all elite athletes, then it is of interest for coaches and athletes. Thus, we report results of an inference statistical approach [40] for the primary outcome variables in Table 3. This analysis supported that no clear beneficial or harmful effect was apparent after 12 weeks of HIT. It should be noted that performance of 100 m and 200 m freestyle may have been impaired in the CON but not in the HIT group whereas VO_{2max} may have decreased in the HIT group but not in the CON group. These observations may be considered in a practical setting depending on the type of swimmer that is exposed to HIT. Apparently, HIT may be of some value to protect against reduced performance in short distance swimmers but based on the possible reduction in VO_{2max}, it can be speculated that HIT would be detrimental for long distance swimmers (i.e. > 800 m) but this remains to be investigated. The possible reduction of VO_{2max} is somewhat supported by the low p-values observed for pre vs. post VO_{2max} and the reduced VO_{2max} normalized to body weight in the HIT group. Another possible concern is that all testing was completed in freestyle for practical reasons. It cannot be ruled out, that for example, breast swimmers benefitted from the training whereas back-strokers did not. However, all swimmers completed more than 50% of the total training volume in freestyle, including the HIT sessions. Thus, this appears a reasonable but negligible concern. It can also be speculated that the CON group achieved optimal adaptations resembling those of HIT by the performed in-water HIT, dry-land resistance training or even less intense but prolonged interval based training that possibly could cause adaptations as fatigue sets in. Even if the CON group somehow did achieve adaptations similar to the HIT group the present findings still demonstrate that a drastic distance reduction for 12 weeks does not compromise performance. Thus, it becomes of interest to investigate if a drastic distance reduction combined with a limited amount of HIT would also be sufficient to sustain performance for a prolonged period of time.

Both genders participated in the present study but the number of subjects was too limited to allow for a separate analysis of possible gender specific adaptation to the intervention. Previously, it has been demonstrated that recreationally active young men and women adapted similar to a 2–3 week period of HIT [41] but it is not known if a gender effect exists in an elite population.

Perspective

The present data demonstrate that it is possible to reduce training volume by 50% without compromising physical capacity. Because time is limited in elite training HIT can be used as a strategy to increase the focus on other types of training because of the long recovery times and reduced time requirement. The present findings indicate that for example technical and tactical focus can be increased for periods of up to 12 weeks during the season by reducing volume and increasing the amount of HIT. In a physiological context, the present data demonstrate that added HIT to a very well trained population all-ready engaging in HIT does not necessarily improve performance as could be expected from previous studies of HIT.

Conclusion

In conclusion, increasing the amount of HIT at the expense of volume for 12 weeks in a group of elite swimmers did neither induce significant improvements nor deterioration of performance or physiological variables.

Acknowledgments

We thank Team Danmark, all participating coaches and swimmers for an invaluable effort.

Author Contributions

Conceived and designed the experiments: NBN AK MJ TL. Performed the experiments: NBN AK MJ TL SJ LJ. Analyzed the data: NBN AK MJ TL SJ LJ. Contributed reagents/materials/analysis tools: NBN AK MJ TL SJ LJ. Wrote the paper: NBN AK MJ TL SJ LJ.

References

1. Gibala MJ, Little JP, MacDonald MJ, Hawley JA (2012) Physiological adaptations to low-volume, high-intensity interval training in health and disease. The Journal of Physiology 590: 1077–1084.
2. Iaia FM, Bangsbo J (2010) Speed endurance training is a powerful stimulus for physiological adaptations and performance improvements of athletes. Scand J Med Sci Sports 20 Suppl 2: 11–23.
3. Burgomaster KA, Howarth KR, Phillips SM, Rakobowchuk M, MacDonald MJ, et al. (2008) Similar metabolic adaptations during exercise after low volume sprint interval and traditional endurance training in humans. J Physiol 586: 151–160.
4. Laursen PB, Shing CM, Peake JM, Coombes JS, Jenkins DG (2002) Interval training program optimization in highly trained endurance cyclists. Med Sci Sports Exerc 34: 1801–1807.
5. Bangsbo J, Gunnarsson TP, Wendell J, Nybo L, Thomassen M (2009) Reduced volume and increased training intensity elevate muscle Na+-K+ pump alpha2-subunit expression as well as short- and long-term work capacity in humans. J Appl Physiol 107: 1771–1780.
6. Iaia FM, Hellsten Y, Nielsen JJ, Fernstrom M, Sahlin K, et al. (2009) Four weeks of speed endurance training reduces energy expenditure during exercise and maintains muscle oxidative capacity despite a reduction in training volume. J Appl Physiol 106: 73–80.
7. Gunnarsson TP, Christensen PM, Holse K, Christiansen D, Bangsbo J (2012) Effect of additional speed endurance training on performance and muscle adaptations. Med Sci Sports Exerc 44: 1942–1948.
8. Howley ET, Bassett DR, Jr., Welch HG (1995) Criteria for maximal oxygen uptake: review and commentary. Med Sci Sports Exerc 27: 1292–1301.
9. Burgomaster KA, Hughes SC, Heigenhauser GJ, Bradwell SN, Gibala MJ (2005) Six sessions of sprint interval training increases muscle oxidative potential and cycle endurance capacity in humans. J Appl Physiol 98: 1985–1990.
10. Burgomaster KA, Heigenhauser GJ, Gibala MJ (2006) Effect of short-term sprint interval training on human skeletal muscle carbohydrate metabolism during exercise and time-trial performance. J Appl Physiol 100: 2041–2047.
11. Shepley B, MacDougall JD, Cipriano N, Sutton JR, Tarnopolsky MA, et al. (1992) Physiological effects of tapering in highly trained athletes. J Appl Physiol 72: 706–711.
12. Allen DG, Lamb GD, Westerblad H (2008) Skeletal muscle fatigue: cellular mechanisms. Physiol Rev 88: 287–332.
13. Laursen PB, Shing CM, Peake JM, Coombes JS, Jenkins DG (2005) Influence of high-intensity interval training on adaptations in well-trained cyclists. J Strength Cond Res 19: 527–533.
14. Dupont G, Akakpo K, Berthoin S (2004) The effect of in-season, high-intensity interval training in soccer players. J Strength Cond Res 18: 584–589.
15. Esfarjani F, Laursen PB (2007) Manipulating high-intensity interval training: effects on VO2max, the lactate threshold and 3000 m running performance in moderately trained males. J Sci Med Sport 10: 27–35.
16. Iaia FM, Thomassen M, Kolding H, Gunnarsson T, Wendell J, et al. (2008) Reduced volume but increased training intensity elevates muscle Na+-K+ pump alpha1-subunit and NHE1 expression as well as short-term work capacity in humans. Am J Physiol Regul Integr Comp Physiol 294: R966–R974.
17. Maglischo, E W. (2003) Swimming Fastest. Champaign, IL, USA: Human Kinetics.
18. Aspenes ST, Karlsen T (2012) Exercise-training intervention studies in competitive swimming. Sports Med 42: 527–543.
19. Sperlich B, Zinner C, Heilemann I, Kjendlie PL, Holmberg HC, et al. (2010) High-intensity interval training improves VO(2peak), maximal lactate accumulation, time trial and competition performance in 9-11-year-old swimmers. Eur J Appl Physiol 110: 1029–1036.
20. Houston ME, Wilson DM, Green HJ, Thomson JA, Ranney DA (1981) Physiological and muscle enzyme adaptations to two different intensities of swim training. Eur J Appl Physiol Occup Physiol 46: 283–291.
21. Faude O, Meyer T, Scharhag J, Weins F, Urhausen A, et al. (2008) Volume vs. intensity in the training of competitive swimmers. Int J Sports Med 29: 906–912.
22. Drenowatz C, Eisenmann JC, Carlson JJ, Pfeiffer KA, Pivarnik JM (2012) Energy expenditure and dietary intake during high-volume and low-volume training periods among male endurance athletes. Appl Physiol Nutr Metab 37: 199–205.
23. Cnaan A, Laird NM, Slasor P (1997) Using the general linear mixed model to analyse unbalanced repeated measures and longitudinal data. Stat Med 16: 2349–2380.
24. Hopkins WG, Marshall SW, Batterham AM, Hanin J (2009) Progressive statistics for studies in sports medicine and exercise science. Med Sci Sports Exerc 41: 3–13.
25. Bickham DC, Bentley DJ, Le Rossignol PF, Cameron-Smith D (2006) The effects of short-term sprint training on MCT expression in moderately endurance-trained runners. Eur J Appl Physiol 96: 636–643.
26. Laursen PB (2010) Training for intense exercise performance: high-intensity or high-volume training? Scand J Med Sci Sports 20 Suppl 2: 1–10.
27. Kohn TA, Essen-Gustavsson B, Myburgh KH (2010) Specific muscle adaptations in type II fibers after high-intensity interval training of well-trained runners. Scand J Med Sci Sports.
28. Figueiredo P, Pendergast DR, Vilas-Boas JP, Fernandes RJ (2013) Interplay of biomechanical, energetic, coordinative, and muscular factors in a 200 m front crawl swim. Biomed Res Int 2013: 897232.
29. Tabata I, Nishimura K, Kouzaki M, Hirai Y, Ogita F, et al. (1996) Effects of moderate-intensity endurance and high-intensity intermittent training on anaerobic capacity and VO2max. Med Sci Sports Exerc 28: 1327–1330.
30. Saltin B, Calbet JA (2006) Point: in health and in a normoxic environment, VO2 max is limited primarily by cardiac output and locomotor muscle blood flow. J Appl Physiol 100: 744–745.
31. Holmer I (1992) Swimming physiology. Ann Physiol Anthropol 11: 269–276.
32. Bangsbo J, Iaia FM, Krustrup P (2007) Metabolic response and fatigue in soccer. Int J Sports Physiol Perform 2: 111–127.
33. Gunnarsson TP, Christensen PM, Thomassen M, Nielsen LR, Bangsbo J (2013) Effect of intensified training on muscle ion kinetics, fatigue development and repeated short term performance in endurance trained cyclists. Am J Physiol Regul Integr Comp Physiol.
34. Nielsen JJ, Mohr M, Klarskov C, Kristensen M, Krustrup P, et al. (2004) Effects of high-intensity intermittent training on potassium kinetics and performance in human skeletal muscle. J Physiol 554: 857–870.
35. Nordsborg N, Ovesen J, Thomassen M, Zangenberg M, Jons C, et al. (2008) Effect of dexamethasone on skeletal muscle Na+,K+ pump subunit specific expression and K+ homeostasis during exercise in humans. J Physiol 586: 1447–1459.
36. Nordsborg N, Mohr M, Pedersen LD, Nielsen JJ, Langberg H, et al. (2003) Muscle interstitial potassium kinetics during intense exhaustive exercise: effect of previous arm exercise. Am J Physiol Regul Integr Comp Physiol 285: R143–R148.
37. Gunnarsson TP, Christensen PM, Thomassen M, Nielsen LR, Bangsbo J (2013) Effect of intensified training on muscle ion kinetics, fatigue development and repeated short term performance in endurance trained cyclists. Am J Physiol Regul Integr Comp Physiol.
38. Harmer AR, McKenna MJ, Sutton JR, Snow RJ, Ruell PA, et al. (2000) Skeletal muscle metabolic and ionic adaptations during intense exercise following sprint training in humans. J Appl Physiol 89: 1793–1803.
39. Degroot M, Massie BM, Boska M, Gober J, Miller RG, et al. (1993) Dissociation of [H+] from fatigue in human muscle detected by high time resolution 31P-NMR. Muscle Nerve 16: 91–98.
40. Hopkins WG, Marshall SW, Batterham AM, Hanin J (2009) Progressive statistics for studies in sports medicine and exercise science. Med Sci Sports Exerc 41: 3–13.
41. Astorino TA, Allen RP, Roberson DW, Jurancich M, Lewis R, et al. (2011) Adaptations to high-intensity training are independent of gender. Eur J Appl Physiol 111: 1279–1286.

12

Left Preference for Sport Tasks Does Not Necessarily Indicate Left-Handedness: Sport-Specific Lateral Preferences, Relationship with Handedness and Implications for Laterality Research in Behavioural Sciences

Florian Loffing[1]*, Florian Sölter[1,2], Norbert Hagemann[1]

1 Institute of Sports and Sports Science, University of Kassel, Kassel, Germany, **2** Institute of Sport and Exercise Sciences, University of Muenster, Muenster, Germany

Abstract

In the elite domain of interactive sports, athletes who demonstrate a left preference (e.g., holding a weapon with the left hand in fencing or boxing in a 'southpaw' stance) seem overrepresented. Such excess indicates a performance advantage and was also interpreted as evidence in favour of frequency-dependent selection mechanisms to explain the maintenance of left-handedness in humans. To test for an overrepresentation, the incidence of athletes' lateral preferences is typically compared with an expected ratio of left- to right-handedness in the normal population. However, the normal population reference values did not always relate to the sport-specific tasks of interest, which may limit the validity of reports of an excess of 'left-oriented' athletes. Here we sought to determine lateral preferences for various sport-specific tasks (e.g., baseball batting, boxing) in the normal population and to examine the relationship between these preferences and handedness. To this end, we asked 903 participants to indicate their lateral preferences for sport-specific and common tasks using a paper-based questionnaire. Lateral preferences varied considerably across the different sport tasks and we found high variation in the relationship between those preferences and handedness. In contrast to unimanual tasks (e.g., fencing or throwing), for bimanually controlled actions such as baseball batting, shooting in ice hockey or boxing the incidence of left preferences was considerably higher than expected from the proportion of left-handedness in the normal population and the relationship with handedness was relatively low. We conclude that (i) task-specific reference values are mandatory for reliably testing for an excess of athletes with a left preference, (ii) the term 'handedness' should be more cautiously used within the context of sport-related laterality research and (iii) observation of lateral preferences in sports may be of limited suitability for the verification of evolutionary theories of handedness.

Editor: David Carrier, University of Utah, United States of America

Funding: This work was supported by a grant from the German Research Foundation (DFG, http://www.dfg.de/en/index.jsp) [HA 4361/5-2]. The funders had no role in study design, data collection and analysis, decision to publish, or preparation of the manuscript.

Competing Interests: The authors have declared that no competing interests exist.

* Email: f.loffing@uni-kassel.de

Introduction

Lateral preference describes humans or 'non-human animals' predominant use of either side of the body for carrying out specific actions. Handedness is the most prominent trait where such preference occurs [1]. While the proportion of human left-handedness varies by geographic region [2,3] and is higher in males compared to females [4,5], overall left-handedness is considerably lower compared to right-handedness in any culture studied so far and such asymmetry seems relatively stable since thousands of years [6,7]. The question of which mechanisms constitute the maintenance of an imbalanced human handedness polymorphism is controversially discussed [8–10]. One suggestion is that left-handedness is associated with both fitness costs (e.g., higher proneness to health-related problems), resulting in frequencies considerably below 50%, and benefits, compensating for some costs and thus preserving left-handedness [11]. From an evolutionary perspective, the fighting hypothesis argues that the costs (potentially) inherent to left-handedness may be offset by negative frequency-dependent selection mechanisms [12]. More specifically, left-handers are assumed to enjoy an advantage in duel-like confrontations because of their relative rarity which, as a result, makes their opponents become less familiar with the left-handers' fighting behaviour. Such fighting advantage in male-male competition, in turn, is thought to have helped left-handers to ensure reproductive success (for a recent critique, e.g. see [13]).

Among other things, elite sporting competition databases have been used to verify the fighting hypothesis [11]. Consistent with its predictions, in professional rankings of interactive sports such as table tennis or fencing, where athletes can directly influence and constrain each other's actions, athletes who use their left hand for tasks like holding a racket or a foil were found overrepresented [12,14,15]. In contrast, no excess of left-handed performers has ever been reported in any non-interactive sport (e.g., darts, snooker, golf) [12,16]. The clear division of sports where left-handers are overrepresented or not suggests that the performance demands inherent to interactive situations (e.g., anticipation of an opponent's action intentions or fast decision-making [17–21]) in combination with frequency-dependent mechanisms favour left-handed performers. In contrast, alternative explanations which propose that mechanisms associated with left-handedness *per se* constitute a left-handers' advantage (e.g., higher aggression [22], less lateralized motor skills [23] or more efficient neural processing [24] in left-handers) are little convincing so far (for a critical review, e.g. see [14]).

The informative value of research on handedness distribution in sports may be partly limited because potentially inappropriate normal population reference values were used. More specifically, in order to determine whether or not there is an excess of left-handed athletes in a sport, observed handedness frequencies are compared with expected frequencies thought to occur in the normal population (e.g., 10–13% left-handers; [12]). However, instead of using reference values that are related to the sport-specific task of interest, estimates of handedness distribution in the normal population were often taken from large surveys [4,5] which reported lateral preferences for unrelated tasks like writing or throwing (for exceptions, e.g. see [16,25,26]). We suppose that reliance on task-*un*related comparative values is questionable, especially if these values are considerably different to the normal population's lateral preferences for the particular sport task of interest. Then, the impact of laterality on sports performance may be over- or underestimated.

Remarkably, the literature almost lacks a comprehensive database of reference values for sport-specific lateral preferences (for an exception see [27]). The above mentioned procedure seems justified either if tasks are very similar [12] or if there is evidence of a close relationship between different items [28,29], as has been reported for throwing a ball and holding a racket [30]. Even in the absence of these two preconditions, as long as unimanually controlled sport tasks are considered (e.g., holding a weapon in fencing), comparative values derived from unrelated but clearly unilateral tasks like writing or throwing may be acceptable.

However, reliance on reference values for unrelated unimanually controlled tasks (e.g., writing or throwing) may be problematic when sport tasks are examined that are not under distinct unilateral control. Examples of such sport tasks are batting in baseball [26] or cricket [31], holding a stick in ice hockey [32], fighting stance in boxing [12] or in related combat sports such as Mixed Martial Arts (MMA) [33,34]. For these tasks, differentiation of athletes into left- vs. right-handers is difficult given that both hands are involved in the control of motor actions (e.g., batting in baseball) or may be used during fights (e.g., in boxing). Considering evidence which suggests that lateral preferences for unilateral and bilateral tasks are not perfectly correlated (e.g., throwing a ball and batting; [26,31]), we expect that task-specific reference values are mandatory particularly when examining bimanually controlled actions.

Moreover, up to now there is very limited understanding of the (strength of) relationship between those preferences and handedness [27,34,35]. Furthering our knowledge about such relationship is important as the detection of inconsistent relationships in particular may have several significant consequences for various domains of laterality research. First, inconsistent relationships would suggest that lateral preferences observed in sports may not allow reliable inferences in support of the fighting hypothesis or other evolutionary models to explain the maintenance of the polymorphism in human handedness. Second, inconsistent relationships between sport-specific lateral preferences and handedness would also question the validity of explanations such as that an excess of left preferences among elite athletes is due to handedness-dependent differences in neurological functioning. Finally, depending on the strength of relationship, it might be advisable that researchers be more cautious with usage of the term 'handedness' when referring to lateral preferences in sports. Such advice could be particularly relevant when dealing with sport tasks for which relationships with handedness are low.

In light of the above issues, the aim of this study was as follows. First, we sought to establish reference values for sport-specific lateral preferences in the normal population. To this end, we designed a paper-based questionnaire which comprised items on 16 different sport tasks that are executed with the hands, either unilaterally (e.g., fencing) or bilaterally (e.g., batting in baseball), the feet (e.g., kicking) or tasks that may be executed in different directions (e.g., rotating left or right when performing a pirouette in figure skating). Albeit we will report the results on all items, our focus is on uni- and bimanual sport tasks. Second, we aimed to identify the relationships between sport-specific lateral preferences and handedness. Therefore, we additionally included an established questionnaire on handedness preferences [36]. To anticipate, we will show that the frequencies of sport-specific left preferences as well as the relationship between lateral preferences and handedness vary considerably across different sport tasks.

Material and Methods

Ethics Statement

The study was approved by the ethics committee at the Department of Social Sciences, University of Kassel (Germany), and was performed in accordance with the ethical standards set out in the Revised Declaration of Helsinki as of November 2008. In the study proposal, the ethics committee was informed that, because our questionnaire did not contain any dubious questions or answers, legal age of participants was not required.

All participants were given written information about the study and they signed written informed consent prior to the completion of the questionnaire. Written information was related to the confidentiality of data, the ensured anonymity of data collection and analysis, the subject's right to withdraw from the study at any stage without any (negative or positive) consequences for the subject and the absence of any potential risks or benefits associated with participation in the study. Data was anonymized upon collection and the authors did not have access to identifying information.

Our sample included five minors (two males, 16 and 17 years old; three females, one 13 and two 17 years old). All participants, including the five minors, were able to comprehend the information provided prior to as well as while filling out the questionnaire. We obtained written informed consent from the minors prior to their participation. However, we did not obtain additional informed consent (neither written nor verbal) from these participants' next of kin, caretakers, or guardians because our research was clearly not suspected to create any distress or harm and only anonymous questionnaires were used. As we understand, this procedure was also in line with the current ethical principles set out by the American Psychological Association (standard 8.05).

Participants

The sample comprised 903 randomly selected individuals (males: $n = 408$, age: 16–77 years, $M = 25.01$ years, $SD = 9.11$;

females: $n = 495$, age: 13–75 years, $M = 22.84$ years, $SD = 6.32$) who were predominantly university students from the University of Kassel (Germany).

Questionnaire

The 16 questions related to sport-specific tasks are summarized in Table 1. For each item, participants were asked to choose their lateral preference out of three alternatives (provided in the following order): 'left', 'no preference' or 'right' (German terms: 'links', 'keine Bevorzugung', 'rechts'). To improve the participants' understanding of the meaning of left vs. right for the respective tasks, each sport-specific question was accompanied by monochrome pictures of a person performing the respective tasks in a left and right orientation (see Table S1). The individual shown on the pictures in Table S1 has given written informed consent (as outlined in PLOS consent form) to publish these images.

In order to examine the relationship between sport-specific lateral preferences and handedness, the questionnaire also included a German version of the Edinburgh Handedness Inventory (EHI) [36]. The EHI comprised ten items such as writing, throwing or holding a spoon. Unlike in the original version of the EHI we provided participants with Likert-like five response alternatives, ordered as follows, of which they had to check one for each item and each alternative was assigned a different score for later analysis (scores were not available to participants): 'exclusively left' (−10), 'rather left' (−5), 'no preference' (0), 'rather right' (+5), or 'exclusively right' (+10) (German terms: 'ausschließlich links', 'eher links', 'keine Bevorzugung', 'eher rechts', 'ausschließlich rechts') [37]. We used these response modes because there is indication that participants do not strictly follow the instructions of placing one or two crosses in a 'left' and/or 'right' column as provided in the initial version of the EHI (e.g., participants just tick a box without differentiating their strength of preference by making one or two crosses) [38]. For each participant, a laterality score (LS) was calculated by summing up the ten items' scores and thus LS ranged from −100 to +100. We calculated LS instead of laterality quotients initially proposed by Oldfield [36], because laterality quotients are only sensitive to the direction of handedness, whereas the LS "is sensitive to both the degree and direction of handedness" (p. 169, [37]; see also for exemplary calculations).

Our questionnaire additionally included a German version of Coren's Lateral Preference Inventory [39], which measures hand, foot, eye and ear preference, as well as questions on the participants' current or past sporting activities. To keep focussed on our study's aim the remaining data will be reported elsewhere.

Results

Overall, differentiation of participants into 'left-handers' (if LS <0) and 'right-handers' (if LS ≥ 0) revealed that our sample comprised 8.86% left-handers and that left-handers were more common in males (10.05%) compared to females (7.88%); however, the sex-dependent difference was not significant, $\chi^2(1, N = 903) = 1.31, p = .25, \omega = 0.04$.

Lateral preferences varied considerably across the different sport-specific tasks and left preferences were higher in males compared to females in 11 out of the 16 tasks (Figure 1; raw data can be accessed in Table S2). To avoid an overestimation of left preferences, we considered responses to all alternatives (i.e., 'left', 'right' and 'no preference') for the calculation of left preference percentages. For tasks that require unilateral control of the hands, left preferences were quite stable, ranging from 7.62% (bowling) to 9.09% (holding a weapon) in males and from 6.26% (holding a weapon) to 7.07% (throwing) in females. However, for tasks requiring bilateral control of the hands, left preferences were clearly higher compared to the former tasks. Here, left preferences ranged from 9.61% (archery) to 23.95%

Table 1. Questions on sport-specific tasks (see also Table S1).

Sport	Task/Item	Question
e.g., darts, team-handball	throwing	Which hand would you use for throwing darts or a ball (e.g., in team-handball)?
fencing	holding a weapon	In which hand would you hold a weapon in fencing?
racket sports	holding a racket	In which hand would you hold a racket (e.g., table tennis, tennis or badminton)?
ninepin, tenpin bowling	bowling	Which hand would you use for bowling (e.g., in ninepin or tenpin)?
billiards	holding a cue	Which hand (rear hand) would you use to hold a cue to play a ball in billiards?
baseball	batting	How would you hold a baseball bat (i.e., which hand is at the top)?
ice hockey	holding a stick	How would you hold a hockey stick (i.e., which hand is at the bottom)?
boxing	stance	Which stance would you choose in boxing to fight an opponent?
golf	holding a golf club	How would you hold a golf club (i.e., which hand is at the bottom)?
target shooting	shooting orientation	Which orientation would you choose for target shooting?
archery	shooting orientation	Which orientation would you choose for doing archery?
soccer	kicking	Which foot would you use for kicking a ball?
long jump	jump off	Which leg would you use to jump off in long jump?
high jump	approaching side *	From which side would you approach the crossbar in high jump?
skateboarding, snowboarding	front foot	Which foot would you stand in front with on a skateboard or snowboard?
e.g., figure skating	rotation direction	Which direction would you prefer when rotating along the vertical axis (e.g., when doing a pirouette in figure skating)?

* *Note:* In high jump, approaching from the left means that an athlete jumps off with his or her right foot (and *vice versa*). All participants were informed in writing about this relationship when filling out the questionnaire. To facilitate understanding of lateral preference for high jump, we will report the preferred foot instead of approach side for this task.

(holding a stick in ice hockey) in males and from 9.31% (holding a cue in billiards) to 34.83% (boxing stance) in females. Similarly, preferences for using the left foot substantially differed as a function of task: 12.07% (kicking) to 66.67% (high jump) in males and 8.28% (kicking) to 58.25% (high jump) in females. With regard to rotating along the vertical axis, 44.94% of male and 39.84% of female participants indicated a left preference.

To determine the relationship between sport-specific lateral preferences and handedness (as represented by LS values obtained from the EHI) we calculated point-biserial correlation coefficients (r_{pb}) for the whole sample and separately for males and females. As is illustrated in Table 2, almost any relationship was statistically significant ($p<.05$); except for rotating along the vertical axis (e.g., in figure skating) overall and in males as well as for skateboarding in males. For all unilateral manual tasks there was very good agreement between sport-specific lateral preferences and handedness. However, the relationship between handedness and tasks that require bimanual control was highly variable depending on the task and relatively low particularly for baseball batting, holding a stick in ice hockey, fighting stance in boxing and golfing. Kicking foot was moderately related to handedness. The lowest relationships were revealed for tasks where an athlete's hands are not primarily involved (i.e., long jump, high jump and skateboarding).

The above patterns in the relationships remain almost identical – irrespective of whether 'no preference' responses on the respective sport tasks are included or not – when participants are first classified into left- ($LS <0$) and right-handers ($LS \geq 0$) [40] and then phi coefficients (Φ) are calculated as measure for the relationship between sport-specific lateral preferences and handedness (see Table S3). The data summarized in Table 3 shows that left-handers (males and females) demonstrated a right preference more often than right-handers demonstrated a left preference across the sport-specific tasks, except for foot preference in high jump. This pattern was particularly evident for unimanually controlled actions (e.g., throwing or holding a racket) for which right-handers clearly preferred the right hand.

Discussion

This study furthers our understanding of sport-specific lateral preferences and their relationship with handedness in the normal population. While the proportion of left-handers in our sample was comparable to previously reported frequencies in males and females [4,5], both sport-specific lateral preferences as well as the relationship between those preferences and handedness varied considerably depending on the task. These findings have several important implications which we will elaborate on in the following.

First, rather than indiscriminately referring to 'handedness' we suggest using more specific and differentiated terminology (e.g., fighting stance or orientation in boxing or MMA [34], shooting side or orientation in ice hockey [32]) when considering athletes' sport-specific lateral preferences. Doing so is necessary because of the inconsistent relationships found between sport-specific lateral preferences and handedness, particularly for bimanually controlled tasks. Athletes who demonstrate a left preference for tasks such as baseball batting or boxing are not necessarily left-handed as determined by handedness preference measures such as the EHI. We anticipate that usage of a more specific and differentiated terminology will reduce researchers' susceptibility to choose task-*un*related reference values (e.g., handedness for throwing) when testing, for example, if there is a higher incidence of left-*oriented* ('southpaw') fighters in boxing [12] or MMA [33]. Our call for more careful use of the term 'handedness' is also motivated by the term's typical use for describing someone's hand preference for *uni*manual, but not for bimanual, tasks [41,42]. As a side note, we acknowledge that some researchers actually determined athletes' handedness through preference questionnaires and therefore the use of the terms left- and right-handedness in the respective works was justified (e.g., in boxing [43] and wrestling [44]). However, the problem is that those studies, in turn, missed to also report the athletes' lateral preferences for the respective domain-specific tasks (e.g., fighting stance) such that it remains unclear whether the differences discovered in fight records were actually due to mechanisms related to handedness, as proposed by the authors, and not to sport-

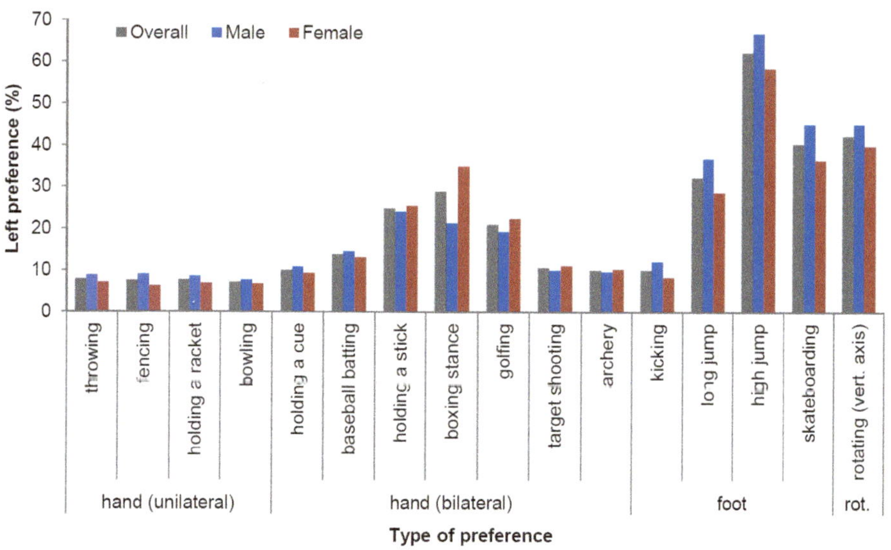

Figure 1. Left preferences for sport-specific tasks overall and differentiated by sex.

Table 2. Relationship between sport-specific lateral preferences and handedness.

		Overall		Male		Female	
Type of preference	**Task**	**N**	r_{pb}	**N**	r_{pb}	**N**	r_{pb}
hand (unilateral)	throwing	888	.812	402	.793	486	.831
	fencing	883	.840	400	.860	483	.816
	holding a racket	890	.851	402	.858	488	.844
	bowling	888	.758	404	.727	484	.791
hand (bilateral)	holding a cue	867	.757	398	.824	469	.690
	baseball batting	847	.461	390	.397	457	.524
	holding a stick	812	.254	365	.175	447	.328
	boxing stance	819	.323	370	.417	449	.276
	golfing	832	.298	381	.232	451	.362
	target shooting	824	.599	383	.668	441	.544
	archery	861	.685	398	.737	463	.645
foot	kicking	834	.557	378	.437	456	.687
	long jump	814	.199	379	$.104^{b}$	435	.292
	high jump	808	−.193	371	−.189	437	−.210
	skateboarding	773	.125	347	$.094^{ns}$	426	$.145^{a}$
rotation	rotating (vertical axis)	753	$.044^{ns}$	329	$-.027^{ns}$	424	$.100^{b}$

Note: For the calculation of r_{pb} we excluded 'no preference' responses for the sport-specific tasks. The majority of relationships were significant with $p<.001$. To facilitate reading the table, only non-significant relationships or significant relationships with *p*-values larger than.001 are indicated as follows: ^{ns} $p>.05$, ^{a} $p<.01$, ^{b} $p<.05$. Please also note that we additionally clustered the participants into left- (LS <0) and right-handers (LS ≥0) and that we used these classifications to determine the relationship between handedness and sport-specific lateral preferences based on the calculation of phi coefficients Φ. In two calculation scenarios, once with inclusion and once with exclusion of 'no preference' responses, similar relationships as those reported above were found (see Table S3 for a summary of the results).

Table 3. Left- and right-handers' lateral preferences for sport-specific tasks.

	Male				Female			
	Left-hander		Right-hander		Left-hander		Right-hander	
Task	L (%)	R (%)	L (%)	R (%)	L (%)	R (%)	L (%)	R (%)
throwing	32 (78.05)	9 (21.95)	4 (1.11)	357 (98.89)	32 (84.21)	6 (15.79)	3 (0.67)	445 (99.33)
fencing	35 (87.5)	5 (12.5)	2 (0.56)	358 (99.44)	28 (82.35)	6 (17.65)	3 (0.67)	446 (99.33)
holding a racket	33 (82.5)	7 (17.5)	2 (0.55)	360 (99.45)	32 (86.49)	5 (13.51)	2 (0.44)	449 (99.56)
bowling	27 (65.85)	14 (34.15)	4 (1.1)	359 (98.9)	29 (76.32)	9 (23.68)	4 (0.9)	442 (99.1)
holding a cue	35 (89.74)	4 (10.26)	9 (2.51)	350 (97.49)	29 (78.38)	8 (21.62)	17 (3.94)	415 (96.06)
baseball batting	23 (58.97)	16 (41.03)	36 (10.26)	315 (89.74)	27 (72.97)	10 (27.03)	37 (8.81)	383 (91.19)
holding a stick	19 (50)	19 (50)	78 (23.85)	249 (76.15)	28 (73.68)	10 (26.32)	96 (23.47)	313 (76.53)
boxing stance	30 (75)	10 (25)	56 (16.97)	274 (83.03)	28 (77.78)	8 (22.22)	143 (34.62)	270 (65.38)
golfing	20 (51.28)	19 (48.72)	58 (16.96)	284 (83.04)	27 (71.05)	11 (28.95)	82 (19.85)	331 (80.15)
target shooting	27 (72.97)	10 (27.03)	13 (3.76)	333 (96.24)	26 (70.27)	11 (29.73)	28 (6.93)	376 (93.07)
archery	30 (75)	10 (25)	9 (2.51)	349 (97.49)	30 (78.95)	8 (21.05)	20 (4.71)	405 (95.29)
kicking	22 (55)	18 (45)	27 (7.99)	311 (92.01)	27 (79.41)	7 (20.59)	14 (3.32)	408 (96.68)
long jump	19 (48.72)	20 (51.28)	130 (38.24)	210 (61.76)	29 (76.32)	9 (23.68)	111 (27.96)	286 (72.04)
high jump (foot)	18 (47.37)	20 (52.63)	252 (75.68)	81 (24.32)	12 (36.36)	21 (63.64)	274 (67.82)	130 (32.18)
skateboarding	24 (63.16)	14 (36.84)	159 (51.46)	150 (48.54)	21 (60)	14 (40)	158 (40.41)	233 (59.59)
rotating (vertical axis)	18 (50)	18 (50)	164 (55.97)	129 (44.03)	17 (58.62)	12 (41.38)	179 (45.32)	216 (54.68)

Note: For each sport-specific task, 'no preference' responses are excluded. Participants were classified as left- and right-handers based on their individual LS values (i.e., left-hander if LS <0 and right-hander if LS ≥ 0). 'L' and 'R' indicate left and right preference for a sport task.

specific lateral preferences in combination with sport-specific performance demands (for a critical review, e.g. see [14]).

Second, in conjunction with being more sensitive to the terminology, our findings highlight the need for task-specific normal population reference values when the aim is to identify if athletes with a left preference are overrepresented. This is a fundamental requirement particularly for sports where actions are bimanually controlled as in baseball or cricket batting, shooting in ice hockey, or fighting in boxing or MMA. Since left preferences were higher for such tasks compared to unimanual tasks (e.g., in our male participants the left preference for boxing was 2.4 times higher than the left preference for throwing), not controlling for task-specific reference values may result in biased results and conclusions. To exemplify, we re-analysed apparently enhanced frequencies of left-oriented performers in the elite domains of baseball (batting: 24.0%, $N=445$, [12]), cricket (batting: 15.6%, $N=371$, [12]), boxing (23.1%, $N=26$, [12]) and MMA (20.4%, $N=245$, [33]; 17.4%, $N=1468$, [34]). Chi-square goodness-of-fit-tests revealed that, when task-specific reference values are considered (i.e., 14.46% and 21.23% left preference in males for batting and fight stance, respectively), a significant excess of left preference was only found for baseball batting (associated with a medium effect size, $\omega=.27$, according to Cohen's conventions [45]). Thus, in contrast to predictions of the fighting hypothesis, left-oriented performers seem not overrepresented in samples taken from combat-like interactive sports such as boxing or MMA.

Third, albeit most relationships between sport-specific lateral preferences and handedness were statistically significant ($p<.05$; see Table 2), the fact that correlations were far from being 'perfect' challenges inferences as to a frequency-dependent maintenance of left-handedness in humans based on sports data. Not every athlete who demonstrates a left or right preference for sport-specific tasks must necessarily be left- or right-handed. A prominent example is the Spanish tennis professional Rafael Nadal, who plays tennis left-handed but is right-handed for most other tasks [46]. Therefore, sports data may be of limited suitability for testing evolutionary theories of handedness [12] or related models [10]. Similarly, the imperfect relationships between sport-specific lateral preferences and handedness cast doubt on alternative explanations like that an excess of performers with a left preference is due to handedness-dependent differences in neurological functioning (e.g., see [24,43] for such argumentation). Generally, our findings demonstrate that it is difficult, if possible at all, to properly attribute increased frequencies or better fight records of athletes who have a sport-specific left preference to mechanisms associated with left-handedness [14,25].

The data presented here might serve as reference values for future research on laterality effects in sports. In this regard, we would like to emphasize that we conservatively estimated the sport-specific left preferences by including all cases into the calculation of frequencies (i.e., 'left', 'right', and 'no preference' answers) instead of considering the number of 'left' and 'right' answers only. Thus, the percentages of sport-specific left preferences found here might even underestimate the "true" ratio of performers with a sport-specific left preference (raw frequencies are available in Table S2). Still, the frequencies identified here clearly show that sport-specific reference values are essential to adequately test observed frequencies of left preferences in sports for potential overrepresentation.

As pointed out earlier, our focus was on uni- or bimanually controlled actions in sports. With regard to non-manual actions, lateral preferences also varied considerably across the different sport tasks and relationships with handedness were moderate to low or even absent (see Table 2). Similar to previous work [27], the majority of participants preferred to use their right foot for kicking a ball or for jumping off in long jump. Also, most participants preferred their left foot for jumping off in high jump, which means that one has to approach the crossbar from the right side (please note that all participants were informed about this relationship in the questionnaire). The left foot preference in high jump appears remarkable in light of the predominance of right preferences for other tasks. A sound theoretical explanation for the occurrence of such left foot preference is missing up to now [47,48], but speculating about it is beyond the scope of this paper. Furthermore, lateral preferences were least asymmetric for skateboarding and rotating along the vertical axis (see Figure 1). This pattern might be explained by task demands. More specifically, more than the other tasks investigated here, both hands and feet are substantially involved in the motor control of skateboarding or rotating along the vertical axis (e.g., in order to balance or to swing before spinning) and thus biased lateral preferences might not evolve to the extent known for other tasks such as throwing or baseball batting.

Finally, we would like to comment on two potential limitations of our work. First, we cannot completely rule out the possibility that some participants were not familiar with carrying out some of the sport tasks (e.g., holding a stick in ice hockey). Motor unfamiliarity might have affected those participants' indication of lateral preference for the respective items; although the direction of such potential biasing effect is unclear (i.e., over- or underestimation of left preferences). Previous work that assessed sport-specific lateral preferences in the normal population based on motor tests, however, found values similar to those reported here [27,49]. Second, we determined our participants' handedness based on a preference questionnaire. While the EHI is one of the most widely used instruments to assess handedness and preference and performance measures of handedness appear highly correlated [42], inclusion of both preference and performance measures may still have resulted in better classification of left- and right-handedness [50]. We acknowledge this aspect as a potential limitation. At the same time, however, we suppose that even if we had included both types of handedness measurements into the protocol, similar varying relationships between sport-specific lateral preferences and handedness, as identified in the present work, would have emerged.

Conclusions

Collectively, we showed that the frequency of the normal population's left preference depends on the sport task and that the relationship between sport-specific lateral preferences and handedness is highly variable. Task-specific reference values are mandatory when testing for an excess of 'left-oriented' athletes in sports. Also, we call for more careful use of the term 'handedness' within research on sport-specific lateral preferences for reasons discussed above. To help unravel the impact of handedness and task-specific lateral preference on high achievement in sports or related behavioural domains, future work is encouraged to include both preference and performance measures as well as to consider the performance demands associated with the domain of interest.

Supporting Information

Table S1 Pictures used to facilitate understanding of left and right for sport-specific tasks.

Table S2 Lateral preferences for sport-specific tasks (raw frequencies).

Table S3 Relationship between sport-specific lateral preferences and handedness.

Acknowledgments

We thank Stefan Kastaun, Benedikt Bussiek and Timo Nocke for their help with data collection.

Author Contributions

Conceived and designed the experiments: FL FS NH. Performed the experiments: FL FS NH. Analyzed the data: FL. Wrote the paper: FL FS NH.

References

1. McManus IC (2002) Right hand, left hand: The origins of asymmetry in brains, bodies, atoms and culture. London: Weidenfeld & Nicolson.
2. Raymond M, Pontier D (2004) Is there geographical variation in human handedness? Laterality 9: 35–51.
3. Faurie C, Schiefenhövel W, Le Bomin S, Billiard S, Raymond M (2005) Variation in the frequency of left-handedness in traditional societies. Current Anthropology 46: 142–147.
4. Gilbert AN, Wysocki CJ (1992) Hand preference and age in the United States. Neuropsychologia 30: 601–608.
5. Peters M, Reimers S, Manning JT (2006) Hand preference for writing and associations with selected demographic and behavioral variables in 255,100 subjects: The BBC internet study. Brain Cogn 62: 177–189.
6. Frayer DW, Lozano M, Bermúdez de Castro JM, Carbonell E, Arsuaga JL, et al. (2012) More than 500,000 years of right-handedness in Europe. Laterality 17: 51–69.
7. Faurie C, Raymond M (2004) Handedness frequency over more than ten thousand years. Proc R Soc Lond B Biol Sci 271: S43–S45.
8. Vallortigara G (2006) The evolutionary psychology of left and right: costs and benefits of lateralization. Dev Psychobiol 48: 418–427.
9. Llaurens V, Raymond M, Faurie C (2009) Why are some people left-handed? An evolutionary perspective. Phil Trans R Soc B 364: 881–894.
10. Abrams DM, Panaggio MJ (2012) A model balancing cooperation and competition can explain our right-handed world and the dominance of left-handed athletes. J R Soc Interface 9: 2718–2722.
11. Faurie C, Raymond M (2013) The fighting hypothesis as an evolutionary explanation for the handedness polymorphism in humans: where are we? Ann N Y Acad Sci 1288: 110–113.
12. Raymond M, Pontier D, Dufour AB, Møller AP (1996) Frequency-dependent maintenance of left handedness in humans. Proc R Soc Lond B Biol Sci 263: 1627–1633.
13. Groothuis TGG, McManus IC, Schaafsma SM, Geuze RH (2013) The fighting hypothesis in combat: how well does the fighting hypothesis explain human left-handed minorities? Ann N Y Acad Sci 1288: 100–109.
14. Loffing F, Hagemann N (2012) Side bias in human performance: A review on the left-handers' advantage in sports. In: Dutta T, Mandal M, Kumar S, editors. Bias in Human Behaviour. Hauppauge, NY: Nova Science. 163–182.
15. Grouios G (2004) Motoric dominance and sporting excellence: Training versus heredity. Percept Motor Skills 98: 53–66.
16. Aggleton JP, Wood CJ (1990) Is there a left-handed advantage in 'ballistic' sports? Int J Sport Psychol 21: 46–57.
17. Hagemann N (2009) The advantage of being left-handed in interactive sports. Atten Percept Psycho 71: 1641–1648.
18. Loffing F, Hagemann N, Strauss B (2010) Automated processes in tennis: Do left-handed players benefit from the tactical preferences of their opponents? J Sports Sci 28: 435–443.
19. Loffing F, Schorer J, Hagemann N, Baker J (2012) On the advantage of being left-handed in volleyball: Further evidence of the specificity of skilled visual perception. Atten Percept Psycho 74: 446–453.
20. Schorer J, Loffing F, Hagemann N, Baker J (2012) Human handedness in interactive situations: Negative perceptual frequency effects can be reversed! J Sports Sci 30: 507–513.
21. Loffing F, Hagemann N (2014) Zum Einfluss des Anlaufwinkels und der Füßigkeit des Schützen auf die Antizipation von Elfmeterschüssen [On the effect of a shooter's approach angle and kicking foot on the anticipation of penalty-kicks]. Zeitschrift für Sportpsychologie 21: 63–73.
22. Dane S, Sekertekin MA (2005) Differences in handedness and scores of aggressiveness and interpersonal relations of soccer players. Percept Motor Skills 100: 743–746.
23. Gorynia I, Egenter D (2000) Intermanual coordination in relation to handedness, familial sinistrality and lateral preferences. Cortex 36: 1–18.
24. Holtzen DW (2000) Handedness and professional tennis. Int J Neurosci 105: 101–119.
25. Wood CJ, Aggleton JP (1989) Handedness in 'fast ball' sports: do left-handers have an innate advantage? BJP 80: 227–240.
26. McLean JM, Ciurczak FM (1982) Bimanual dexterity in major league baseball players: a statistical study. The New England Journal of Medicine 307: 1278–1279.
27. Oberbeck H (1989) Seitigkeitsphänomene und Seitigkeitstypologie im Sport [Phenomena and profiles of sidedness in sports]. Schorndorf: Hofmann.
28. Loffing F, Schorer J, Cobley SP (2010) Relative Age Effects are a developmental problem in tennis: but not necessarily when you're left-handed! High Ability Studies 21: 19–25.
29. Loffing F, Hagemann N, Strauss B (2012) Left-handedness in professional and amateur tennis. PLoS ONE 7: e49325.
30. Peters M, Murphy K (1992) Cluster analysis reveals at least three, and possibly five distinct handedness groups. Neuropsychologia 30: 373–380.
31. Brooks R, Bussière LF, Jennions MD, Hunt J (2004) Sinister strategies succeed at the cricket World Cup. Proc R Soc Lond B Biol Sci 271: S64–S66.
32. Puterman J, Schorer J, Baker J (2010) Laterality differences in elite ice hockey: An investigation of shooting and catching orientations. J Sports Sci 28: 1581–1593.
33. Pollet TV, Stulp G, Groothuis TGG (2013) Born to win? Testing the fighting hypothesis in realistic fights: Left-handedness in the ultimate fighting championship. Anim Behav 86: 839–843.
34. Baker J, Schorer J (2013) The Southpaw Advantage? – Lateral Preference in Mixed Martial Arts. PLoS ONE 8: e79793.
35. Mikheev M, Mohr C, Afanasiev S, Landis T, Thut G (2002) Motor control and cerebral hemispheric specialization in highly qualified judo wrestlers. Neuropsychologia 40: 1209–1219.
36. Oldfield RC (1971) The assessment and analysis of handedness: The Edinburgh inventory. Neuropsychologia 9: 97–113.
37. Schachter SC (2000) The quantification and definition of handedness: implications for handedness research. In: Mandal MK, Bulman-Fleming MB, Tiwari G, editors. Side bias: A neuropsychological perspective. Dordrecht: Kluwer. 155–174.
38. Fazio R, Coenen C, Denney RL (2011) The original instructions for the Edinburgh Handedness Inventory are misunderstood by a majority of participants. Laterality 17: 70–77.
39. Coren S (1993) The lateral preference inventory for measurement of handedness, footedness, eyedness, and earedness: Norms for young adults. BPS 31: 1–3.
40. Büsch D, Hagemann N, Bender N (2010) The dimensionality of the Edinburgh Handedness Inventory: An analysis with models of the item response theory. Laterality 15: 610–628.
41. Annett M (1970) A classification of hand preference by association analysis. BJP 61: 303–321.
42. Brown SG, Roy EA, Rohr LE, Bryden PJ (2006) Using hand performance measures to predict handedness. Laterality 11: 1–14.
43. Gursoy R (2009) Effects of left- or right-hand preference on the success of boxers in Turkey. Br J Sports Med 43: 142–144.
44. Ziyagil MA, Gursoy R, Dane S, Yuksel R (2010) Left-handed wrestlers are more successful. Percept Motor Skills 111: 65–70.
45. Cohen J (1988) Statistical power analysis for the behavioral sciences. Hillsdale, NJ: Erlbaum.
46. Gorney C (17 June 2009). Ripped. (Or Torn Up?). The New York Times. Available: http://www.nytimes.com/2009/06/21/magazine/21nadal-t.html?pagewanted=all&_r=0. Accessed 25 June 2014.
47. Friberg O, Kvist M (1988) Factors determining the preference of takeoff leg in jumping. Int J Sports Med 09: 349–352.
48. Miyaguchi K, Demura S (2010) Specific factors that influence deciding the takeoff leg during jumping movements. Journal of Strength and Conditioning Research 24: 2516–2522.
49. Oberbeck H (1992) Seitigkeitstypologie im Leistungssport [Sidedness profiles in competitive sports]. Leistungssport 22: 35–40.
50. Corey DM, Hurley MM, Foundas AL (2001) Right and left handedness defined: a multivariate approach using hand preference and hand performance measures. Neuropsychiatry, Neuropsychology and Behavioral Neurology 14: 144–152.

13

Optimizing the Prediction Process: From Statistical Concepts to the Case Study of Soccer

Andreas Heuer[1,2]*, **Oliver Rubner**[1,2]

1 Institute of Physical Chemistry, WWU Muenster, Muenster, Germany, **2** Center of Nonlinear Science CeNoS, WWU Muenster, Muenster, Germany

Abstract

We present a systematic approach for prediction purposes based on panel data, involving information about different interacting subjects and different times (here: two). The corresponding bivariate regression problem can be solved analytically for the final statistical estimation error. Furthermore, this expression is simplified for the special case that the subjects do not change their properties between the last measurement and the prediction period. This statistical framework is applied to the prediction of soccer matches, based on information from the previous and the present season. It is determined how well the outcome of soccer matches can be predicted theoretically. This optimum limit is compared with the actual quality of the prediction, taking the German premier league as an example. As a key step for the actual prediction process one has to identify appropriate observables which reflect the strength of the individual teams as close as possible. A criterion to distinguish different observables is presented. Surprisingly, chances for goals turn out to be much better suited than the goals themselves to characterize the strength of a team. Routes towards further improvement of the prediction are indicated. Finally, two specific applications are discussed.

Editor: Dominik Wodarz, University of California Irvine, United States of America

Funding: The authors acknowledge support by Deutsche Forschungsgemeinschaft and Open Access Publication Fund of University of Muenster. The funders had no role in study design, data collection and analysis, decision to publish, or preparation of the manuscript.

Competing Interests: The authors have declared that no competing interests exist.

* Email: andheuer@uni-muenster.de

Introduction

Panel data analysis deals with a regression procedure where individual subjects as well as information at different times is taken into account [1]. The update of estimators with time can be related to Bayesian approaches [2,3] as explicitly discussed, e.g., in [4]. For Gaussian statistics there exists a direct connection between Bayesian inference and a regression analysis; see, e.g., [5]. Actually, Bayesian inference to soccer has recently been discussed in Ref. [6].

Of key interest is the knowledge about the quality of the estimator. Here we simplify the general result by using the assumption that the underlying property of the subject does not change between the final measurement and the prognosis time interval. This does not necessarily hold for the time of earlier measurements. However, due to the random noise, by which the most recent measurement may be disturbed, it may still be favorable to take into account older pieces of information. Having an explicit expression of the estimator quality it is possible to judge the relevance of the available information for the prediction process in a detailed manner. Furthermore, we can define the limit of optimum prediction and judge, how far a specific prediction procedure differs from this limit.

We apply this approach to the prediction of soccer matches but we expect that it may have a broader applicability for many different types of sports and beyond where the future achievements of, generally speaking, different subjects is constant between the most previous measurement and the near future.

To set the present approach into perspective, we would like to summarise some specific approaches for soccer prediction. In one type of models [7–10] appropriate parameters are introduced to characterise the properties of individual teams such as the offensive strength. Of course, the characterisation of team strengths is not only restricted to soccer; see, e.g., [11]. The specific values of these parameters can be obtained via Monte-Carlo techniques. These models can then be used for prediction purposes and allow one to calculate probabilities for individual match results. A key element of these approaches is the Poissonian nature of scoring goals [12–14]. Beyond these goals-based prediction properties also results-based models are used. Here the final result (home win, draw, away win) is predicted from comparison of the difference of the team strength parameters with some fixed values [15]. The quality of both approaches has been compared and no significant differences have been found [16]. Going beyond these approaches additional covariates can be included. For example home and away strengths are considered individually or the geographical distance is taken into account [16]. Recently, also the ELO-based ratings have been used for the purpose of forecasting soccer matches [17]. Recent studies suggest that statistical models are superior to lay and expert predictions but have less predictive power than the bookmaker odds [17–20]. This observation strongly suggests that either the information, used by the bookmakers, is more powerful or, alternatively, the inference process, based on the same information, is more efficient. Probably, both aspects may play a role.

The structure of this paper is as follows. First, we introduce the statistical background of prediction. In particular we show that under the general assumptions, mentioned above, the quality of the estimation can be determined in simple analytical terms. Then this general scheme is applied to the prediction of soccer matches, using the German premier league (Bundesliga) as an example. It can be shown that all assumptions, used in the previous Section, are fulfilled to a very good approximation. Furthermore, it is shown that chances for goals possess a very high information content about the individual team strengths and are, thus, chosen for the respective covariates. Subsequently, the theoretical results are compared with the explicit bivariate regression analysis. The specific setting is chosen such that one wants to predict the outcome of the second half of a season, based on knowledge of a variable number of matches from the first half of the same season as well as all matches of the previous season. In particular we discuss the dependence of the prediction quality on the number of matches, taken into account. Furthermore, it is shown, how the present concepts can be applied to the prediction of single matches. We end with a discussion.

The Statistical Background of Prediction

Variables

We consider two successive time intervals, in which we measure the independent variables X and Y. For the later application to soccer this might be the accumulated goal difference during the previous season and during the present season, measured individually for each team. Here we consider differences in order to capture both the offensive and defensive strength. Specifically, we perform this analysis after half of the present season is over. Naturally, this can be easily generalized to other situations. The aim is to predict the goal difference Z, i.e. the dependent variable, of each team during the second half of the season. This setup is sketched in Fig.1. The prediction quality can be explicitly expressed and compared with the theoretical optimum.

Regression

First, we briefly review some key relations of regression analysis. We start with the linear relation $Z = bY$ for the independent variable Y and the dependent variable Z. Note that we assume all variables fulfill the condition that their first moment is zero. Generalisation is, of course, straightforward. The regression problem requires the minimisation of $\langle (Z-\hat{Z})^2 \rangle$ with respect to b where $\hat{Z} = bY$ is the predictor of Z. Substituting the resulting value of $b_{opt} = corr(Y,Z)\sqrt{Var(Z)/Var(Y)}$ yields for the optimum quadratic variation, denoted $\chi^2(Y)$,

$$\chi^2(Y) = Var(Z)\left[1 - [corr(Y,Z)]^2\right] \tag{1}$$

where $Var(Z)$ denotes the variance of the distribution of Z and

$$corr(Y,Z) = \frac{\langle YZ \rangle}{\sqrt{Var(Y)Var(Z)}} \tag{2}$$

is the Pearson correlation coefficient between the variables Y and Z. Eq.1 has a simple intuitive interpretation: The higher the correlation between the variables Y and Z, the better the predictability of Z in terms of Y.

For the present work we are mainly dealing with the bivariate regression $\hat{Z} = aX + bY$. Via normal equations, one can obtain general expressions for the regression coefficients a and b. Interestingly, the prediction quality of the bivariate prediction can be analogously expressed to Eq.1 and reads

$$\chi^2(X,Y) = \chi^2(Y)\left[1 - [corr(X-Y, Z-Y)]^2\right] \tag{3}$$

where the partial correlation coefficient

$$corr(X-Y,Z-Y) = \frac{corr(X,Z) - corr(X,Y)corr(Y,Z)}{\sqrt{1-corr(X,Y)^2}\sqrt{1-corr(Y,Z)^2}} \tag{4}$$

is used and $\chi^2(Y)$ is defined as in Eq.1. The second factor on the right-hand side of Eq.3 explicitly contains the additional information of the variable X as compared to Y. One can easily show that in agreement with expectation Eq.3 is completely symmetric in X and Y.

Here we present a straightforward derivation of Eq.3. Let $d_{Y\,Z}$ denote the solution of the regression problem $Z = dY$. Accordingly, $d_{Y\,X}$ is the solution of the regression problem $X = dY$. In a next step one defines the new variables $\tilde{Z} = Z - d_{Y\,Z}Y$ and $\tilde{X} = X - d_{Y\,X}Y$. For these new variables the correlation with Y is explicitly taken out. A straightforward calculation shows that the Pearson correlation coefficient $corr(\tilde{X},\tilde{Z})$ is exactly given by the partial correlation coefficient $corr(X-Y,Z-Y)$.

Now we consider the regression problem of interest $Z = aX + bY$. In a first step it is formally rewritten as

$$Z - d_{Y\,Z}Y = a(X - d_{Y\,X}Y) + (b - d_{Y\,Z} + a d_{Y\,X})Y. \tag{5}$$

Using the above notation and introducing the new regression parameter $\tilde{b}$ we abbreviate this relation via

$$\tilde{Z} = a\tilde{X} + \tilde{b}Y. \tag{6}$$

By construction the observable Y is uncorrelated to $\tilde{X}$ and $\tilde{Z}$. Therefore the independent variable Y does not play any role for the prediction of $\tilde{Z}$ so that effectively one just has a single-variable regression problem. Therefore one can immediately write

$$\chi^2(X,Y) = Var(\tilde{Z})\left[1 - [corr(\tilde{X},\tilde{Z})]^2\right]. \tag{7}$$

The first factor is identical to $\chi^2(Y)$ whereas the Pearson correlation coefficient in the second factor is identical to $corr(X-Y,Z-Y)$. This concludes the derivation of Eq.3.

Prediction for individual subjects/teams

As introduced, the variables X, Y, Z denote the output of a team or, more generally, of some subject during three successive time intervals. For the first time interval, the outcome of team i is

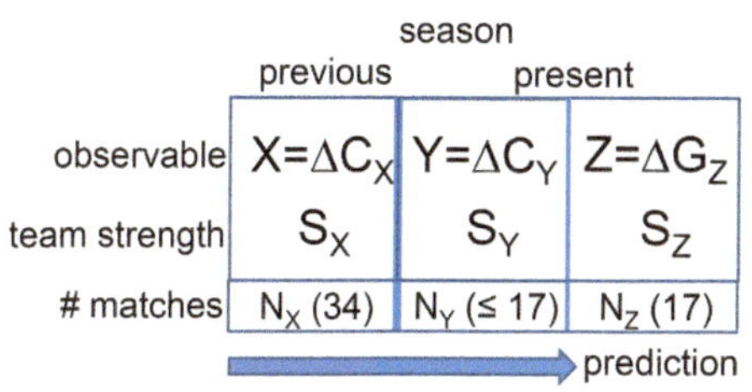

Figure 1. Schematic representation of the general prediction setup.

denoted x_i. Conceptually, this value has contributions from the true underlying team strength $s_{X,i}$ as well as from random non-predictable effects $\epsilon_{X,i}$, i.e.

$$x_i = s_{x,i} + \epsilon_{x,i}. \tag{8}$$

Thus, only in the absence of random effects the team strength $s_{X,i}$ could be directly identified with the outcome x_i. In what follows we use the terminology of soccer but this approach can be directly applied to other cases where the observable is the sum of the properties of the respective subject and some random effects.

Following the previous discussion we only consider observables X for which the first moment disappears after averaging over all teams. Naturally, the same holds for the team strength observable S_X. Squaring Eq.8 and averaging over all teams yields

$$Var(X) = Var(S_X) + Var(\epsilon_x). \tag{9}$$

Analogous relations hold for $Var(Y)$ and $Var(Z)$.

For the evaluation of the prediction quality Eq.3 one needs to calculate individual correlations such as $corr(Y,Z)$. A straightforward calculation yields

$$corr(Y,Z) = \frac{corr(S_Y,S_Z)}{\sqrt{1+Var(\epsilon_Y)/Var(S_Y)}\sqrt{1+Var(\epsilon_Z)/Var(S_Z)}}. \tag{10}$$

Again, analogous expressions hold for $corr(X,Z)$ and $corr(X,Y)$.

Eq.10 allows one to identify two distinct reasons why the correlation of Y and Z is smaller than unity. First, the team strength may change between the two time intervals, i.e. $corr(S_Y,S_Z)<1$. Second, the random effects, which influence the observables Y and Z, may play an important role $(Var(\epsilon_Y), Var(\epsilon_Z)>0)$.

The subsequent discussion is based on the mathematical identity

$$\frac{corr(X,Y)}{corr(X,Z)corr(Y,Z)} = \frac{corr(S_X,S_Y)}{corr(S_X,S_Z)corr(S_Y,S_Z)}\left(1+\frac{Var(\epsilon_Z)}{Var(S_Z)}\right). \tag{11}$$

As a first step of simplification we want to estimate the team strength S_Z rather than Z itself. Then the prediction quality is denoted by $\tilde{\chi}^2(X,Y)$. All relations remain identical except $Var(\epsilon_Z)=0$ in the evaluation of quantities, occurring in Eq.3. Naturally, one has the simple relation

$$\chi^2(X,Y) = \tilde{\chi}^2(X,Y) + Var(\epsilon_Z). \tag{12}$$

As the second step we consider the special case that the team strengths are the same in the second and third time interval, belonging to Y and Z, respectively. Actually, it has been already shown in Ref. [21] that apart from short-time fluctuations the team strength remains constant during the course of a season. As a consequence one has $S_Y \approx S_Z$, i.e. nearly the same team strength in the first and the second half of a season. Mathematically, we assume a strict equality. The corresponding empirical result will be discussed further below. A mathematical consequence is (see below for specific data) $corr(S_X,S_Y) = corr(S_X,S_Z)$. Under this assumption, Eq.11 can be rewritten as

$$corr(X,Y) = corr(X,S_Z)corr(Y,S_Z). \tag{13}$$

Inserting this relation into Eq.3 for the prediction quality of S_Z the general expression simplifies significantly and one obtains

$$\tilde{\chi}^2(X,Y) = Var(S_Z)\frac{(1-[corr(Y,S_Z)]^2)(1-[corr(X,S_Z)]^2)}{1-[corr(X,Y)]^2}. \tag{14}$$

This is the key relation to be used when estimating the quality of the prediction. Apart from the assumption of constant properties during the final two time intervals, this relation is generally valid.

Application to the Case of Soccer Prediction: Concepts

General

Our general goal is the prediction of the future results of soccer matches. Specific data are taken for the German premier league (Bundesliga), employing information about all matches between the seasons 1995/96 and 2010/11. During a season a team has 34 matches.

Our goal is the prediction of the aggregated results z_i of each team i of the second half of a season, based on knowledge about N_Y match results y_i from the first half of the season as well as the $N_X = 34$ results x_i from the previous season. As the dependent variable z_i we choose the goal difference but a similar analysis could be also performed for points; see again Fig.1. Of course, due to the generality of our approach also different prediction problems can be handled. For the explicit calculations of the goal differences we correct for the home advantages [5] so that the statistical properties are independent of the home advantage.

Disentangling random and systematic effects

For our analysis it is essential to decompose the variables X,Y and Z into its systematic parts $(S_{X,Y,Z})$ and its random contributions $(\epsilon_{X,Y,Z})$; see Eq.8. As mentioned above, z_i will be identified as the goal difference of team i after N_Z matches, normalised by N_Z. In case of matches under identical conditions the random effects are averaged out as reflected by the standard scaling relation $Var(\epsilon_Z) \propto 1/N_Z$ where the proportionality constant is denoted V_Z. Thus, we have

$$Var(\epsilon_Z) = \frac{V_Z}{N_Z}. \tag{15}$$

By studying the dependence of $Var(Z)$ on N_Z the systematic and random contributions to $Var(Z)$, as expressed in Eq.9, can be identified. Of course, analogous relations hold for X and Y.

Strictly speaking, the scaling with the inverse number of the matches breaks down for N_Z close to unity because then different strenghts of the opponents no longer average out. In practice it turns out that for $N_Z > 4$ the difference of the N_Z opponents has sufficiently averaged out. This dependence on the number of considered matches has been explicitly analysed in Ref. [5,22]. For the present set of data we obtain $Var(S_Z) = 0.21$ and $V_Z = 2.95$. Actually, V_Z is very close to the total number of goals per match (2.85). This expectation is compatible with the assumption of independent Poisson processes.

Choice of observables

The goal is to predict the goal difference Z or, alternatively, the team strength S_Z. A natural choice for the independent variables X and Y are the goal differences in the respective time intervals. In what follows, goal differences are denoted as ΔG. However, as will be shown below, this choice is far from optimum. Generally speaking, one aims for observables which contain as much information as possible about the team strength.

How to capture the information content of a given observable? For this discussion we restrict ourselves to the prediction problem $Y \rightarrow Z$ to be solved via a simple univariate regression as summarised above (see Eq.1). For this analysis we use $N_Y = N_Z = 17$, i.e. all matches from the first and second half of the season, respectively. The quality of the prediction is captured by $corr(Y,Z)$. The larger the value $corr(Y,Z)$, the better the prediction and thus the higher the information content of Y about the team strength. From the empirical data we obtain $corr(Y = \Delta G_Y, Z = \Delta G_Z) = 0.56$.

Can one increase $corr(Y,Z)$ significantly beyond the value of 0.56 by using other observables? The scoring of goals is the final step in a series of match events. One may thus hope that there exist other match characteristics which are even more informative about the team strength. A possible candidate is the number of chances for goals. They are provided by a professional sports journal (www.kicker.de) for all seasons, considered in this work. We denote the chances for goals as $C_\pm$ and the goals as $G_\pm$. The sign indicates whether it refers to the considered team (+) or the opponent of that team (−).

Next we define the scoring efficiencies $p_\pm$ via the relation

$$G_\pm = C_\pm \cdot p_\pm . \qquad (16)$$

Here, $p_+ (= G_+/C_+)$ denotes the probability that the team is able to convert a chance for a goal into a real goal and $1 - p_-$ that the team manages to not concede a goal after a chance for a goal of the opponent. Averaging over all teams and seasons one obtains $\langle p_\pm \rangle = 0.24$. Thus, every forth chance for a goal ends up in a goal.

In Fig.2 the actual scoring efficiencies p_+ after a season are shown together with the respective values of ΔC. Very clearly, the goal efficiencies are widely distributed between approx. 15% and 35%. On average, better teams with a larger value of ΔC have a slightly better efficiency to score goals and more likely avoid to concede goals (correlation coefficients ± 0.26). Despite this small correlation, the large scatter of $p_\pm$ cannot be explained in terms of ΔC.

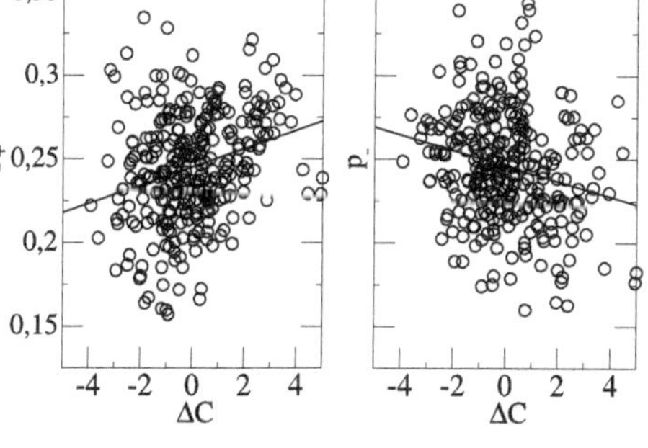

Figure 2. The efficiency factors $p_\pm$ as a function of the differences of the chances for goals ΔC.

This large unexplained variance seems to imply that the scoring efficiencies strongly vary from team to team in an a priori unknown way. As a consequence the chances for goals would hardly contain additional information about the expected number of goals, which a team is going to score in the future. In particular, the estimation of the team strength, which is defined on the basis of goals, would hardly be improved by taking into account the chances for goals.

With the definition $\Delta C = C_+ - C_-$ this statement is equivalent to the presence of a weak correlation between ΔC_Y and ΔG_Z. However, this preliminary conclusion is wrong. Rather the correlation coefficient turns out to be $corr(Y = \Delta C_Y, Z = \Delta G_Z) = 0.65$ which is much larger than the value of $corr(Y = \Delta G_Y, Z = \Delta G_Z) = 0.56$. Stated differently, the chances for goals are by far more informative for the prediction of the team strength than the goals themselves!

Why chances for goals are so informative

This observation could be rationalized under the hypothesis that the scoring efficiencies are very similar for all teams. Qualitatively, one can argue in this limit that random effects are stronger for goals than for chances for goals, since the number of goals is typically smaller than the number of chances for goals. To quantify this aspect, we consider a simple example of a fictive coin-tossing tournament where the head appears with probability p which in this simple example is given by $1/2$. A team is allowed to toss the coin M times per round. In the first round this results in g_1 times tossing the head. Thus, in the first round one has observed the number of tosses M as well as the number of heads g_1. In the relation to soccer M would correspond to the number of chances for goals and g_1 to the number of goals in that match. In order to keep the argument simple we assume that M is a constant whereas in a real soccer match M can vary. How to predict the expected number of heads g_2 in the next round? Here we consider two different approaches. (1) The prediction is based on the achievement of the first round, i.e. on the value of g_1. Then the best prediction is $g_2 = g_1$. The variance of the statistical error of the prediction can be simply written as $\sum_{g_1,g_2} p(g_1)p(g_2)(g_1 - g_2)^2$ where $p(g)$ is the binomial distribution. A straightforward calculation yields for this variance a value of $2Mp(1-p)$. (2) The prediction is based on the knowledge of tossing attempts M. If furthermore the value of p is known the optimum prediction is, of course, pM. The variance of the statistical error is given by the binomial distribution, i.e. by $Mp(1-p)$. Stated differently, knowing the number of attempts to reach a specific goal (here tossing a head) is more informative than the actual number of successful outcomes as long as the probability p is well known. Note that in this limit the common value of the scoring efficiency is very well determined because it results from averaging over all teams.

This hypothesis seems to contradict the results Fig.2, as presented above. However, a priori the large fluctuations of $p_\pm$ in Fig.2 do *not* necessarily contradict the presence of a rather uniform value of $p_\pm$ for all teams. Rather, this apparent disagreement can be easily resolved by discussing in more detail the possible reasons for the strong fluctuations of $p_\pm$ when comparing different teams. In general, these fluctuations are a superposition of two effects: (i) true differences between teams and (ii) statistical fluctuations, reflecting the random effects in the 34 soccer matches of the season. In analogy to the previous discussion both effects can be disentangled by studying the dependence of the variance of $p_\pm$ on the number of matches N, which has been used for the averaging. The results of this analysis is shown in Fig. 3. One can see that the extrapolation to large N, i.e. the systematic

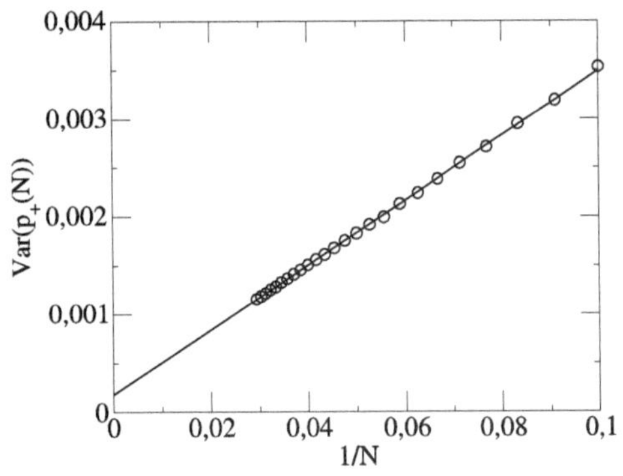

Figure 3. The variance of the distribution of scoring efficiencies in dependence of the number of match days.

team-specific variance of $p_{\pm}$, yields a value (0.0002) which is much smaller than the variance for $N = 34$ (0.0012), i.e. after averaging over a whole season. Thus, the large fluctuations in Fig.2 are mainly of statistical nature and the efficiency to score a goal from a chance for a goal is basically the same for all teams! We note in passing that to a large extend the residual variance of 0.0002 can be explained via the above-mentioned effects that better teams have a slightly higher scoring efficiency.

Based on this intriguing result we will identify X and Y as the differences of the chances of goals in the respective time intervals, denoted ΔC_X and ΔC_Y. In analogy to Eq.9 and Eq.15 we can identify the disentanglement into systematic and random contributions. The results are listed in Tab.1.

As expected the statistical characterisation of the random components of X (complete season) and Y (first half of a season) are very similar because both deal with chances for goals. The small remaining differences express the fact that the statistical properties of the first and the second half of the season are slightly different [22]. Finally, we note in passing (data not shown) that knowledge of the goal differences of $2N$ matches has the same information content as knowing the chances of goals of just (approx.) N matches.

General statements about the degree of predictability

In the explicit form of $corr(Y,Z)$ (see Eq.10) all terms on the left and right side except for $corr(S_Y,S_Z)$ have been quantified so far, either via the information in Tab.1 or via explicit determination of $corr(Y=\Delta C_Y, Z=\Delta G_Z)$, yielding $corr(Y=\Delta C_Y, Z=\Delta G_Z) = 0.65$ (with the choice $N_Y = N_Z = 17$). This allows one to determine the correlation between the team strength in the first half and the second half of the league. We obtain $corr(S_Y,S_Z) = 1.00$. This has two important implications. First, the variation of the team strength during a single season is basically absent, as already reported in [5]. Second, the team strength as defined via the chances for goals (corresponding to S_Y) is, apart from a proportionality factor, basically identical to the definition of the team strength as defined via the goals (corresponding to S_Z). Both results are very promising with respect to the ability to predict soccer matches. In particular, the key approximation, entering Eq.14, is indeed very well fulfilled.

We mention in passing [22] that a closer analysis reveals that the team strength fluctuates with a small amplitude of approx. $A = 0.17$ and with a decorrelation time of approx. 7 matches. Since we average over a larger number of matches and, furthermore, restrict ourselves to the prediction of the total second half, these temporal fluctuation are to a large extent averaged out and do not show up in the present statistical analysis.

In case that the team strength S_Y is perfectly known, i.e. $Y = S_Y$, Eq.10 yields (using $\epsilon_Y = 0$) $corr(S_Y,Z) = 1/\sqrt{1 + V_Z/[17 Var(S_Z)]} = 0.74$. One may compare this limit of optimum prediction with the case where Y was calculated based on the the chances for goals (correlation of 0.65) or based on the goals (correlation of 0.56). This clearly reveals that using the chances for goals instead of the goals yields a significant step towards the theoretical optimum.

The final unknown in our prediction scheme are values of $corr(S_X,S_Y)$ and $corr(S_X,S_Z)$ which can be determined in analogy to $corr(S_Y,S_Z)$. Explicit calculation yields $corr(S_X, S_Z) = 0.88$ and $corr(S_X,S_Y) = 0.86$. Both values are identical within statistical errors ($corr(S_X,S_Z) - corr(S_X,S_Y) = 0.02 \pm 0.02$). This is compatible with the observation that the team strength does not vary within a season but vary within the summer break. For future purposes we use the average value of $corr(S_X,S_{Y,Z}) = 0.87$ for the characterization of the correlation of the team strength between two seasons.

Table 1. The different systematic and random contributions of the observables, relevant for this work.

	$Var(S_i)$	V_i
$X : \Delta C_X$	2.32	14.1
$Y : \Delta C_Y$	2.66	14.2
$Z : \Delta G_Z$	0.21	2.95

Application to the Case of Soccer Prediction: Results

Prediction of team strength

To check our analytical results we perform an explicit multivariate regression analysis to estimate Z based on knowledge of X and Y by using standard algorithms. To capture the dependence on the information content of the first half of the present season we also vary the number of considered matches N_Y. To improve the statistical quality of the data for $N_Y < 17$ we always average over different random selections of N_Y matches from the first half of the season. For the determination of ΔC_X we choose all matches, i.e. $N_X = 34$ (thus taking the whole season). To check the relevance of the information from the previous season we alternatively set $X = 0$, i.e. ignore the information from the previous season.

One technical aspect needs to be mentioned. In a given season two or three teams have just been promoted. Thus, no data about the previous season are available. Therefore, we set the value of x_i for the differences of the chances for goals for the promoted team to a constant value x_{prom}. This value is determined by the condition that the resulting average value x_i (averaged over all teams of the present season) is zero.

The numerical results are shown in Fig.4. We start with the case $X = 0$. One can see that (trivially) for $N_Y = 0$ the standard deviation in the estimation of the team strength is identical to the standard deviation of the S_Z-distribution because no team-specific information has been used. The longer the season, the more information is available to distinguish between stronger and weaker teams. Using the information of the complete first half of the season ($N_Y = 17$) the statistical uncertainty decreases to 0.22.

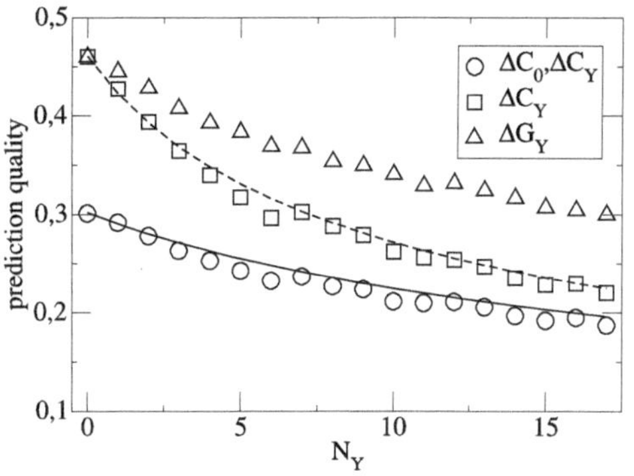

Figure 4. The prediction quality of the team strength, determined via $\sqrt{\tilde{\chi}^2(X,Y)}$, as a function of the number of match days N_Y. Different choices of variables are shown. For the second and third case (ΔG_Y and ΔC_Y, respectively) the information from the previous season is neglected. The solid lines are based on the explicit formulas for the prediction quality.

We have repeated the same calculation by identifying Y with the goal differences ΔG_Y. The prediction quality is significantly worse and one obtains an uncertainty of 0.30 rather than 0.22 after $N_Y = 17$ matches.

When additionally incorporating the information from X, the statistical uncertainty is already quite small at the beginning of the season (0.3). Of course, when increasing N_Y it further decreases. Even after 17 matches the additional gain of using X is significant (0.19 vs. 0.22). Thus, despite the slight decorrelation of the team strength during the summer break it is advantageous to take into account the information from the previous season even after half of the present season has been played.

Furthermore, we compare in Fig.4 the actual uncertainty of the prediction of Z with the theoretical expectation as expressed by Eq.12 and Eq.14. One finds a very close agreement with the actual data. This serves as a consistency check of our whole procedure and just reflects the fact that the assumptions, underlying the derivation of Eq.14, are fulfilled very well.

Finally, we explicitly apply this formalism to the prediction of a specific season of the Bundesliga. We aim to predict the goal difference of the 2nd half based on previous information. The regression problem reads $\hat{\Delta G_Z} = a(N_Y)\Delta C_X + b(N_Y)\Delta C_Y(N_Y)$ where the weighting factors depend on the number of matches, included from the first half of the present season. They are listed in Tab.2 for different values of N_Y. Naturally, for $N_Y = 0$ the estimation is only based on ΔC_X. Here the regression coefficient can be also calculated analytically using the values, mentioned in this work. Specifically, one gets $a(N_Y = 0) = 17 corr(\Delta C_X, \Delta G_Z)/Var(\Delta C_X) = 17 corr(S_X, S_Z)\sqrt{Var(S_X)Var(S_Z)}/Var(\Delta C_X) = 17 \cdot 0.88 \cdot \sqrt{2.32 \cdot 0.21}/(2.32 + 14.1/34) \approx 3.8$ which is very close to the numerically determined value of 3.71. As expected, more information during the present season, i.e. larger N_Y, leads to a stronger weighting of ΔC_Y. After $N_Y = 12$ matches the information contents of the previous season is basically equal to that of the first matches of the present season.

Table 2. The two regression parameters as a function of N_Y.

N_Y	$a(N_Y)$	$b(N_Y)$
0	3.71	0
4	3.20	0.82
8	2.60	1.70
12	2.23	2.30
17	1.86	2.77

Based on these regression parameters we explicitly predict the goal difference of the second half for the two cases $N_Y = 0$ and $N_Y = 17$. We present data for the season 2007/08. Both predictions for ΔG_Z are listed in Tab.3 together with the actual values of ΔG_Y and ΔG_Z during that season.

One can see that for most cases the prediction before the season and in the middle of the season agree quite well, i.e. no dramatic reevaluations of the team strength as compared to the previous year was necessary. Notable exceptions are München (estimation of +10 before the season and +21 after half of the season) and Leverkusen (increase from +2 to +9). Obviously, this reevaluation reflects that the fact that both teams played much better during the first half of that season (goal differences of +23 and +16 for München and Leverkusen, respectively) than expected beforehand.

The final column also contains information about the logarithm of the market value (taken from www.transfermarkt.de) as an independent variable for a trivariate regression problem. The scaling of the team strength with the logarithm of the market value has been explicitly shown in previous work [22]. The resulting modifications in the estimation of ΔG_Z are small but significant. When averaging over all years between 2001/02 and 2010/11, for which the market value is available, it turns out that the prediction quality improves by 0.02 for $N_Y = 17$. Thus, relative to 0.19 a further significant improvement can be achieved.

Prediction of single matches

Please note that the estimation of ΔG_Z is the basis for many other types of prediction. Since ΔG_Z is nothing else than the team strength, this value can be directly taken to estimate individual matches. For example, on the 18th match day of the season 2007/08 Cottbus was playing vs. Leverkusen. As shown in Refs. [21,22] the expected goal difference during a match of team i and j in the Bundesliga is given by the difference of the team strength of both teams plus some team-independent contribution, reflecting the home advantage. Nonlinear effects can be neglected. For this specific match the expected outcome was (using the final column in Tab.3): $(-12)/17 - (+8)/17 + 0.3 = -0.9$, using the home advantage of approx. 0.3 during that season. Thus, the best estimation for the resulting goal difference of that match, based on the available information used in this work, is -0.9. Actually, the final result was 2:3.

Here is a brief summary of the different prediction steps, following the general procedure in [21] and in agreement with previous work (e.g.[10]).

1. Calculation of the team strength via a linear regression approach. As main parameters enter ΔC_X, ΔC_Y, and the logarithm of the market value of the team at the beginning of the season. Naturally, for a match on the M-th match day one uses $N_Y = M - 1$. Minor further improvements can be reached by introducing an index for promoted teams and by taking into account short-time fluctuations of the team strength by using the results of the last seven matches as an individual parameter [22]. In total, this ends up in a five-dimensional regression analysis. The regression parameter have been obtained from comparison of all seasons between 1995/96 and 2010/11, excluding the season which predictions are performed.

Table 3. The predictions of the goal difference of the second half of the Bundesliga-season 2007/08 for each team, based on the differences of chances for goals ΔC_X of the previous season (3rd column) or, additionally, on the differences of chances for goals ΔC_Y of the first 17 matches of the present season (4th column).

	$17\Delta G_Y$	$17\Delta G_Z$	$17\Delta G_{Z,est}(N_Y=0)$	$17\Delta G_{Z,est}(N_Y=17)$	$17\Delta G_{Z,est}(N_Y=17)$ **plus market value**
B. München	23	24	10	21	23
Bremen	18	12	11	15	14
Hamburg	11	10	3	9	10
Leverkusen	16	1	2	9	8
Schalke	9	14	8	12	11
Karlsruhe	−2	−13	−8	−6	−7
Hannover	−1	−1	3	−1	−2
Stuttgart	−1	1	9	5	6
Frankfurt	−4	−3	2	−3	−4
Dortmund	−4	−8	0	0	2
Wolfsburg	0	12	−4	−5	−2
Hertha	−5	0	−5	−8	−5
Bochum	−2	−4	−1	−4	−7
Bielefeld	−19	−6	−6	−11	−10
Rostock	−10	−12	−8	−11	−13
Nürnberg	−7	−9	1	1	1
Cottbus	−10	−11	−8	−10	−12
Duisburg	−12	−7	−8	−13	−12

The estimation in the final column also involves information about the market value. The actual goal differences of the first half of that season and the second half are included in the first two columns, respectively.

2. Calculation of the sum of goals by a corresponding regression analysis, taking into account the goals, scored in the present season so far, and the goals of the previous season [21]. However, for the calculation of the outcome of individual matches this step is by far less important than the estimation of the team strength.

3. Estimation of the team-independent home advantage in the corresponding season in analogy to the previous step [22].

4. Calculation of the expectation value of goals of both teams from steps 1–3.

5. Estimating possible final scores by assuming independent Poisson processes.

6. Correcting for the effect that draws are more likely than expected on the expense of matches with goal differences ± 1 [23].

Note that in earlier work goals rather than chances for goals were employed. We would like to stress again that the critical part of this endeavor is the determination of the team strength as described in this work.

To characterize the quality of the present approach we have compared the predictions of single matches with odds from Oddset, using data between the seasons 2002/03 and 2006/07, where the odds were available to us. Specifically, we used the scaled inverse odds as an estimate of the respective probabilities for a win of the home team, a draw, or a win for the away team. An objective measure is the parameter

$$K = -\langle \ln(\text{probability for win, draw, loss})\rangle \tag{17}$$

where the probability for the actual outcome is taken as the argument of the logarithm. One can show that the value of K is a

Table 4. The K-value for the regression model during the seasons 2002/03 and 2006/07 as well as for the Oddset-odds.

	first 10 matches of season	**all 34 matches**
Only home advantage	1.073	1.057
+ matches of present season	1.054	1.013
+ matches of previous season	1.027	1.004
+ market value	1.019	1.000
Oddset	1.025	1.012
Difference	0.006 ± 0.009	0.012 ± 0.004

The impact of adding additional information to the model is listed.

minimum if the predicted probabilities for a win, a draw, and a loss are identical to the true probabilities. Analogous measures can be already found in literature, e.g. [10,24]. One can see in Tab.4 the additional consideration of new information indeed gives rise to a lower value of K. Furthermore, restricting the choice of matches to those taking place during the first 10 match days, the prediction becomes worse (larger K). In particular, the additional impact of the market value is larger, if restricting oneself to the first 10 matches of the season. When averaging over all matches in these seasons [22], it turns out that the K-value of the present approach is smaller than the K-value for the Oddset-odds by 0.012 ± 0.004. Thus, the comparison yields a highly significant improvement of the present model as compared to the Oddset-odds. The size of this improvement is non-negligible if compared to the variations of K when adding different pieces of information; see Tab.4.

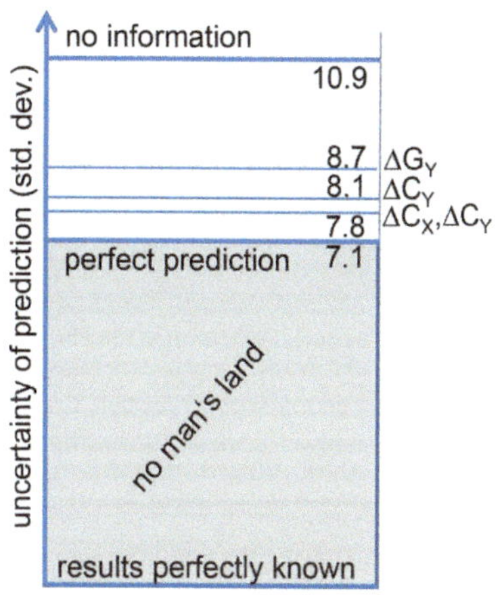

Figure 5. The uncertainty of the prediction of the goal difference of the second half when using the complete information of the first half ($N_Y = 17$). Different choices of variables are shown. Furthermore, the limit of perfect predictability is indicated.

Discussion

The main goal of this work is to provide a theoretical framework which allows one to determine the quality of the prediction. Conceptually, it is related to the Bayesian approach because it takes into account the impact of additional information as well as the impact of decorrelations on the estimation of future events. As a formal framework we have used a multivariate regression approach.

The prediction of soccer results is a particularly nice case study of this approach due to the availability of well-defined data and due to the popular interest in this matter. Beyond the application of the analytical results it turned out to be essential to search for observables (here: chances for goals) with a high information content.

One interesting question arises: is the residual statistical error of S_Z for $N_Y = 17$ small or large? This question may be discussed from two different perspectives. First, one may want to predict the outcome of the second half of the league. Then the uncertainty is given by $17\sqrt{\chi^2(X,Y)} = 17\sqrt{\tilde{\chi}^2(X,Y) + V_Z/17}$. These values are plotted for different prediction scenarios in Fig.5. One can see how the additional information decreases the uncertainty of the prediction. Most importantly, the *no man's land* below an uncertainty of $\sqrt{17V_Z} = 7.1$ cannot be reached by any type of prediction. The art of approaching this perfect prediction thus resorts to decrease the present value of 7.8 to a value closer to 7.1. Second, one may be interested in the prediction of a single match. This case is somewhat different. Since the team fluctuations are very difficult to predict, the fluctuation amplitude $A = 0.17$ (see above) serves as a scale for estimating the highest possible quality of match prediction. If the uncertainty is much smaller than A any further improvement would be irrelevant due to the non-predictable fluctuations of the team strength. However, in the present case the statistical error after $N_Y = 17$ is close to A so that a further reduction of $\tilde{\chi}^2(X,Y)$ would still be relevant for prediction purposes of individual matches.

Repeating this analysis for the prediction of the points in the second half of the season the statistical uncertainty of the estimation corresponds to approx. 6 points (standard deviation). This corresponds to lose rather than to win two matches or vice versa.

Note that the chances for goals are not a completely objective observable because finally also the subjective judgement of a sports journalist may influence its estimates. In this sense the high information content of chances for goals indicates that the subjective component is quite small and the general definition is very reasonable. Of course, in the future one may look for strictly objective match observables taken by commercial companies to further improve the information content. In any event, the chances for goals are by far more informative than the actual results, as typically taken for prediction purposes.

As demonstrated above, the present results can be directly applied to the prediction of individual soccer matches. The reason is that the team strength, as estimated via the above regression analysis, is the key input for the formalism of single-match prediction, as outlined in Ref. [21,22].

Of course, it is conceivable that the general ideas can be used for different applications under the condition that very recent (exact but noisy) and more previous information (slightly changed but low noise level) is present. Note that the type of data is identical to panel data, popular in socio-economic studies. Popular cohort studies deal with the time-evolution of the income or the health situation (see, e.g., [25-27]). For the testing of stochastic concepts sports data are, of course, particularly suited, because of the easily accessible and reliable data basis.

Acknowledgments

We gratefully acknowledge helpful discussions with D. Riedl, B. Strauss, and J. Smiatek.

Author Contributions

Conceived and designed the experiments: AH OR. Performed the experiments: AH OR. Analyzed the data: AH OR. Contributed reagents/materials/analysis tools: AH OR. Wrote the paper: AH OR.

References

1. Woolridge JM (2002) Econometric analysis of cross section and panel data. Cambridge: MIT Press.
2. Goldstein M, Wooff D (2005) Statistical Models: Theory and Practice. Cambridge University Press.
3. Freedman D (2007) Bayes Linear Statistics, Theory and Methods. Wiley.
4. Laird N, Ware J (1982) Random-effects models for longitudinal data. Biometrics 38: 963–974.

5. Heuer A, Rubner O (2009) Fitness, chance and myths: an objective view on soccer results. Er Phys J B 67: 445–458.
6. Constantinou A, Fenton NE, Neil M (2012) pi-football: A Bayesian network model for forecasting Association Football match outcomes. Knowl-Based Syst 36: 322–339.
7. Lee A (1997) Modelling scores in the premier league: is manchester united really the best? Chance 10: 15–19.
8. Dixon M, Coles S (1997) Modelling association football scores and inefficiencies in a football betting market. Appl Statist 46: 265–280.
9. Dixon M, Robinson M (1998) A birth process model for association football matches (pages 523538). The Statistician 47: 523–538.
10. Rue H, Salvesen O (2000) Prediction and retrospective analysis of soccer matches in a league. The Statistician 49: 399–418.
11. Sire C, Redner S (2009) Understanding baseball team standings and streaks. Eur Phys J B 67: 473–481.
12. Maher M (1982) Modelling association football scores. Statistica Neerlandica 36: 109–118.
13. Bittner E, Nussbaumer A, Janke W, Weigel M (2007) Self-affirmation model for football goal distributions. Europhys Lett 78: 58002.
14. Bittner E, Nussbaumer A, Janke W, Weigel M (2009) Football fever: goal distributions and non-gaussian statistics. Eur Phys J B 67: 459–471.
15. Koning R (2000) Balance in competition in dutch soccer. The Statistician 49: 419–431.
16. Goddard J (2005) Regression models for forecasting goals and match results in association football. International Journal of Forecasting 21: 331–340.
17. Hvattum LM, Arntzen H (2010) Using elo ratings for match result prediction in association football. International Journal of Forecasting 26: 460–470.
18. Andersson P, Edman J, Ekman M (2005) Predicting the world cup 2002 in soccer: Performance and confidence of experts and non-experts. International Journal of Forecasting 21: 565–576.
19. Song CU Boulier BL, Stekler HO (2007) The comparative accuracy of judgmental and model forecasts of american football games. International Journal of Forecasting 23: 405–413.
20. Forrest D, Simmons R (2000) Forecasting sport: the behaviour and performance of football tipsters. International Journal of Forecasting 16: 317–331.
21. Heuer A, Mueller C, Rubner O (2010) Soccer: is scoring goals a predictable poissonian process? Europhys Lett 89: 38007.
22. Heuer A (2012) Der perfekte Tipp: Statistik des Fussballspiels. Wiley–VCH.
23. Heuer A, Rubner O (2012) How does the past of a soccer match influence its future? PLoS ONE 7/11: e47678.
24. Goddard J, Asimakopoulos I (2004) Football results and the efficiency of fixed-odds betting. J Forecast 32: 51–66.
25. Judge T, Hurst C (2008) How the rich (and happy) get richer (and happier): Relationship of core self-evaluations to trajectories in attaining work success. Journal of Applied Psychology 93: 849–863.
26. Schnitzlein D (2014) How important is the family? evidence from sibling correlations in permanent earnings in the usa, germany, and denmark. J Popul Econ 27: 69–89.
27. Ambrey C, Fleming C (2014) The causal effect of income on life satisfaction and the implications for valuing non-market goods. Economics Letters 123: 131–134.

Speed Trends in Male Distance Running

Timothy N. Kruse[1], Rickey E. Carter[2], Jordan K. Rosedahl[2], Michael J. Joyner[3]*

1 The University of Washington School of Medicine, 1959 N. E. Pacific Street, Seattle, WA, 98195, United States of America, **2** Department of Health Sciences Research, Mayo Clinic, 200 First Street SW, Rochester, MN, 55905, United States of America, **3** Department of Anesthesiology, Mayo Clinic, 200 First Street SW, Rochester, MN, 55905, United States of America

Abstract

The major cycling "Grand Tours" have shown an attenuation of performance over the last decade. This has been interpreted as circumstantial evidence that newer anti-doping strategies have reduced the use of performance-enhancing drugs. To examine this idea under more controlled conditions, speed trends for world class 5000 m, 10000 m, and marathon performances by men from 1980 to 2013 were analyzed. We obtained comprehensive records from the International Association of Athletics Federations, Association of Road Racing Statisticians, and the Track and Field All-time Performances database webpages. The top 40 performances for each event and year were selected for regression analysis. For the three distances, we noted cumulative performance improvements in the 1990s thru the mid-2000s. After the peak speed years of the mid 2000 s, there has been limited improvement in the 5000 m and 10,000 m and world records set during that time remain in place today, marking the longest period of time between new records since the early 1940s. By contrast marathon speed continues to increase and the world record has been lowered four times since 2007, including in 2013. While the speed trends for 5000 m and 10000 m track results parallel those seen in elite cycling, the marathon trends do not. We discuss a number of explanations other than improved anti-doping strategies that might account for these divergent findings.

Editor: Maria F. Piacentini, University of Rome, Italy

Funding: This work was supported by the National Institutes of Health grants R25 GM075148 and UL1 TR000135. The funders had no role in study design, data collection and analysis, decision to publish, or preparation of the manuscript.

Competing Interests: The authors have declared that no competing interests exist.

* Email: Joyner.Michael@Mayo.edu

Introduction

The use of performance-enhancing drugs (doping) can be dated back to the ancient Olympics [1], [2]. Since then athletes have used a wide range of substances including red wine, caffeine, nitroglycerin, cocaine, opiates, amphetamines, growth hormone, blood transfusions, anabolic steroids, and erythropoietin (EPO) in an effort to gain a physiological advantage [3]. Because performance-enhancing drugs compromises the idealized principles of pure competition, the World Anti-Doping Agency (WADA) was created in 1999 [4]. Since the formation of WADA, it has developed widely applied policies and drug testing protocols (including regular out of competition testing) in an attempt to stop the apparently wide spread doping in elite sports competition [5].

If recent improvements in athletic performance have been driven by doping, then improved doping control might be reflected by a leveling off or declining performances in sports where doping is thought to be ubiquitous. In recent analyses of major cycling races including the Tour de France, Giro d'Italia, Vuelta A España, the average speed has been leveling off or declining [6], [7] since the introduction of improved techniques to detect use of exogenous EPO in 2005 [4]. However, the analysis of cycling is confounded by varying race distances, yearly changes in course, and weather. Endurance running eliminates many of these confounding factors. The tracks and courses are identical from year to year. For the two shorter distances, there are numerous competitive opportunities per year and at least some would likely have nearly ideal environmental conditions.

With this information as a background, we tested the hypothesis that elite distance running times would show a pattern of leveling in the middle 2000 s similar to that seen in cycling. Such a finding could be explained by improved doping control. We also discuss alternate explanations including that humans are reaching the biological limits of performance and the potential role technical innovations in training and equipment [8], [9]. Finally, any potential explanation might also be confounded by changes in the economic landscape associated with world class distance running.

Materials and Methods

We obtained the top male performances from 1980–2013, by year, in major endurance running races (5000 m, 10000 m on the track; marathon on road courses) from the International Association of Athletics Federations (IAAF: http://www.iaaf.org/home), Association of Road Racing Statisticians (ARRS: http://www.arrs.net), and the Track and Field all-time Performances database websites (http://www.alltime-athletics.com/index.html) [10], [11], [12].

The 1980–2013 epoch was selected because besides new performance-enhancing drugs (PEDs), a case can be made that potentially transformative changes in training or equipment has not occurred. For example, by 1980 high volume and high intensity training had been widely adopted by top competitors for several decades and athletes from East Africa had been participating at the international level since the early 1960s. High quality synthetic tracks were also widely available by 1980 and carbohydrate loading was widely practiced in the marathon and it is unclear if technical changes in shoes have had a measureable impact on performance. While ideas about training have been refined the extent to which these have been uniformly adopted by elite athletes, especially the East Africans, is not known [13], [14], [15].

Beyond these training and globalization related factors, professionalism also emerged during the 1980s. We also restricted our analysis to men because women were not routinely permitted to participate in long distance racing until the 1970s and performances dropped dramatically in the early years of widespread competition by women. While the gap in world records has been steady since that time women still lag in competitive depth in many events [16], [17].

Finally, the first synthetic EPO (Epogen) was approved by the FDA in 1989 and within a few years it was clear that EPO can have profound effects on maximal oxygen transport (VO2 max) [18] in humans and was being used to enhance athletic performance by the early 1990s. Additionally, because EPO and related analogues are injectable the logistical challenges of traditional blood doping (autologous red cell transfusions) are eliminated [19].

The abstracted data consisted of the total number of performances below 2012's Olympic A standard: 5000 m-13:20, 10,000 m-27:45, and also performances under 2:10:00 for the marathon (the Olympic A standard was 2:15 in 2012, a time that equals an estimated 29.22 10,000 m [20]). Performances below these standards were considered 'elite'. To study the speed tends more formally, the 40 fastest athlete performances (the fastest performance of the 40 fastest athletes) were recorded per year and event for regression modeling (described below). Age and country of residence at time of race were also abstracted.

Initial data summaries included the frequency tabulation elite performances by event and distance. To analyze the changes in speed trends over the study period, we used regression techniques consisting of quadratic splines (cubic B-splines with 3 equally spaced interior knots) against our years of interest using the top 40 athlete performances per year. These generalized regression models allowed for flexibility of estimating the change in performance over time while providing traditional measures of model fit (e.g., R-square value). It was hypothesized that different regression profiles would be observed between the top 40 finishing times and the fastest yearly performances, so the percentage difference in speed of the fastest performance relative to the 40th fastest time per year was also modeled using regression splines and locally weighted smoothers (LOESS). When reporting measures of model fit for the cubic B-splines regression models (i.e., change in speed as a function of year), the omnibus F test for the regression model and R-square were reported. The LOESS curves, which were used for illustrative purposes of changes in pacing based on the relative placing, were not summarized using traditional regression summaries such as R-square on account of their intended visual utilization.

Cubic B-spli ne regression analyses were conducted using The SAS System (v9.3, Cary, NC) using PROC ORTHOREG. LOESS smoothing was conducted using PROC SGPLOT using default parameters.

Results

The number of performances below the 2012 Olympic A qualifying standard plus sub 2:10:00 for each distance increased over the 1980–2013 (Figure 1a–c). The world record for the 5000 m was set in 2004 while the 10000 m world record was set in 2005; these records stand today, which is the longest gap between world records since the 1940s. The number of performances below the 2012 Olympic A qualifying standard for the 5000 m and 10,000 m also appears to have leveled off since the middle 2000 s. Similarly the number of athletes breaking 2:10:00 for the marathon has also leveled off. 2:10:00 was chosen as a comparable standard for the marathon because this time is considered generally similar to or slightly slower than the A standards for shorter distances based on various empirical point tables, scoring systems and time conversion programs [20].

All three regression splines presented in Figures 2a–c were statistically significant ($p<0.0001$ for each). Furthermore, year alone explained a large percentage of the variation in the speed trends (R-square: 53%, 37% and 69% for 5000 m, 10000 m and marathon, respectively). Consistent with these overall model estimates, the 5000 m and 10000 m had significant increases in speed during the 1990s whereas the marathon showed an increase over the entire three plus decades (Figures 2a–c). In particular, the 5000 m the speed trend levels off starting around 2000. The marathon and 10000 m times do not show this as a pronounced tendency.

Figures 3a–c explores the speed trends using an alternative classification approach to provide additional insights into the temporal effects. The fastest performance of the year is plotted alone and summarized using a LOESS smoother. Speed trends of the mean top 10, mean top 20 and mean top 40 athlete performances are superimposed in these same figures. With the 5000 m and 10000 m, there is a pronounced 'outlying' effect of the top performance from 1995 to late 2010. The marathon, however, displays no attenuation of the increased speed over the epoch sampled and the relative speed of the fastest annual time does not appear to be an outlier (i.e., the figure lines appear as roughly parallel).

To better quantify the observations made from Figure 3, the percentage changes in speeds over time were examined and found to be consistent with the differential findings of the top performance vs. the 40th fastest athlete performance. The degree to which the fastest times were relatively fast (compared to other years) was observed during the 2000s in the 5000 m and 10000 m distances. The regression spline analyses supported these findings that the fastest relative times for the 5000 m and 10000 m varied over the epoch (5000 m: $p=0.048$, R-square = 32%; 10000 m: $p=0.0007$, R-square = 51%). As illu strated in Figure 3c, trends for the marathon distance were not clearly identified in the data ($p=0.29$, R-square = 19%).

Discussion

The speed and performance trends for top 5000 m and 10000 m distance running performers on the track show a period of increased speed among the fastest runners to the mid-2000 s with an attenuation of speed in either all (5000 m) or the fastest performances (10000 m) after this period of time. For the marathon, all indices of speed show a nearly linear increase in speed with an increased number of elite performances over the three plus decades we sampled. We believe there are a number of possible explanations for these findings.

First, the findings for the 5000 m can be interpreted as consistent with the hypothesis that improved drug testing has

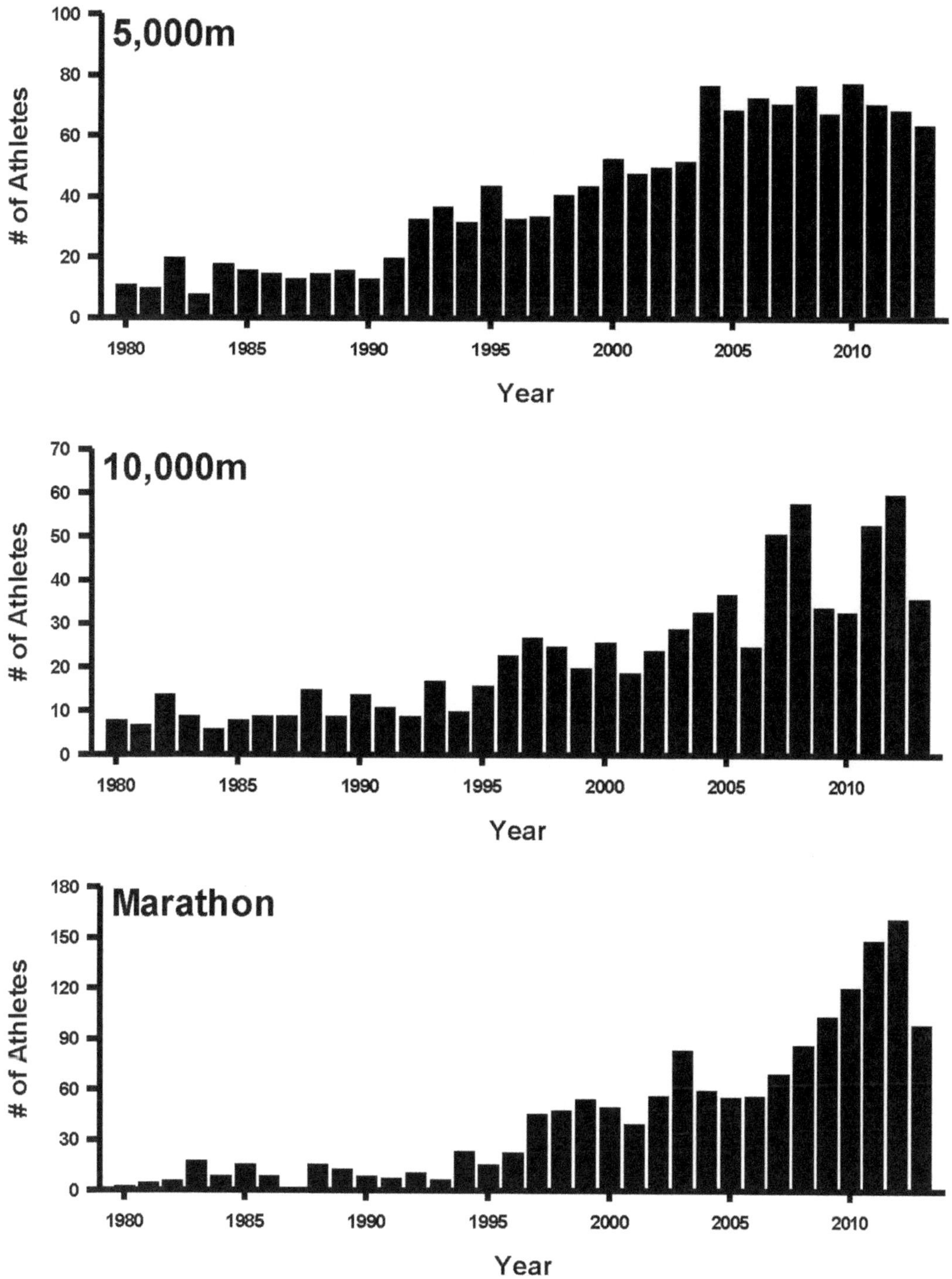

Figure 1. Total number of elite performances by year. Times under 13:20 for the 5000 m, 27:45 for the 10000 m, and 2:10 for the marathon.

limited the ability of elite athletes to manipulate their oxygen transport systems with EPO (or other techniques to improve oxygen transport during exercise) since the middle 2000 s. These observations are also broadly consistent with recent speed trends in elite cycling races [6], [7]. This interpretation can also be applied to the 10000 m results, but only when considering the fastest times. By contrast, the data for the marathon shows continued improvements in running speed during the same time period along with more total elite performances and world records. These observations challenge the idea that the speed leveling seen in the 5000 m on the track and in the so-called "Grand Tours" of cycling is due primarily to better drug testing and the reduced use of performance enhancing drugs.

A second possible interpretation is that world class performances are leveling off and reaching a physiological upper limit as has been postulated for equine and canine athletes [8], [9,], [21]. In the case of the marathon a number of empirical estimates and physiological modeling suggest the record is relatively slow in comparison to the 5,000 m and 10,000 m times and is merely catching up by comparison [20], [22], [23]. In this context, it is

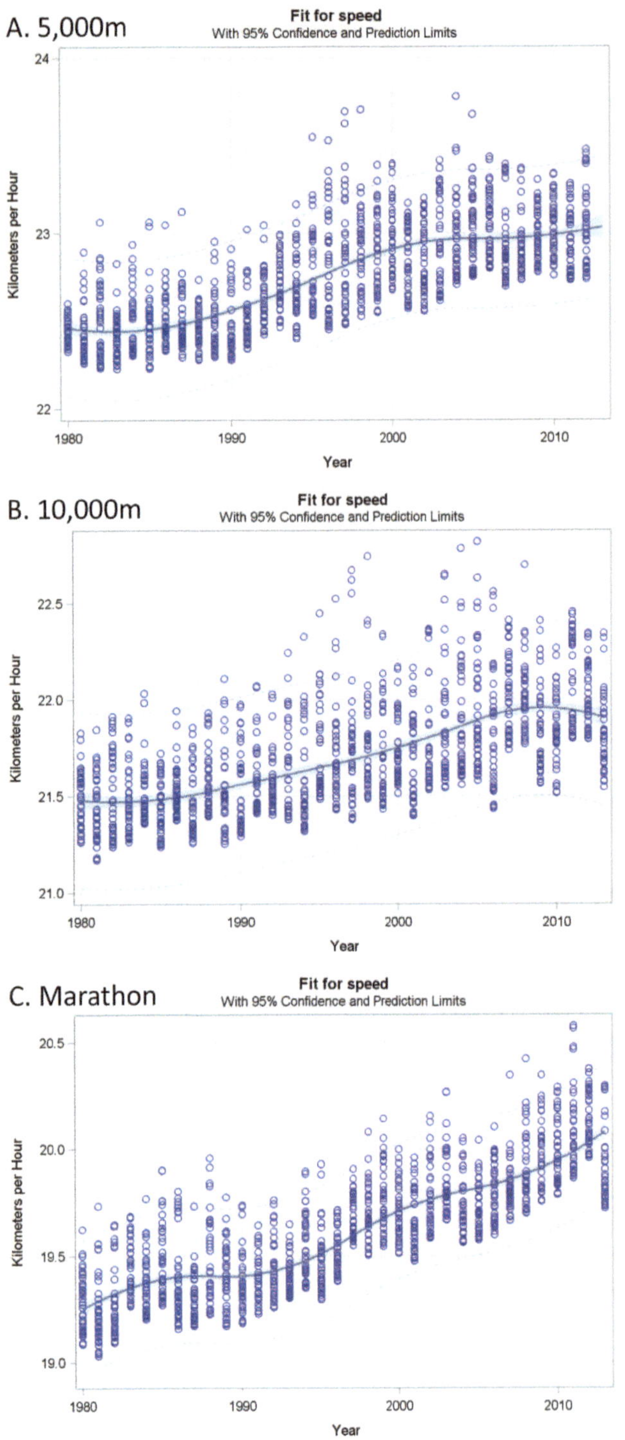

Figure 2. Top 40 athlete performances of the 5000 m, 10000 m, and marathon (circles). The solid line is a quadratic spline fit with three equally spaced knots (points of inflection).

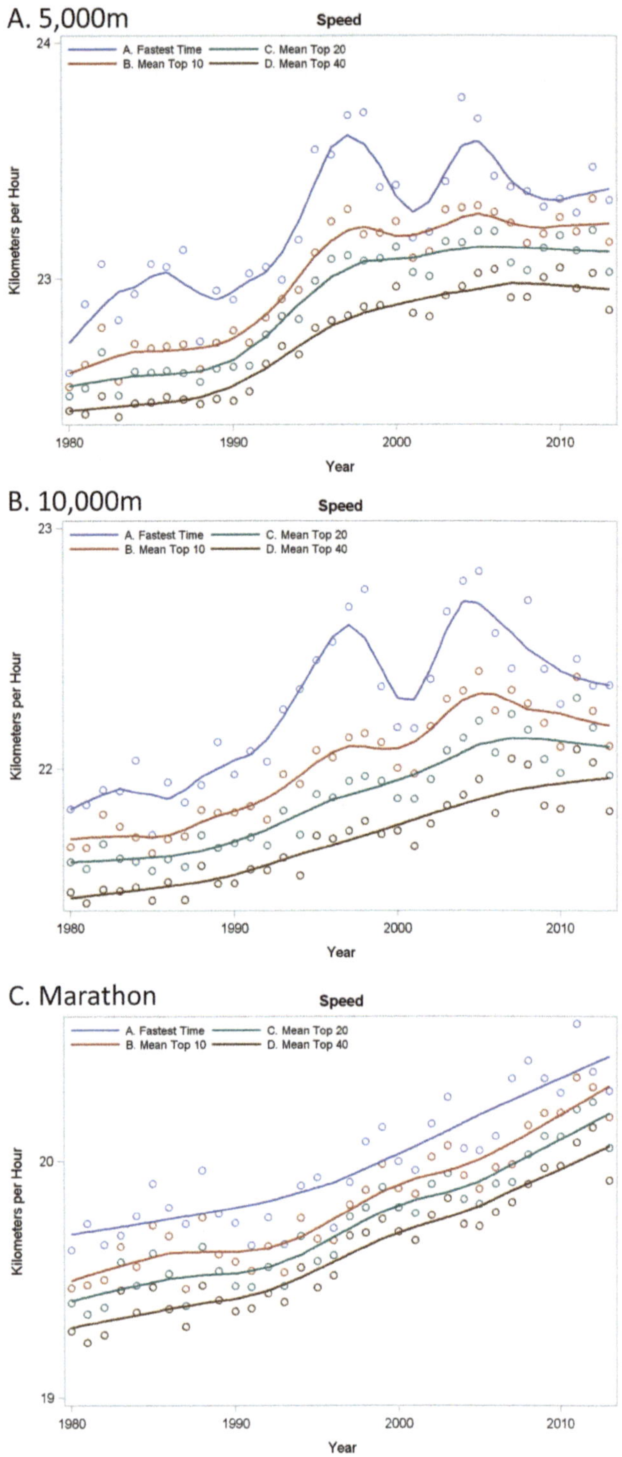

Figure 3. LOESS smoothers fit through the fastest yearly performance by year for the 5000 m (A), 10000 m (B) and marathon (C). In addition, the mean speed for the top 10, top 20 and top 40 athlete performances are also plotted for reference.

interesting to note that top speeds have not fallen for the shorter races but only leveled off.

The third element of any interpretation focuses on the changing financial incentives in professional distance running. Prize money for top marathon performances has increased. Specifically, in 1980 the highest total payout for any marathon was $50,000; just over two decades later the first million dollar race was run [24]. These incentives could be attracting a stronger pool of competitors to "move up" and focus on the marathon and forgo record setting attempts at shorter distances. This could lead to more competitive races among top runners at the major marathons. Second the highest profile marathon races are now being staged in a way designed for world record attempts that include the use of pacers. Along these lines, the use of pacers has been wide spread for races on the track for many years, and many top athletes have bonus plans and other financial incentives from sponsors that reward fast times at the shorter distances. There are a number strengths and limitations to this study. A major strength of our data set and analysis is that it includes standardized distances and courses with numerous competitive opportunities at the shorter two distances when environmental conditions are likely to be optimal. By contrast, a limitation to our analysis is that we have no idea if improved approaches to training or equipment (shoes and tracks) might have contributed to the trends we report. However, we favor the interpretation that the entire epoch we have analyzed has been relatively stable from a technical perspective. This includes widespread use of high volume and high intensity training, widespread availability of synthetic tracks, and adequate footwear. Additionally, while ideas about training have been refined it is not known if how uniformly these have been adopted by elite athletes, especially the East Africans [13], [14], [15]. This perspective contrasts to the major improvements in equipment for cycling that includes use of advanced materials and improved aerodynamic designs to construct faster bikes.

A final concern whenever the topic of doping is raised is discussed relates to what might be called the continuous "cat and mouse" game between those trying to enforce the rules with improved testing and those trying to circumvent them. This has engendered speculation that micro-doses of EPO can be titrated by athletes in a way to achieve high levels of performance and yet avoid a positive drug test [19], [25], [26]. There is also widespread speculation about the use less or undetectable compounds and so-called designer performance enhancing drugs. Advocates of these points of view have argued that while doping is considered widespread the number of positive tests in major competitions is quite low [5]. The counter argument is that the low number of positive results demonstrates that the testing is working and deterring doping. The lack of hard data on the true incidence of doping and how it has or has not been influenced by improved testing is unknown and a major limitation to any discussion on this topic. However, it is clear that anonymous questionnaire based surveys suggest the true incidence of doping it is much higher (14–39%) than ~2% rate of positive tests suggests [27]. This is clearly an area of sports sociology that requires increased attention.

It should also be noted that the sociology surrounding the doping phenomenon along with the ongoing incentives to dope are complex. In this context, strategies beyond testing alone will be required to improve the efficacy of doping control. A comprehensive discussion of this complex topic is beyond the scope of our analysis, but there has been much thoughtful discussion of related topics [28], [29], [30], [31], [32], [33], [34].

Conclusion

In summary, our analysis demonstrates that speed trends for elite distance running are divergent depending on distance and have event specific patterns. Thus, any generalizations about performances in world class competition providing evidence that drug testing is or is or is not "working" need to be viewed with caution. Further caution is required given the many caveats and potential factors that could explain our findings.

Acknowledgments

We would like to thank IAAF, Peter Larsson, and Ken Young for compiling the data. This work was supported by the National Institutes of Health grants R25 GM075148 and UL1 TR000135.

Author Contributions

Conceived and designed the experiments: TNK MJJ REC. Performed the experiments: TNK MJJ. Analyzed the data: TNK MJJ REC JKR. Contributed reagents/materials/analysis tools: TNK MJJ REC JKR. Contributed to the writing of the manuscript: TNK MJJ REC.

References

1. Conti AA (2010) Doping in sports in ancient and recent times. Med Secoli 22: 181–190.
2. Papagelopoulos PJ, Mavrogenis AF, Soucacos P (2004) Doping in ancient and modern Olympic Games. Orthopedics 27: 1226–1231.
3. Gaudard A, Varlet-Marie E, Bressolle F, Audran M (2003) Drugs for increasing oxygen transport and their potential use in doping - A review. Sports Med 33: 187–212, doi:10.2165/00007256-200333030-00003.
4. World Anti-Doping Agency (2010) A Brief History of Anti-Doping.
5. International Olympic Committee (2014) The Fight Against Doping and Promotion of Athletes' Health.
6. El Helou N, Berthelot G, Thibault V, Tafflet M, Nassif H, et al. (2010) Tour de France, Giro, Vuelta, and classic European races show a unique progression of road cycling speed in the last 20 years. J Sports Sci 28: 789–796, doi:10.1080/02640411003739654.
7. Perneger TV (2010) Speed trends of major cycling races: does slower mean cleaner? Int J Sports Med 31, 261–264, doi:10.1055/s-0030-1247593.
8. Berthelot G, Tafflet M, El Helou N, Len S, Escolano S, et al. (2010) Athlete atypicity on the edge of human achievement: performances stagnate after the last peak, in 198. PLoS One 5: e8800, doi:10.137/journal.pone.0008800.
9. Berthelot G, Thibault V, Tafflet M, Escolano S, El Helou N, et al. (2008) The citius end: world records progression announces the completion of a brief ultra-physiological quest. PLoS One 3: e1552, doi:10.1371/journal.pone.0001552.
10. Home of World Athletics (2014) International Association of Athletics Federation. Available: http://www.iaaf.org/records/toplists. Accessed 15 May 2014.
11. Young K (13 June 2014) Yearly Rankings- Marathon. Association of Road Racing Statisticians. Available: http://www.arrs.net. Accessed 15 May 2014.
12. Larsson P (16 Jun 2014) Men's standard events. Track & Field All-time Performances Homepage. Available: http://www.alltime-athletics. com/index. html. Accessed 15 May 2014.
13. Billat V, Lepretre PM, Heugas AM, Laurence MH, Salim D, et al. (2003) Training and bioenergetic characteristics in elite male and female Kenyan runners. Med Sci Sports Exerc 35: 297–304.
14. Wilber RL, Pitsiladis YP (2012) Kenyan and Ethiopian distance runners: what makes them so good? Int J Sports Physiol Perform 7: 92–102.
15. Bourne ND (2008) Fast science: A history of training theory and methods for elite runners through 1975, Doctor of Philosophy Thesis, University of Texas.
16. Thibault V, Guillaume M, Berthelot G, Helou NE, Schaal K, et al. (2010) Women and men in sport performance: the gender gap has not evolved since 1983. J Sports Sci Med 9: 214–223.
17. Hunter SK, Stevens AA, Magennis K, Skelton KW, Fauth M (2011) Is there a sex difference in the age of elite marathon runners? Med Sci Sports Exerc 43: 656–664, doi:10.1249/MSS.0b013e3181fb4e00.
18. Joyner MJ (2003) VO2MAX, blood doping, and erythropoietin. Br J Sports Med 37: 190–191.
19. Lundby C, Achman-Andersen NJ, Thomsen JJ, Norgaard AM, Robach P (1985) Testing for recombinant human erythropoietin in urine: problems associated with current anti-doping testing. J Appl Physiol 105: 417–419, doi:10.1152/japplphysiol.90529.2008.
20. Hill R (1 Jun 2014) Race Conversion. Hill Runner. Available: http://www.hillrunner.com/calculators/raceconversion.php. Accessed 17 May 2014.
21. Denny MW (2008) Limits to running speed in dogs, horses and humans. J Exp Biol 211: 3836–3849, doi:10.1242/jeb.024968.
22. Joyner MJ, Ruiz JR, Lucia A (2011) The two-hour marathon: who and when? J Appl Physiol (1985) 110: 275–277. doi:10.1152/japplphysiol. 00563.2010.
23. Joyner MJ (1991) Modeling: optimal marathon performance on the basis of physiological factors. J Appl Physiol (1985) 70: 683–687.
24. Miller T, Lawrence G, McKay J, Rowe D (2001) Globalization and Sports. (SAGE).
25. Jelkmann W, Lundby C (2011) Blood doping and its detection. Blood 118: 2395–2404, doi:10.1182/blood-2011-02-303271.
26. Lonnberg M, Lundby C (2013) Detection of EPO injections using a rapid lateral flow isoform test. Anal Bioanal Chem 405: 9685–9691, doi:10.1007/s00216-013-6997-8.

27. de Hon O, Kuipers H, van Bottenburg M (2014) Prevalence of doping use in elite sports: a review of numbers and methods. Sports Med Aug 29 [Epub ahead of print].
28. Delanghe JR, Joyner MJ (2008) Testing for recombinant human erythropoietin. J Appl Physiol (1985) 105: 395–396, doi:10.1152/japplphysiol.90746.2008.
29. D'Angelo C, Tamburrini C (2010) Addict to win? A different approach to doping. J Med Ethics 36: 700–707.
30. Baron DA, Martin DM, Abol Magd S (2007) Doping in sports and its spread to at-risk populations: an international review. World Psychiatry Off J World Psychiatr Assoc WPA 6: 118–123.
31. Tokish JM, Kocher MS, Hawkins RJ (2004) Ergogenic aids: a review of basic science, performance, side effects, and status in sports. Am J Sports Med 32: 1543–1553.
32. Haugen KK (2004) The performance-enhancing drug game. J Sports Econ 5: 67–86.
33. Noakes TD (2004) Tainted glory–doping and athletic performance. N Engl J Med 351: 847–849.
34. Strelan P, Boeckmann RJ (2006) Why drug testing in elite sport does not work: perceptual deterrence theory and the role of personal moral beliefs. J Appl Soc Psychol 36: 2909–2934.

15

Genotype by Sex and Genotype by Age Interactions with Sedentary Behavior: The Portuguese Healthy Family Study

Daniel M. V. Santos[1]*, Peter T. Katzmarzyk[2], Vincent P. Diego[3], John Blangero[3], Michele C. Souza[1], Duarte L. Freitas[4], Raquel N. Chaves[5], Thayse N. Gomes[1], Fernanda K. Santos[1], José A. R. Maia[1]

1 Centre of Research, Education, Innovation and Intervention in Sport, Faculty of Sports, University of Porto, Porto, Portugal, **2** Pennington Biomedical Research Center, Louisiana State University System, Baton Rouge, Louisiana, United States of America, **3** Texas Biomedical Research Institute, San Antonio, Texas, United States of America, **4** Sport and Physical Education Department, University of Madeira, Funchal, Portugal, **5** Physical Education Department, Federal University of Technology - Parana, Campus Curitiba, Curitiba/PR, Brasil

Abstract

Sedentary behavior (SB) expression and its underlying causal factors have been progressively studied, as it is a major determinant of decreased health quality. In the present study we applied Genotype x Age (GxAge) and Genotype x Sex (GxSex) interaction methods to determine if the phenotypic expression of different SB traits is influenced by an interaction between genetic architecture and both age and sex. A total of 1345 subjects, comprising 249 fathers, 327 mothers, 334 sons and 325 daughters, from 339 families of The Portuguese Healthy Family Study were included in the analysis. SB traits were assessed by means of a 3-d physical activity recall, the Baecke and IPAQ questionnaires. GxAge and GxSex interactions were analyzed using SOLAR 4.0 software. Sedentary behaviour heritability estimates were not always statistically significant ($p > 0.05$) and ranged from 3% to 27%. The GxSex and GxAge interaction models were significantly better than the single polygenic models for TV (min/day), EEsed (kcal/day), personal computer (PC) usage and physical activty (PA) tertiles. The GxAge model is also significantly better than the polygenic model for Sed (min/day). For EEsed, PA tertiles, PC and Sed, the GxAge interaction was significant because the genetic correlation between SB environments was significantly different from 1. Further, PC and Sed variance heterogeneity among distinct ages were observed. The GxSex interaction was significant for EEsed due to genetic variance heterogeneity between genders and for PC due to a genetic correlation less than 1 across both sexes. Our results suggest that SB expression may be influenced by the interactions between genotype with both sex and age. Further, different sedentary behaviors seem to have distinct genetic architectures and are differentially affected by age and sex.

Editor: Antonio Gonzalez-Bulnes, INIA, Spain

Funding: This work was supported by the FCT – Fundação para a Ciência e a Tecnologia (www.fct.pt): PTDC/DES/67569/2006 FCOMP-01-0124-FEDEB-09608. The funders had no role in study design, data collection and analysis, decision to publish, or preparation of the manuscript.

Competing Interests: The authors have declared that no competing interests exist.

* Email: d.monteiro.santos13@gmail.com

Introduction

Sedentary behaviors, i.e. sitting or reclining, have been increasingly linked with poor health status, and are associated with chronic diseases such as type 2 diabetes, and overall mortality [1]. Furthermore, there is reliable evidence showing that the hazardous effects of sedentary lifestyles are observed across different age groups and in both sexes [1–3]. In a recent 5-year follow-up study it was observed that adolescents who engaged in excessive screen viewing had significantly lower quality of life scores [2]. In addition, evidence from longitudinal studies during adulthood show associations of sedentary behavior with site-specific cancers (ovarian, endometrial and colon), cardiovascular disease and type 2 diabetes [1]. During later life, some sedentary behaviors, such as television viewing, have been linked with lower cognitive performance [3].

In a review of the genetic basis of physical activity and sedentary behavior, Santos et al. [4] observed heritability estimates for sedentary behavior and physical inactivity phenotypes ranging from 0.00 in twins [5] to 0.60 in nuclear families [6]. Recently, in a sample of 1654 middle-aged twins, den Hoed et al. [7] found that genetic factors explained 31% of the variance in time spent in sedentary behaviors. Further, Simonen et al. [8] reported a heritability estimate of 25% in Canadian nuclear families for physical inactivity [9]. Given that there are few such studies focusing on the heritability of sedentarism, the exploration of the genetic architecture of different indicators of sedentary behavior in nuclear families will add to the ongoing debate about the regulation of sedentarism. Furthermore, information about sex and age effects on the genetic regulation of sedentary behavior is almost nonexistent.

The main purposes of the present study, using a nuclear family design, are to estimate the magnitude of genetic factors responsible for the variation in distinct sedentary behavior phenotypes, and to study potential Genotype-by-Sex and Genotype-by-Age interactions influencing these sedentary behaviors. We hypothesize that SB is genetically driven and that GxSex and GxAge interactions will have a significant influence in SB phenotype expression.

Materials and Methods

The Healthy Family Study, from the Portuguese *Famílias Saudáveis* (FAMS), investigates the relationship among metabolic syndrome indicators, physical activity, physical fitness and body composition in nuclear families. Children and adolescents aged ≤ 18 years were recruited in schools from Azores and Madeira archipelagos, and the northern and central regions of mainland Portugal, and were approached to freely participate in the study with their siblings and parents. School officers provided family lists, and families with at least two siblings were initially invited. However, given that families with 3 or more children are scarce in the Portuguese population [10], and to improve statistical power, one-offspring families were randomly ascertained with respect to phenotype and recruited to the study. Subjects with chronic diseases, physical handicaps or psychological disorders were excluded as these conditions might impair their daily routines, namely their physical activities within schools and/or sports clubs. The ethics committee of the College of Sport, University of Porto, approved the study, and written informed consent was obtained from all subjects including the legal representatives of the children involved.

Data Collection

The standardized procedures of Lohman et al. [11] were used to measure height with a Siber Hegner anthropometer (GMP instruments), and weight with a Tanita scale (model BC-418 MA).

Using a 3-d physical activity diary (B3DAR) [9], a trained technician interviewed each subject, recording the dominant activity for each 15-min period during 24 h by using a list of categorized activities. Categories from 1 to 9 refer to increasing levels of energy expenditure (METs) of each activity. Sedentary behaviors, such as sleeping or sitting, are listed in categories 1 to 3 and indicate low/very low METs. The number of 15-min periods for these three categories was first summed over the 3-day period and divided by 3 which resulted in minutes in sedentary behavior per day (Sed). Total energy expenditure in sedentary behaviors (TEESB) was then calculated by weighting each category for its own approximate median energy cost (kcal/kg/15 min). This value was then summed and multiplied by the subjects body weights. Total daily sedentary energy expenditure [EEsed (kcal/day)] was then calculated by dividing TEESB by 3.

The Baecke questionnaire is a self-administered questionnaire aiming to analyze 3 different dimensions of habitual physical activity: (i) sports physical activity (SPA), (ii) leisure physical activity (LPA) and (iii) work/school physical activity (WPA). It is a Likert scale-based questionnaire that refers to the past 12 months, and includes 16 questions divided into 3 distinct sections: questions 1-8 assess work or school physical activity; questions 9–12 assess sports activities and exercise programs; and questions 13–16 assess leisure and locomotive activities. The sums of the specific scores of each section constitute the physical activity level for WPA, SPA and LPA, respectively. The sum of these 3 scores constitutes the habitual or total physical activity level (TPA). Sports were subdivided into three levels of energy expenditure according to Durnin and Passmore [12]; the low level for sports such as, billiards, sailing, bowling, golf (average energy expenditure 3 kcal/min); the middle level for sports such as, badminton, cycling, dancing, swimming and tennis (average energy expenditure 5 kcal/min); and the high level for sports such as boxing, football, basketball, rugby and rowing (average energy expenditure 7 kcal/min). A question about the total time per day the subject used a personal computer (PC) was applied to further classify sedentary behavior. Also, subjects were considered sedentary, light active and high active, depending upon if they were in the first, second, or third tertile of TPA.

The International Physical Activity Questionnaire (IPAQ) [13] was conceived to obtain comparable estimates of PA across countries. We applied the IPAQ short version (IPAQs), which is suitable for use in national and regional surveillance systems. Subjects were asked to recall the time spent in vigorous (activities in which the heart rate increases dramatically), moderate (activities in which the heart rate increases moderately, except walking) and low (activities such as walking) intensity activities performed in the last seven days at home/work, during leisure time and transportation. For this particular paper, IPAQ was used to assess time (minutes per day) watching TV (TV) and sitting.

Statistical Analysis

Descriptive analysis. Descriptive analyses were performed in PEDSTATS v0.6.12 and group comparisons were made in PEPI 4.0.

Univariate genetic procedures. Univariate quantitative genetic procedures as implemented in SOLAR v4.1 [14] under a special class of the multivariate linear model, namely the variance components (VC) approach, were used to estimate additive genetic and environmental VCs for each of the SB traits. Prior to all modeling, age, age-squared, sex, age-by-sex, and age-squared-by-sex were used as covariates in a preliminary VC model. Residuals were thus derived for each trait and were normalized using an inverse normal transformation, as previously advocated [15,16]. Assuming that dominance and epistasis are negligible, comparisons of individual phenotype y define the covariance of the basic polygenic model as:

$$Cov(y_i,y_j)=2\phi_{ij}\sigma_g^2+\sigma_e^2\delta_{ij} \qquad \text{(Eq.1)}$$

where i and j index individuals, $2\phi_{ij}$ gives the expected coefficient of relationship, σ_g^2 is the additive genetic variance, σ_e^2 is the environmental variance, and δ_{ij} isdefined as 1 when individuals i and j are the same, and 0 otherwise. This model is used to estimate heritability, which is given as:

$$h^2=\frac{\sigma_g^2}{\sigma_g^2+\sigma_e^2}=\frac{\sigma_g^2}{\sigma_p^2}, \qquad \text{(Eq.2)}$$

where σ_p^2 is the total phenotypic variance. Heritability estimates (h^2) were computed using a maximum likelihood approach to estimate variance components under the standard polygenic model as implemented in SOLAR v.4.3.1 software [14].

Gene-by-Sex and Gene-by-Age interactions. To test for GxSex and GxAge interactions, basic initial hypotheses were formulated regarding the variance/covariance relationship of a SB indicator between family members with different gender or age. For the GxSex model we treated sex as a discrete environment (male or female), and for the GxAge model we treated the age continuum as a continuous environment. As regards Genotype by Environment (GxE) interaction in general, the fundamental null hypothesis is that the expression of a polygenotype (i.e., aggregate of all genotypes related to the expression of a phenotype) is independent of the environment. It can be shown from first principles that if there is no GxSex or GxAge interaction, the same SB trait measured in subjects with different genders or ages will have a genetic correlation of 1.0 and the genetic variance will be homogeneous across both genders or across all ages [17,18]. On the contrary, if GxSex or GxAge interactions are present, the genetic correlation will be significantly less than 1.0 and/or the genetic variance will not be the same in different genders or ages.

The basic polygenic model can be extended to account for GxSex interaction by allowing for sex-specific additive genetic and environmental variances denoted by σ^2_{gf}, σ^2_{gm}, σ^2_{ef}, and σ^2_{em}, where f and m index females and males, respectively, and for an across-sex genetic correlation denoted by $\rho_{g(f,m)}$. Under the GxSex model, the two null hypotheses are $\sigma^2_{gf}=\sigma^2_{gm}=\sigma^2_g$ and $\rho_{g(f,m)}=1$.

Under the GxAge interaction model, variance and correlation are modeled as continuous functions of age. For the genetic variance function (and similarly for the environmental variance function) variance is modeled using an exponential function to ensure positivity, which is required since any variance is a squared term [17,18]:

$$\sigma^2_g = \exp[\alpha_g + \gamma_g(age_i - \overline{age})], \qquad \text{(Eq.3)}$$

where α_g and γ_g are parameters to be estimated, and age_i is the age of the i-th individual standardized against the sample mean,. An additional justification for the exponential function is suggested by the alternative name of this approach, namely the log-linear model of the variance:

$$\ln \sigma^2_g = \alpha_g + \gamma_g(age_i - \overline{age}) \qquad \text{(Eq.4)}$$

That is, on taking the natural logarithm of the variance modeled as an exponential function, we have the equation of a line. In this form, the variance homogeneity null hypothesis obviously holds for a slope-term equal to 0: $\gamma_g=0$. For the genetic correlation function, we modeled the genetic correlation as an exponential decay function of the pair-wise age differences for the i-th and j-th individuals:

$$\rho_g = \exp(-\lambda|age_i - age_j|), \qquad \text{(Eq.5)}$$

where λ is a parameter to be estimated. Here we also have an elegant re-expression of the interaction null hypothesis, in this case regarding the genetic correlation, in that a genetic correlation equal to 1 is equivalent to $\lambda=0$. This is because for $\lambda=0$, we have $\rho_g = \exp(\lambda|age_i - age_j|) = e^0 = 1$.

For reasons detailed in Diego et al. [17], the likelihood ratio test statistic (LRT) to test $\sigma^2_{gf}=\sigma^2_{gm}=\sigma^2_g$ or γ_g under the GxSex or GxAge interaction models is distributed as χ^2_1, a chi-square random variable with 1 degree of freedom (d.f.), and the LRT to test $\rho_{g(f,m)}=1$ and $\lambda=0$ is distributed as $(\frac{1}{2}\chi^2_o + \frac{1}{2}\chi^2_1)$, a 50:50 mixture of chi-square random variable with a point-mass at 0, denoted byχ^2_o, and a chi-square with 1 d.f. Prior to examination of these hypotheses, we first confirmed if the overall GxSex and GxAge interaction models provided a better fit to the data than the standard so-called polygenic models. The LRT for this comparison can be shown to be distributed as $(\frac{1}{2}\chi^2_2 + \frac{1}{2}\chi^2_3)$[19].

We also performed a post-hoc power analysis to determine the power in our sample to detect GxSex and GxAge interaction effects. Power is defined as the probability of correctly rejecting the null hypothesis, and is computed as the probability integral from the point on the alternative distribution corresponding to the nominal significance level or alpha (on the null distribution) to the upper limit of the alternative distribution at positive infinity. Since the total probability of any distribution is 1, power can be conveniently computed as:

$$\Pr\left(\sigma^2_{gf} \neq \sigma^2_{gm}\right) \text{or}$$

$$\Pr(\rho_{g(f,m)}<1) = \int_{\chi^2_{\alpha;\upsilon,\xi=0}}^{\infty} d\chi^2_{\upsilon,\xi} = \int_0^{\infty} d\chi^2_{\upsilon,\xi} - \int_0^{\chi^2_{\alpha;\upsilon,\xi=0}} d\chi^2_{\upsilon,\xi} \qquad \text{(Eq.6)}$$

$$= 1 - \int_0^{\chi^2_{\alpha;\upsilon,\xi=0}} d\chi^2_{\upsilon,\xi} = 1-\beta$$

where the distribution under the alternative hypothesis is the non-central chi-square distribution, denoted by $\chi^2_{\upsilon,\xi}$, υ is the degrees of freedom (d.f.) parameter, ξ is the non-centrality parameter (NCP), $\chi^2_{\alpha;\upsilon,\xi=0}$ is the point on the non-central chi-square distribution corresponding to the $100(1-\alpha)$ percentage point on the distribution under the null hypothesis, and

$$\beta = \int_0^{\chi^2_{\alpha;\upsilon,\xi=0}} d\chi^2_{\upsilon,\xi} \qquad \text{(Eq.7)}$$

is the probability of making a type II error. We used a similar approach to that used by Blangero et al. [15].

Results

Table 1 presents basic descriptive information. Some relatives were not able to fully engage in the data collection procedures (fathers = 32.5%; mothers = 3.6%; sons = 1.5%; daughters = 4.1%). As such, a total of 1345 subjects, comprising 249 fathers, 327 mothers, 334 sons and 325 daughters, from 339 families were included. The average family size was 3.97 subjects.

As assessed by the Baecke questionnaire, no differences were observed for PC usage between fathers and mothers ($\chi^2 = 0.401$, p = 0.05), sons and daughters ($\chi^2 = 3.322$, p = 0.07), and between parents and offspring ($\chi^2 = 3.413$, p = 0.07). As for the IPAQ phenotypes, offspring spend more time watching TV (p<0.01) and sitting (p<0.001) than parents. Mothers spend less time watching TV (p<0.01) and no significant differences were observed between fathers and mothers sitting time. Parents' energy expenditure in SB is higher than offsprings' (p<0.001), even though time spent in sedentary behaviors as assessed by the B3DAR was higher in offspring (p<0.001).

Heritability estimates presented in Table 2 varied in their magnitude (from 0.03 to 0.27) and significance. Time spent in sedentary behaviors was the most heritable trait with a value of 27%. followed by PA tertiles with and heritability estimate of 23%. On the other hand. PC usage assessed in an ordinal 5 point scale. sitting time (min) and TV watching (min) from the IPAQ were not significantly heritable.

To test for the influence of age and sex on the expression of SB indicators, the polygenic model was compared to its alternative models (GxSex and GxAge) by means of a log-likelihood ratio test (see Table 3). The GxSex and GxAge interaction models are significantly better than the polygenic model for TV (min/day),

Table 1. Sample descriptive statistics.

	Father	Mother	Son	Daughter
	Mean ± Std.Dev.	Mean ± Std.Dev.	Mean ± Std.Dev.	Mean ± Std.Dev.
Age (yrs)	45.93±4.38	43.55±4.41	14.68±2.85	14.33±2.84
Height (cm)	170.39±6.67	158.62±5.76	162.41±13.36	155.93 ± 9.85
Weight (kg)	80.19±12.73	67.22±10.23	57.69±16.83	52.81±12.86
BMI (kg/m^2)	27.62±3.98	26.72±3.92	21.47±4.23	21.47±3.99
Sitting (min/day)	291.26±211.77	306.85±284.20	345.06 ± 273.54	364.07±218.09
TV (min/day)	97.85±±75.14	75.74 ± 59.20	137.35±130.01	113.47±105.65
Sed (min/day)	1040.85±186.28	950.80±180.26	1233.14±112.22	1232.21±110.25
EEsed (kcal/day)	2099.57±536.17	2063.79±485.44	1583.31±479.51	1485.95±386.64
	%	%	%	%
PC <30 min	39.7%	43.8%	16.5%	25.8%
30 min - 60 min	13.8%	14.3%	27.0%	27.2%
60 min - 90 min	6.9%	5.8%	20.9%	19.8%
90 min - 120 min	5.8%	5.4%	15.2%	11.1%
> 120 min	33.9%	30.8%	20.4%	16.1%

Legend: TV – television viewing; Sed – minutes spent in sedentary behaviors as assessed by B3DAR; EEsed – energy expenditure in sedentary behaviors as assessed by B3DAR; PC – daily personal computer usage (ordinal variable).

EEsed (kcal/day), PC (ordinal variable) and PA tertiles (see Table 4). Further, GxAge is also significantly better than the polygenic model for Sed (min/day). These results only mean that the GxSex and GxAge interaction models fit the data better than the polygenic model for these SB traits.

In order to assess if there is GxAge and/or GxSex interactions, each of the full models were compared to its constrained alternatives (i.e. setting $\gamma_g=0$ or $\lambda=0$ for GxAge and $\sigma^2_{gf}=\sigma^2_{gm}=\sigma^2_g$ or $\rho_{g(f,m)}=1$ for GxSex) for Tv, Sed, EEsed, PC, sitting and PA tertiles.

Figure 1 shows the results for those traits (PC, Sed, EE and PA tertiles) that showed significant variance heterogeneity and a correlation function that is significantly different from 1 in the GxAge model. For EEsed and PA tertiles significant GxAge interaction was due to rejection of the genetic correlation hypothesis ($p<0.05$). For PC and Sed, both null hypotheses, i.e., genetic correlation (ρ_g) equals 1 and variance homogeneity, were significantly rejected. Figure 1a highlights that, for PC and Sed genetic variance increases with age. Concomitantly, Figure 1b displays that, for EEsed, PA tertiles, PC and Sed, the genetic correlation decreases with increasing differences between family members' ages.

Figure 2 illustrates that GxAge interaction for PC and Sed, is a joint function of genetic variance heterogeneity and a genetic correlation function not equal to one. Thus, we express them jointly as a covariance function in the vertical axis.

Figure 3 shows that the additive genetic effects in EEsed is greater in males than in females, suggesting that the expression of EEsed is under more genetic control in boys than in girls. That is, there is significant GxSex interaction for EEsed due to genetic variance heterogeneity. We also found significant GxSex interaction for PC due to a genetic correlation less than 1 across the sexes ($\rho_g=-0.85$; $p=0.009$).

The power analysis results for the GxSex model are presented in Table 5. Taking 80% power as the criterion for sufficient power to detect a GxSex effect, we found that we did not have sufficient

Table 2. Heritability estimates (h^2) and % of variance accounted for by covariates of different sedentary phenotypes in the Portuguese Healthy Families Study.

Trait	h^2	Std. Error	p-value	% variance accounted for by covariates[1]
TV (min/day)	0.05	0.06	0.235	6.00
Sed (min/day)	0.27	0.06	<0.001*	41.00
EEsed (kcal/day)	0.19	0.07	0.003*	33.00
PC	0.04	0.07	0.265	1.00
Sitting (min/day)	0.03	0.09	0.344	1.00
PA Tertiles	0.23	0.06	<0.001*	0.00

Significant estimates are labeled with an *.
Legend: Tv – television viewing; Sed – minutes spent in sedentary behaviors as assessed by B3DAR; EEsed – energy expenditure in sedentary behaviors as assessed by B3DAR; TV – television viewing (ordinal variable); PC – personal computer usage (ordinal variable).
[1]Covariates - age, age^2, sex and their interactions.

Table 3. Results of log-likelihood ratio tests (LRT) and respective p-values contrasting a polygenic model vs a GxSex model for each of the SB indicators.

Trait	Polygenic LnL	GxSex LnL	LRT	p-value
TV (min/day)	−358.811	−346.953	23.715	<0.001*
Sed (min/day)	−457.404	−456.522	1.764	0.302
EEsed (kcal/day)	−457.592	−453.058	9.066	0.009*
PC	−421.924	−417.977	7.895	0.015*
Sitting (min/day)	−338.818	−337.030	3.577	0.124
PA Tertiles	−489.192	−468.144	42.097	<0.001*

Significant estimates are labeled with an *.
Legend: TV – television viewing; Sed – minutes spent in sedentary behaviors as assessed by B3DAR; EEsed – energy expenditure in sedentary behaviors as assessed by B3DAR; PC – personal computer usage (ordinal variable).

power in the sample for any of the traits. However, power is highest for the two traits for which at least one of the null hypotheses were rejected. For EEsed we found evidence of GxSex interaction due to variance heterogeneity, and the power to detect GxSex interaction due to variance heterogeneity is highest for this trait. Similarly, for PC we found evidence of GxSex interaction due to a genetic correlation less than 1, and the power to detect this particular interaction effect was highest for PC.

The power analysis results for the GxAge model are presented in Table 6. Unlike our power to detect GxSex interaction effects, we had for the most part ample power to detect GxAge interaction effects in regard to rejection of both null hypotheses of variance homogeneity and a genetic correlation equal to 1. It should be noted that sufficient power to reject either null hypothesis when they are false does not necessarily mean that they are false.

Discussion

The novelty of these results presented in this study is the estimation of heritability for a set of distinct SB markers in nuclear families as well as the application of genotype x environment interaction models to better understand how SB is influenced by age and sex. It should be emphasized that the heritabilities varied from 3% (sitting) to 27% (Sed), which means that these phenotypes have distinct genetic contributions. This is quite relevant to understanding the mechanisms that lead to distinct sedentary behaviors and suggests that even though some behaviors are under some genetic regulation, others seem to be just an adaptation to the contemporary way of living. The only result that could be compared with other studies is from the 3-d diary, that yielded an heritability estimate of 27% for sedentary behavior which is in agreement with previous data from the Quebec Family Study [8] showing that 25% of the variance in the same phenotype was due to genetic factors.

Some studies have used accelerometry to quantify sedentary behavior [5,20] in genetic studies. For example, the *Viva La Familia* study [20] demonstrated a heritability estimate of 57% for the percentage of wake time in activities with an energy expenditure of ≤ 0.01 kcal/kg/min. More recently, an adult twin study [5] yielded an heritability estimate of 0 for sedentary time defined as <100 counts/min. Further, a robust analysis of 1654 twins made by den Hoed et al. [7] showed that 35% of the variance in SB assessed by accelerometry and heart rate monitors was due to genetic factors. This obvious disparity in the results may be due to different sample sizes, design, distinct markers of SB and cut-points used and/or different statistical procedures and corresponding statistical adjustments for diverse covariates. However, we argue that these discrepancies may be related to an imprecise definition of SB and the use of distinct markers that may not measure the same thing. In fact, sedentarism has been defined as a group of behaviors that occur whilst sitting or lying down while awake and typically require very low energy requirements [21]. This definition has led to the emergence of several markers (e.g., television viewing, computer usage, time seated during work or in school) expressed in different units (e.g., minutes, METs, or ordinal scales) that map different facets of

Table 4. Results of log-likelihood ratio tests (LRT) and respective p-values contrasting a polygenic model vs a GxAge model for each of the SB indicators.

Trait	Polygenic LnL	GxAge LnL	LRT	p-value
Tv (min/day)	−358.811	−329.454	58.715	<0.001*
Sed (min/day)	−457.404	−396.015	122.778	<0.001*
EEsed (kcal/day)	−457.592	−429.013	57.157	<0.001*
PC	−421.924	−406.722	30.405	<0.001*
Sitting (min/day)	−338.818	−336.627	4.383	0.167
PA Tertiles	−489.192	−481.619	15.147	0.001*

Significant estimates are labeled with an *.
Legend: TV – television viewing; Sed – minutes spent in sedentary behaviors as assessed by B3DAR; EEsed – energy expenditure in sedentary behaviors as assessed by B3DAR; PC – personal computer usage (ordinal variable).

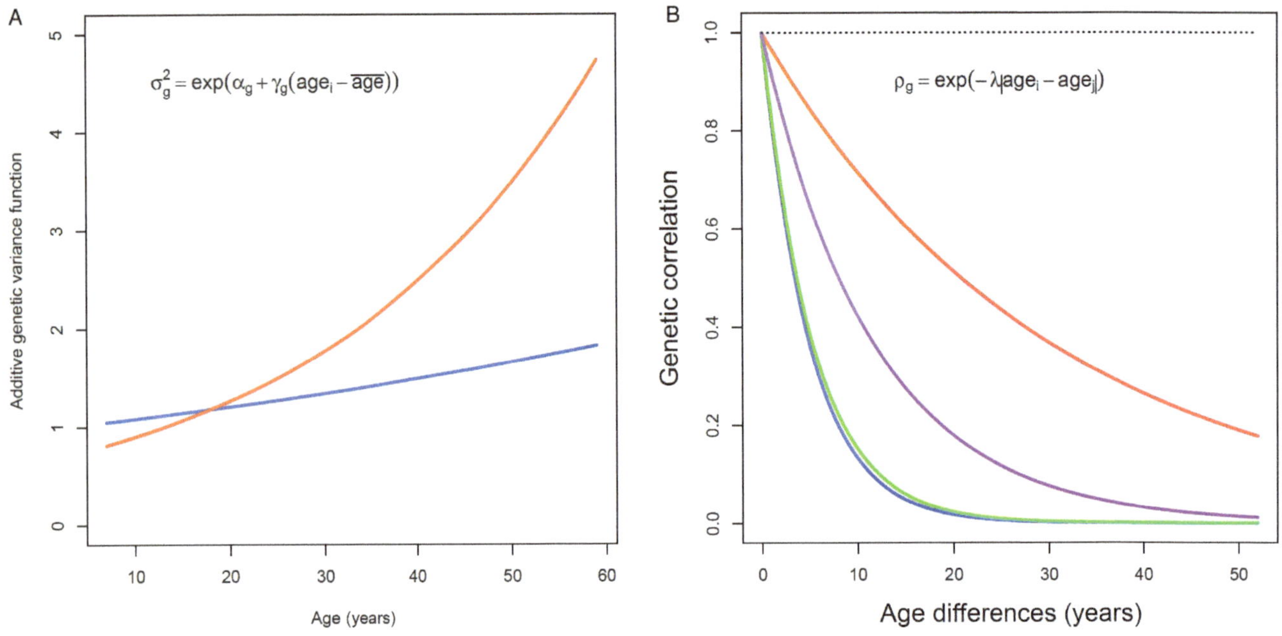

Figure 1. Genotype X Age genetic variance (a) and Genotype X Age genetic correlation (b). Legend: Blue – PC; Red – Sed; Green – EE; Purple – PA tertiles.

sedentarism, that may hinder our understanding of the putative mechanisms that regulate sedentary behaviors. Therefore, it may not be advisable to compare the heritability of different indicators, as these are not the same phenotypes and any comparison has a degree of associated bias.

The growing interest in the association between SB and health has led researchers to examine the influence of age and sex in the expression of distinct sedentary behaviors. Specifically, Genotype x Sex and Genotype x Age interaction analyses can be very helpful to disentangle these issues and are a sophisticated way to analyze the association of age and gender with SB. We found that the GxSex interaction model was a significantly better predictor of TV, EEsed, PC and PA tertiles than the polygenic model, meaning that there is variability in the expression of these behaviors that may be explained by differences between males and females in the genetic regulation of SB. Given the consistently higher additive genetic variance in males, our interpretation of these results is that the genetic regulation of energy expenditure in sedentary behaviors is stronger in males than in females. Once again, we were not able to find any study comparable to ours, namely because our model does not include any 'family/shared' factors as a source of environmental variation. However, previous work [22]

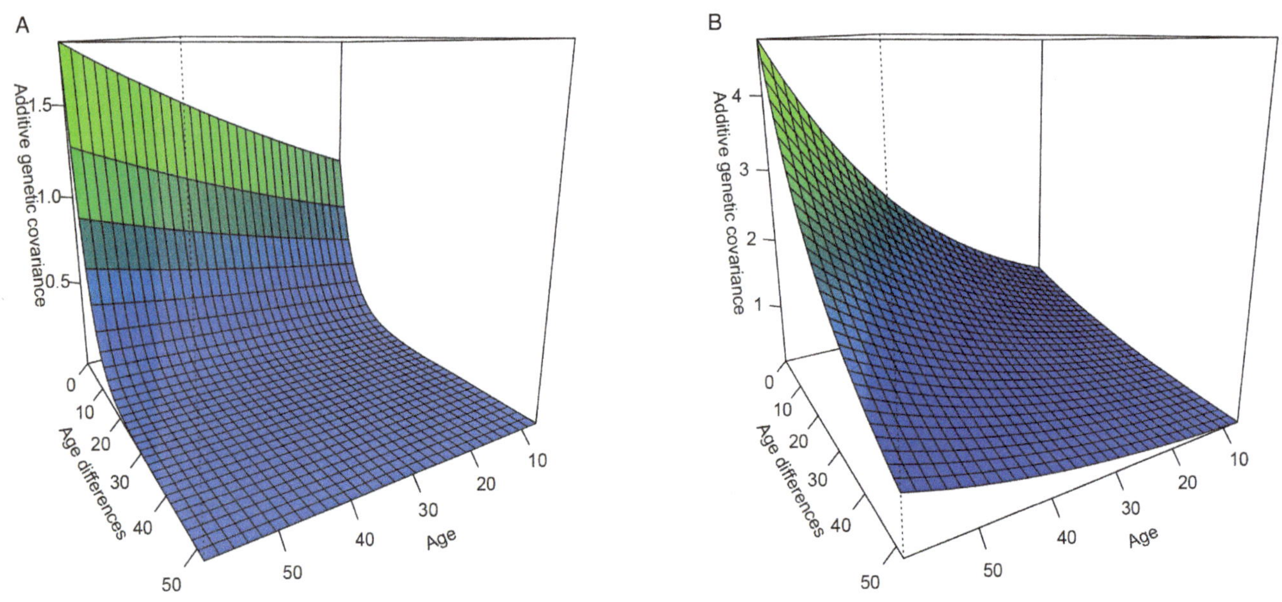

Figure 2. Genotype X Age for PC (A) and Sed (B).

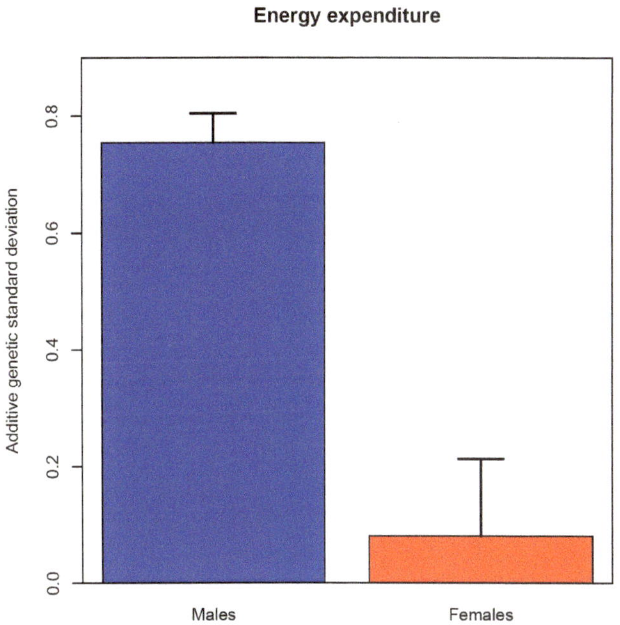

Figure 3. Genotype X Sex genetic variance for EEsed.

has shown that the household effect under the polygenic model and under a similar GxSex model failed to be significant for any of their PA traits. Recently, in a sample from the Netherlands Twin Registry (NTR) (aged 12–20 y), SB was defined as an overall score of weekly frequency of television viewing, playing electronic games, and computer or internet use, and the results showed that SB was significantly higher for boys than girls ($\chi^2 = 755.56$; $P < 0.05$), highlighting the presence of sex differences in the expression of SB. However, in 2010, another study with the NTR found that irrespective of age, sedentarism is more prevalent in females when using a distinct marker of SB (subjects were sedentary if total weekly MET score was lower than 5.0, i.e., the energy expenditure due to PA was lower than 1 kcal·kg^{-1}·h^{-1}). Once again, this seems to be quite difficult to understand, as even within the same sample and the same research group, SB results can be so diverse. This is why SB may not be a one-dimensional phenotype *per se*. Rather, it is a multi-dimensional behavior, characterized by low energy expenditure that is quite diverse in their structure, levels and patterns. Our results raise new questions regarding daily activities and/or routines, because evidence shows that males tend to be more active than females [23,24]. So, if males are more prone to suffer from environmental exposures that lead to SB, how come they are more active than females? It has been shown that SB may coincide with sports activities. For instance, elite athletes present long periods of sedentariness in their daily routines while recovering from their highly intense training sessions [25]. In this case, we might speculate that the environment that leads males to more intense activities is also the force leading to increased levels of sedentarism.

In regard to the influence of age on SB, the GxAge interaction model was a significantly better predictor of TV viewing, EEsed, PC, Sed and PA tertiles than the polygenic model, meaning that the expression of SB could be age-specific. In this case, the age effect is not simply the accumulation of habits and experiences as people get older, but mainly the way by which our genetic background probably deals with those routines. To the best of our knowledge, this kind of analysis has never been performed on SB and is of utmost importance because it can help to explain why some people tend to become sedentary as age increases. Typically, it is expected that people become more sedentary as they move from childhood to adolescence, adulthood and finally late adulthood. This has been attributed to changes in lifestyle between these life stages. For instance, adolescent development is known for being highly dependent upon peer approval, as engaging in sports or leisure's activities is dependent upon being part of a team or club [26,27], and is also influence by physical ability as being successful in a sport is a highly significant environmental factor contributing to increased levels of physical activity [28]. Moving to adulthood, people tend to spend more time seated due to their job responsibilities and during late adulthood people's low fitness levels determine the increase of sedentarism [29,30]. However, this study attempts to understand if SB is not only a function of the environmental changes that most people (at least in developed countries) experience throughout a lifespan but also if those changes can be distinctly integrated by different subjects. The current study found that SB expression is influenced by a mediation effect of age through genetic regulation which might explain why some people are not sedentary even at older ages.

Some limitations of the present study must be addressed: (i) our sample is not representative of the general Portuguese population, (ii) the relatively young and healthy sample of families may limit the generalizability of the results to older individuals, (iii) the usage of self-reporting SB is doomed to diminished reliability when compared to more objective measures which may influence heritability estimates, and (iv) the lack of information about resting metabolic rate may influence the EEsed and Sed results, although previous work [31,32] with this 3-d diary never considered this possibility. Further, the lack of sufficient power in the sample to estimate GxSex interactions for any of the traits is a serious weakness. Still, our sample is made of 339 families, which is in line with previous analysis performed with 319 families from

Table 5. Power to detect GxSex interaction effects.

Trait	σ^2_{gf}	σ^2_{gm}	Power	$\rho_{g(f,m)}$	power
EEsed	0.08066	0.75473	0.72809	1	0.1
PC	0.53845	0.53375	0.05008	−0.84644	0.77167
Sed	0.63816	0.39684	0.21	0.97973	0.10011
Sit	0.30612	0.01312	0.0801	1	0.1
PA tertiles	0.38023	0.47452	0.07131	0.86639	0.10578
TV	0.20082	0.63	0.36311	0.98777	0.10001

Table 6. Power to detect GxAge interaction effects.

Trait	γ_g	power	λ	Power
EEsed	0.02159	1	0.12883	1
PC	0.0107	0.90895	0.20179	1
Sed	0.03388	1	0.03327	1
Sit	−0.00512	0.96473	0.63717	0.9894
PA tertiles	−0.01939	1	0.08582	0.79523
TV	0.00651	1	0.03306	1

the Viva la Familia Study (30) and 207 families from the Quebec Family Study [8]. Moreover, the reliance on different markers of SB, the use of state-of-the-art statistical procedures and the novelty of the analytical strategy are strengths of the present study.

In conclusion, the present results highlight that, in our sample, 3 to 27% of the variation in sedentary behaviors is due to a genetic component adding to the known fact that sedentarism is a multifaceted and variable construct that is highly dependent upon measurement strategy. Further, our results suggest that SB expression may be influenced by the interactions between genes with both sex and age, which helps to understand some of the observed variation in these traits' expression. However, it must be acknowledged that different sedentary behaviors have distinct genetic foundations and are affected differently by age and sex, which should motivate efforts to develop better assessment tools that can be more easily comparable.

Acknowledgments

We thank the participants in The Healthy Family Study.

Author Contributions

Conceived and designed the experiments: DS JARM VPD PTK. Performed the experiments: DS JARM RNC MCS TNG FKS. Analyzed the data: DS JARM VPD. Wrote the paper: DS JARM PTK VPD DLF. Designed the software used in analysis: JB.

References

1. Thorp AA, Owen N, Neuhaus M, Dunstan DW (2011) Sedentary behaviors and subsequent health outcomes in adults a systematic review of longitudinal studies, 1996–2011. American journal of preventive medicine 41: 207–215.
2. Gopinath B, Hardy LL, Baur LA, Burlutsky G, Mitchell P (2012) Physical activity and sedentary behaviors and health-related quality of life in adolescents. Pediatrics 130: e167–174.
3. Kesse-Guyot E, Charreire H, Andreeva VA, Touvier M, Hercberg S, et al. (2012) Cross-sectional and longitudinal associations of different sedentary behaviors with cognitive performance in older adults. PloS one 7: e47831.
4. de Vilhena e Santos DM, Katzmarzyk PT, Seabra AF, Maia JA (2012) Genetics of physical activity and physical inactivity in humans. Behavior genetics 42: 559–578.
5. Fisher A, van Jaarsveld CH, Llewellyn CH, Wardle J (2010) Environmental influences on children's physical activity: quantitative estimates using a twin design. PloS one 5: e10110.
6. Butte NF, Cai G, Cole SA, Comuzzie AG (2006) Viva la Familia Study: genetic and environmental contributions to childhood obesity and its comorbidities in the Hispanic population. The American journal of clinical nutrition 84: 646–654; quiz 673–644.
7. Hoed M, Brage S, Zhao JH, Westgate K, Nessa A, et al. (2013) Heritability of objectively assessed daily physical activity and sedentary behavior. The American journal of clinical nutrition 98: 1317–1325.
8. Simonen RL, Perusse L, Rankinen T, Rice T, Rao DC, et al. (2002) Familial aggregation of physical activity levels in the Quebec Family Study. Med Sci Sports Exerc 34: 1137–1142.
9. Bouchard C, Tremblay A, Leblanc C, Lortie G, Savard R, et al. (1983) A method to assess energy expenditure in children and adults. The American journal of clinical nutrition 37: 461–467.
10. Rosa MJV, Chitas P (2010) Portugal: os números. Lisboa.
11. Lohman TG, Roche AF, Martorel R (1988) Anthropometric Standardization Reference Manual. Illinois: Human Kinetics Books Champaign.
12. Durnin JVGA, Passmore R (1967) Energy, work and leisure. London: Heinemann Educational Books, Lda.
13. Craig CL, Marshall AL, Sjostrom M, Bauman AE, Booth ML, et al. (2003) International physical activity questionnaire: 12-country reliability and validity. Med Sci Sports Exerc 35: 1381–1395.
14. Almasy L, Blangero J (1998) Multipoint quantitative-trait linkage analysis in general pedigrees. American journal of human genetics 62: 1198–1211.
15. Blangero J, Diego VP, Dyer TD, Almeida M, Peralta J, et al. (2013) A kernel of truth: statistical advances in polygenic variance component models for complex human pedigrees. Advances in genetics 81: 1–31.
16. Diego VP, Rainwater DL, Wang XL, Cole SA, Curran JE, et al. (2007) Genotype x adiposity interaction linkage analyses reveal a locus on chromosome 1 for lipoprotein-associated phospholipase A2, a marker of inflammation and oxidative stress. American journal of human genetics 80: 168–177.
17. Diego VP, Almasy L, Dyer TD, Soler JM, Blangero J (2003) Strategy and model building in the fourth dimension: a null model for genotype x age interaction as a Gaussian stationary stochastic process. BMC genetics 4 Suppl 1: S34.
18. Blangero J (2009) Statistical genetic approaches to human adaptability. 1993. Human biology 81: 523–546.
19. Diego VP (2005) Genotype × Age Interaction, and the Insulin-Like Growth Factor I Axis in the San Antonio Family Heart Study: A Study in Human Senescence. New York: Graduate School of Binghamton University. pp. 317.
20. Cai G, Cole SA, Butte N, Bacino C, Diego V, et al. (2006) A quantitative trait locus on chromosome 18q for physical activity and dietary intake in Hispanic children. Obesity (Silver Spring) 14: 1596–1604.
21. Pate RR, O'Neill JR, Lobelo F (2008) The evolving definition of "sedentary". Exercise and sport sciences reviews 36: 173–178.
22. Horimoto AR, Giolo SR, Oliveira CM, Alvim RO, Soler JP, et al. (2011) Heritability of physical activity traits in Brazilian families: the Baependi Heart Study. BMC medical genetics 12: 155.
23. Klinker CD, Schipperijn J, Christian H, Kerr J, Ersboll AK, et al. (2014) Using accelerometers and global positioning system devices to assess gender and age differences in children's school, transport, leisure and home based physical activity. The international journal of behavioral nutrition and physical activity 11: 8.
24. Casper JM, Harrolle MG, Kelley K (2013) Gender differences in self-report physical activity and park and recreation facility use among Latinos in Wake County, North Carolina. Annals of behavioral medicine: a publication of the Society of Behavioral Medicine 45 Suppl 1: S49–54.
25. Judice PB, Silva AM, Magalhaes JP, Matias CN, Sardinha LB (2014) Sedentary behaviour and adiposity in elite athletes. Journal of sports sciences 32: 1760–1767.
26. Salvy SJ, Bowker JW, Roemmich JN, Romero N, Kieffer E, et al. (2008) Peer influence on children's physical activity: an experience sampling study. Journal of pediatric psychology 33: 39–49.
27. (2004) Children's peer relations: From development to intervention. Washington, DC, US: American Psychological Association. xvi, 289 p.
28. Katzmarzyk PT, Malina RM (1998) Contribution of organized sports participation to estimated daily energy expenditure in youth. Pediatr Exerc Sci 10: 378–386.
29. Christensen U, Stovring N, Schultz-Larsen K, Schroll M, Avlund K (2006) Functional ability at age 75: is there an impact of physical inactivity from middle age to early old age? Scandinavian journal of medicine & science in sports 16: 245–251.

30. Gretebeck RJ, Ferraro KF, Black DR, Holland K, Gretebeck KA (2012) Longitudinal change in physical activity and disability in adults. American journal of health behavior 36: 385–394.
31. Loos RJ, Rankinen T, Tremblay A, Perusse L, Chagnon Y, et al. (2005) Melanocortin-4 receptor gene and physical activity in the Quebec Family Study. International journal of obesity 29: 420–428.
32. Simonen RL, Rankinen T, Perusse L, Leon AS, Skinner JS, et al. (2003) A dopamine D2 receptor gene polymorphism and physical activity in two family studies. Physiology & behavior 78: 751–757.

16

Relationships between Training Load, Salivary Cortisol Responses and Performance during Season Training in Middle and Long Distance Runners

Carlos Balsalobre-Fernández*, Carlos Mª Tejero-González, Juan del Campo-Vecino

Department of Physical Education, Sport and Human Movement, Autonomous University of Madrid, Madrid, Spain

Abstract

Purpose: Monitoring training from a multifactorial point of view is of great importance in elite endurance athletes. This study aims to analyze the relationships between indicators of training load, hormonal status and neuromuscular performance, and to compare these values with competition performance, in elite middle and long-distance runners.

Method: Fifteen elite middle and long-distance runners (12 men, 3 women; age = 26.3±5.1 yrs) were measured for training volume, training zone and session rate of perceived exertion (RPE) (daily), countermovement jump (CMJ) and salivary free cortisol (weekly) for 39 weeks (i.e., the whole season). Competition performance was also observed throughout the study, registering the season best and worst competitions.

Results: Season average salivary free cortisol concentrations correlate significantly with CMJ ($r = -0.777$) and RPE ($r = 0.551$). Also, weekly averages of CMJ significantly correlates with RPE ($r = -0.426$), distance run ($r = -0.593$, $p < 0.001$) and training zone ($r = 0.437$, $p < 0.05$). Finally, it was found that the CMJ (+8.5%, $g = 0.65$) and the RPE (−17.6%, $g = 0.94$) measured the week before the best competition performance of the season were significantly different compared with the measurement conducted the week before the season's worst competition performance.

Conclusions: Monitoring weekly measurements of CMJ and RPE could be recommended to control training process of such athletes in a non-invasive, field-based, systematic way.

Editor: Pedro Tauler, University of the Balearic Islands, Spain

Funding: The authors have no support or funding to report.

Competing Interests: The authors have declared that no competing interests exist.

* Email: carlos.balsalobre@uam.es

Introduction

Although training volume is not directly related to performance of elite endurance athletes [1–3], it seems clear that such athletes need to train several hours per week during their training cycle to increase their performance [4–6]. Specifically, elite distance runners may run a lot of km throughout the season, with weekly amounts totaling up to 230 km or more in the case of marathon runners [7]. Thus, monitoring the training process of such athletes is essential in order to observe their adaptation to training load and to avoid overtraining syndrome [8–10]. Although the assessment of physiological parameters such as maximal oxygen uptake or blood cell count is of great importance in endurance sports [11,12], their invasive, laboratory-based nature complicate regular measurement during daily training. Therefore, the use of some indicators that could, systematically and without disturbing the athletes, facilitate in-the-field monitoring of the training processes required.

The most common variable used on a daily basis to monitor the training process in running is the training load [9]. Specifically, training volume, intensity and session-RPE are the most used indicators of the training load because they can be assessed every day without disturbing the athletes and have shown significant relationships with performance or fatigue [13,14]. For example, Esteve-Lanao et al. [13] recorded training volume and intensity of sub-elite cross-country runners for 6 months, discovering that the time expended training at low intensities (below the ventilator threshold) was significantly related to performance in a cross-country competition. Similarly, Garcin et al. [14] measured session-RPE in 8 young, elite middle-distance runners for 8 weeks, proving that this indicator of training load was able to detect states of overreaching. Meanwhile, the measurement of the vertical jump score as an indicator of neuromuscular performance has been used to assess fatigue in different kinds of athletes [15–17]. For example, it has been shown that the decrease in the countermovement jump (CMJ) score after a set of full-squats performed until failure correlates highly with blood lactate concentrations ($r = 0.97$, $p < 0.001$) [17]. With respect to distance runners, it has been observed that a marathon competition significantly impairs the height reached in the CMJ [18]. Finally, the measurement of salivary free cortisol (hormone related with fatigue and stress) is commonly used to monitor the effects of training in several sports, due to its non-invasive, field-based nature [19,20]. Moreover, it seems that cortisol levels are related to neuromuscular performance in well-trained strength athletes [21,22]. For example, it has been demonstrated that changes in salivary free cortisol levels after 15 weeks of training are related to changes in the power clean mean power production over the same period in young elite wrestlers [23]. However, as far as we know, the relationship between salivary free cortisol levels and neuromuscular performance has not been studied on high-level middle and long-distance runners throughout a whole season.

Thus, although the measurement of the training load, salivary free cortisol or CMJ are very common to monitor training process in different kinds of athletes [7,24,25], any relationships between such variables in high-level distance runners, as well as their impact on the performance of such athletes, is, as far as we know, unknown. Therefore, the objectives of this investigation are: (1) to disclose the relationships between training load (measured using daily km run totals, training zone and session-RPE), salivary free cortisol and CMJ scores throughout a whole season in elite middle and long-distance runners; and (2) to compare the values of the study variables measured just before the season-best competition performance with the values measured just before the season-worst competition performance. As such, and according to the above, our study hypotheses are that: (a) weekly values of training load, salivary free cortisol and CMJ measured throughout the season are significantly related; and (b) the values of these variables measured just before the season-best competition performance are significantly different compared with those measured just before the season-worst competition performance.

Materials and Methods

Subjects

The participants in this study were 15 high-level middle and long-distance runners from the High Performance Sports Center Madrid (12 men, 3 women; age = 26.3±5.1 yrs), with personal bests in outdoor 1500-metres between 3:38–3:58 min. (men) and 4:12–4:23 min. (women). See Table 1 for more details.

Ethics statement

The study protocol complied with the Declaration of Helsinki for Human Experimentation and was approved by the ethics committee at the Autonomous University of Madrid (approval number CEI-45 889). Written informed consent was obtained from each subject before participation.

Design

Athletes were assessed for CMJ score, salivary free cortisol levels and training load throughout a whole season (October–July, 39 weeks). CMJ and cortisol were measured once a week, while training load, assessed by session rate of perceived exertion (session-RPE), km run and training zone were measured daily. Competition performance was observed throughout the whole season, registering the season best (SB) and worst (SW) results (i.e., fastest and slowest times in competitions). Correlations between the variables evaluated in this investigation and differences in CMJ, cortisol and training load just before the SB and SW events were then analyzed. See Figure 1 for more information about the training load variation throughout the season.

Table 1. Characteristics of the participants (average ± SD).

	Age (yrs.)	Height (cm)	Weight (kg)	PB in outdoor 1500 m (min:s)	PB in urban 10 km (min:s)	Average CMJ (cm)	Average Session-RPE (0–10)	Average weekly km run	Average weekly training zone	Average salivary free cortisol (ng/mL)
Men	25.7±5.4^N	1.79±0.04^N	63.9±3.1^N	3:43±0:6^N	30:33±0:43^N	30.3±4.8^N	5.7±0.4^N	85.4±5.8^N	1.8±0.06^N	11.9±2.3^N
Women	29.0±2.0^N	1.67±0.05^N	52.0±3.6^N	4:18±0:5^N	34:50±1:32^N	27.9±1.4^N	6.1±0.3^N	83.2±7.0^N	1.8±0.5^N	12.4±2.1^N

^{N} = Normally distributed variable (Kolmogorov-Smirnov test, $p>0.05$). Abbreviations: PB = personal best; CMJ = countermovement jump; Session-RPE = session rate of perceived exertion.
Note: Training zones ranges from 1–3 according to session average running pace. Zone 1 = 3:45–3:10 min/km; Zone 2 = 3:10–2:50 min/km; Zone 3 = 2:50 min/km to full sprint.

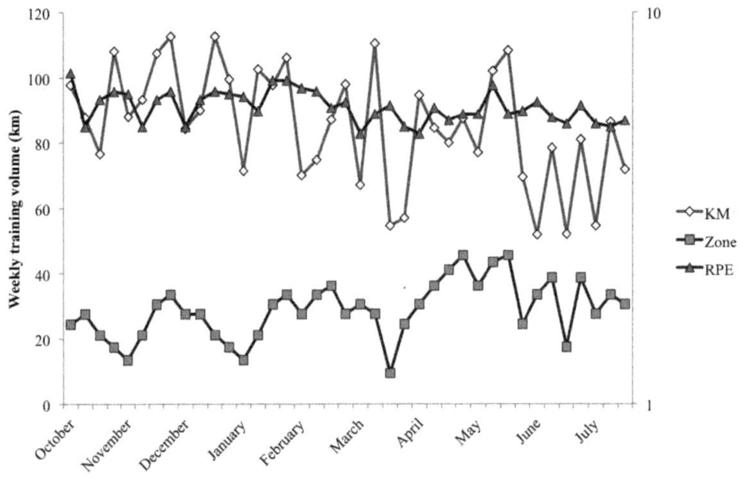

Figure 1. Training load variation throughout the whole season. Weekly training volume, training zone and session-RPE are represented. Training volume is represented on the left Y-axis (in km.), while training zone and session-RPE are represented on the right Y-axis with a logarithmic scale. Abbreviations: KM = weekly average km run; Zone = weekly average training zone; RPE = weekly average session-RPE.

Methodology

Training load. Training load was measured daily throughout the whole season using daily session-RPE, km run and training zone parameters. Session-RPE was assessed after each training session using the Borg 0–10 scale by asking, "How hard was the training session, with 0 being very, very light and 10 extremely heavy?". Kilometres run and training zone were recorded using the coach's endurance training programmes designed for each athlete. When an athlete coudln't fulfil his or her training programme, the km run and training zone values of the what the athlete did complete were recorded. Every training session was classified in one of 3 training zones according to the characteristics of the principle part of the session: Zone 1 included long-distance continuous training, or interval training with long sets (4–6 km), at paces of between 3:45-3:10 min/km; Zone 2 included middle-distance interval training (sets of 1–3 km) at paces between 3:10-2:50 min/km; and Zone 3 included short-distance and sprint interval training (sets of 200–600 m) at paces ranging from 2:50 min/km to full sprint.

Salivary-free cortisol. To establish the basal cortisol level (in ng/mL), athletes collected a saliva sample immediately after they woke up (i.e., 1–2 min after waking up), with an empty stomach, once a week throughout the whole season using Salivette tubes (Sarstedt, Germany). Athletes chewed the cotton inside the Salivette tube for 60 seconds after they rinsed their mouth with water, then they stored the sample at −20°C for 1 hour before subsequently bringing it to the laboratory for analysis. All measurements were performed on the same day of the week, at the same time and under the same environmental conditions. All the subjects woke up almost at the same time of the day (8:30–9 a.m.) since they lived in the same area and trained together. The samples were then stored at −20°C according to the manufacturer's instructions. All samples were analyzed at the Biochemical Laboratory of the Polytechnic University of Madrid (Official Lab. Number 242 in the Region of Madrid) using Free Cortisol in Saliva ELISA Assay kits (Demeditec Diagnostics, Germany). The coefficient of variation (CV) of the measurements was CV = 4.3–5.6%.

CMJ. The CMJ scores were measured once a week throughout the whole season, on the same day that saliva samples were collected and just before beginning the training session. An Optojump infrared (IR) platform (Microgate, Italy) was used for the assessment. The CMJ was performed with hands on hips, knees straight in the flight phase while trying to jump as high as possible. All measurements were taken on the same day of the week, at the same time and under the same spatial and environmental conditions. The average of 3 attempts was recorded. The reliability of the measurements was calculated using the intraclass correlation coefficient (ICC = 0.979–0.990, $p < 0.001$).

Statistical analysis

To analyze the relationship between the variables, we used the Pearson correlation coefficient, unilateral contrast. For the comparison of means, we used the paired samples t-test. For the calculation of the effect size (ES), we used the Hedge's g. Effects sizes below 0.5 were considerate *low,* and ES between 0.5–1.0 were considerate *moderate to high* [26]. The level of significance was set at 0.05. All calculations were performed using IBM SPSS Statistics 22 software (IBM Co., USA).

Results

Significant correlations were found between season average CMJ and cortisol ($r = -0.777$, $p<0.001$), CMJ and session-RPE ($r = -0.489$, $p = 0.049$) and session-RPE and cortisol ($r = 0.551$, $p = 0.025$) values. Analysis of the average weekly values of the variables throughout the whole season showed that CMJ scores correlate significantly with session-RPE ($r = -0.426$, $p = 0.012$), cortisol ($r = 0.556$, $p<0.001$), km run ($r = -0.593$, $p<0.001$) and training zone ($r = 0.437$, $p = 0.007$). Also, km run correlates significantly with session-RPE ($r = 0.444$, $p = 0.009$) and cortisol levels ($r = -0.366$, $p = 0.017$). See Table 2 for more details.

Comparing the values for the variables measured the week before the season-best (SB) and season-worst (SW) competition performances, it was found that the CMJ scores prior to the SB was significantly higher than the CMJ score prior to the SW (+ 8.5%, $g = 0.65$, $p<0.001$). The session-RPE for the week before the SB was significantly lower than the session-RPE for the week before the SW (−17.6%, $g = 0.94$, $p = 0.022$). There were no significant differences between salivary free cortisol, km run or

Table 2. Pearson correlation coefficient (r) between study variables.

	Session-RPE		Cortisol		Km run		Training zone	
	Season average	Weekly average	Season average	Weekly average	Season average	Weekly average	Season average	Weekly average
CMJ	**−0.489***	**−0.426***	**−0.777****	**0.556****	0.133	**−0.593****	−0.231	**0.437***
Session-RPE	–	–	**0.551***	−0.037	0.168	**0.444***	−0.130	−0.080
Cortisol	–	–	–	–	−0.051	−0.366	−0.228	0.171
Km run	–	–	–	–	–	–	**−0.599***	−0.044

Season average: correlations between average variables for the group throughout the whole season; Weekly average: correlations between average variables of the group for every week of the season. CMJ = countermovement jump score; Session-RPE = rate of perceived exertion of the training session; km run = total weekly km run.
*p<0.05;
**p<0.001.

training zone values measured before SB and SW. See Table 3 for more details.

Discussion

The results of our study have revealed that noteworthy relationships exist between salivary free cortisol and CMJ scores assessed throughout a whole season in elite middle and long-distance runners. Also, moderate relationships between session-RPE and salivary-free cortisol were found. Firstly, our data demonstrates a significant trend in which athletes with higher [average] cortisol levels measured throughout the season were those with lower CMJ scores. It worth to mention that females and males salivary free cortisol were equivalent throughout the season, despite some studies have reported hormonal differences between sexes [27,28]. It has previously been demonstrated that post-exercise blood lactate and ammonia concentrations are negatively and significantly related to the height jumped in the CMJ performed just after an intensive exercise session, so greater CMJ decreases correspond to a higher level in such physiological markers [17]. In highly-trained strength athletes, it was observed that salivary cortisol is negatively and significantly related to neuromuscular performance [14,22]. For example, Kraemer et al. [22] studied the changes on cortisol and performance of a group of highly-trained soccer players throughout a season, and they showed that salivary cortisol levels measured before training have a significant correlation with the vertical jump height scores recorded on the same day ($r = -0.59$, $p<0.05$). That study concludes that athletes starting the season with elevated cortisol values may experience significant reductions on performance during the season. Our study expands the knowledge in this respect, demonstrating that subjects with higher long-term salivary free cortisol levels significantly tend to be those with lower CMJ scores throughout the season. However, when correlations between weekly average cortisol and CMJ values were analyzed, a significant trend was observed in which the weeks with higher salivary free concentrations were those in which higher CMJ scores were recorded. Thus, despite athletes with higher [average] cortisol levels throughout the season had significantly lower CMJ [average] values, it seems that weeks with higher cortisol concentrations produce a potentiation of CMJ performance. Although some investigations have studied the relationships between salivary cortisol concentrations and force production [23] or vertical jump [21], they used strength-related athletes and measured the variables less frequently (6 times during a season). However, we are not aware of studies which analyze the relationship between weekly salivary free cortisol concentrations and CMJ height measurements throughout a whole season in elite middle and long-distance runners. Further research is needed to clarify the nature of the relationship between salivary cortisol concentrations and CMJ performance in elite middle and long-distance runners.

Furthermore, training load was also shown to correlate significantly with salivary cortisol levels and CMJ scores. Specifically, weekly values for session-RPE, km run and training zone correlate significantly with CMJ scores, in such a way that in weeks with lower rates of perceived exertion, less km run and with higher training zone (i.e., more Zone 3 sessions) correspond with those weeks with higher CMJ performance. Similarly, our data shows that athletes with higher average season-long, session-RPE values significantly tend to be those who trained more km and had higher average season-long salivary cortisol concentrations. Some authors have proposed that elite athletes endurance training must consist of lower training volume to produce the desired

Table 3. Comparison of variables measured the week before the season best (SB) and season worst (SW) competition performances.

Variables	SAv	SB	SW	Hedge's g	95% CI	%
	Av ± SD	Av ± SD	Av ± SD			
CMJ (cm)	29.8 ± 4.6^N	32.5 ± 4.5^N	29.7 ± 4.0^N	0.65	[1.9, 3.6]	+8.5**
Session-RPE (0–10)	5.8 ± 4.5^N	5.6 ± 1.3^N	6.6 ± 0.8^N	0.94	[−1.9, −0.2]	−17.6*
Salivary free cortisol (ng/mL)	12.0 ± 2.2^N	15.7 ± 7.3^N	12.1 ± 6.7^N	0.52	[−1.2, 8.3]	+22.9
Km run	84.9 ± 5.9^N	75.8 ± 24.4^N	87.2 ± 22.8^N	0.48	[−26.8, 4.2]	−15.0
Training zone	1.8 ± 0.8^N	1.9 ± 0.4^N	2.0 ± 0.4^N	0.21	[−0.4, 0.2]	−5.2

^{N} = Normally distributed variable (Kolmogorov-Smirnov test, $p > 0.05$);
*$p < 0.05$;
**$p < 0.001$.
Abbreviations: SAv = average value for the season; SB = value measured the week before the season best competition performance; SW = value measured the week before the season worst competition performance; Av = average value; SD = standard deviation; 95% CI = 95% confidence interval of the differences between SB and SW values; % = percentage difference between SB and SW; CMJ = countermovement jump score; Session-RPE = rate of perceived exertion of the training session; km run = total weekly km run.

adaptations [1,29]. For example, it has been proven in elite kayakers that a 1-year traditional endurance training programme produces lower increases in physical fitness than a 1-year block-periodisation endurance training programme with 50% less volume [1]. Similarly, it has been shown that resistance training performed until failure produces higher fatigue accumulation and lower increases in performance than an identical training regime in which half of the possible repetitions per set were executed [29]. Therefore, results in our study show that training with a higher volume and greater session-RPE correlate significantly with higher salivary cortisol concentrations and a lower performance in the CMJ.

Moreover, when analyzing the difference between the training load, salivary free cortisol and CMJ values measured the week before the season best and season worst competition performances, it is observed that, before the SB, athletes achieved higher CMJ scores than before the SW. Also, the CMJ before the SB was significantly higher than the season average, while the CMJ measured before the SW did not vary from the season average. Meanwhile, session-RPE measured before the SB was significantly lower than that measured before the SW. Furthermore, session-RPE before the SB was lower (although not significantly) than the season average, while the session-RPE before the SW was significantly higher than the season average. There were no significant differences in the other variables, although athletes trained 11.4 km less the week before the SB than before the SW performances. That is to say, the week before the best competition performance of the season, athletes trained with significantly lower session-RPE, achieved higher CMJ scores and ran more than 11 km less in comparison with the SW performance. In this sense, it was previously demonstrated that the reduction of training volume near to an important competition could improve physical performance of highly-trained athletes [30,31].

In summary, the weekly assessment of training load (using daily session-RPE, km run and training zone), salivary free cortisol and CMJ scores may help to control the training process of elite middle and long-distance runners using simple, non-invasive, systematic, field-based methods throughout a whole season. For the very first time, this study analyzes the relationships between training load, salivary free cortisol concentrations and CMJ scores measured throughout 39 weeks of training by such athletes.

Practical Applications and Conclusions

This study reveals the significant relationships between average season values for CMJ scores, salivary free cortisol levels and session-RPE-athletes with higher salivary cortisol concentrations demonstrated a significant correlation with a tendency for lower CMJ scores and higher session-RPE values-. When observing the weekly average of the group, it was observed that the weeks in which higher CMJ scores were achieved significantly correspond to those with lower volume (km), higher training zone and lower session-RPE values. Finally, it was proven that CMJ scores were significantly higher and session-RPE values were significantly lower the week before the season best competition performance in comparison with the week before the season worst competition performance. The results of our study agree with those in other investigations which propose that training with lower volumes and less fatigue-inducing sessions are more effective in terms of increasing performance. Monitoring training load through daily session-RPE and weekly CMJ measurements could help control the training process of elite middle and long-distance runners. Furthermore, such variables can be measured throughout a whole season without interfering with the athlete's training using simple, non-invasive, field-based methods.

Acknowledgments

Firstly we would like to thank the coach and their athletes for their involvement in this study throughout an entire season of training. We would also like to thank the personnel of the Biochemical Laboratory of the Polytechnic University of Madrid for their contributions.

Author Contributions

Conceived and designed the experiments: CBF JDCV. Performed the experiments: CBF JDCV. Analyzed the data: CBF CMTG JDCV. Contributed reagents/materials/analysis tools: CBF CMTG. Contributed to the writing of the manuscript: CBF CMTG.

References

1. García-Pallarés J, García-Fernández M, Sánchez-Medina L, Izquierdo M (2010) Performance changes in world-class kayakers following two different training periodization models. European Journal Of Applied Physiology 110: 99–107.
2. Legaz Arrese A, Serrano Ostariz E, Casajus Mallen JA, Munguia Izquierdo D (2005) The changes in running performance and maximal oxygen uptake after long-term training in elite athletes. Journal of Sports Medicine & Physical Fitness 45: 435–440.
3. Wilber RL, Pitsiladis YP (2012) Kenyan and Ethiopian Distance Runners: What Makes Them So Good? International Journal of Sports Physiology & Performance 7: 92–102.
4. Enoksen E, Tjelta AR, Tjelta LI (2011) Distribution of Training Volume and Intensity of Elite Male and Female Track and Marathon Runners. International Journal of Sports Science & Coaching 6: 273–294.
5. Ingham SA, Fudge BW, Pringle JS (2012) Training Distribution, Physiological Profile, and Performance for a Male International 1500-m Runner. International Journal of Sports Physiology & Performance 7: 193–195.
6. Leif Inge T (2013) A Longitudinal Case Study of the Training of the 2012 European 1500 m Track Champion. International Journal of Applied Sports Sciences 25: 11–18.
7. Stellingwerff T (2012) Case Study: Nutrition and Training Periodization in Three Elite Marathon Runners. International Journal of Sport Nutrition & Exercise Metabolism 22: 392–400.
8. O'Connor PJ (2007) Monitoring and Titrating Symptoms. Sports Medicine 37: 408–411.
9. Borresen J, Lambert MI (2009) The Quantification of Training Load, the Training Response and the Effect on Performance. Sports Medicine 39: 779–795.
10. Meeusen R, Duclos M, Foster C, Fry A, Gleeson M, et al. (2013) Prevention, diagnosis, and treatment of the overtraining syndrome: joint consensus statement of the European College of Sport Science and the American College of Sports Medicine. Med Sci Sports Exerc 45: 186–205.
11. Billat V, Lepretre PM, Heugas AM, Laurence MH, Salim D, et al. (2003) Training and bioenergetic characteristics in elite male and female Kenyan runners. Medicine & Science in Sports & Exercise 35: 297–304.
12. Auersperger I, Knap B, Jerin A, Blagus R, Lainscak M, et al. (2012) The Effects of 8 Weeks of Endurance Running on Hepcidin Concentrations, Inflammatory Parameters, and Iron Status in Female Runners. International Journal of Sport Nutrition & Exercise Metabolism 22: 55–63.
13. Esteve-Lanao J, San Juan AF, Earnest CP, Foster C, Lucia A (2005) How Do Endurance Runners Actually Train? Relationship with Competition Performance. Medicine & Science in Sports & Exercise 37: 496–504.
14. Garcin M, Fleury A, Billat V (2002) The ratio HLa:RPE as a tool to appreciate overreaching in young high-level middle-distance runners. International Journal of Sports Medicine 23: 16–21.
15. Cormack SJ, Newton RU, McGuigan MR (2008) Neuromuscular and Endocrine Responses of Elite Players to an Australian Rules Football Match. International Journal of Sports Physiology & Performance 3: 359–374.
16. Jiménez-Reyes P, Cuadrado-Peñafiel V, González-Badillo JJ (2011) Application of the Counter Movement Jump Test to Monitor Training Load in Sprint Sessions. Culture, Science & Sport 7: 105–112.
17. Sanchez-Medina L, González-Badillo JJ (2011) Velocity Loss as an Indicator of Neuromuscular Fatigue during Resistance Training. Medicine & Science in Sports & Exercise 43: 1725–1734.
18. Petersen K, Hansen C, Aagaard P, Madsen K (2007) Muscle mechanical characteristics in fatigue and recovery from a marathon race in highly trained runners. European Journal Of Applied Physiology 101: 385–396.
19. McLean BD, Coutts AJ, Kelly V, McGuigan MR, Cormack SJ (2010) Neuromuscular, Endocrine, and Perceptual Fatigue Responses During Different Length Between-Match Microcycles in Professional Rugby League Players. International Journal of Sports Physiology & Performance 5: 367–383.
20. Papacosta E, Nassis GP (2011) Saliva as a tool for monitoring steroid, peptide and immune markers in sport and exercise science. Journal of Science & Medicine in Sport 14: 424–434.
21. Crewther BT, Lowe TIM, Weatherby RP, Gill N, Keogh J (2009) Neuromuscular performance of elite rugby union players and relationships with salivary hormones Journal of Strength & Conditioning Research 23: 2046–2053.
22. Kraemer WJ, French DN, Paxton NJ, Häkkinen K, Volek JS, et al. (2004) Changes in exercise performance and hormonal concentrations over a big ten soccer season in starters and nonstarters. Journal of Strength & Conditioning Research 18: 121–128.
23. Passelergue PA, Lac G (2012) Salivary hormonal responses and performance changes during 15 weeks of mixed aerobic and weight training in elite junior wrestlers. Journal of Strength & Conditioning Research 26: 3049–3058.
24. McGuigan MR, Egan AD, Foster C (2004) Salivary cortisol responses and perceived exertion during high intensity and low intensity bouts of resistance exercise. Journal of Sports Science & Medicine 3: 8–15.
25. Gorostiaga EM, Grandados C, Ibanez J, Gonzalez-Badillo JJ, Izquierdo M (2006) Effects of an Entire Season on Physical Fitness Changes in Elite Male Handball Players. Medicine & Science in Sports & Exercise 38: 357–366.
26. Rhea MR (2004) Determining the magnitude of treatment effects in strength training research through the use of the effect size. Journal of Strength & Conditioning Research 18: 918–920.
27. Obmiński Z (2008) Blood Cortisol Responses to Pre-Competition Stress in Athletes: Sex-Related Differences. Research Yearbook 14: 103–108.
28. Tyndall GL, Kobe RW, Houmard JA (1996) Cortisol, testosterone, and insulin action during intense swimming training in humans. European Journal of Applied Physiology & Occupational Physiology 73: 61–65.
29. Izquierdo-Gabarren M, De Txabarri Expósito RG, García-Pallarés J, Sánchez-Medina L, De Villarreal ESS, et al. (2010) Concurrent Endurance and Strength Training Not to Failure Optimizes Performance Gains. Medicine & Science in Sports & Exercise 42: 1191–1199.
30. Bosquet L, Montpetit J, Arvisais D, Mujika I (2007) Effects of Tapering on Performance: A Meta-Analysis. Medicine & Science in Sports & Exercise 39: 1358–1365.
31. Knicker AJ, Renshaw I, Oldham ARH, Cairns SP (2011) Interactive Processes Link the Multiple Symptoms of Fatigue in Sport Competition. Sports Medicine 41: 307–328.

17

Changes in Morphological and Elastic Properties of Patellar Tendon in Athletes with Unilateral Patellar Tendinopathy and Their Relationships with Pain and Functional Disability

Zhi Jie Zhang[1,2], Gabriel Yin-fat Ng[1], Wai Chun Lee[1], Siu Ngor Fu[1]*

1 Department of Rehabilitation Sciences, The Hong Kong Polytechnic University, Hung Hom, Kowloon, Hong Kong, **2** Guangdong-Hongkong Joint Sports Rehabilitation and Research Center, Guangdong Provincial Work Injury Rehabilitation Hospital, Guangzhou, China

Abstract

Background: Patellar tendinopathy (PT) is one of the most common knee disorders among athletes. Changes in morphology and elasticity of the painful tendon and how these relate to the self-perceived pain and dysfunction remain unclear.

Objectives: To compare the morphology and elastic properties of patellar tendons between athlete with and without unilateral PT and to examine its association with self-perceived pain and dysfunction.

Methods: In this cross-sectional study, 33 male athletes (20 healthy and 13 with unilateral PT) were enrolled. The morphology and elastic properties of the patellar tendon were assessed by the grey and elastography mode of supersonic shear imaging (SSI) technique while the intensity of pressure pain, self-perceived pain and dysfunction were quantified with a 10-lb force to the most painful site and the Victorian Institute of Sport Assessment-patella (VISA-P) questionnaire, respectively.

Results: In athletes with unilateral PT, the painful tendons had higher shear elastic modulus (SEM) and larger tendon than the non-painful side ($p<0.05$) or the dominant side of the healthy athletes ($p<0.05$). Significant correlations were found between tendon SEM ratio (SEM of painful over non-painful tendon) and the intensity of pressure pain ($rho = 0.62$; $p = 0.024$), VISA-P scores ($rho = -0.61$; $p = 0.026$), and the sub-scores of the VISA-P scores on going down stairs, lunge, single leg hopping and squatting (*rho* ranged from -0.63 to -0.67; $p<0.05$).

Conclusions: Athletes with unilateral PT had stiffer and larger tendon on the painful side than the non-painful side and the dominant side of healthy athletes. No significant differences on the patellar tendon morphology and elastic properties were detected between the dominant and non-dominant knees of the healthy control. The ratio of the SEM of painful to non-painful sides was associated with pain and dysfunction among athletes with unilateral PT.

Editor: François Hug, The University of Queensland, Australia

Funding: The authors have no support or funding to report.

Competing Interests: The authors have declared that no competing interests exist.

* Email: amy.fu@polyu.edu.hk

Introduction

Patellar tendinopathy (PT) is a common and often chronic knee disorder among competitive athletes [1]. Its prevalence has been reported to be as high as 30% to 45% in athletes involved in jumping sports [2]. Subjects with PT are characterized with localized pain at the proximal patellar tendon associated with jumping and squatting activities that load the tendon [3]. Since the primary function of tendon is to transmit tensile loading, any change in its morphology and elastic properties may affect its function during normal activities.

Tendinopathy results in disruption and disorganization of the tendon fibers [4], along with increases in tendon thickness [3,5] and cross-sectional area (CSA) of the structure affected [6]. Based on ultrasound imaging, Cook et al. [7] observed hypoechoic changes in human tendons with tendinopathy. The authors thereby recommended the use of ultrasonography in addition to clinical examination to confirm the diagnosis of PT. Alteration in the elastic properties of patellar tendon, however, have not been adequately described. In individuals with PT, the tendon was found to be more elastic in one study [8] but no difference was reported in another 2 studies [9–10] when compared with controls. In those studies, tendon stiffness was assessed using ultrasound imaging with dynamometry. This technique measures the elastic properties of the whole tendon during ramped maximum voluntary isometric contraction. Clinically, pathological lesions in PT typically occur at about 5 mm from the apex of the patella [3,11], therefore site-specific evaluation at the pathological region might shed light on the changes on tissue elastic properties associated with tendinopathy.

Recently, strain imaging has been used to assess regional tendon elastic properties [12–13]. A compressive force is applied either manually or by the emission of low radiofrequency impulses via an ultrasound probe to the tendon surface causing tendon displacement. Tissue elasticity is graded as either soft, intermediate or hard and expressed in colour-coded images (elastogram) [12]. Based on this technique, the common extensor tendon was found softer in subjects with lateral epicondylitis [13] but harder among those with Achilles tendinopathy [12] than healthy controls. To date, regional-specific evaluation on tendon elasticity associated with tendinopathy is scarce and findings are conflicting. In addition, the strain imaging technique provides qualitative but not quantitative information of tissue elasticity [14–15]. Thus, the magnitude of changes could not be quantified.

The supersonic shear imaging (SSI) technique provides quantitative values of tendon elastic properties at a selected area of interest [16–20]. It relies on measuring the speed of propagation of shear waves generated by acoustic radiation force and to estimate the shear elastic modulus of soft tissues [20]. Our recent findings indicated that the patellar tendon shear elastic modulus measured using SSI has good intra- and inter-rater reliability and is correlated with the Young's modulus of the tissue [17]. Based on this technique, decreases in tendon elastic modulus in acute ruptured Achilles tendon in human subjects [18] and in partial tendon tears in a porcine model [19] were reported. These studies provide the evidence base on the feasibility of using SSI for measuring tendon elastic properties. However, these findings cannot be generalized to tendon with tendinopathy because this condition is a degenerative process [21]. In addition to interruption of tendon fibrils [22], changes in fiber type [23] and increases in collagen cross-link concentration [24] were detected in tendon with tendinopathy. Based on the SSI technique, quantitative regional-specific tendon elasticity could be measured and compared between subjects with and without patellar tendinopathy. Such information could increase our understanding in regional changes on tissue elastic properties as well as the magnitude of changes.

There is also a question of how the changes in tendon morphological and/or elastic properties in individuals with PT relate to their perceived pain and dysfunctions. Increased tendon thickness has been reported to be associated with greater pain among athletes with PT [25]. To date, the relationship between elastic properties of tendon and self-perceived pain in individuals with PT has not been investigated. In view that pain and decrease in functional strength in the tendons could mean an end to the athletic career of a sportsman, it is therefore important to find out how changes in tendon morphology and mechanical properties are related to the disability and dysfunctions in people with PT, so that appropriate remedial measures can be developed.

The objectives of this study were to 1) compare the elastic modulus of patellar tendon between dominant and non-dominant sides among healthy subjects; 2) compare tendon on the painful and non-painful side of the same subject and also with healthy control subjects and; 3) determine whether changes in tendon shear elastic modulus were related to pain and dysfunction.

Materials and Methods

Ethics statement

This study was approved by the Human Subject Ethics Subcommittee of the administrating institution. The experimental procedures were conducted in accordance with the Declaration of Helsinki. The procedures of the study were fully explained to the participants and they provided their informed written consent before testing.

Study population

Subjects were recruited from the volleyball, basketball and handball teams of local universities and the community. Only males were recruited, because PT is more prevalent in male than female athletes [2]. The inclusion criteria were as follows: 1) between 18 and 35 years of age; 2) had unilateral pain in the inferior pole of patella or the proximal part of patellar tendon; 3) pain duration ≥3 months; 4) maximum intensity of pain in the previous week ≥3 using a visual analogue scale (VAS) with 0 as no pain and 10 as the worst pain; 5) VISA score ≤80 [26]; 6) no history of corticosteroid injection or surgery to the lower limb. All recruited subjects were physically assessed by an experienced physical therapist (WCL) who has 13 years of clinical experience and then ultrasonography examination was conducted by another physical therapist (ZJZ) who has 3 years of experience in ultrasound scanning. The subject was diagnosed as having PT based on the clinical examination and ultrasonography findings that included the following: 1) local tenderness in the inferior pole of patella, or the proximal part of patellar tendon; 2) pain aggravation during single leg squatting and jumping [27]; 3) thickening of proximal part of patellar tendon with area of hypoechoic signals [6]. Twenty healthy athletes, with similar age and training hours but without clinical symptoms or abnormal ultrasound-based images of the patellar tendon, were recruited as the controls for this study.

All subjects filled in a form recording their age, weight, height and training duration per week. Subjects with PT completed the Victorian Institute of Sport Assessment-patella (VISA-P) questionnaire. The leg of dominance was determined by asking the subject to kick a ball [28].

Ultrasound Examination

An Aixplorer ultrasound unit (Supersonic Imaging, Aix-en-Provence, France) in conjunction with a 50-mm linear-array transducer at 4–15 MHz frequency was used in this study [20]. B-mode was used to measure the tendon thickness and CSA. Shearwave mode was used to measure the shear elastic modulus of the patellar tendon at its proximal part. This location was selected because the pathological changes with diagnostic imaging for PT are most commonly found in the proximal part of the patella at about 5 mm distal to the apex of the patella [6]. The musculoskeletal acquisition mode was used to measure the elastic modulus of patella tendon with the temporal averaging (persistence) and spatial smoothing set to medium and 6, respectively. The elastic modulus measurements were taken at 1 Hz.

Each participant was examined in supine lying with 30° of knee flexion [29]. The knee was supported on a firm towel and a custom-made ankle stabilizer to keep the leg in neutral alignment on the coronal and transverse planes. Prior to testing, the subject was allowed to have 5 minutes of rest in a comfortable position in order to unload the tension on the patellar tendon [13]. The room temperature was controlled at 25°C.

Measurement of patellar tendon thickness and CSA

The thickness and CSA in the inferior pole of patella were measured by grey scale mode (B-mode) of the Aixplorer ultrasound unit. The inferior pole of patella was identified by palpation of the examiner. The transducer was lightly located at the inferior pole of the patella and the transducer was placed longitudinally on the patellar tendon. B- mode was activated to capture the image of the patellar tendon and stored for off-line measurements. The transducer was then turned by 90° so that a transverse view of the proximal insertion of the patellar tendon could be captured and stored for off-line analysis. Three images were obtained for measuring the thickness and CSA [30]. Both knees were evaluated for all the subjects.

After obtaining the ultrasound images, off-line measurements were performed. The tendon thickness was measured using the distance measurement software in the ultrasound machine. Measurements were taken from the inferior pole of patella vertically to the superior border of the patella tendon (Fig. 1A) using a trackball. The CSA of the patellar tendon (Fig. 1B) was measured by the tracing measurement software which allows the examiner to trace the outer margin of the tendon through the trackball, and the tracing measurement software was used to calculate the total area traced. The mean from the 3 measurements were used for statistical analysis.

Eleven healthy sedentary subjects were assessed twice with one week apart for test-retest reliability of patellar tendon thickness and CSA measurements. The inter-rater coefficient of correlation of tendon thickness and CSA were 0.94 (CV = 18.75%) and 0.98 (CV = 32.30%), respectively.

Measurement of patellar tendon elastic modulus

B-mode was used to locate and align the patellar tendon longitudinally with the transducer. When a clear image of the patellar tendon was captured, the shear wave elastography mode was then activated. The transducer was stationed on the skin with light pressure on top of a generous amount of coupling gel, perpendicularly on the surface of the skin. The transducer was kept stationary for 8–12 seconds during the acquisition of the SSI map [16]. A total of 3 images were captured for the tendon on each knee for off-line analysis.

Off-line analysis was conducted and the procedures have been described in our recent paper [16]. The region of interest (ROI) was first defined by a rectangular box of 13.5 mm × 12.5 mm (biggest size provided from the manufacturer) distal to the apex of the patella and with the patellar tendon located within its centre part. In the painful tendon, the circular quantification box (Q-Box) was centered where hypoechogenicity, disruption or fragmentation

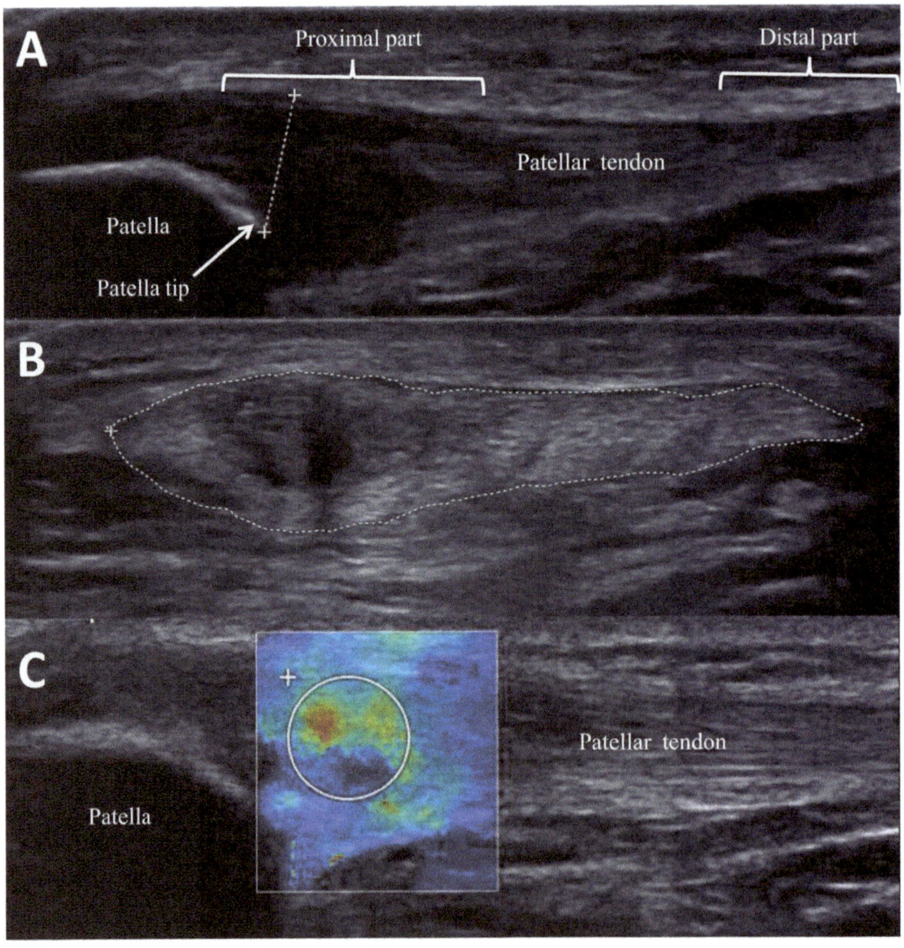

Figure 1. Sonography images of the patellar tendon (A) Thickness of the patellar tendon (dotted line) was measured from the superior border of the patellar tendon to the tip of the patellar. (B) Cross-sectional area of the patellar tendon was measured by tracing the outer margin of the patellar tendon (dotted circle) (C) Shear elastic modulus of the patellar tendon was quantified by the elastography. The white circle delineates the area of interest.

Table 1. Demography comparison between athletes with and without unilateral PT.

Variables	Control group (n = 20)	PT group (n = 13)	*P* Value
Age, y	24.9±4.4	22.9±4.6	0.222
Weight, kg	73.4±7.9	76.2±6.3	0.280
Height, cm	181.7±6.0	180.0±5.7	0.425
BMI, kg/m^2	22.2±2.1	23.6±2.4	0.094
Sport-specific training, h/wk	7.5±3.7	5.4±2.5	0.102
Injury duration, y		1.7±1.6	
Dominate/non-dominate side (painful side)		8/5	

Values shown as mean± standard deviation; PT = patellar tendinopathy; BMI = body mass index.

of collagen fiber, or focal sonolucent were observed. Similar to a previous study [11], the pathological lesions in our subjects were detected an average of 4.6 mm (ranged from 3–7 mm) distal to the apex of the patella (Fig.1C). The diameter of the Q-Box was determined by the width of the tendon. In the non-painful tendon, the Q-Box was centered at the proximal part of the patellar tendon with consistent images and at about 5 mm from the apex of the patella. Young's modulus (E) was estimated by the SSI system based on the following equation. $E = 3\rho c^2$, where ρ is the density (constant and equal to 1000 kg/m^3) and c is the velocity of the shear wave propagation based on the assumption that the tissue is isotropic. A higher Young's modulus indicates greater stiffness [20]. The mean and maximum values of Young's modulus within the Q-Box were computed and displayed in kPa at the right bottom corner of the computer screen. The mean tendon shear elastic modulus was calculated by dividing the Young's modulus generated from the system by 3 [31]. The SSI has excellent test-retest reliability on patellar tendon shear elastic modulus (ICC: 0.98; coefficient of variation: 29.53%) [17].

The ratio of mean shear elastic modulus, tendon thickness and CSA between the painful and non-painful knee was calculated as elastic ratio, thickness ratio and CSA ratio in athletes with unilateral PT.

Clinical Evaluation

Pressure pain was measured by a hand-held algometer (manufactured by pdt, Rome, Italy). Pain was provoked through a rubber disc at the end of the algometer. The participant was positioned in supine lying with 30° of knee flexion on the couch. The most painful area on the proximal patellar tendon was determined by palpation and then a 10lb force was applied via the algometer onto this area. The intensity of pain being provoked was reported using a visual analogue scale (VAS) from 0 to 10, with 0 indicating no pain, and 10 indicating the worst pain during testing. The VAS scale is a reliable and valid scale in the evaluation of patients with anterior knee pain [32].

The VISA-P questionnaire is used to assess the severity of symptoms and functional ability in subjects with PT [33]. The questionnaire comprises 8 questions with 4 on self-perceived pain associated with a functional activity, 2 on the ability in performing functional activities, and 2 on the ability to play sport. Self-perceived pain or abilities are rated on a 10-point Likert scale with 0 being the worst pain or lowest ability and 10 as the least pain and highest ability. The total score of the questionnaire is 100 and the final score would quantify the functional level. The VISA-P questionnaire has been used for studies on PT in various athletic populations [2,34].

Statistical Analysis

Independent *t* tests were performed to compare the demographic data between athletes with and without PT. After the normality distributions were confirmed using the Shapiro-Wilk tests, paired *t*-tests were used to compare the outcome measures (thickness, CSA and shear elastic modulus of patellar tendon) between the dominant and non-dominant sides in the healthy athletes, and also the painful and non-painful sides in athletes with unilateral PT. Univariate analysis of covariance tests were used to compare between the affected side in athletes with PT and the dominant side of the controls with demographic factors that demonstrated significant group difference as covariates. Spearman's rank correlation tests were used to examine the thickness ratio, CSA ratio and elastic ratio with the pressure pain, individual and total scores of the VISA-P questionnaire. SPSS version 17.0 (SPSS Inc, Chicago, IL) was used to perform statistical analyses. A

Table 2. Comparisons of the shear elastic modulus, thickness and CSA between painful and non-painful sides in athletes with unilateral PT.

Variables	Painful side (n = 13)	Non-painful side (n = 13)	*P* Value
Shear elastic modulus, kPa	43.6±17.9	25.8±10.6	0.008*
Thickness, mm	6.9±1.8	4.6±0.6	0.001*
CSA, cm^2	1.7±0.4	1.4±0.3	0.002*

Values shown as mean± standard deviation; PT = patellar tendinopathy; CSA = cross sectional area. *$P<0.05$.

Table 3. Side-to-side comparisons of the shear elastic modulus, thickness and CSA in healthy athletes.

Variables	Dominant side (n = 20)	Non-dominant side (n = 20)	*P* Value
Shear elastic modulus, kPa	27.5±11.3	27.9±8.4	0.868
Thickness, mm	5.6±1.2	5.3±1.0	0.095
CSA, cm^2	1.4±0.3	1.4±0.3	0.917

Values shown as mean± standard deviation; CSA = cross sectional area.

p value of <0.05 was considered as significant for each of the measurements.

Results

Participant's demographic data

Participants' age, height, weight, BMI and training intensity in the two groups are shown in Table 1. No significant differences were found between the two groups in age, height, weight, BMI and training intensity ($p>0.05$), but a medium trend was found in BMI between the 2 groups ($p = 0.094$; Cohen's $d = 0.52$).

Side-to-side differences on thickness, CSA and shear elastic modulus

In athletes with unilateral PT, B-mode ultrasound measurements revealed significant differences between the painful and non-painful sides in patellar tendon thickness ($p = 0.001$) and CSA ($p = 0.002$) (Table 2). On average, the painful tendons were thickened by 33.3% and enlarged by 12.5% in CSA than the non-painful side. The shear elastic modulus in the painful side (mean: 43.6 kPa) was significantly higher than the non-painful side (mean: 25.8 kPa) by 40.8% ($p = 0.008$).

Side-to-side differences on the outcome measures were not observed in healthy athletes. There were no significant differences on the patellar tendon morphology and elastic properties between the dominant and non-dominant sides ($p>0.05$) despite a trend of increase in patellar tendon thickness in the dominant than the non-dominant leg ($p = 0.095$) (Table 3). The mean tendon thickness, CSA and shear elastic modulus were 5.6 mm, 1.4 cm^2 and 27.5 kPa in the dominant leg; 5.3 mm, 1.4 cm^2, and 27.9 kPa in the non-dominant leg.

Comparison of shear elastic modulus, thickness and CSA between healthy athletes and athletes with unilateral PT

Group differences were observed on the patellar tendon morphology and elastic properties between athletes with PT and without PT. The mean group differences on the patellar tendon thickness and CSA were 1.3 mm and 0.3 cm^2, respectively (Table 4). The shear elastic modulus was increased from 27.5 kPa to 43.6 kPa (by 36.9%, $p = 0.003$) in the painful tendon among athletes with PT when compared with the controls.

Relationships between changes in tendon morphology, elastic properties, pressure pain and dysfunctions

Table 5 shows the relationships between changes in tendon properties, pressure pain and dysfunctions. Significant negative correlation was found between elastic ratio and VISA-P scores (*rho* $= -0.61$; $p = 0.026$) (Fig. 2A). Significant positive correlation was found between elastic ratio and pressure pain (*rho* $= 0.62$, $p = 0.024$) (Fig. 2B) and negative relationships were established between elastic ratio and self-perceived pain based on the subscores from the VISA-P questionnaire (*rho* ranged from -0.63 to -0.67; $p<0.05$) (Fig. 2C, 2D, 2F, 2G, 2H) except for the knee extension (*rho* $= -0.26$, $p = 0.394$) (Fig. 2E). A higher ratio, greater differences between the painful and non-painful tendon, was associated with greater intensity of pain with pressure and when performing forward lunge, going down stairs and single leg hopping; as well as greater dysfunctions. Similar relationships could not be detected with thickness ratio and CSA ratio.

Discussion

The present study revealed changes in patellar tendon morphology and elastic properties in athletes with unilateral PT lasting from 3 months to 6 years. The painful tendons were thicker and larger in size with an increase in stiffness when compared with the non-painful side and healthy control subjects. This study also established associations between elastic properties of patellar tendon and intensity of pressure- and activity-related pain, as well as dysfunctions in basketball and volleyball players with unilateral PT.

Morphological changes such as thickening and larger CSA in pathological tendons, have been reported [3,5,6] and the changes

Table 4. Comparisons of the shear elastic modulus, thickness and CSA of the patellar tendon on the painful side of athletes with unilateral PT and dominant side of the healthy athletes.

Variables	Control group (n = 20)	PT group (n = 13)	*P* Value
Shear elastic modulus, kPa	27.5±11.3	43.6±17.9	0.003*
Thickness, mm	5.6±1.2	6.9±1.8	0.019*
CSA, cm^2	1.4±0.3	1.7±0.4	0.032*

Values shown as mean ± standard deviation; PT = patellar tendinopathy; CSA = cross sectional area.*$P<0.05$.

Table 5. Spearman's rank correlations between the ratio of tendon thickness, CSA and shear elastic modulus of the painful and non-painful side with intensity of pressure pain, individuals and total VISA-P scores.

		Morphology		Elastic properties
Pain		Thickness ratio	CSA ratio	Elastic ratio
	Pressure pain	0.53	−0.04	0.62*
	Downstairs	−0.28	−0.22	−0.65*
	Knee extension	0.02	0.42	−0.26
	Single leg hopping	−0.30	−0.13	−0.64*
	Lunge	−0.11	−0.07	−0.67*
Ability				
	Prolong sitting	−0.46	−0.15	−0.63*
	Squatting	−0.14	−0.00	−0.64*
Dysfunction				
	VISA-p score	−0.25	−0.07	−0.61*

Abbreviations: CSA = cross sectional area; VISA-P = Victorian Institute of Sports Assessment-patella Questionnaire; *$P<0.05$.

were about 22.7% in thickness [5] and 15.8% in CSA [6] in the proximal part of the patellar tendon. Cook et al. [7] even advocates the use of ultrasound imaging together with clinical examination in making diagnosis of tendinopathy. In this study, patients were confirmed to have PT based on both clinical examination and ultrasound imaging, it is therefore not surprising to find differences on the size and CSA of the pathological tendons from the unaffected side or the patellar tendon of the healthy controls. In the present study, the tendon size was increased by 35.7% and the CSA was enlarged by 21.4% in the pathological tendons. These changes could be explained by an increase in ground substance [35], collagen fiber disorganization [4], and hypercellularity [36].

One of the main findings from this study was the change in tendon elastic properties in athletes with unilateral PT using supersonic shear imaging technique. The painful tendons were stiffer than the non-painful side as well as the dominant side of the healthy controls. The measurements were made on the proximal portion of the tendon where pain was elicited on palpation and perceived during functional activities of the lower limb. Patellar tendon elastic properties were previously quantified by ultrasonography with dynamometry. Kongsgaard et al. [9] did not find any difference in the tendon stiffness between 9 healthy individuals and 8 subjects with patellar tendinopathy. A later study by Couppé et al. [10] also reported no difference on the tendon stiffness between the painful and non-painful sides of 7 badminton players with unilateral PT and also compared with 9 control subjects. Based on a relatively larger sample, Helland et al. [8] found significantly lower tendon stiffness (by 21.4%) in the patellar tendon in 13 volleyball players with PT when compared with 15 controls. In these studies, elastic properties of the whole tendon were measured so as to unveil the entire physical properties of the tendon. We were more interested to investigate regional-specific changes around the pathological region, where pain is normally elicited.

Similar to our study, regional-specific increase in tendon stiffness was reported in subjects with chronic pain in the Achilles tendons by Sconfienza et al [12]. The stiffness of Achilles tendons was assessed by ultrasound sonoelastography at the myotendinous junction, tendon body and calcaneal enthesis. Loss of elasticity was detected in the tendon body but not in the myotendinous junction or calcaneal enthesis when compared with control. On the contrary, De Zordo reported decrease in tendon stiffness at the common extensor origin in patients with lateral epicondylitis [13]. More study is required to examine whether tendinopathy associated changes in elastic properties would be different in the lower and upper limb tendons.

The study from Sconfienza et al. [12] observed lower elastic values in areas with fragmentation and loss of fibrillar texture. In our study, the tendon shear elastic modulus was measured at the proximal part of the patellar tendon in area of hypoechoic or fragmentation signals based on ultrasound imaging. On the contrary, lower tendon stiffness was detected in subjects with acute Achilles tendon rupture [18] and in partial tendon tears in a porcine model [19]. Chen et al. [18] commented that the shearwave images could not be registered in areas with hematoma. The elastic value was dramatically reduced to 0 thus lowering the mean value. Furthermore, changes that occur in tendons with tendinopathy but not in tendons with acute rupture include transition of collagen fibers between Type I and Type III [23,37]; disorganization of collagen fibers [4], increase in collagen cross-links [24] and formation of scar tissues [38]. These changes would likely increase tissue elastic modulus. Biochemical and histological tests are suggested to assess changes on collagen fibers, extracellular matrix and tendon elastic modulus.

The patellar tendon is short and thick where considerable force is transmitted. An inextensible tendon would have the most efficient force transmission. This tendon also serves other important functions such as energy storage/release upon loading and unloading and protection from muscle fiber injury [39]. To serve these functions, the patellar tendon exhibits spring-like characteristic, due to the presence of elastic components. Increased tendon stiffness in athletes with PT might be suitable for rapid and effective force transmission but could affect its function as mechanical buffer and elastic saving for economy of motion.

Besides measuring tendon elastic properties at rest, we also correlated the resting tendon elastic properties with pain and dysfunctions. Significant correlations were found between pain and dysfunctions with modulation on the tendon elastic properties but not with tendon morphology (thickness and CSA). Patients with PT are characterized with pain at the proximal patellar

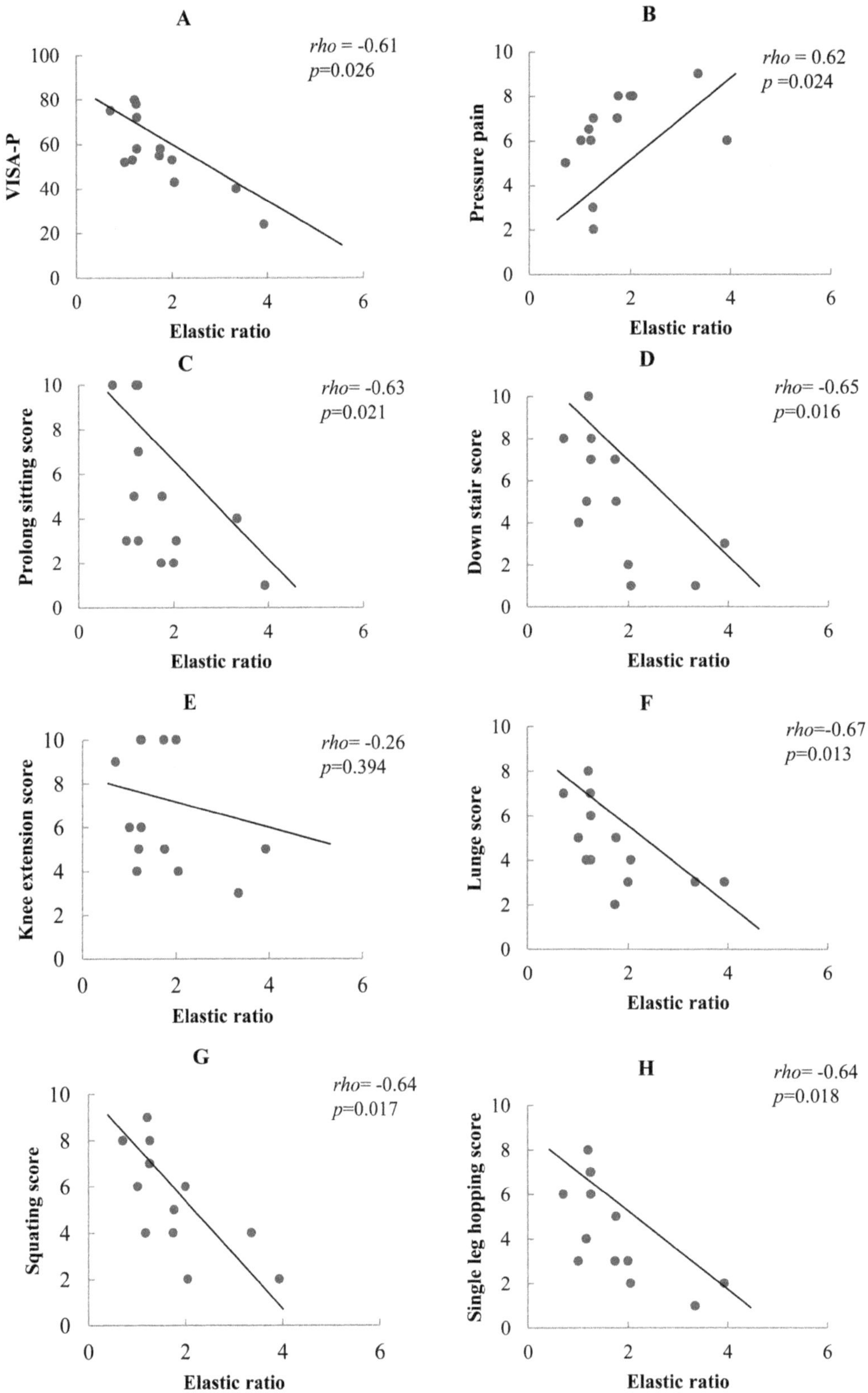

Figure 2. Correlations between elastic ratio and clinical variables. (Pressure pain, individual and total score from VISA-P, Victorian Institute of Sport Assessment- Patella).

tendon associated with activities that load the tendon [3]. The present findings provide evidence that a greater increase in stiffness of the painful tendon, i.e. greater ratio on the shear elastic modulus between the painful and non-painful side, are associated with the self-perceived pain with local pressure and during tendon-loading activities. Most importantly, the dysfunctions as reflected from the VISA-P scores are related with the modulation in the tendon elastic properties. Tendon pain is closely linked to loading while excessive energy storage and release (over stretch) to the tendon would most commonly provoke pain [40]. We could not establish a relationship between the change in tendon morphology with pain or dysfunction. Malliaras et al. [25] found that hypoechoic area and diffuse thickening in patellar tendon were more likely to be painful. However, Warden et al. [41] and the present study could not establish a relationship between the CSA of patellar tendon and the VISA-P scores in athletes with unilateral PT.

Interestingly, there was not a significant side-to-side difference in the shear elastic modulus, thickness and CSA of patellar tendon between the dominant and non-dominant sides among healthy athletes. Such observations are partially in agreement with the findings from Couppé et al [42]. The authors found similar shear elastic modulus between the dominant and non-dominant legs. The thickness and CSA of patellar tendon, however, were found to be significantly thicker and larger in the leading leg in fencers and badminton players when compared with the other leg. A proposed explanation for this finding is the unilateral/asymmetrical training in these athletes. In our study, we recruited athletes in volleyball, basketball and handball that are generally regarded as bilateral sports.

Limitations of the present study

The prevalence of PT is reported to be between 30% and 45% in the jumping athletes [2], but many of them suffered from bilateral PT. During the study period, 13 subjects with unilateral PT were recruited. Despite this small sample size, statistical significant difference was established on patellar tendon shear elastic modulus and thickness between athletes with and without PT. We also detected correlations between the tendon elastic modulus and the intensity of pain and functional scores. Such findings illustrated influence of tendon stiffness on pain and function. However, further study with larger number of subjects and in female athletes are suggested to support the present findings. Also, we conducted evaluation of tendon elastic properties on the proximal patellar tendon that does not represent the entire tendon. This is valid because the pathological changes in patellar tendon occurred mostly in the inferior pole of patella or proximal part of the tendon [6]. However, further study measuring tendon elastic modulus at different portions of the tendon would provide information on whether changes are isolated at the pathological region. In addition, ultrasound imaging was used to determine pathological lesions that had not been verified with histological tests. The present study was a cross-sectional study, we could not determine whether a stiffer proximal patellar tendon was the cause or consequence of the PT. Finally, only male athletes were recruited in this study, thus the findings from this study may not be generalized to female basketball, handball and volleyball players.

Conclusions

The present study revealed changes in both morphology and elastic properties at the painful part of patellar tendon in athletes with unilateral PT. The affected tendons are stiffer, thicker and have larger cross-sectional area than the non-painful side and the tendon of healthy controls. In addition, the ratio of the painful and non-painful tendon elastic properties is associated with the intensity of pressure pain and VISA-p scores in athletes with unilateral PT.

Acknowledgments

Thanks are due to Dr Raymond Chung for his statistical advice.

Author Contributions

Conceived and designed the experiments: SNF. Performed the experiments: ZJZ WCL. Analyzed the data: SNF ZJZ. Contributed reagents/materials/analysis tools: SNF GYFN. Wrote the paper: ZJZ SNF GYFN. Manuscript editing: GYFN SNF.

References

1. Witvrouw E, Bellemans J, Lysens R, Danneels L, Cambier D (2001) Intrinsic risk factors for the development of patellar tendinitis in an athletic population. A two-year prospective study. Am J Sports Med 29: 190–195.
2. Lian ØB, Engebretsen L, Bahr R (2005) Prevalence of jumper's knee among elite athletes from different sports: a cross-sectional study. Am J Sport Med 33: 561–567.
3. Cook JL, Khan KM, Kiss ZS, Griffiths L (2000) Patellar tendinopathy in junior basketball players: a controlled clinical and ultrasonographic study of 268 patellar tendons in players age 14–18 years. Scand J Med Sci Sports 10: 216–220.
4. Maffulli N, Testa V, Capasso G, Ewen SW, Sullo A, et al. (2004) Similar histopathological picture in males with Achilles and patellar tendinopathy. Med Sci Sports Exerc 36: 1470–1475.
5. Gisslen K, Gyulai C, Soderman K, Alfredson H (2005) High prevalence of jumper's knee and sonographic changes in Swedish elite junior volleyball players compared to matched controls. Br J Sports Med 39: 298–301.
6. Kulig K, Landel R, Chang YJ, Hannanvash N, Reischl SF, et al. (2013) Patellar tendon morphology in volleyball athletes with and without patellar tendinopathy. Scand J Med Sci Sports 23: e81–88.
7. Cook JL, Khan KM, Harcourt PR, Kiss ZS, Fehrmann MW, et al. (1998) Patellar tendon ultrasonography in asymptomatic active athletes reveals hypoechoic regions: a study of 320 tendons. Clin J Sport Med 8: 73–77.
8. Helland C, Bojsen-Møller J, Raastad T, Seynnes OR, Moltubakk MM, et al. (2013) Mechanical properties of the patellar tendon in elite volleyball players with and without patellar tendinopathy. Br J Sports Med 47: 862–868.
9. Kongsgaard M, Qvortrup K, Larsen J, Aagaard P, Doessing S, et al. (2010) Fibril morphology and tendon mechanical properties in patellar tendinopathy: effects of heavy slow resistance training. Am J Sports Med 38: 749–756.
10. Couppé C, Kongsgaard M, Aagaard P, Vinther A, Boesen M, et al. (2012) Differences in tendon properties in elite badminton players with or without patellar tendinopathy. Scand J Med Sci Sports 23: e89–95.
11. Fredberg U, Stengaard-Pedersen K (2008) Chronic tendinopathy tissue pathology, pain mechanisms, and etiology with a special focus on inflammation. Scand J Med Sci Sports 18: 3–15.
12. Sconfienza LM, Silvestri E, Cimmino MA (2010) Sonoelastography in the evaluation of painful Achilles tendon in amateur athletes. Clin Exp Rheumatol 28: 373–378.
13. De Zordo T, Lill SR, Fink C, Feuchtner GM, Jaschke W, et al. (2009) Real-time sonoelastography of lateral epicondylitis: comparison of findings between patients and healthy volunteers. AJR Am J Roentgenol 193: 180–185.
14. Itoh A, Ueno E, Tohno E, Kamma H, Takahashi H, et al. (2006) Breast disease: clinical application of US elastography for diagnosis. Radiology 239: 341–350.
15. Klauser AS, Faschingbauer R, Jaschke WR (2010) Is sonoelastography of value in assessing tendons? Semin Musculoskelet Radiol 14: 323–333.
16. Kot BCW, Zhang ZJ, Lee AWC, Leung VYF, Fu SN (2012) Elastic Modulus of Muscle and Tendon with Shear Wave Ultrasound Elastography: Variations with Different Technical Settings. PLoS ONE 7: e44348.
17. Zhang ZJ, Fu SN (2013) Shear Elastic Modulus on Patellar Tendon Captured from Supersonic Shear Imaging: Correlation with Tangent Traction Modulus Computed from Material Testing System and Test-Retest Reliability. PLoS ONE 8: e68216.
18. Chen XM, Cui LG, He P, Shen WW, Qian YJ, et al. (2013) Shear wave elastographic characterization of normal and torn achilles tendons: a pilot study. J Ultrasound Med 32: 449–455.
19. Dewall RJ, Jiang J, Wilson JJ, Lee KS (2014) Visualizing tendon elasticity in an ex vivo partial tear model. Ultrasound Med Biol 40(1): 158–167.

20. Bercoff J, Tanter M, Fink M (2004) Supersonic shear imaging: A new technique for soft tissues elasticity mapping. IEEE Trans Ultrason Ferroelectr Freq Control 51: 396–409.
21. Khan KM, Cook JL, Bonar F, Harcourt P, Astrom M. (1999) Histopathology of common tendinopathies. Update and implications for clinical management. SportsMed 27: 393–408.
22. Maffulli N, Testa V, Capasso G, Ewen SW, Sullo A, et al. (2004) Similar histopathological picture in males with Achilles and patellar tendinopathy. Med Sci Sports Exerc 36: 1470–1475.
23. Ireland D, Harrall R, Curry V, Holloway G, Hackney R, et al. (2001) Multiple changes in gene expression in chronic human Achilles tendinopathy. Matrix Biol 20: 159–169.
24. Kongsgaard M, Kovanen V, Aagaard P, Doessing S, Hansen P, et al. (2009) Corticosteroid injections, eccentric decline squat training and heavy slow resistance training in patellar tendinopathy. Scand J Med Sci Sports 19: 790–802.
25. Malliaras P, Purdam C, Maffulli N, Cook JL (2010) Temporal sequence of grey scale ultrasound changes and their relationship with neovascularity and pain in the patellar tendon. Br J Sports Med 44: 944–947.
26. Zwerver J, Hartgens F, Verhagen E, van der Worp H, van den Akker-Scheek I, et al. (2011) No effect of extracorporeal shockwave therapy on patellar tendinopathy in jumping athletes during the competitive season: a randomized clinical trial. Am J Sports Med 39: 1191–1199.
27. Lian ØB, Holen K, Engebretsen L, Bahr R (1996) Relationship between symptoms of jumper's knee and the ultrasound characteristics of the patellar tendon among high level male volleyball players. Scand J Med Sci Sports 6: 291–296.
28. Bjornaraa J, Di Fabio RP (2011) Knee kinematics following ACL reconstruction in females; the effect of vision on performance during a cutting task. Int J Sports Phys Ther 6: 271–284.
29. Bensamoun SF, Ringleb SI, Littrell L, Chen Q, Brennan M, et al. (2006) Determination of thigh muscle stiffness using magnetic resonance elastography. J Magn Reson Imaging 23: 242–247.
30. Nyland J, Fried A, Maitra R, Johnson DL, Caborn DN (2006) Wrist circumference is related to patellar tendon thickness in healthy men and women. Clin Imaging 30: 335–338.
31. Royer D, Gennisson JL, Deffieux T, Tanter M (2011) On the elasticity of transverse isotropic soft tissues (L). J Acoust Soc Am 129: 2757–2760.
32. Crossley KM, Bennell KL, Cowan SM, Green S (2004) Analysis of outcome measures for persons with patellofemoral pain: which are reliable and valid? Arch Phys Med Rehabil 85: 815–822.
33. Visentini PJ, Khan KM, Cook JL, Kiss ZS, Harcourt PR, et al. (1998) The VISA score: an index of severity of symptoms in patients with jumper's knee (patellar tendinosis). Victorian Institute of Sport Tendon Study Group. J Sci Med Sport 1: 22–28.
34. Frohm A, Saartok T, Edman G, Renström P (2004) Psychometric properties of a Swedish translation of the VISA-P outcome score for patellar tendinopathy. BMC Musculoskelet Disord 5: 49.
35. Sharma P, Maffulli N (2005) Tendon injury and tendinopathy: healing and repair. J Bone Joint Surg Am 87: 187–202.
36. Kader D, Saxena A, Movin T, Maffulli N (2002) Achilles tendinopathy: some aspects of basic science and clinical management. Br J Sports Med 36: 239–249.
37. Goncalves-Neto J, Witzel SS, Teodoro WR, Carvalho-Junior AE, Fernandes TD, et al. (2002) Changes in collagen matrix composition in human posterior tibial tendon dysfunction. Joint Bone Spine 69: 189–194.
38. Hooley CJ, Cohen RE (1979) A model for the creep behaviour of tendon. Int J Biol Macromol 1: 123–132.
39. Magnusson SP, Hansen P, Kjaer M (2003) Tenodn properties in relation to muscular activity and physical training. Scand J Med Sci Sports 13: 211–223.
40. Lichtwark GA, Wilson AM (2005) In vivo mechanical properties of the human Achilles tendon during one-legged hopping. J Exp Biol 208(24): 4715–4725.
41. Warden SJ, Kiss ZS, Malara FA, Ooi AB, Cook JL, et al. (2007) Comparative accuracy of magnetic resonance imaging and ultrasonography in confirming clinically diagnosed patellar tendinopathy. Am J Sports Med 35: 427–436.
42. Couppé C, Kongsgaard M, Aagaard P, Hansen P, Bojsen-Moller J, et al. (2008) Habitual loading results in tendon hypertrophy and increased stiffness of the human patellar tendon. J Applied Physiol 105: 805–810.

18

Technical Performance Reduces during the Extra-Time Period of Professional Soccer Match-Play

Liam D. Harper, Daniel J. West, Emma Stevenson, Mark Russell*

Health and Life Sciences, Northumbria University, Newcastle-upon-Tyne, United Kingdom

Abstract

Despite the importance of extra-time in determining progression in specific soccer tournament matches, few studies have profiled the demands of 120-minutes of soccer match-play. With a specific focus on the extra-time period, and using a within-match approach, we examined the influence of prolonged durations of professional soccer match-play on markers of technical (i.e., skilled) performance. In 18 matches involving professional European teams played between 2010 and 2014, this retrospective study quantified the technical actions observed during eight 15-minute epochs (E1: 00:00–14:59 min, E2: 15:00–29:59 min, E3: 30:00–44:59 min, E4: 45:00–59:59 min, E5: 60:00–74:59 min, E6: 75:00–89:59 min, E7: 90:00–104:59 min, E8: 105:00–119:59 min). Analysis of players who completed the demands of the full 120 min of match-play revealed that the cumulative number of successful passes observed during E8 (61±23) was lower than E1–4 (E1: 88±23, $P = 0.001$; E2: 77±21, $P = 0.005$; E3: 79±18, $P = 0.001$; E4: 80±21, $P = 0.001$) and E7 (73±20, $P = 0.002$). Similarly, the total number of passes made in E8 (71±25) was reduced when compared to E1 (102±22, $P = 0.001$), E3 (91±19, $P = 0.002$), E4 (93±22, $P \leq 0.0005$) and E7 (84±20, $P = 0.001$). The cumulative number of successful dribbles reduced in E8 (9±4) when compared to E1 (14±4, $P = 0.001$) and E3 (12±4, $P \leq 0.0005$) and the total time the ball was in play was less in E8 (504±61 s) compared to E1 (598±70 s, $P \leq 0.0005$). These results demonstrate that match-specific factors reduced particular indices of technical performance in the second half of extra-time. Interventions that seek to maintain skilled performance throughout extra-time warrant further investigation.

Editor: Oyvind Sandbakk, Norwegian University of Science and Technology, Norway

Funding: The authors have no support or funding to report.

Competing Interests: The authors have declared that no competing interests exist.

* Email: mark.russell@northumbria.ac.uk

Introduction

Soccer is a high-intensity intermittent sport which is normally played over 90 min. However, when scores are tied at the end of certain matches in soccer tournaments (e.g., FIFA World Cup, UEFA Champions League, FA Cup etc.), an extra-time period, consisting of two additional 15-min periods of play, follows the end of normal time. Notably, between 1986 and 2010, 33 matches have required that extra-time be played in FIFA World Cup competitions. In the 2014 FIFA World Cup, of the matches played in the knockout stages, 50% required extra-time to be played. Although the physiological and performance responses to the normal duration (i.e., 90 min) of soccer match-play have been extensively researched [1,2,3,4,5], comparable data during the extra-time period is lacking. This is somewhat surprising considering the role that this additional period of play has in determining success in tournament situations.

The ability to maintain skill proficiency during soccer match-play is considered an important factor in overall player performance and match success [6]. However, soccer-specific exercise appears to influence skilled performances executed during normal durations (i.e., 90 min) of match-play. For example, using a within-subject study design, Russell et al., [7] observed reductions in total possessions and the number of ball distributions in the second versus the first half of English Championship matches. Further analysis across 15-min intervals revealed that the total number of ball possessions and distributions reduced in the final 15 min when compared with the opening phase of play. Although self-pacing strategies [8] and tactical modifications [9] have been suggested to explain such changes, these data support studies where the accumulated effects of match-related fatigue have been proposed to explain decrements in short passing performance during Italian Serie A matches [4] and the increased number of goals conceded in the final 15 min of match-play [10].

Interestingly, the decrement in skill performance observed throughout soccer-specific exercise appears to differ according to the skill being performed. For example, Rampinini et al. [4] identified that three quarters of the technical measures examined were similar between halves in Serie A players who experienced physical fatigue decrements. Russell et al. [7] also identified no changes in five of the seven indices of technical performance (i.e., number of touches taken per possession, number of challenges, percentage of challenges won, length of forward distributions and percentage success of distributions) examined throughout match-play. Therefore, it appears that the technical response to the normal duration of soccer match-play is not uniform. However, it is plausible that the prolonged duration of games that enters in to the extra-time period elicit different technical responses compared to those observed during 90 min. No data is currently available that has profiled the skill response associated with soccer matches where the extra-time period has been played.

Therefore, using performance analysis techniques, the aim of this study was to examine the influence of prolonged durations of actual soccer match-play (i.e., those matches which required extra-time to be played) on markers of technical performance. We hypothesised that extra-time would influence technical performance; specifically, by reducing certain indices of performance.

Methods

Participants

Eighteen matches that required an extra-time period to be played were included in the analyses. Only outfield players that completed the full 120 min of the match (i.e., 90 min plus 30 min extra-time) were analysed. Using a within-match approach, the technical actions elicited during matches involving professional European clubs (ranging from the third tier of their domestic league to top tier and International teams) were analysed (15 ± 1 players per match). Written informed consent was obtained from the professional soccer clubs who supplied footage to be analysed for the purpose of the study. The study was approved by the Faculty of Health and Life Sciences Ethics Committee of Northumbria University in Newcastle upon Tyne, UK.

Match Analysis Procedures

In agreement with the experimental design used by previous authors [7], skill-related performances were analysed retrospectively during competitive matches played since 2010 using existing footage obtained from television recordings (8 matches) and footage supplied following correspondence with specific clubs (10 matches). To minimise variation, each match was manually coded (Sportstec Gamebreaker, Sportstec, New South Wales, Australia) by one experienced performance analyst according to operational definitions detailed by Rampinini et al. [4] and Opta Sports Data (http://www.optasports.com/news-area/blog-optas-event-definitions.aspx). A total of 17 technical variables (Table 1) were analysed for each match.

In order to investigate the transient effects of 120 min of soccer match-play on technical performance, all matches were divided into eight 15 min epochs (i.e., E1: 00:00–14:59 min, E2: 15:00–29:59 min, E3: 30:00–44:59 min, E4: 45:00–59:59 min, E5: 60:00–74:59 min, E6: 75:00–89:59 min, E7: 90:00–104:59 min, E8: 105:00–119:59 min). To ensure that the duration of each epoch was standardised, data collected in injury time was not

Table 1. Operational definitions of the technical variables analysed (derived from Rampinini, et al. [4] and Opta Sports Data).

Variable		Operational definition
Passing	Successful passes	A pass that is performed with the foot or head that is received successfully by a teammate
	Unsuccessful passes	A pass that is performed with the foot or head that is not received successfully by a teammate (i.e., is instead either intercepted by an opposition player or leaves the field of play)
	Total passes	Sum of successful and unsuccessful passes
	Pass accuracy (%)	Successful passes divided by total passes, multiplied by 100
Dribbling	Successful dribbles	A situation when a player takes control of the ball and is able to keep possession of the ball before performing another action such as a pass or shot
	Unsuccessful dribbles	A situation when a player takes control of the ball and is subsequently dispossessed by an opposing player or dribbles the ball out of play
	Total dribbles	Sum of successful and unsuccessful dribbles
	Dribble accuracy (%)	Successful dribbles divided by total dribbles, multiplied by 100
Shooting	Shots on target	Any goal attempt that: a) Goes into the net b) Would have gone into the net but for being stopped by a goalkeeper's save c) Would have gone into the net but for being stopped by a defender who is the last man.
	Shots off target	Any goal attempt where the ball is going wide of the target, misses the goal or hits the woodwork
	Total shots	Sum of shots attempted
	Shot accuracy (%)	Shots on target divided by total shots, multiplied by 100
Crossing	Successful crosses	A long pass using the foot that is performed by a player within the last 35 m of the pitch and which is directed into the penalty area and is received by a teammate
	Unsuccessful crosses	A long pass using the foot that is performed by a player within the last 35 m of the pitch and which is directed into the penalty area and is not received by a teammate but is instead controlled or cleared by an opposition player or goes out of play for a goal-kick or throw in
	Total crosses	Sum of successful and unsuccessful crosses
	Cross accuracy (%)	Successful crosses divided by total crosses, multiplied by 100
Time-in-play		The amount of time in seconds per 15 min epoch that the ball is within the field of play. A ball is deemed out of the field of play in the cases of a(n): goal kick, free kick, throw in, penalty, corner, goal celebration, substitution, extraordinary circumstances (e.g., pitch invasions). In these occurrences, the clock is restarted when the ball re-enters the field of play or in the case of goal celebrations, when the subsequent kick-off is taken by the team that conceded the goal.

Table 2. Test-retest reliability data (intraclass correlation coefficients) for the technical variables examined.

Variable	E1	E6	E8
Successful passes	0.993*	0.999*	0.998*
Unsuccessful passes	0.961*	0.982*	0.997*
Total passes	0.969*	0.998*	0.998*
Pass accuracy (%)	0.982*	0.950*	0.938*
Successful dribbles	0.916*	0.954*	0.999*
Unsuccessful dribbles	0.927*	0.885*	0.827*
Total dribbles	0.892*	0.977*	0.982*
Dribble accuracy (%)	0.929*	0.648	0.715
Shots on target	1.000*	0.615	0.432*
Shots off target	0.851*	0.956*	0.956*
Total Shots	0.937*	1.000*	0.906*
Shot accuracy (%)	0.964*	1.000*	0.135
Successful crosses	0.962*	1.000*	0.968*
Unsuccessful crosses	0.852*	0.982*	1.000*
Total crosses	0.692*	0.977*	0.993*
Cross accuracy (%)	0.946*	0.999*	0.938*
Ball time in play	0.999*	0.968*	0.978*

Where E1 = 00:00–14:59 min, E6 = 75:00–89:59 min, E8 = 105:00–119:59 min.
*represents significance at $P \leq 0.05$ level.

included in the analyses. The intra-observer reliability of measurements was assessed by repeated coding of all variables on two occasions for selected epochs in six randomly chosen matches (Table 2). To minimise learning effects, coding during the retest was performed in a blind fashion and 4 weeks separated the test and retest measurements.

Statistical Analysis

The appropriateness of statistical methods to analyse data yielded from multiple matches has been debated [11,12]. To minimise the influence of dependence in the data sets, given that each match has distinct characteristics, we have used a within-match design; therefore, the data presented (means ± SD) reflects the cumulative totals of technical actions performed within each match per epoch. Due to violations of normality, differences between time-points were investigated using Friedman's repeated-measures analysis of variance on ranks tests. Where appropriate, post-hoc analyses were applied using Bonferroni-corrected Wilcoxon's signed rank tests. Statistical significance was set at $P \leq 0.05$. Effect sizes (ES) for statistical differences were determined according to Field [13] with values of 0.2, 0.5, and >0.8 considered to reflect small, medium, and large differences respectively [14]. Test-retest reliability was assessed using intra-class coefficient (ICC) calculations. All statistical analyses were conducted using SPSS Version 21.0 (IBM, Armonk, NY, USA).

Results

Extra-time influenced 4 of the 17 technical variables analysed (Table 3). Specifically, the number of successful passes observed during E8 was lower than E1 (−31%, $P = 0.001$, ES = 0.52), E2 (−22%, $P = 0.005$, ES = 0.42), E3 (−24%, $P = 0.001$, ES = 0.50), E4 (−25%, $P = 0.001$, ES = 0.53) and E7 (−17%, $P = 0.002$, ES = 0.48). Similarly, the total number of passes made in E8 was reduced when compared to E1 (−30%, $P = 0.001$, ES = 0.52), E3 (−21%, $P = 0.002$, ES = 0.49), E4 (−21%, $P \leq 0.0005$, ES = 0.54) and E7 (−15%, $P = 0.001$, ES = 0.50). Furthermore, dribbling success in E8 was reduced when compared to E1 (−32%, $P = 0.001$, ES = 0.50) and E3 (−24%, $P \leq 0.0005$, ES = 0.59). The time the ball was in play was less in E8 compared to E1 (−16%, $P < 0.0005$, ES = 0.55). All other technical variables analysed, including shooting and crossing indices, were similar between extra-time and the rest of the match.

Discussion

The aim of this observational study was to identify the influence of the extra-time period on the technical requirements elicited during professional soccer match-play. In agreement with our hypothesis, we demonstrated using a within-match study design, that indices of technical performance, namely passing and dribbling, reduced in the last 15-min of extra-time. To our knowledge, this is the first study to report data concerning the influence of extra-time on professional soccer match-play; therefore such data can be used as a benchmark for future work. Given the importance of this additional competitive period in deciding success and progression in soccer tournament scenarios, this data is likely to be of interest to those responsible for the technical preparations of soccer players.

Passing performance (i.e., the number of successful and total passes) reduced by more than 20% during E8 when compared to the first half of match-play. However, the accuracy of passing remained unchanged during this time (Table 1). Although changes in formation appear to influence passing frequency [15], our data may also indicate that the effects of match-related fatigue observed during the extra-time period of actual match-play impairs the ability to get involved with the ball rather than a player's passing proficiency *per se* [4]. Unfortunately, physical performance measures are unavailable to substantiate this speculation and

Table 3. Technical performance variables (mean ± SD) as a function of timing throughout matches.

Variable	Timing throughout match								Time effect		Post-hoc differences ($P \leq 0.007$) compared to E7 and E8
	E1	E2	E3	E4	E5	E6	E7	E8	Chi Square ($X^2_{(7)}$)	*P* value	
Passing											
Successful passes	88±23	77±21	79±18	80±21	66±20	65±17	73±20	61±23	32.91	<0.0005	E8 vs. E1, E2, E3, E4, E7
Unsuccessful passes	14±5	12±5	11±4	13±4	10±3	10±5	11±4	11±5	22.97	0.002	
Total passes	102±22	89±21	91±19	93±22	76±21	76±21	84±20	71±25	37.23	<0.0005	E8 vs. E1, E3, E4, E7
Pass accuracy (%)	85±7	86±7	87±5	86±4	86±6	86±5	87±6	84±7	4.10	0.769	
Dribbling											
Successful dribbles	14±4	13±5	12±4	13±5	11±4	12±4	11±3	9±4	15.79	0.027	E8 vs. E1, E3
Unsuccessful dribbles	5±3	5±2	4±1	4±3	4±2	5±2	4±2	5±2	7.20	0.408	
Total dribbles	18±4	18±6	16±5	17±5	15±4	16±4	15±3	15±5	13.12	0.069	
Dribble accuracy (%)	72±15	74±12	76±9	72±18	72±14	71±16	72±12	64±16	8.17	0.318	
Shooting											
Shots on target	1±1	1±1	1±1	1±1	2±1	1±1	1±1	1±1	11.45	0.120	
Shots off target	2±1	2±1	2±2	2±2	2±1	3±2	2±1	2±1	11.57	0.116	
Total shots	3±2	2±1	3±2	4±2	4±2	4±2	3±2	3±1	12.57	0.083	
Shot accuracy (%)	37±37	37±32	30±28	39±32	44±28	22±27	36±27	31±26	7.44	0.384	
Crossing											
Successful crosses	1±1	1±1	2±1	1±1	1±1	2±1	2±1	2±1	5.44	0.606	
Unsuccessful crosses	3±2	4±2	3±3	5±2	4±3	4±2	4±2	4±2	11.95	0.102	
Total crosses	5±2	5±2	5±3	6±3	6±3	6±3	6±2	6±3	5.17	0.640	
Cross accuracy (%)	29±27	15±15	37±28	22±25	31±29	29±25	28±21	27±19	10.48	0.163	
Time in play (s)	598±70	554±81	554±52	553±60	493±83	502±81	551±65	504±61	27.66	<0.0005	E8 vs. E1

Where E1 = 00:00–14:59 min, E2 = 15:00–29:59 min, E3 = 30:00–44:59 min, E4 = 45:00–59:59 min, E5 = 60:00–74:59 min, E6 = 75:00–89:59 min, E7 = 90:00–104:59 min, E8 = 105:00–119:59 min.

further research is needed to provide further information regarding the extra-time responses of soccer players.

Although direct comparison of our data to that reported in other performance analysis studies is limited, our findings support, and extend, previously published data identifying decrements of both physical [4,16] and technical [4,7] markers in the latter stages of normal time (i.e., 90 min). In players who were deemed to be fatigued, Rampinini et al. [4] reported between-half reductions of ~12–16% in the number of technical involvements performed per player in the Italian Serie A league. In combination with our observations, it therefore appears that the proficiency, and number, of specific technical actions reduces as a match progresses.

Match-related fatigue could plausibly explain our observations but it is important to note that the reductions in the physical performances observed in midfield players was not previously accompanied by reduced technical performance [16]. To date, the effects of 120 min of soccer-specific exercise remain to be fully elucidated using controlled and repeatable experimental procedures (e.g., Soccer Match Simulation; [17]). Notably, the lack of differences observed during E8 relative to the technical performances observed in E6 means that the transient changes observed during extra-time, at least in the variables assessed in this study, appear to be similar to those elicited in the latter stages of normal time (e.g., E6). It is therefore plausible that interventions that seek to counteract the deleterious effects of match-related fatigue during games that last 90 min, may also be efficacious during extra-time. However, this supposition is yet to be examined.

In previous studies where soccer match-play has been subdivided into smaller segments, statistical artefacts have been proposed to explain the identification of transient reductions in performance when compared to the opening phase of play [9]. A desire to enforce tactical superiority [9] and residual ergogenic effects resulting from the warm-up [7] have been cited to artificially elevate the pace of play in the initial stages of a match and thereby influence subsequent comparisons to observations made during this interval. In the absence of appropriate methods of data analysis that overcome such approaches, it is important to note that the transient changes identified in E8 in this study were rarely yielded from comparison to E1 alone. In combination with the medium effect sizes for the majority of differences observed, we propose that the transient changes identified are reflective of the demands of the extra-time period and not a reflection of statistical artefacts.

Not all of the technical actions examined demonstrated a uniform response to exercise when match-play was separated into 15-min epochs; for example, ~23% of the variables examined exhibited transient changes. These findings support our previous data, albeit during 90 min of English Championship match-play, where only two of the seven technical measures examined (namely total number of possessions and distributions performed) reduced in the last 15 min [7]. However, contrary to previous literature [4,16], we observed a reduction in the number of successful dribbles performed in the final 15 min of extra-time. As far as we are aware, and while acknowledging the differential effects of soccer-specific exercise on technical performance [5], no study has previously identified transient changes in dribbling performance throughout actual match-play. We attribute the identification of this finding to the longer duration of exercise examined in this study. Such data is likely to have important implications for the tactics employed by teams competing in the extra-time period.

The precise mechanisms regulating performance throughout soccer-specific exercise remain to be established and are likely to be multifaceted in nature. Notwithstanding the influence of previously mentioned factors, such as team tactics [9] and self-pacing strategies [8], it must be noted that a greater degree of variation is observed in technical performance measures [18,19] when compared to physical performance. Furthermore, although it has previously been proposed that a lack of sensitivity exists in the gross measures derived from computerised time-motion analysis studies [16], we have again used performance analysis techniques, albeit with a within-match rather than within-player study design, and observed differences in the cumulative technical responses observed during 15 min epochs in matches involving professional soccer players. Furthermore, we have also demonstrated the test-retest reliability of such measures over different assessment periods.

When interpreting the current findings, a number of limitations should be considered. Firstly, it is prudent to note that this data represents a within-match rather than a within-player approach. The low occurrence of games requiring extra-time, the number of eligible games that footage was available for, and the number of repeated player observations, would have yielded data with extremely low statistical power if a within-player approach has been adopted. While acknowledging this limitation, we believe that we are the first group to present data relating to the technical responses observed during the extra-time period in soccer. Additionally, our findings support previously published data, especially in relation to the transient variations observed [4]. Secondly, as the ball was in play for longer in E8 than E1 (note that this was the only variable to show differences between E8 and E1 alone), one could argue that the differences observed were reflective of an interaction with this variable. However, as aforementioned, the reductions in performance observed in E8 were yielded from comparison to other epochs in addition to E1; therefore, it is unlikely that such differences reflect the time that the ball was in play. Finally, this study was a descriptive study; therefore, it was not possible to determine the cause of temporal changes in the performance of technical actions but we acknowledge the potential role of match-specific factors such as game context (e.g., score line, venue, team/opposition quality etc.) and the area of the pitch in which technical actions are performed (e.g. attacking and defensive third) [20,21].

Conclusions

In summary, this study presents novel findings describing temporal patterns in the technical actions observed during 120 min of professional soccer match-play. We provide evidence demonstrating that the number of successful and total passes, number of successful dribbles and the time that the ball was in play, reduced by more than 20% in matches that required extra-time to be played; particularly in the last 15-min of extra-time. Although the current study was unable to elucidate the specific reasons for these findings, coaches and conditioning staff could use this information to inform team tactics and technical training sessions. Implementation of strategies that seek to minimise such occurrences (e.g., substitutions, aerobic and anaerobic conditioning programs and nutritional supplementation protocols [22] etc.) should be considered; however, the efficacy of such strategies remains to be confirmed when 120 min of actual match-play is performed.

Author Contributions

Conceived and designed the experiments: MR DW ES LH. Performed the experiments: MR DW ES LH. Analyzed the data: MR DW ES LH. Contributed reagents/materials/analysis tools: MR DW ES LH. Contributed to the writing of the manuscript: MR DW ES LH.

References

1. Di Salvo V, Baron R, Tschan H, Calderon Montero FJ, Bachl N, et al. (2007) Performance characteristics according to playing position in elite soccer. Int J Sports Med 28: 222–227.
2. Mohr M, Krustrup P, Bangsbo J (2003) Match performance of high-standard soccer players with special reference to development of fatigue. J Sports Sci 21: 519–528.
3. Rahnama N, Reilly T, Lees A, Graham-Smith P (2003) Muscle fatigue induced by exercise simulating the work rate of competitive soccer. J Sports Sci 21: 933–942.
4. Rampinini E, Impellizzeri FM, Castagna C, Coutts AJ, Wisloff U (2009) Technical performance during soccer matches of the Italian Serie A league: effect of fatigue and competitive level. J Sci Med Sport 12: 227–233.
5. Russell M, Benton D, Kingsley M (2011) The effects of fatigue on soccer skills performed during a soccer match simulation. Int J Sports Physiol Perform 6: 221–233.
6. Lago-Penas C, Lago-Ballesteros J, Dellal A, Gomez M (2010) Game-related statistics that discriminated winning, drawing and losing teams from the Spanish soccer league. J Sports Sci Med 9: 288–293.
7. Russell M, Rees G, Kingsley MI (2013) Technical demands of soccer match play in the english championship. J Strength Cond Res 27: 2869–2873.
8. Edwards AM, Noakes TD (2009) Dehydration: cause of fatigue or sign of pacing in elite soccer? Sports Med 39: 1–13.
9. Weston M, Batterham AM, Castagna C, Portas MD, Barnes C, et al. (2011) Reduction in physical match performance at the start of the second half in elite soccer. Int J Sports Physiol Perform 6: 174–182.
10. Reilly T (2003) Motion analysis and physiological demands. In: Williams AM, Reilly T, editors. Science and Soccer. London: Routledge. 59–72.
11. Wilkinson M, Akenhead R (2013) Violation of statistical assumptions in a recent publication? Int J Sports Med 34: 281.
12. Aughey RJ, Varley MC (2013) Acceleration profiles in elite Australian soccer. Int J Sports Med 34: 282.
13. Field A (2009) Discovering statistics using SPSS. London: Sage publications.
14. Cohen J (1988) Statistical power analysis for the behavioral sciences. New Jersey: Lawrence Erlbaum.
15. Bradley PS, Carling C, Archer D, Roberts J, Dodds A, et al. (2011) The effect of playing formation on high-intensity running and technical profiles in English FA Premier League soccer matches. J Sports Sci 29: 821–830.
16. Carling C, Dupont G (2011) Are declines in physical performance associated with a reduction in skill-related performance during professional soccer match-play? J Sports Sci 29: 63–71.
17. Russell M, Rees G, Benton D, Kingsley M (2011) An exercise protocol that replicates soccer match-play. Int J Sports Med 32: 511–518.
18. Ali A, Williams C, Hulse M, Strudwick A, Reddin J, et al. (2007) Reliability and validity of two tests of soccer skill. J Sports Sci 25: 1461–1470.
19. Russell M, Benton D, Kingsley M (2010) Reliability and construct validity of soccer skills tests that measure passing, shooting, and dribbling. J Sports Sci 28: 1399–1408.
20. Mackenzie R, Cushion C (2013) Performance analysis in football: a critical review and implications for future research. J Sports Sci 31: 639–676.
21. Taylor JB, Mellalieu SD, James N, Shearer DA (2008) The influence of match location, quality of opposition, and match status on technical performance in professional association football. J Sports Sci 26: 885–895.
22. Russell M, Kingsley M (2014) The efficacy of acute nutritional interventions on soccer skill performance. Sports Med 44: 957–970.

19

Nonlinear Pedagogy: An Effective Approach to Cater for Individual Differences in Learning a Sports Skill

Miriam Chang Yi Lee[1]*, Jia Yi Chow[1], John Komar[2], Clara Wee Keat Tan[1], Chris Button[3]

1 Physical Education and Sports Science, National Institute of Education, Nanyang Technological University, Singapore, Singapore, **2** CETAPS, Faculty of Sports Sciences, University of Rouen, Rouen, France, **3** School of Physical Education, Sport and Exercise Sciences, University of Otago, Dunedin, New Zealand

Abstract

Learning a sports skill is a complex process in which practitioners are challenged to cater for individual differences. The main purpose of this study was to explore the effectiveness of a Nonlinear Pedagogy approach for learning a sports skill. Twenty-four 10-year-old females participated in a 4-week intervention involving either a Nonlinear Pedagogy (i.e.,manipulation of task constraints including equipment and rules) or a Linear Pedagogy (i.e., prescriptive, repetitive drills) approach to learn a tennis forehand stroke. Performance accuracy scores, movement criterion scores and kinematic data were measured during pre-intervention, post-intervention and retention tests. While both groups showed improvements in performance accuracy scores over time, the Nonlinear Pedagogy group displayed a greater number of movement clusters at post-test indicating the presence of degeneracy (i.e., many ways to achieve the same outcome). The results suggest that degeneracy is effective for learning a sports skill facilitated by a Nonlinear Pedagogy approach. These findings challenge the common misconception that there must be only one ideal movement solution for a task and thus have implications for coaches and educators when designing instructions for skill acquisition.

Editor: Donald A. Robin, University of Texas Health Science Center at San Antonio, Research Imaging Institute, United States of America

Funding: This paper was funded by a research grant from the Office of Education Research (OER 15/09 CJY), National Institute of Education, Nanyang Technological University, Singapore. The funders had no role in study design, data collection and analysis, decision to publish, or preparation of the manuscript.

Competing Interests: The authors have declared that no competing interests exist.

* Email: miriamlee.cy@gmail.com

Introduction

Motor skill acquisition during childhood forms the foundation for lifelong participation in sport, essential for long-term health and fitness benefits [1]. Learning a sports skill is a complex process that involves a multitude of factors. At the level of the learner, every individual is unique with differences in characteristics such as genetic composition, social-economic backgrounds, prior experiences, and learning styles [2]. A key challenge for movement practitioners is to cater for this abundance of individual characteristics during practice. Clearly, an instructional approach underpinned by a robust theoretical framework is essential for effective acquisition of a sports skill.

Traditionally, practitioners (e.g., coaches, teachers, etc.) have adopted approaches which are prescriptive and repetitive, utilizing technical demonstrations that provide learners with a "visual template or criterion model" for the desired skill [3]. The underlying assumption that has fuelled such pedagogies is that an ideal movement pattern exists for a task and that the practitioner's role is to help learners to recreate that pattern [3]. Furthermore, some theorists have suggested that learning is a gradual, linear process offering the 'power law' as supportive evidence [4,5], although this viewpoint is not without its critics [6]. An increasing amount of evidence from the Dynamical Systems Theory (DST) perspective challenge these traditional assumptions about skill acquisition [3,7,8].

From the DST viewpoint, the learning process does not generally follow continuous linear progressions of behaviour but rather involves sudden discontinuous changes over time [9]. Learners should be conceived as nonlinear dynamical systems, comprising numerous component parts that interact and self-organize to form stable patterns. The emergence of self-organized functional movement solutions is faciliated through the interaction of performer, task and environment constraints which act as boundaries to shape goal-directed behaviours. Unlike tradtional approaches in motor learning, there is no central controller (e.g., an authoritative coach) that determines how movement behaviors should be produced to meet task goals [7]. Chow et al. [10] were the first to propose the use of the umbrella term "Nonlinear Pedagogy" to capture how practitioners can benefit from these contemporary theoretical concepts.

Grounded in the constraints-led approach, Nonlinear Pedagogy (referred to from here as NP) advocates the manipulation of key constraints that form boundaries for the learner to explore functional movement solutions [11,12]. Thus, NP provides a framework for pedagocial principles that can be used to account for the nonlinear behavioural changes typically observed in learning movement skills. It provides a theoretical impetus for practitioners to incorporate "representativeness, manipulation of constraints, attentional focus, functional variability, and the maintenance of pertinent information-movement couplings" to effectively design motor learning interventions [13]. Firstly, NP emphasizes the importance of a representative learning design in which learning is situated in real-game contexts. When placed in representative learning environments, information-movement couplings relevant to the desired sports skill are presented to the learner, providing functional affordances (i.e., opportunities for action) for the individual. NP also advocates the manipulation of task constraints such as instructions, rules of the activity, and equipment (e.g., racquets, balls, court size), to encourage learners to explore various movements solutions most suitable for themselves. In addition, just as instructions based on external focus of attention seem to reduce the conscious processing of information in skill acquisition [14], NP focuses on movement outcomes rather than movement form. At this juncture, it is important to highlight that while the NP approach may encompass practical features similar to external focus of attention, NP is underpinned by key aspects from DST and thus the guiding principles for implementation of the two approaches are not the same. Lastly, NP embraces functional movement variability in developing a coordinated movement, since movement variability is a critical feature of learning in human movement systems.

When it comes to teaching sports skills, NP provides the appropriate framework for practitioners to cater for individual complexities and dynamic learning environments. In NP, learners are encouraged to experiment with different movement patterns and adapt individual coordinative structures to achieve functional movement solutions [15]. This process, known as degeneracy, is crucial in skill acquisition as it empowers the individual with a variety of movement possibilities that may be recruited to suit task and environmental demands. According to Bernstein [16], learners form functional muscle-joint linkages, known as coordinative structures, to deal with the numerous component parts present in the human movement system. Every time a new movement task is performed, these coordinative structures are reassembled temporarily and flexibility, adapting the various component parts to suit the specific task condition [17]. Degeneracy is the ability for complex neurobiological systems (i.e., learners in this case) to achieve different solutions for the same task goals and provides the individual with an improved capacity to deal with information-rich dynamic environments [7,18]. Previous studies have shown that there are individual differences in the acquisition of coordination and control even when presented with the same task [19,20].

It seems reasonable to expect that the NP approach would produce a greater variety of movement solutions compared to the traditional instructional approach for acquisition of sports skills. Traditional motor learning pedagogies involve instructions that are prescriptive, repetitive, and drill-like with a strong focus on "criterion model" technique, labelled as Linear Pedagogy (LP) in this study. While learners taught with a LP approach are expected to reproduce movement patterns that are more similar to the "criterion model", the NP approach is likely to produce a greater variety of movement patterns that are more suited to the individual. A recent study provides initial evidence that learners taught with a NP approach were able to develop functional 'personal patterns of coordination' which were more biomechanically efficient in breastroke swimming indicated by a longer gliding time and a coordination pattern closer to anti-phase with learning [21]. There are also examples in the literature to indicate that explorative instructions (e.g., analogy, external focus of attention and manipulation of task constraints) tend to produce better results than instructions that are generally prescriptive and drill-like [14,22,23]. These studies suggest that explorative instructions, which contain features of NP, could result in greater performance benefits although more evidence is still required.

It is unclear how a NP approach adopted within a controlled school setting will influence motor skill acquisition. The purpose of this study was to investigate the effectiveness of a NP approach, in relation to a LP approach. It was predicted that: 1) The LP group would produce higher movement criterion scores, indicating a movement pattern that is more similar to the "criterion model"; 2) The NP group would result in a greater number of movement clusters, indicating the presence of degeneracy; 3) Both groups would improve in performance accuracy scores although the NP group would produce higher scores as a result of the expression of degenerate behavior.

Methods

Participants

24 right-handed female participants aged 9 to 10 years were selected for this study and randomly assigned to either the NP or the LP group. Three participants did not complete the study due to various reasons, leaving 11 participants in the NP group (mean weight = 31.33 ± 2.72 kg; mean height = 133.00 ± 2.30 cm) and 10 participants in the LP group (mean weight = 31.97 ± 2.16 kg; mean height = 140.70 ± 2.17 cm). All participants were novices with limited experience in playing any racquet sports. Prior to the start of the study, written informed parental consent and participant assent was obtained. Ethics approval was granted by the Nanyang Technological University Institutional Review Board.

Task

Participants within each experimental group were required to learn the tennis forehand groundstroke in a modified tennis setting. The task involved a modified tennis ball being played to the participants by the experimenter. The goal was to return the ball using a forehand groundstroke over the net to several pre-assigned targets on the court.

Procedures

The present study consisted of a pre-intervention session, followed by a 4-week intervention (eight sessions, each lasting 15 minutes), a post-intervention session and a retention session conducted four weeks after the intervention.

1. Testing procedures. The pre, post and retention sessions comprised the same procedures administered at the respective time points of the study. At the start of the testing sessions, a demonstration video of the experimental task was shown to participants. Following this, reflective markers were placed on 17 anatomical landmarks namely: the acromion process, medial and lateral epicondyles, medial and lateral styliod process, illac crests, and greater trochanter on the left and right sides, as well as three markers on the left upper arm, right forearm, and right upper back to assist in identification of the left and right segments [24]. Five reflective markers were also placed at positions corresponding to 2-, 3-, 4-, 8-, and 10'o-clock on the racquet face to identify the racquet head segment. The markers were required to build a 3D-model of the body segments and racquet to obtain kinematic movement data of each participant.

After 10 warm-up trials consisting of hitting over the net (0.8 m) with no accuracy demands, participants performed 10 forehand trials aimed at a target on the court (target 1; referred to as specific target trials) followed by 15 forehand trials aimed at three different targets (target 2, 3 and 4; referred to as multiple target trials) requiring them to vary their shots in a pre-assigned sequence (See Figure 1). During these trials, a modified-tennis ball (Gamma foam ball) was played by the feeder to land in front of the participants. A live feeder was preferred over a machine feed as it allowed participants to utilize the cues from the movement of the racquet, similar to returning a tennis shot in an authentic tennis game [25]. To ensure that the feed was consistent, the ball had to land within a marked out feeding zone (0.7 m×0.5 m). A trial in which the feed was not of acceptable accuracy was repeated and the consistency of the feed was later validated by an expert tennis coach.

2. Interventions. Following the pre-test, the participants underwent a 4-week practice intervention, with 15 minute lessons twice a week, to learn a forehand groundstroke taught using either the NP or LP approach. For both the NP and LP groups, each practice session consisted of 80 forehand groundstroke trials with instructions from either the NP or LP approach. The volume of practice for both groups was comparable with a total of 120 minutes of practice over 4 weeks comprising 640 practice trials. The intervention was developed by the research team and verified by two academics knowledgeable in the area of NP and LP approaches respectively, but external to this research. Both NP and LP interventions were delivered by the same researcher according to the instructions and activity plans developed prior to the intervention phase.

The NP and LP interventions were designed on the understanding that learners could be viewed as either nonlinear or linear systems respectively. The key differences between the nonlinear and linear systems are explained as follows (for detailed justification, see Chow et al. [26]). Firstly, small changes to practice task constraints, such as instructions or equipment, may lead to non-proportionate changes in performance for nonlinear

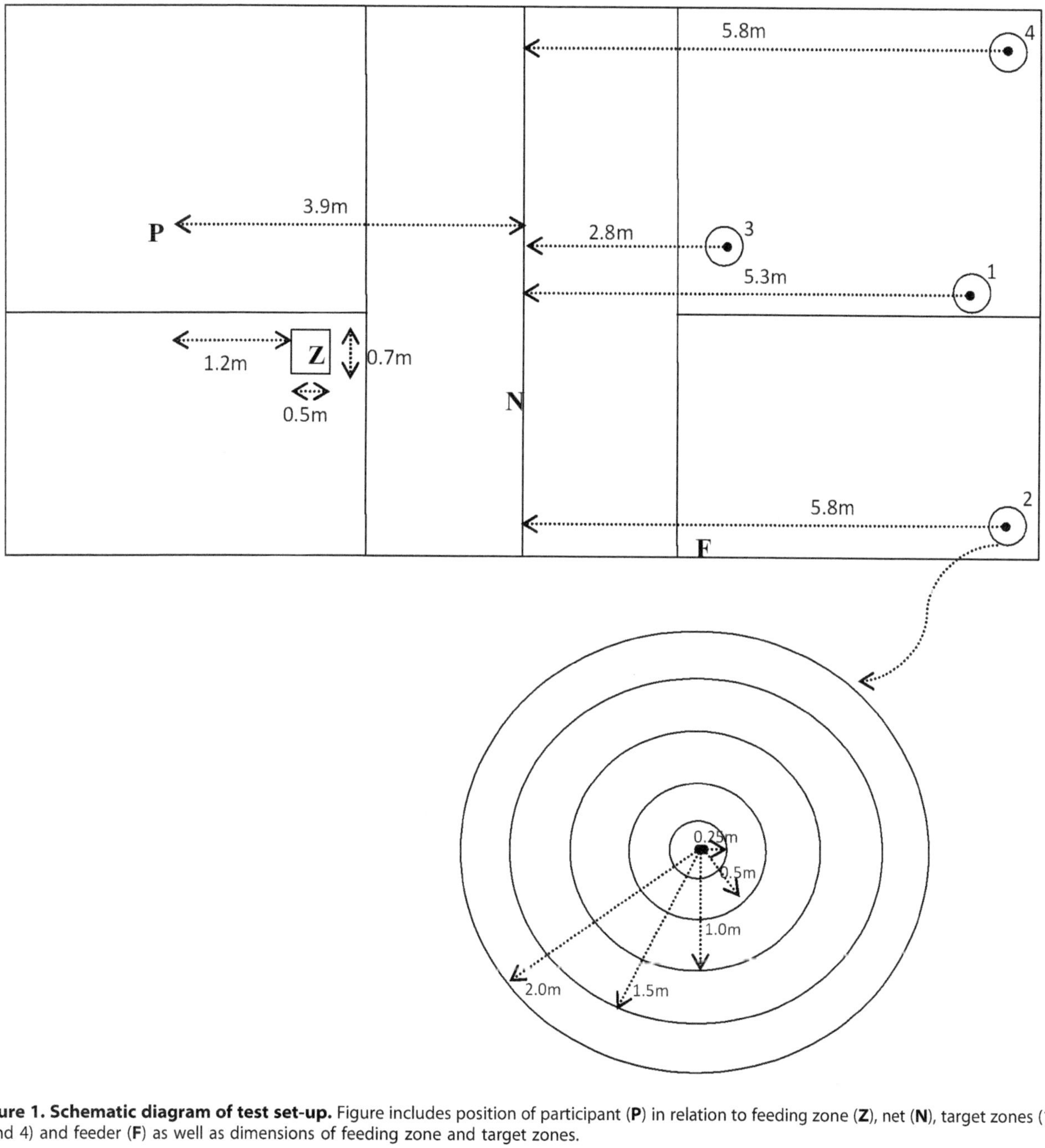

Figure 1. Schematic diagram of test set-up. Figure includes position of participant (**P**) in relation to feeding zone (**Z**), net (**N**), target zones (1, 2, 3 and 4) and feeder (**F**) as well as dimensions of feeding zone and target zones.

systems, while in linear systems it is assumed that a change in practice task leads to a proportionate change in performance. Another difference describes how nonlinear systems are multi-stable (i.e., one cause may result in multiple possible behavioral effects) whereas linear systems are mono-stable (i.e., one cause will result in a single behavioral effect). Multi-stability can be facilitated through the manipulation of a relevant task constraint in NP. Parametric control is the third characteristic of nonlinear systems whereas linear systems involve a centralized control (e.g., top-down, prescriptive approach in LP). Lastly, variability or noise can play a functional role in the likelihood of nonlinear systems transiting between multiple states (i.e., exploration of multiple solutions) whereas in linear systems, noise is seen to play a detrimental role and produces undesired output variability.

Essentially, NP addresses the nonlinearity in learners through the manipulation of constraints, mainly task constraints, creating boundaries for the learner to explore and discover functional movement solutions. The manipulation of task constraints in the NP condition included the manipulation of net height, target area, court size, and rules to achieve specific task goals. In addition, instructions were outcome-focused such as "Hit ball flight like shape of a rainbow"; "Call out color and hit to zone"; "Hit to baseline zone". These conditions also encouraged functional variability such as the use of a variety of balls and racquets, and hitting to different target zones. An important attribute of the NP approach was the application of Newell's [27] stages of learning (Coordination, Control, and Skill) that focuses on individual learning rates for learning a movement skill. Within each stage of learning, the milestones for teaching net-barrier games were adapted from Hopper [28]: 'consistency' (contact with ball, hit over net, hit within opposite court), 'accuracy' (hit to target), 'depth' (hit to baseline), and 'spin' (develop topspin). Participants from this group were provided with instructions according to their individual progression which was assessed during the last 10 trials of each session. If a participant achieved a score of 8 or more, determined from pilot sessions, the participant progressed to the next milestone.

In contrast, LP comes from a traditional perspective that views learners as linear systems and that all learners should aspire towards a common, idealized motor pattern. LP instructions involved a "centralized control" where practitioners instruct what is considered as the ideal movement pattern for a task through the use of prescriptive cues and repetitive drills, leaving negligible opportunity for exploration (see Chow [13] for brief discussion on NP and traditional pedagogical approaches that typifies 'LP'). The LP condition in this study consisted of prescriptive tennis forehand groundstroke technique instructions and repetitive practice drills. The forehand cues provided were according to the different phases of a forehand stroke: 1) Preparation: "Shake hands with racquet", "Racquet in front, feet shoulder-width apart"; 2) Pre-execution: "Turn shoulders to side and bring racquet back", "Move to ball and step"; 3) Execution: "Moving racquet low to high, contact ball in front of forward foot"; 4) Follow through: "Follow through and end swing above opposite shoulder" [29]. The tennis cues, which are common in a traditional tennis lesson, were developed and verified by an expert tennis coach who was blinded to the purpose of this study. At the start of the practice session and at intervals of every 15 trials, the forehand stroke was demonstrated according to the cues and participants had to perform a shadow drill following the experimenter.

Apparatus and measurements

1. Performance accuracy scores. Performance accuracy scores were determined based on a 6-point rating scale according to the landing position of the ball for the assigned target of the respective trial (6 points = on target; 4 to 1 points given according to distance away from center of target; 0 = out of target). The suitability of the position of the target zone and the scoring system was confirmed during pilot sessions prior to the study. Such scoring scales were also used in previous studies to investigate learning a sports skill in soccer kicking [19] and basketball shooting [30].

2. Movement criterion scores. Movement performance of the forehand groundstroke were captured by a digital video (DV) camera (Canon, Legria HF S100) positioned approximately 5 m to the right side of the participant and fixed to a 1.2 m high tripod. Qualitative forehand movement performance was rated according to a movement checklist which consisted of the critical features of a traditional tennis forehand stroke [29]. The critical features on the movement checklist were validated by an expert tennis coach. The movement performance was rated for the 10 specific and 15 multiple target trials in each test session, according to the frequency each critical feature was observed (0 = never; 1 = sometimes; 2 = always). A total score (maximum score = 20) was given for the specific and multiple target trials respectively for each participant, with a higher score indicating a movement pattern to be more similar to the "criterion model" of the forehand stroke. All trials were rated by a trained research assistant who was blinded to the study. Intraclass correlation coefficient (ICC = 0.938) of forty randomly selected trials rated by an expert tennis coach and the research assistant indicated a high reliability for the movement criterion score ratings.

3. Kinematic movement pattern. The 22 spherical reflective markers (19 mm) placed on the assigned landmarks were captured by 7 infrared cameras (Hawk Digital Camera, Motion Analysis Corporation) and recorded at 200 Hz on the cortex software (Motion Analysis Corporation, SantaRosa, CA, USA). Capture of the reflective markers enabled a 3D model for each participant to be built and subsequently the kinematic data for the relevant joint angles to be determined. The displacement of the markers in 3D space was processed using the cortex software for all 10 specific target trials pre, post and retention tests. After visual inspection, a low pass Butterworth digital filter at a frequency of 10 Hz was applied [31]. Visual 3D software (C-Motion Inc) was then used to construct a 6-segment upper body model (upper arm, forearm, thorax and pelvis) and the racquet head segment. 3D kinematic variables and joint angles were calculated from the respective segments for each individual participant.

Based on previous tennis studies examining the forehand tennis strokes, 12 time-continuous kinematics variables were chosen for further analysis: Right and left elbow flexion/extension, right and left shoulder flexion/extension, abduction/adduction and internal/external rotation, thorax and pelvis rotation, separation angle (difference between hip and shoulder rotation angle) and racquet rotation angle (information about racquet horizontal displacement in the transverse plane) [32,33,34]. The 'start' of each forehand swing was defined as the point preceding any backward movement of the racquet in the y-direction (front/back direction) and the 'end' was determined as the furthest racquet horizontal displacement in the transverse plane. All trials were normalized to 100 data points between the 'start' to the 'end' for simultaneous comparison across trials and individuals [35]. The normalized time-continuous kinematic data was subsequently used for cluster analysis (see section on 'Inter-individual cluster analysis').

Data analysis

1. Statistical analysis (performance accuracy and movement criterion scores). This study followed a 3 (time:

pre, post, retention)×2 (intervention: NP and LP group) factorial design. A mixed-design ANOVA was used to determine differences within and between groups for two dependent variables: performance accuracy scores and movement criterion scores. Any violation in sphericity was corrected using Greenhouse-Geisser epsilon (ε). Fishers LSD *post hoc* test was used to further analyze significant main effects and interactions to determine the location of differences within (time) and between (intervention) factors. Statistical difference was accepted at $p<0.05$ and effect size was calculated using partial eta squared (η_p^2).

2. Inter-individual cluster analysis (movement clusters). Cluster analysis is typically used to examine changes in movement patterns and to determine the presence of movement variability. In particular, cluster analysis is used to group individual trials based on kinematic or kinetic variables (rather than performance scores) so that natural groupings can be observed in the data [36]. According to Rein et al. [37] cluster analysis invovles three main steps: 1) Data pre-processing (selection and processing of appropriate kinematic variables), 2) Cluster analysis, and 3) Cluster validation. The application of cluster analysis methods has been commonly used to examine movement pattern variability in variety of movement skills such as swimming [38], walking [39], kicking [40] and throwing [41]. Therefore, cluster analysis was deemed suitable as no *a priori* knowledge was available on possible groupings between individuals or trials.

In this study, cluster analysis was used to identify the presence of degeneracy for learning a tennis forehand stroke. Specifically, cluster analysis determined the number of movement clusters found in each group for specific target trials following procedures used by Komar and colleagues [38]. A greater number of movement clusters indicated the presence of degeneracy in a given data set. It was expected that the NP approach would produce a greater number of movement clusters following the intervention as this approach facilitated exploration, while the LP approach was likely to display fewer movement cluster as all participants were taught to conform to an idealized motor pattern.

The 12 time-continuous kinematics variables of participants were selected as input variables into a cluster analysis using the Fisher-EM algorithm [42]. This kind of algorithm is based on a probabilistic model which projects the data in a latent subspace at each iteration in such a way that emerging clusters maximize the Fisher information (i.e. maximize the inter-cluster distance while minimizing the intra-cluster distance). Cluster analysis was run for each respective test session (pre, post or retention), for each intervention group (NP or LP) seperately (i.e., six data sets). Each data set comprised 100 trials (10 participants×10 trials). Subsequently, the Bayesian Information Criterion (BIC) index was used as a model-selection criterion to validate the number of clusters found in each respectively data set. Cluster analysis was performed for a potential number of cluster from 2 to 12 and represented in a vector containing the BIC index ($\times10^5$) for [2,3,4,5,6, 7,8,9,10,11,12] number of clusters. The number of clusters which corresponded to the first local maximum represented the ideal number of clusters that best fitted the data set (i.e., that shows the highest ratio between inter-cluster distance and intra-cluster distance) [43].

In addition to the Fisher-EM algorithm, the dimension of the latent subspace where the clustering was performed could be modulated by a "sparsity" parameter. The sparsity index which corresponded to the "weight" of each point into the clustering was also calculated for each kinematic variable. The average sparsity index for each kinematic variable (i.e., from 100 data points) indicated which variable was most discriminative. A higher sparsity value indicated that the respective kinematic variable had a higher percentage contribution to the clustering. Mean movement patterns for kinematic variables, selected based on sparsity values, were displayed on angle-plots for each movement cluster. Movement clusters were indicated as C1...C7 for each respective data set. The mean movement pattern of each cluster was determined from the kinematic data of the trials assigned to a particular cluster. The number of trials and distribution of participants found in each cluster was also displayed in a bar chart to examine the changes in the composition of the movement clusters over time.

Results

Performance accuracy scores

For specific target trials, a main effect for time was observed, F (2,38) = 3.386, $p=0.044$, $\eta_p^2=0.151$. *Post hoc* analysis showed that performance accuracy scores were significantly different (p = 0.019) from pre (NP = 0.62±0.53; LP = 0.65±0.59) to post test (NP = 0.95±0.44; LP = 1.10±0.78). A main effect for time was also observed for multiple target trials F (2,38) = 3.616, $p=0.037$, $\eta_p^2=0.160$. *Post hoc* analysis showed that performance accuracy scores were significantly different ($p=0.013$) from pre (NP = 0.56±0.56; LP = 0.68±0.39) to retention test (NP = 1.05±0.49; LP = 0.93±0.72). The time×intervention interaction was not significant for specific (F(2, 38) = 0.079, $p>0.05$, $\eta_p^2=0.004$) and multiple trials (F(2, 38) = 0.600, p>0.05, $\eta_p^2=0.031$). In addition, no significant differences ($p>0.05$) were observed between the intervention groups for both specific and multiple target trials.

Movement criterion scores

For specific target trials, mean movement criterion scores showed a main effect for time (F(2,38) = 42.559, $p<0.001$, $\eta_p^2=0.691$) and intervention (F(1,19) = 5.313, $p<0.001$, $\eta_p^2=0.219$), with a significant time×intervention interaction (2,38) = 12.217, $p<0.001$, $\eta_p^2=0.391$). Figure 2A shows the nature of the interaction effect. *Post hoc* analysis showed that both the NP and LP group increased significantly in movement criterion scores from pre to post (LP: $p<0.001$; NP: $p=0.049$) and from pre to retention (LP: $p<0.001$; NP: $p=0.012$), with significantly higher scores for the LP group at post (NP = 9.27±3.35; LP = 14.60±3.92; $p=0.003$) and retention tests (NP = 9.91±3.53; LP = 13.90±3.73; $p=0.021$).

For multiple target trials, mean movement criterion scores showed a main effect for time (F(1.20,22.73) = 37.845, $p<0.001$, $\eta_p^2=0.666$, ε = 0.598) and intervention (F(1,19) = 6.085, $p=0.023$, $\eta_p^2=0.243$), with a significant time×intervention interaction (F(1.20,22.73) = 15.377, $p<0.001$, $\eta_p^2=0.447$, ε = 0.598). Figure 2B shows the nature of the interaction effect. *Post hoc* analysis showed that movement criterion scores changed only for the LP group with a significant increase from pre to post ($p<0.001$) and from pre to retention test ($p<0.001$), and a significant decrease from post to retention test ($p<0.001$). In addition, the movement criterion scores were significantly higher for the NP group at pre-test (NP = 6.91±2.071; LP = 4.80±1.62; $p=0.018$), but resulted in significantly higher scores for the LP group at post (NP = 8.91±3.11; LP = 14.60±3.72; $p=0.001$) and retention tests (NP = 9.00±2.97; LP = 12.60±3.60; $p=0.021$).

Movement clusters

One participant in the NP group was excluded from the movement cluster analysis due to issues with the calibration during data collection, thus only 10 participants from each group were included for cluster analysis.

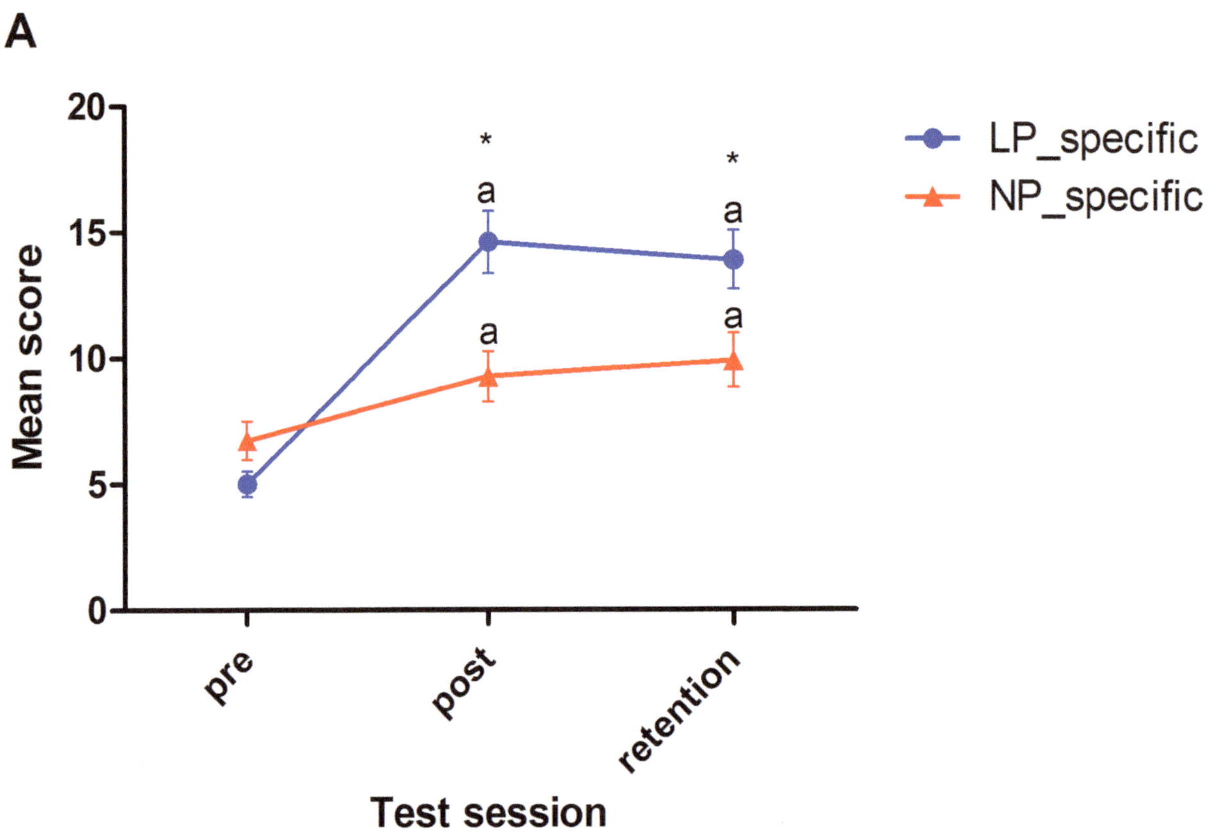
A
20
15
10
5
0
Mean score
*
a
*
a
a
a
LP_specific
NP_specific
pre
post
retention
Test session

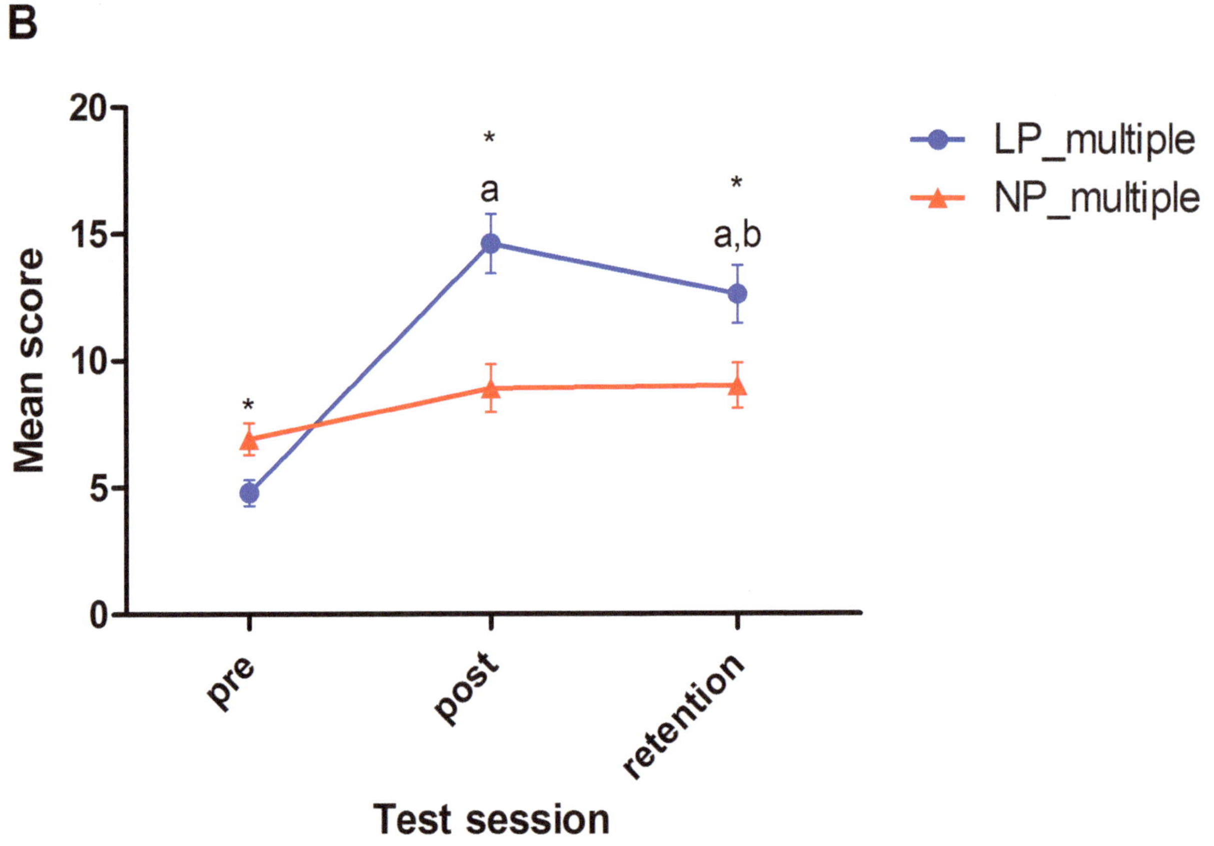
B
20
15
10
5
0
Mean score
*
a
*
a,b
*
LP_multiple
NP_multiple
pre
post
retention
Test session

Figure 2. Mean movement criterion scores for (A) specific and (B) multiple target trials at pre, post and retention tests. (a) indicates significant differences from pre-test ($p<0.05$), (b) indicates significant differences from post-test ($p<0.05$) and (*) indicates significant differences between groups ($p<0.05$). Error bars represent Standard Error Measure (S.E.M) (n = 21).

1. Cluster validation. Fisher-EM clustering for the kinematic variables at pre-test showed that the first local maximum of the BIC index corresponded with 4 clusters for both NP (BIC index $(\times 10^5) = [-5.19, -5.16, \boldsymbol{-5.14}, -5.14, -5.13, -5.18, -5.15, -5.20, -5.19, -5.20, -5.22]$) and LP (BIC index $(\times 10^5) = [-5.21, -5.17, \boldsymbol{-5.13}, -5.14, -5.12, -5.13, -5.17, -5.17, -5.18, -5.18, -5.22]$). In addition, the first local maximum of the BIC index corresponded with 7 clusters for NP (BIC index $(\times 10^5) = [-5.31, -5.29, -5.27, -5.25, -5.25, \boldsymbol{-5.24}, -5.28, -5.28, -5.29, -5.32, -5.34]$) and 3 clusters for LP (BIC index $(\times 10^5) = [-5.33, \boldsymbol{-5.28}, -5.30, -5.27, -5.26, -5.26, -5.26, -5.26, -5.30, -5.31, -5.32]$) at post-test, followed by 5 clusters for NP (BIC index $(\times 10^5) = [-5.28, -5.26, -5.24, \boldsymbol{-5.21}, -5.22, -5.23, -5.24, -5.26, -5.27, -5.27, -5.31]$) and 7 clusters for LP (BIC index $(\times 10^5) = [-5.32, -5.27, -5.26, -5.25, -5.24, \boldsymbol{-5.23}, -5.27, -5.28, -5.26, -5.27, -5.30]$) at retention test.

The higher sparsity values indicate that the respective kinematic variable represents a higher percentage contribution to the clustering. Right and left elbow flexion/extension, right and left shoulder internal/external rotation, and racquet rotation angle were the five kinematic variables with higher sparsity values (Table 1). From here, two of the kinematic variables were selected for examination of the mean movement patterns to discriminate the movement clusters. The right shoulder rotation was selected as it had the highest sparsity among the right-sided joint angles and racquet rotation angle was chosen as it provided information about the racquet position.

2. Mean movement patterns for each cluster. The movement patterns within each group showed changes following the 4-week intervention, although both groups changed in different ways. At post-test, the LP group displayed movement patterns that were relatively uniform across all participants in C1 to C3 (i.e., cluster 1 to cluster 3). For example, Figure 3E shows that the LP group generally displayed consistent patterns for shoulder rotation at post-test: internal rotation at the start of the swing (preparation phase), followed by external rotation at backswing and internal rotation at the end of the swing (follow through). Figure 4E shows that for the LP group at post-test, both C1 and C2 exhibited a racquet rotation angle close to 0° at the start of the swing (preperation phase), followed by C1 to C3 displaying angles close to 180° at backswing, ending with angles close to −90° and below at the end of swing (follow through). On the other hand,the NP group did not show such consistency but displayed greater variabilty from cluster to cluster in terms of the general movement pattern and the range of motion of the forehand swing at post-test. For example, the angles that occurred at backswing and at the end of the swing varied from C1 to C7 as seen in Figure 3B and 4B.

At retention test, the movement patterns in the LP group changed drastically displaying a greater variety of kinematic movement patterns for the forehand stroke (Figure 3F and 4F). The NP group continued to display a variety of movement patterns at retention test as seen in Figure 3C and 4C.

3. Distribution of trials across clusters. Each movement cluster in Figure 5 corresponded to the movement cluster in Figure 3 and 4 for each respective data set. For example, C1 in Figure 5A comprised 30 trials from which the mean movement pattern was determined for C1 in Figure 3A and 4A. Figure 5A and 5D shows that the distribution of trials in the movement clusters was similar in both NP and LP group at pre-test. For example, the cluster with the most number of trials at pre-test (C2 in Figure 5A and Figure 5D), consisted of 39 and 44 trials from seven participants for NP and LP groups respectively, while the smallest cluster (C4 in NP and C3 in LP) only comprised 10 trials from one participant. Following the intervention, the number of trials and distribution of participants in each cluster changed considerablly at post-test. The distribution of participants across the clusters was more varied in the NP group with some of the same partcipants distributed across several clusters (Figure 5B). In the LP group, most of the participants were found in C1 and C2 with the highest number of the trials assigned to C2 (41 trials) followed by C1 (32 trials) (Figure 5E). At retention test, the distribution of trials changed again especially for the LP group in which partiticipants were spread throughout the 7 clusters (Figure 5F).

Discussion

The purpose of this study was to investigate the effectiveness of a NP approach for learning a tennis forehand stroke in a controlled setting. Based on previous literature, it was predicted that while the NP group would perform better in accuracy scores, it would produce lower movement criterion scores and display a greater variety of movement patterns to achieve the task goal, as compared to the LP group, indicating the presence of degeneracy.

Following the 4-week intervention, both NP and LP groups improved in performance accuracy scores just as well. Improvements in accuracy scores for the NP group occurred despite an intervention that encouraged learners to explore functional movement solutions, without involving prescriptive, repetitive instructions. Perhaps the NP approach required a longer intervention time to be most effective and for the children to discover more fully the functional movement solutions for themselves. Even though the initial prediction was not met, the results provide evidence that it is not necessary for learners to achieve the "criterion model" in order to be successful and that the NP approach, which encourages exploration and variability, is effective [3,19].

Information about how similar participants' forehand stokes were to the "criterion model" was indicated by the movement criterion scores. Movement criterion was measured against a scoring scale in which a higher score indicated a more ideal movement form according to the "criterion model" of the forehand stroke typically taught by coaches. For both the specific and multiple target tasks, the LP group displayed significantly higher movement criterion scores at post and retention tests, providing evidence that the LP group performed more closely to the "criterion model". On the other hand, the NP group only showed changes in movement criterion scores at post and retention tests for specific trials but not for multiple target trials, suggesting the presence of degeneracy. Participants from the NP group were able to adapt to the constraints of the tasks and adjust their hitting patterns accordingly. Furthermore, any changes in the forehand stroke for the NP group were different from what is typically deemed as the ideal forehand stroke, perhaps representing movement patterns that were more individualized.

Table 1. Mean sparsity index (%) for each kinematic variable.

	NP				LP			
	Pre	**post**	**ret**	**Avg[a]**	**pre**	**post**	**Ret**	**Avg[a]**
Right elbow (flex/ext)	7.44	8.29	8.56	**8.10**	8.69	9.08	7.22	**8.33**
Left elbow (flex/ext)	7.28	8.38	9.23	**8.30**	10.01	11.71	8.51	**10.08**
Right shoulder (flex/ext)	6.05	6.86	6.89	6.60	6.46	4.11	8.86	6.48
Right shoulder (abd/add)	6.12	7.68	6.58	6.79	8.49	5.95	7.54	7.33
Right shoulder (int/ext rotation)	13.70	13.89	14.69	**14.09**	12.92	13.99	16.31	**14.41**
Left shoulder (flex/ext)	5.79	6.48	7.62	6.63	6.22	6.99	7.12	6.78
Left shoulder (abd/add)	6.65	6.77	8.80	7.40	6.38	6.70	5.87	6.32
Left shoulder (int/ext rotation)	15.77	14.39	12.56	**14.24**	15.13	16.62	12.76	**14.84**
Separation angle	6.23	4.93	4.33	5.16	4.55	3.10	5.83	4.49
Thorax rotation	5.86	5.62	5.88	5.78	5.00	7.32	4.89	5.74
Pelvis rotation	6.72	5.78	5.56	6.02	4.59	5.46	5.70	5.25
Racquet rotation angle	12.41	10.94	9.31	**10.88**	11.57	8.95	9.39	**9.97**
Total[b]	100	100	100	100	100	100	100	100

[a]Refers to the average of the mean sparsity (%) for each kinematic variable for the NP and LP group.
[b]Refers to the sum of all 12 kinematic variables' mean sparsity (%) for each test session.

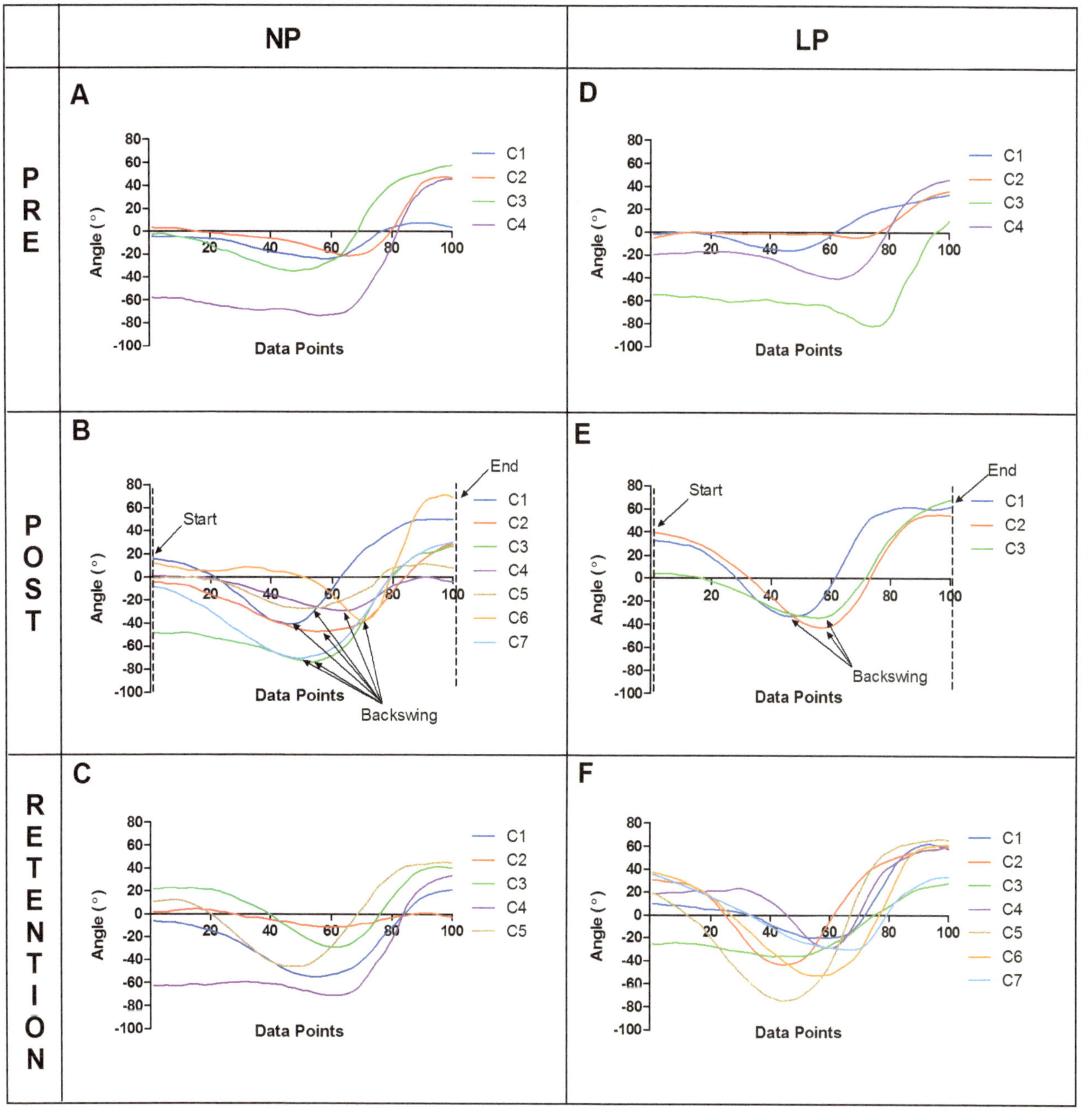

Figure 3. Mean right shoulder internal/external rotation angle. Mean kinematic data normalized to 100 data points for movement clusters found in specific target trials for the six data sets: NP - pre (A), post (B), retention (C); LP - pre (D), post (E), retention (F). C1, C2...C7 represent movement clusters found within each data set. Positive angles indicate internal rotation and negative angles indicate external rotation. The "Backswing" is approximated based on the point where the external rotation was the greatest.

Inter-individual cluster analysis provided a more in-depth understanding of the movement pattern changes that occurred following the 4-week intervention for specific target trials. As predicted, there were more movement clusters in the NP group (7 clusters) than in the LP group (3 clusters) at post-test, verifying that the presence of degeneracy is stronger in the NP group. Even though the NP group showed a greater variety of movement patterns as a result of more opportunities to explore, participants in this group improved their accuracy scores just as well as the LP group. This is consistent with previous studies [19,30,44] and provides evidence that there is more than one ideal way of hitting the ball to achieve the same task successfully.

An interesting observation was that the number of movement clusters for the LP group increased to 7 clusters at retention test. This greater variety of movement patterns at retention test coincided with the significant decrease in movement criterion scores from post to retention test for the multiple target trials, suggesting that learning the "criterion model" was not permanent. After a period without intervention, learners in the LP group seemed to incline towards a preferred stable state which was more appropriate for their individual composition. As learners in the LP

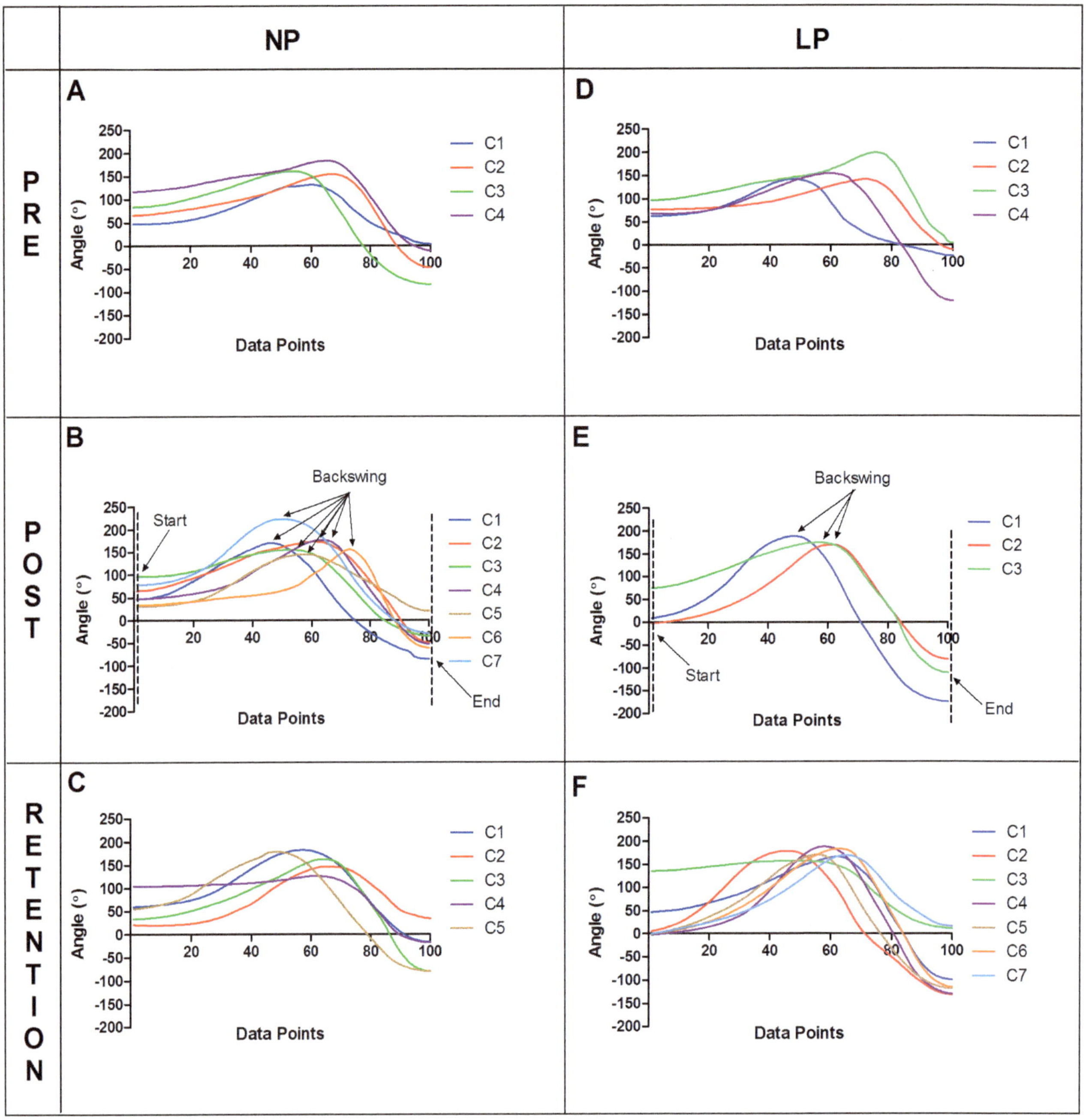

Figure 4. Mean racquet rotation angle. Mean kinematic data normalized to 100 data points for movement clusters found in specific target trials for the six data sets: NP - pre (A), post (B), retention (C); LP - pre (D), post (E), retention (F). C1, C2...C7 represent movement clusters found within each data set. An angle of 0° indicated that the racquet was pointing towards the net while an angle of 180° indicated that the racquet was pointing towards the baseline (typically at or near backswing). The "Backswing" is approximated based on the point where the racquet rotation was the greatest.

group started to use movement patterns that they were more comfortable with, performance accuracy scores for the multiple target trials also improved during the retention test.

At post-test, the two more dominant clusters found in the LP group (i.e., C1 followed by C2) displayed characteristics that closely mimicked the given forehand cues in the LP instructions. For example, the racquet rotation angle was close to 0° at the start of the swing (preparation phase) indicating that the racquet head was pointing towards the net (Figure 4E), followed by an external rotation at backswing and an internal rotation of the right shoulder at the end of the swing (follow through) as the racquet ended above the left shoulder (Figure 3E). In accordance with traditional methods of skill acquisition, if the prescribed "criterion model" was the idealized motor pattern for performing the forehand stroke, all participants found in the dominant clusters should show better performance accuracy scores (see William & Hodges [3]). In terms of accuracy scores, two of the highest scoring LP participants (LP1 = 2.1 points; LP10 = 2.0 points) were found in C1 and C2 at

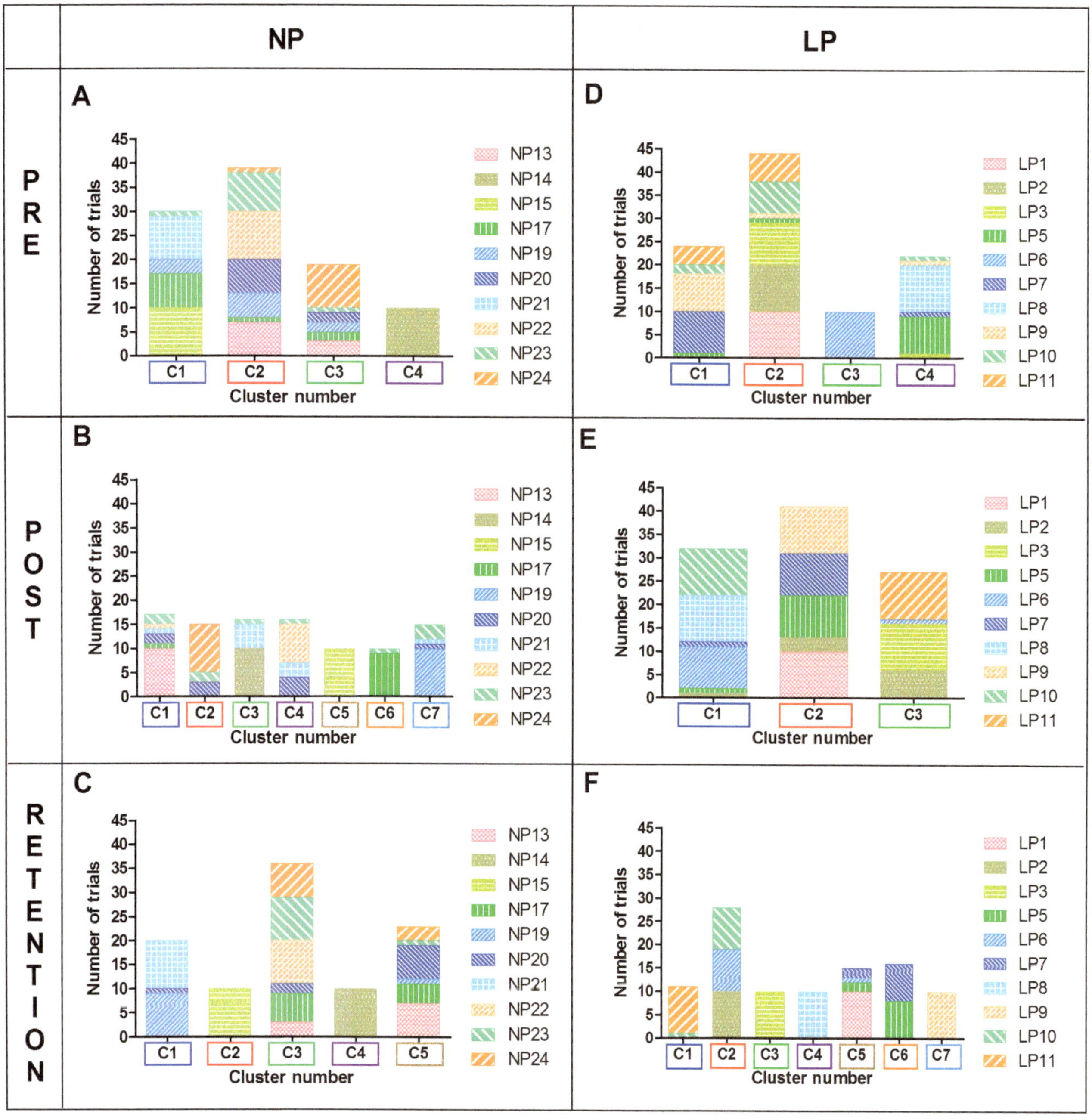

Figure 5. Number of trials and distribution of participants in each cluster. Each bar represents the number of trials and distribution of participants found in each movement cluster for specific target trials in the six data sets: NP - pre (A), post (B), retention (C); LP - pre (D), post (E), retention (F). C1, C2...C7 represent movement clusters found within each data set. Participants are labelled as LP1...LP11 (for LP group) and NP13...NP24 (for NP group).

post-test for specific target trials (Figure 5E). At the same time, the participants in the LP group who performed the worst (LP5 = 0.2 points; LP6 = 0.0 points; LP8 = 0.3 points) in terms of accuracy scores had trials that were also found predominantly in C1 and C2 (Figure 5E). This meant that even though these learners were able to perform the stroke in the "ideal" way, their performance accuracy scores showed otherwise. Furthermore, these three participants had among the highest scores for movement criterion scores (LP5 = 19; LP6 = 20; LP8 = 17) implying that their movement patterns were "almost perfect" or "perfect" in the case of LP6. LP6 was a typical example in which achieving the ideal movement technique, taught in a prescriptive and repetitive approach, resulted in a possible over conscious control of movement [15] or freezing of coordinative structures [46], leading to detrimental accuracy performance at post-test.

The NP participants on the other hand were not concerned with achieving the "right" movement pattern but displayed a greater variety of movement solutions putatively more functional for the individual learner. The highest scoring participant for performance accuracy in the specific target trials at post-test was NP17 (score = 2.0) found predominantly in C6 (Figure 5B). This participant had a movement crietrion score of 12 indicating that the movement patterns utilized were different from the "criterion model". Visual inspection of C6 in Figure 3B and 4B showed that the movemement patterns of NP17 were quite distinct from the movement patterns of the other movement clusters found within the NP group as well as compared to the LP group (Figure 3E and 4E). Another participant, NP23, who also achieved among the highest performance accuracy scores (score = 1.4) in the NP group had trials found in six of the seven movement clusters, displaying distinct movement pattern characteristics from NP17 (Figure 5B). The presence of degeneracy is evident among these two highest scoring NP participants as different methods of achieving the same task goals were used by both participants and even within participant for the case of NP23. Research from an ecological dynamics perspective on skilled performance in sport has demonstrated the relationship between performance accuracy and functional variability, highlighting that degeneracy plays a functional role in helping performers to adapt to ever-changing task demands during practice and performance [21,47,48]. Further investigation showed that two participants from the NP group with the lowest accuracy scores (NP20 = 0.4; NP21 = 0.6) had trials spread among five of the seven clusters and were in transition from the coordination to control stage of learning. Similar to previous studies, perhaps this greater variability may represent exploratory behavior as the novice learners attempted to search for stable and functional states of coordination [40].

The results in this study show that movement variability is not necessarily detrimental but rather an essential process of acquiring a new skill. It provides new empirical evidence that there are multiple ways of achieving a task goal and challenges the common misconception that learners must achieve the "ideal" movement pattern to be successful. This study also supports that degeneracy is beneficial in learning a sports skill and verifies that this exploratory process is effectively facilitated by the NP approach [49]. In essence, the NP approach was able to cater for individual learning differences such that each child did not have to conform to a pre-determined movement pattern but were provided suitable boundaries to explore and discover unique functional movement solutions. Indeed, the NP approach prepares the individual with a variety of movement solutions to cope with a dynamic sporting environment.

From a practical viewpoint, practitioners should be less concerned if learners are not performing the "correct" movement pattern but emphasize instructions that focus on ensuring representativeness, establishing information-movement couplings, movement outcomes, functional movement variability and the manipulation of constraints so that learners can explore and discover effective movement solutions. While there may be concerns in the implementation of the NP approach such as 'whether exploratory learning is time consuming', 'whether the practitioner has the right level of expertise and competency', and 'whether this approach is actually impactful' [13], this study provides empirical evidence that NP is effective and is an instructional approach worth pursuing.

Conclusions

While this study serves as a useful starting point to appreciate the potential benefits of NP at the individual level, further evidence and investigation is necessary. In particular, we signal the need for more representative learning designs such as that adopted in the present study to protect the practical significance of the research. Future studies should investigate how NP can be an optimal approach relative to training both in a game and team/class setting. What are the interactions that occur between teammates in terms of movement displacement? Will the dynamic interactions between other players and teammates escalate the 'chaos' present in a NP approach to a degree which contributes constructively to learners or is it destructive? How will NP affect motivation in a learning environment? There are potentially many logistical barriers for teachers to overcome in implementing NP amongst large groups of learners but in our opinion they are worth tackling and are not insurmountable. The road ahead may be challenging, but nevertheless this journey could help ensure individuals better prepare for a lifetime of physical activity and fulfilment from sports.

Acknowledgments

A special thanks to the chidren who participated in this study, for making this research possible.

Author Contributions

Conceived and designed the experiments: ML JC CT CB. Performed the experiments: ML JC CT. Analyzed the data: ML JC JK. Contributed reagents/materials/analysis tools: ML JC JK. Contributed to the writing of the manuscript: ML JC JK CT CB.

References

1. Barnett L, Van Beurden E, Morgan P, Brooks L, Beard J (2008) Does childhood motor skill proficiency predict adolescent fitness? Medicine and Science in Sports and Exercise 40: 2137.
2. Thelen E, Smith LB, Karmiloff-Smith A, Johnson MH (1994) A dynamic systems approach to the development of cognition and action: MIT Press.
3. Williams AM, Hodges NJ (2005) Practice, instruction and skill acquisition in soccer: Challenging tradition. Journal of Sports Sciences 23: 637–650.
4. Crossman ERFW (1959) A theory of acquisition of speed-skill. Ergonomics 1: 153–166.
5. Snoddy GS (1926) Learning and stability. Journal of Applied Psychology 10: 1–36.
6. Newell KM (1986) Constraints on the development of coordination. Motor development in children: Aspects of coordination and control: 341–360.
7. Davids K, Button C, Bennett S, editors (2008) Dynamics of skill aquisition: a constraints-led approach. 1st ed. USA: Human kinetics.
8. Ovens A, Hopper T, Butler J, editors (2013) Complexity thinkingin physical education. London, England: Routledge.
9. Kelso JAS, editor (1995) Dynamic Patterns: The self-organization of brain and behaviour: MIT Press.
10. Chow JY, Davids K, Button C, Shuttleworth R, Renshaw I, et al. (2007) The role of Nonlinear Pedagogy in Physical Education. Review of Educational Research 77: 251–278.
11. Chow JY, Davids K, Button C, Renshaw I, Shuttleworth R, et al, editors (2009) Nonlinear Pedagogy: Implications for Teaching Games for Understanding. Ottawa, Canada: Physical Health Education Association.
12. Renshaw I (2010) A constraints-led perspective to understanding skill acquisition and game play: a basis for integration of motor learning theory and physical education praxis? Physical Education and Sport Pedagogy 15: 117–137.
13. Chow JY (2013) Nonlinear Learning Underpinning Pedagogy: Evidence, Challenges, and Implications. Quest 65: 469–484.
14. Wulf G, McConnel N, Gärtner M, Schwarz A (2002) Enhancing the learning of sport skills through external-focus feedback. Journal of Motor Behavior 34: 171–182.
15. Tan CWK, Chow JY, Davids K (2012) 'How does TGfU work?': examining the relationship between learning design in TGfU and a nonlinear pedagogy. Physical education and sport pedagogy 17: 331–348.
16. Bernstein N, editor (1967) The co-ordination and regulation of movements. New York: Pergamon Press.
17. Davids K, Glazier P, Araujo D, Bartlett R (2003) Movement systems as dynamical systems: the functional role of variability and its implications for sports medicine. Sports Medicine 33: 245–260.
18. Edelman GM, Gally JA (2001) Degeneracy and complexity in biological systems. Proceedings of the National Academy of Sciences 98: 13763.
19. Chow JY, Davids K, Button C, Koh M (2008) Coordination changes in a discrete multi-articular action as a function of practice. Acta Psychologica 127: 163–176.

20. Seifert L, Wattebled L, Herault R, Poizat G, Adé D, et al. (2014) Neurobiological Degeneracy and Affordance Perception Support Functional Intra-Individual Variability of Inter-Limb Coordination during Ice Climbing. PLoS ONE 9: e89865.
21. Komar J, Chow J-Y, Chollet D, Seifert L (2013) Effect of Analogy Instructions with an Internal Focus on Learning a Complex Motor Skill. Journal of Applied Sport Psychology 26: 17–23.
22. Farrow D, Reid M (2010) The effect of equipment scaling on the skill acquisition of beginning tennis players. Journal of Sports Sciences 28: 723–732.
23. Liao C-M, Masters RSW (2001) Analogy learning: A means to implicit motor learning. Journal of Sports Sciences 19: 307–319.
24. Rab G, Petuskey K, Bagley A (2002) A method for determination of upper extremity kinematics. Gait & Posture 15: 113–119.
25. Knudson DV, Blackwell JR (2005) Variability of impact kinematics and margin for error in the tennis forehand of advanced players. Sports Engineering 8: 75–80.
26. Chow JY, Davids K, Hristovski R, Araújo D, Passos P (2011) Nonlinear pedagogy: Learning design for self-organizing neurobiological systems. New Ideas in Psychology 29: 189–200.
27. Newell K, editor (1985) Coordination, control and skill. Amsterdam: Elsevier Science. 295–317 p.
28. Hopper T (1998) Teaching Games Centred Games Using Progressive Principles Of Play. CAHPERD 64: 4–7.
29. ASEP editor (2008) Coaching youth tennis. 4th ed. Champaign, IL: Human Kinetics.
30. Rein R, Davids K, Button C (2010) Adaptive and phase transition behavior in performance of discrete multi-articular actions by degenerate neurobiological systems. Experimental Brain Research 201: 307–322.
31. Fleisig G, Nicholls R, Elliott B, Escamilla R (2003) Kinematics used by world class tennis players to produce high-velocity serves. Sports Biomechanics 2: 51–64.
32. Elliott B (2006) Biomechanics and tennis. British Journal of Sports Medicine 40: 392–396.
33. Landlinger J, Lindinger S, Stoggl T, Wagner H, Muller E (2010) Kinematic differences of elite and high-performance tennis players in the cross court and down the line forehand. Sports Biomechanics 9: 280–295.
34. Takahashi K, Elliot B, Noffal G (1996) The role of upper limb segment rotations in the development of spin in the tennis forehand. Australian journal of Science and Medicine in Sport 28: 106–113.
35. Button C, MacLeod M, Sanders R, Coleman S (2003) Examining movement variability in the basketball free-throw action at different skill levels. Research Quarterly for Exercise and Sport 74: 257–269.
36. Webb LM (1993) Statistical pattern recognition. Chichester, England: Wiley.
37. Rein R, Button C, Davids K, Summers J (2010) Cluster analysis of movement patterns in multiarticular actions: A tutorial. Motor Control 14: 211–239.
38. Komar J, Herault R, Seifert L (2014) Key point selection and clustering of swimmer coordination through Sparse Fisher-EM. arXiv preprint arXiv: 14011489.
39. Toro B, Nester CJ, Farren PC (2007) Cluster analysis for the extraction of sagittal gait patterns in children with cerebral palsy. Gait & Posture 25: 157–165.
40. Chow JY, Davids K, Button C, Rein R (2008) Dynamics of movement patterning in learning a discrete multiarticular action. Motor Control 12: 219–240.
41. Schorer J, Baker J, Fath F, Jaitner T (2007) Identification of interindividual and intraindividual movement patterns in handball players of varying expertise levels. Journal of Motor Behavior 39: 409–421.
42. Bouveyron C, Brunet-Saumard C (2013) Discriminative variable selection for clustering with the sparse Fisher-EM algorithm. Computational Statistics: 1–25.
43. Ludden TM, Beal SL, Sheiner LB (1994) Comparison of the Akaike Information Criterion, the Schwarz criterion and the F test as guides to model selection. Journal of pharmacokinetics and biopharmaceutics 22: 431–445.
44. Barris S, Farrow D, Davids K (2014) Increasing Functional Variability in the Preparatory Phase of the Takeoff Improves Elite Springboard Diving Performance. Research Quarterly for Exercise and Sport 85: 97–106.
45. Wulf G, McNevin N, Shea CH (2001) The automaticity of complex motor skill learning as a function of attentional focus. The Quarterly Journal of Experimental Psychology: Section A 54: 1143–1154.
46. Hodges NJ, Hayes S, Horn R, Williams AM (2005) Changes in coordination, control and outcome as a result of extended practice on a novel motor skill. Ergonomics 48: 1672–1685.
47. Phillips E, Portus M, Davids K, Renshaw I (2012) Performance accuracy and functional variability in elite and developing fast bowlers. Journal of Science and Medicine in Sport 15: 182–188.
48. Davids K, Button C, Araújo D, Renshaw I, Hristovski R (2006) Movement models from sports provide representative task constraints for studying adaptive behavior in human movement systems. Adaptive Behavior 14: 73–95.
49. Renshaw I, Davids K, Shuttleworth R, Chow JY (2009) Insights from ecological psychology and dynamical systems theory can underpin a philosophy of coaching. International Journal of Sport Psychology 40: 540–602.

20

Effectiveness of a Video-Feedback and Questioning Programme to Develop Cognitive Expertise in Sport

Luis García-González[1]*, M. Perla Moreno[2], Alberto Moreno[2], Alexander Gil[2], Fernando del Villar[2]

1 Faculty of Health and Sport Sciences, University of Zaragoza, Huesca, Spain, **2** Faculty of Sport Sciences, University of Extremadura, Cáceres, Spain

Abstract

The importance within sport expertise of cognitive factors has been emphasised in many research studies. Adaptations that take place in athletes' long-term memories are going to condition their decision-making and performance, and training programmes must be developed that improve these adaptations. In our study, we provide a tactical-cognitive training programme based on video-feedback and questioning in order to improve tactical knowledge in tennis players and verify its effect when transferred to athletes' decision-making. 11 intermediate tennis players participated in this study (12.9 ± 0.7 years old), distributed into two groups (experimental, $n = 5$; control, $n = 6$). Tactical knowledge was measured by problem representation and strategy planning with a verbal protocol. Decision-making was measured by a systematic observation instrument. Results confirm the effectiveness of a combination of video-feedback and questioning on cognitive expertise, developing adaptations in long-term memory that produce an improvement in the quality of tactical knowledge (content, sophistication and structure). This, in turn, is transferred to the athletes' decision-making capacity, leading to a higher percentage of successful decisions made during game play. Finally, we emphasise the need to develop effective programmes to develop cognitive expertise and improve athletes' performance, and include it in athletes' formative stages.

Editor: José César Perales, Universidad de Granada, Spain

Funding: Funded by Ministry of Science and Innovation (Spain) with the research project DEP2011-29527 "Thinking and action. Development of a knowledge-stimulation programme during competition, to improve individual tactical performance of athletes" (http://www.idi.mineco.gob.es/portal/site/MICINN/). The funders had no role in study design, data collection and analysis, decision to publish, or preparation of the manuscript.

Competing Interests: The authors have declared that no competing interests exist.

* E-mail: lgarciag@unizar.es

Introduction

We can find many research studies within the field of expert performance that emphasise the influence of cognitive elements on sport expertise (see [1–3] for a review). From the cognitive psychology approach, expertise level in a certain sport depends on inner mental representations and on the cognitive processes that lie between stimulus interpretation and action selection [4]. The athlete's limited knowledge will determine cognitive processes such as decision-making in sport [5].

There is a strong interrelationship between the different elements that comprise cognitive expertise. Knowledge structures stored in our memory are a constraint to decision-making [6]. The greater and more varied this knowledge is, the better the anticipation and decision-making will be in athletes [7–8]. Knowledge has an influence on other cognitive processes, such as directing attention, visual behaviour, anticipation as well as response selection, decision-making and execution or performance. Likewise, the knowledge accessed and the use of strategies and tactics will depend on the context determined by the environment, the athlete and the task [9]. Furthermore, the development of procedural knowledge will permit the development of processes that determine when intuitive decisions are necessary and when deliberate decisions are more adequate [10], as both deliberate decisions and intuitive decisions exist within a continuum of consciousness [11].

Related to deliberate decision-making and with reference to knowledge and internal processes, as the sport expertise level increases, we can find greater development of specific adaptations and structures, stored in the long-term memory (LTM). Thus, when a decision has to be made during a real match situation, an expert tennis player will make a better decision, because of two specialised adaptations of LTM: i) action plan profiles, which are rules stored in the LTM, and are used to make the current environmental conditions coincide with the motor actions, including cognitive skills, to supervise current conditions; ii) and current event profiles, which are tactical scripts that guide the construction and constant change of important concepts, which are going to be taken into account in subsequent actions (e.g. updating information about the opponent's strong points during a game). Current event profiles are constructed on the basis of previous competitions, previous experiences, or with cognitive skills to collect data as the competition advances (for further review of this model, [6,9,12–13]). Both profiles are predicted to allow players easy access to and retrieval of important information to make decisions during competition and to compensate or make adjustments during time-constrained moments [6].

The schemes related to decision-making (e.g., action plan profiles) will allow players to quickly and efficiently plan and programme responses [14]. The use of the Long-Term Working Memory [15] can also be important because it is an additional mechanism to access relevant tactical information by means of adaptations in the LTM. These adaptations enable information to be coded and recovered [9]. Specialised profiles in the LTM (e.g., action plan profiles and current event profiles) will make access to relevant tactical information easier. This will also help athletes take better and more successful decisions in real game play situations [6,12–13].

These recovery structures will enable the information to be classified and stored, in order to carry out a superior representation about game scenarios, facilitating recognition and anticipation vis-à-vis game events [16]. A dynamic coding of the environment will integrate recovery structures in "real time" where experts can anticipate future events, predict results and develop proactive and reactive behaviours by developing action plans [17].

Research within the expert-novice approach may help understand and comprehend sport expertise and expert performance [18]. Research carried out in tennis, within the expert-novice paradigm, presents remarkable differences in content, sophistication and conceptual structure of the expert players' knowledge. Knowledge is greater, more varied and sophisticated. Furthermore, these developed concepts are related to each other and favour greater knowledge structuring [6,13,19–22]. In addition, better tennis playing is caused by better temporal processing [23]. Consequently, it is possible to find a considerable relationship between expertise level, knowledge, tactical decision-making skills and performance in sport [24–25]. All these cognitive characteristics enable expert tennis players to make more suitable decisions based on superior mental representations [6], it being necessary to develop the different cognitive processes related to performance. The superior expertise level of expert athletes is made evident through their mental representations and their cognitive processes (e.g. decision-making). These elements indicate performance in sport [4].

In open sports, the knowledge basis changes when the expertise level increases, developing different modifications in content, sophistication and knowledge structure: a) action plans without a hierarchically defined structure are replaced by conditions and actions that act as decision rules; b) weak or unsuitable conditions and actions become tactical and associated conditions and actions; c) approaches to global sport situations, with minimum processing of relevant task elements, are replaced by more tactical approaches, with relevant information (including past events and current facts); d) processing environmental events or superficial characteristics is replaced by the in-depth processing of information [13,22,26].

One of the difficulties found here is the lack of research about how to produce these adaptations, apart from those developed through hours of practice. The last step in the expert performance approach establishes the need to examine the acquisition of identified expertise characteristics using training interventions [27]. That is why we wonder: Which activities may favour the development of LTM adaptations to improve cognitive skills (e.g., tactical knowledge and decision-making)?

There are some activities directly related to performance improvement, such as video training or individual instructions [28,29]. Specific research on the development of cognitive factors is much more limited, although we find some approaches to develop factors related to cognitive expertise (see [30] for a review).

To develop tactical-decisional skills and cognitive skills in sport, the main goals are to promote and construct tactical experiences. Vickers [31] develops a Decisional Training Model (DTM), and points to the use of tools such as video-feedback and questioning [30–32]. The use of video-feedback is also recommended to analyse tactical behaviour (own and opponent's) during competition, to develop situation profiles, to develop tactical knowledge in athletes, or to improve the recognition of contextual factors [10,33]. Consequently, video-feedback seems to be a useful tool to develop cognitive expertise, although the help of an expert in its use and interpretation is recommended to find benefits. Showing videos to athletes about themselves has limited results, because recorded events happen too fast and there is a lot of available information [31]. On the other hand, when the athlete's attention is directed by a supervisor towards specific signs through questioning, results are significantly positive [31,34]. However, there is a little research in the combined use of both decisional tools (i.e., video-feedback and questioning). This combination of tools for training could be defined as an explicit learning strategy. This explicit learning, defined as an intentional acquisition which produces verbalisable knowledge, may be focused on which signals could be used and how to use them to get results or to make decisions in sport [35–36]. Furthermore, decisional learning, which begins through deliberate, intentional and explicit procedures, may become automated and intuitive with time [37].

The use of video-feedback and questioning programmes is recommended for the cognitive development of athletes, especially at lower performance levels, where this could be more effective [38–39]. That is why our interest lies in examining and confirming the effect of a combined video-feedback and questioning programme on the cognitive expertise and decision-making of tennis players. The basic hypothesis suggests that the application of a tactical-cognitive training programme based on video-feedback and questioning will have a significant positive effect on the tactical knowledge of tennis players, on its content, sophistication and conceptual structure. In addition, an improvement of athletes' cognitive expertise will produce an increase in decision-making skills with a higher percentage of successful decisions made during real game play.

Methods

Participants

11 male players took part in this research, and they were divided into two groups: control ($n=6$) and experimental ($n=5$). One player, who was initially included in the experimental group, comprised of six players, was removed because of an injury produced during this study. All athletes belonged to the Under-14 category. To ensure that all players would be exposed to the same formative process, all players belonged to the same club, to the same training group, they had the same trainer and all of them trained 4 hours per week. All of them had the same classification according to the ITF (International Tennis Federation), by means of the International Tennis Number (ITN). They were also included in level 5-Intermediate.

The subdivision into two groups (experimental and control) was done according to the evaluation of the decision-making level, by means of the observation protocol of Nielsen & McPherson [24]. This evaluation was done in 4 complete matches, as a pre-test, and before the start of the intervention (see Figure S1). Another criterion to form the groups was tactical knowledge obtained in the pre-test. Tests for variance homogeneity were performed on all the aforementioned variables by means of the Levene test. Levene's statistic was not significant in problem representation variables ($p > .05$ in all variables), planning strategies variables ($p > .05$ in all variables) or decision-making ($p > .05$). This showed the equivalence of groups before starting the intervention.

Characteristics such as age, years of practice and years of competition in tennis of each group are included in Table 1.

The research has been developed under the recommendations of the Helsinki Declaration. Before starting the research, participants and their parents were informed about this study. Participants and their parents signed an informed consent as

Table 1. Characteristics of participants in every group.

Variables	Control Group (n = 6)		Experimental Group (n = 5)	
	M	SD	M	SD
Age	12.83	0.75	13.00	0.71
Years of practice in tennis	6.50	1.05	6.80	0.83
Years of competition in tennis	3.67	0.52	3.60	0.54

required by the Helsinki Declaration (2008) and the local ethics committee. The University of Extremadura Ethics Committee has also approved this research project.

Intervention Programme

The independent variable was the tactical-cognitive training programme using video-feedback and questioning. The basis of this programme was the analysis by the players of their own decisions, by means of video-feedback and helped by the trainer with questioning. They had to visualise successful and unsuccessful decisions taken about their own actions. By viewing their actions, athletes should identify the main reasons why they took those decisions at the time. The aim of the supervisor taking part in video feedback and questioning sessions was to guide the analysis of the game situation through open questioning, but not intervening directly or giving answers to the proposed questions.

The specific characteristics of the programme were: i) supervision of 6 actions (3 successful decisions and 3 unsuccessful decisions). The order of these actions was random in every session, to prevent players from knowing if the action to be supervised was right or wrong; ii) individual analysis for every selected decision, by means of videos, showing the development of the whole point. The supervisor pointed out which action was being analysed within the whole point.

The entire set of 6 actions to be analysed comprised one complete video-feedback session. The intervention structure was similar to other intervention studies carried out on team sports [40–41]. Every action was supervised by means of the following structure:

Step 1. The images were viewed two consecutive times. The expert completed information with some contextual details: moment of the point in the game (e.g., fifth game of the match), scoreboard before the point (e.g., winning 3–2, score 15–40).

Step 2. Self-analysis and initial reflection of the player, where the athlete explained and initially assessed what had happened.

Step 3. Player and expert analyse together. They make a sequential analysis of the causes and reasons for the decision taken. A detailed analysis was conducted of the game context, possible solutions, decision taken, consequences and possible alternatives. All these aspects were analysed according to the tactical elements that characterise tennis shots such as: type of shot (forehand, backhand), effect (flat, topspin, backspin or slice), direction (down the line, cross-court, to the centre), depth (short, medium, long), height (high, medium or low trajectory) and hitting power. For a better understanding of the process, Table 2 shows every phase in detail, with its main aspects.

Variables

The dependent variables of this study were tactical knowledge and decision-making of tennis players. By means of tactical knowledge, we purported to assess the level of cognitive expertise of these players. The analysis of tactical knowledge was conducted by means of problem representation and strategy planning [19–21] during a real game situation. By means of decision-making skills we want to reflect the cognitive expertise and tactical skills of athletes in real game play. Decision-making skills in tennis are defined as the adaptation of the selected shot to the specific conditions of the game situation, based on an observation instrument [24] and they are measured by the percentage of successful decision-making over the total of decisions made. This percentage was calculated for each complete match played for the pre-test (4 matches) and the post-test (4 matches) (see Figure S1).

Instruments

Tactical knowledge. The verbal protocol validated for tennis in previous studies [6,13,19–21,42] was used to evaluate tactical knowledge as a reflection of cognitive expertise.

This instrument, which measures tactical knowledge, consists of carrying out interviews during the action, and then coding this interview by means of a system of categories structured into 3 levels (conceptual content, conceptual sophistication and conceptual structure), both in problem representation and in strategy planning.

Interview procedures: the interview comprises two questions developed to access the problem representation and the strategy planning of tennis players, following the very same procedure as in other similar studies [6,21,42]. Interviews were collected during a real game situation and they were carried out on the actual court where players were competing, during a full set. Prior studies indicated that the athletes' performance was not affected by the application of interviews [24]. Before beginning this process, participants were familiarised with the data collection situation. The researcher explained to players that they did not have any time limitation to answer and they had to answer the questions asked as accurately as they could, reporting the information about previous and current thoughts. Two previous interviews were carried out following the explanation and before the start of the measurement in order to verify that the athletes responded accurately and with no time constraint. After that, they carried out a 10-minute warm-up before starting the game, as established by the Spanish Tennis Federation rules. During the pauses between two points, players answered two questions. The first question of the verbal protocol was asked immediately after ending every point: *'What were you thinking about while playing this point?'* (Recall Interview-RI [6,42]). This question requires players to remember their thoughts about the previous point. Verbalisations made with this question will assess problem representation. The second question is: *'What are you thinking about now?'* (Planning Interview-PI [6,21]). This was asked immediately after the RI and immediately before playing the following point. By means of this question, players inform about their current thoughts, possibilities about subsequent points, and also assess their planning. Answers

Table 2. Sequence for the analysis of every game action.

STEP 1 - WATCHING selected images :	
1.1.- Watching the full point and the selected action to be analysed.	
1.2.-Waiting moment to favour stimulated remembering.	
1.3.- New watching of the same action and contextualization of that point (scoreboard).	
Observations: The expert completes information with data such as game order in which the point is framed (e.g., fifth game of the match) and scoreboard before the beginning of the point (e.g., winning 2-1, 40-30).	
STEP 2 - SELF-ANALYSIS and player's reflection:	
2.1.- Explanation and valuation of the analysed point. Global analysis of his action and initial analysis of the decision made	
STEP 3 - COMBINED ANALYSIS player-expert:	
Sequential analysis of the causes and reasons of the decision through questioning	
3.1.- Analysis of the decision context	Scoreboard, opponent's placement, player's placement, ball placement and direction, shot executed by the rival, etc. These context conditions were analysed as constraints to decision-making.
3.2.- Valuation of possible solutions	Type of shot (forehand, backhand), effect shot (flat, topspin, backspin or slice), direction (down the line, cross-court, to the centre), depth (short, medium, long), height (high, medium or low trajectory) and shot power that might be done. Valuation of the best resources of every shot characteristic taking into account the decision context.
3.3.- Analysis of the selected response	Type of shot (forehand, backhand), effect shot (flat, topspin, backspin or slice), direction (down the line, cross-court, to the centre), depth (short, medium, long), height (high, medium or low trajectory) and shot power selected Analysis of the characteristics of the shot selected respect to the decision context.
3.4.- Analysis of the execution of the decision	Analysis of the result of the selected action. Differentiation between decision and execution. The player must differentiate between tactical intention and execution outcome.
3.5.- Analysis of the result of the decision	Main consequences on the opponent and on the player. In a successful decision, players have to identify some good consequences (e.g., displacement of the opponent, entire space to send the next shot, etc.). In an unsuccessful decision, players have to identify some bad consequences (e.g., their displacement, loss of initiative, etc.).
3.6.- Global analysis of the action. Proposal of alternatives (if needed)	Comparison with the analysis done in step 2. Reinforcement of decision-making or proposal of alternatives (only when analysing an error). If the decision-making analysed was successful, the player has to reinforce why the decision made was successful. If the decision-making analysed was unsuccessful, the player has to search for the best alternative after analysing context and possible solutions, and justify why this is the best.

obtained in this case assess the strategy planning. Likewise, this procedural knowledge assessment method is developed in performance environments where athletes have to respond to real competition situations, which permits enhancing the validity of the data [43].

Coding system: 16 interviews were selected at random for every individual from the total number of interviews carried out in a real game situation, following the same criteria as in previous research studies [6]. After transcribing the interviews, these two questions were separated. Within the coding process, they were firstly divided into concepts or information units, and later they were coded by means of a system of categories into three levels of analysis. The first level of analysis is *Conceptual Content* (comprised of *Main concept categories* and *Subconceptual categories*). The second level of analysis is *Conceptual Sophistication*, and the third level of analysis is *Conceptual Structure* (see [6] for a review).

Within the quantitative analysis of verbal reports, in order to analyse the first level (conceptual content: total and variety of concepts), the total value as well as of a variety of each one of the main conceptual categories (goal, condition, action, and regulatory concepts) was obtained. For conceptual sophistication (level 2) all the verbalised concepts were analysed at all the levels of goals, conditions and actions concepts. The conceptual structure (level 3) was assessed by means of the total number of linkages and the total number of structures found (double and triple).

Reliability of the coding system: in order to code interviews, only one coder was used, who underwent coding training taught by one of the researchers. Coder had a Sport Sciences Degree, specific training as a tennis coach (Level 2 in the Spanish Tennis Federation), and also specific training in coding. Reliability was calculated for all three levels of analysis in every question (RI and PI). To obtain the required coding reliability, 10 training sessions were held sequentially with the coder and at different moments in time. Reliability between coders (researcher-coder) was calculated using Cohen's Kappa index, obtaining values of up to.75 [44] to ensure reliability. Temporal reliability was also ensured, coding the same interviews 10 days later with a test-retest reliability of up to.80.

Decision-making. To assess decision-making in tennis players, an observation instrument was used to test tactical skills in real game play [24]. This has already been used for other studies, applied to tennis players with different expertise [24,42,45]. The decision-making section on "game play" taken from this instrument, which assesses all shots made after serve, was used. This is a useful instrument to assess expertise and performance differences, complying with the recommendation of Travassos et al. [43] about the need to perform sporting actions under *in situ* conditions to assess expertise effect.

The instrument evaluates decision-making skills in every action as 'successful decisions' (value 1) and 'unsuccessful decisions' (value 0), by means of criteria that assess the player's intention (offensive or defensive) according to: opponent's position, player's position, ball trajectory, and the intention of putting pressure on the opponent (trying to displace the opponent, keeping him/her on the baseline, playing to his/her weak side, etc.) or defending (recovering position after a forceful shot by the opponent) [24].

Decision-making skills were assessed by means of the percentage of successful decisions (value 1) made during the match. Filming and observation conditions proposed by Nielsen and McPherson [24] were taken into account in order to apply the observation instrument.

Inter- and intra- observer's reliability: To correctly observe all the matches of every player, 2 experienced observers were selected. Observers were external to the study, they had a Sport Sciences Degree, with specific training as tennis coaches (Level 2 in the Spanish Tennis Federation) with at least five years' experience as coaches at this level, and also specific training in systematic observation processes through a Master Course. Cohen's Kappa statistic was calculated for inter- and intra-observers reliability. Values achieved were higher than.81 in inter-observers' reliability, and higher than.84 for intra-observers' reliability in all observers. Values over.75 establish very good/ almost complete concordance [44].

Procedures

In order to carry out this study, a quasi-experimental design was developed with two groups: control and experimental. A total of 18 matches were carried out for each tennis player. Tactical knowledge was measured before and after applying the intervention programme (pre-test and post-test), selecting 16 random interviews out of all the interviews held for every individual participating in this study. Decision-making measures were assessed during 4 matches before (pre-test) and 4 matches after (post-test) applying the intervention programme (see Figure S1).

As shown in Figure S1, the 18 matches played by all the players were distributed in three phases. The first 4 matches were used as a pre-test of the decision-making variable. After these 4 matches, the pre-test of the tactical knowledge was carried out (problem representation and strategy planning) in a real game situation, as explained above. After performing the pre-test of all the variables, the players were divided into two groups (experimental and control). The following 10 matches (from match 5 to match 14) the intervention was carried out with the experimental group, developing the intervention programme based on video-feedback and questioning for 10 sessions after each one of the matches. All the players developed the same number of matches and training sessions. Finally, the final 4 matches (from match 15 to match 18) were used to make the post-test measurement of the decision-making variable. The post-test of tactical knowledge (problem representation and strategy planning) was carried out after the 18 matches.

Furthermore, during the entire time the research lasted, the athletes did their on-court training as usual, regardless of the group they belonged to. This training lasted for 4 hours a week spread out over 3 days. The athletes from the control group and from the experimental group accumulated a total of 72 hours' training throughout the entire research. All players trained at the same time and with the same coach. The eleven players competed in 18 matches (1 match per week) during the research. Only the players from the experimental group received the intervention programme explained above, which lasted for a maximum of 40 minutes per session and per player. Thus, the tennis players in the control group accumulated 72 hours' training and 18 competition matches, and the tennis players from the experimental group accumulated 72 hours' training, 18 competition matches and a maximum of 7 hours' intervention programme.

To obtain a competition structure that would guarantee a continuous weekly intervention by means of video-feedback and questioning, and on a real game situation, we developed a round-robin structure, in which each player meets all other players in turn. They had to play one match every week. By means of this system, it was possible to play 18 matches on a continuous basis. Thus, the experimental group could carry out 10 video-feedback sessions, one after every match played.

Matches were played on Sundays. The video-feedback programme was applied the following day, within 24 hours after competition and before the first training session of the week.

The on-court trainer was not informed about the specific objectives of the programme in order not to influence this process.

Data analysis

Results were obtained by parametric and non-parametric statistics because the values were achieved by means of the Shapiro-Wilks test (for samples with less than 30 individuals) indicating data normality in decision-making and non-normality in tactical knowledge variables.

Mean and standard deviation was used to describe variables, and also mean ranks were reported to tactical knowledge variables. To analyse the effect of the intervention programme four 2×2 Mixed MANOVAs (Test-time x Group) were used for tactical knowledge variables, following the procedures established by Thomas, Nelson & Thomas [46] and Thomas & Thomas [47] to use multivariate analyses with non-parametric variables. These variables were grouped to perform MANOVAs into: i) Concept content-total; ii) Concept content-variety; iii) Concept Sophistication; and iv) Concept Structure. In 2×2 Mixed MANOVAs, a repeated measure factor (pre-test and post-test) and a Group factor (Experimental and Control group) were used. Later, univariate ANOVAs were reported to test differences in every tactical knowledge variable. These analyses follow the method of Puri & Sen [48] Rank-Order General Linear Method. This method maintains good power and protects against type I errors, having to develop three steps: a) change data to ranks (mean ranks reported in descriptive statistics); b) use standard parametric procedures with ranked scores; c) calculate the L-statistic instead of F [46-47,49].

The L-statistic for all MANOVAs = $[(N-1)\ r^2]$, where r^2 = Pillai's trace. Univariate analyses of variances (ANOVAs) were conducted to individually test differences in variables. The L-statistic for all *post-hoc* ANOVAs = $[(N-1)\ r^2]$, where $r^2 = SS_{Between}/SS_{Total}$. All the MANOVAs performed meet the requirements and assumptions of MANOVA designs about normality (in ranked data) and multicollinearity. For repeated measures, the sphericity assumption was met in all variables, with a value of 1.0 in the Huynh-Feldt epsilon [46]. These non-parametric procedures have been used in other studies to test differences in tactical knowledge in tennis (e.g., [6]).

In addition, a 2×2 Mixed ANOVA (Test-time x Group) was conducted to assess the effect of the intervention programme on the decision-making variable, using a repeated measures factor (Test-time: pre-test and post-test) and a Group factor (Experimental and Control). The estimation of the Effect Size was included in Mixed ANOVA for decision-making, by means of partial squared Eta (η_p^2) to improve the assessment of the differences found, because it eliminates the influence of the sample size.

Alpha was set at 0.05, and 95% Confidence Interval for differences (Diff. 95% CI) was reported. The IBM SPSS Statistics v.19.0 statistical program was used for data analysis.

Results

Problem representation

To test the effect of the intervention programme on problem representation, a 2×2 Mixed MANOVA was performed on Concept Content-total, Concept Content-variety, Concept Sophistication and Concept Structure. In each Mixed MANOVA, multivariate contrasts were reported and univariate contrasts were included in Tables 3 and 4 to show variables differences (see also Appendix S1).

There was no significant main effect for Group in Concept Content-total variables interaction in pre-test ($L(3) = 2.15$; $p > .05$; see Table 3). In contrast, in post-test, there was a significant main effect for Group in Concept Content-total variables interaction ($L(3) = 8.74$; $p < .05$). Univariate follow-up analyses of Concept Content-total variables in post-test (Table 4) show significant differences between experimental and control group in Total of concepts ($p < .01$) and Total regulatory concepts ($p < .05$) with higher values in the experimental group.

No significant main effect was found for Group in Concept Content-variety variables interaction in pre-test ($L(3) = 2.47$; $p > .05$; see Table 3). In post-test, there was no significant main effect, either, of Concept Content-variety variables ($L(3) = 6.36$; $p > .05$; see Table 4).

No significant main effect was found for Group in Concept Sophistication variables interaction in pre-test ($L(3) = 6.20$; $p > .05$; see Table 3). In contrast, in post-test, there was a significant main effect for Group in Concept Sophistication variables interaction ($L(3) = 9.35$; $p < .05$). Follow-up univariate analysis of Concept Sophistication variables in post-test (Table 4) show significant differences between experimental and control group in Goal Concepts Level 2 ($p < .05$), Condition Concepts Level 3 ($p < .01$) and Action Concepts Level 3 ($p < .01$) with higher values in the experimental group.

The MANOVA for Concept Structure showed no significant main effect for Group in Concept Structure variables interaction in pre-test ($L(2) = 0.75$; $p > .05$; see Table 3). In contrast, in post-test, there was a significant main effect for Group in Concept Structure variables interaction ($L(2) = 7.79$; $p < .05$). Follow-up univariate analysis of Concept Structure variables in post-test (Table 4) showed significant differences between experimental and control group in number of linkages ($p < .01$) and triple concepts ($p < .01$) with higher values in the experimental group.

Planning strategy

The same analyses were performed in planning strategy. Multivariate contrasts for each Mixed MANOVA were reported,

Table 3. Mean, standard deviation, mean rank and univariate contrast in problem representation variables for pre-test.

Variables	Control group ($n=6$)			Experimental group ($n=5$)			$L_{(1)}$	p	Diff. 95% CI [LO,HI]
	M	SD	MR	M	SD	MR			
Concept Content (total)									
Total concepts	43.33	11.74	5.50	45.60	6.23	6.60	0.30	>.05	[-5.8,3.6]
Total goals	18.33	8.26	5.83	17.60	7.92	6.20	0.03	>.05	[-5.1,4.4]
Total conditions	10.50	8.07	5.17	12.80	6.91	7.00	0.84	>.05	[-6.4,2.7]
Total actions	11.67	5.46	6.58	9.20	4.21	5.30	0.41	>.05	[-3.4,5.9]
Total regulatory	2.67	2.07	5.00	4.80	3.11	7.20	1.23	>.05	[-6.6,2.2]
Concept Content (variety)									
Variety goals	6.17	1.33	6.83	5.20	1.64	5.00	0.93	>.05	[-2.5,6.2]
Variety conditions	4.83	2.86	5.33	5.80	1.48	6.80	0.54	>.05	[-6.1,3.2]
Variety actions	4.50	1.64	6.50	4.20	1.09	5.40	0.33	>.05	[-3.4,5.6]
Variety regulatory	1.67	1.03	4.83	2.60	0.89	7.40	1.95	>.05	[-6.5,1.4]
Concept sophistication									
Goal hierarchies									
1-Selves & opponent	5.50	4.76	4.83	9.80	6.14	7.40	1.64	>.05	[-6.9,1.8]
2-Win attributes	3.17	1.72	6.58	2.60	1.34	5.30	0.44	>.05	[-3.2,5.8]
Condition qualities									
2-Appropriate-one feature	6.33	4.41	6.25	5.80	3.27	5.70	0.08	>.05	[-4.2,5.3]
3-Appropriate-two features	1.67	1.51	6.00	1.60	1.52	6.00	0.00	>.05	[-4.7,4.7]
Action qualities									
2-Appropriate-one feature	6.50	2.88	6.33	5.00	2.91	5.60	0.14	>.05	[-4.0,5.5]
3-Appropriate-two features	2.33	2.25	6.00	2.00	1.58	5.90	0.01	>.05	[-4.5,4.9]
Concept structure									
N° linkages	22.50	8.45	5.25	25.20	6.91	6.90	0.68	>.05	[-6.2,2.9]
Double-concept linkages	7.67	1.97	6.25	1.64	13.5	5.70	0.08	>.05	[-4.1,5.2]
Triple-concept linkages	5.00	2.28	5.25	1.82	10.5	6.90	0.70	>.05	[-6.2,2.9]

MR = Mean Rank.

Table 4. Mean, standard deviation, mean rank and univariate contrasts in problem representation variables for post-test.

Variables	Control group ($n=6$)			Experimental group ($n=5$)			$L_{(1)}$	*p*	Diff. 95% CI [LO,HI]
	M	SD	MR	M	SD	MR			
Concept Content (total)									
Total concepts	38.83	8.97	3.50	75.80	25.81	9.00	7.53	**<.01**	[-7.9, -3.1]
Total goals	15.83	7.00	4.50	25.80	10.23	7.80	2.71	>.05	[-7.4,0.8]
Total conditions	9.00	7.72	4.42	24.00	16.98	7.90	3.04	>.05	[-7.5,0.5]
Total actions	10.17	3.71	4.50	16.60	6.69	7.80	2.76	>.05	[-7.3,0.7]
Total regulatory	2.50	2.81	4.17	8.20	5.54	8.20	4.11	**<.05**	[-7.7, -0.4]
Concept Content (variety)									
Variety goals	5.50	1.38	4.75	7.20	1.79	7.50	1.98	>.05	[-6.9,1.4]
Variety conditions	4.67	3.72	4.75	7.80	2.28	7.50	1.90	>.05	[-7.0,1.5]
Variety actions	4.50	2.07	5.25	5.60	1.14	6.90	0.71	>.05	[-6.1,2.8]
Variety regulatory	1.67	1.51	4.17	3.80	1.30	8.20	4.17	**<.05**	[-7.6, -0.4]
Concept sophistication									
Goal hierarchies									
1-Selves & opponent	6.00	4.00	3.92	13.40	3.85	8.50	5.28	**<.05**	[-7.8, -1.3]
2-Win attributes	3.00	2.37	5.67	3.20	1.64	6.40	0.14	>.05	[-5.4,3.9]
Condition qualities									
2-Appropriate-one feature	5.83	5.11	4.92	10.20	7.22	7.30	1.45	>.05	[-6.7,1.9]
3-Appropriate-two features	1.50	1.97	3.67	9.20	6.42	8.80	6.81	**<.01**	[-7.8, -2.5]
Action qualities									
2-Appropriate-one feature	6.67	2.34	6.17	7.20	4.76	5.80	0.03	>.05	[-4.3,5.0]
3-Appropriate-two features	1.50	1.05	3.58	7.40	3.21	8.90	7.11	**<.01**	[-7.9,2.8]
Concept structure									
N° linkages	20.50	4.09	3.50	47.80	17.30	9.00	7.57	**<.01**	[-7.8,,3.1]
Double-concept linkages	8.50	2.07	7.58	5.80	2.39	4.10	3.04	>.05	[-0.5,7.5]
Triple-concept linkages	4.67	2.25	3.50	12.60	2.88	9.00	7.64	**<.01**	[-7.8, -3.2]

MR = Mean Rank.

and univariate contrasts were included in Tables 5 and 6 to show variables differences (see also Appendix S1).

There was no significant main effect for Group in Concept Content-total variables interaction in pre-test (L(3) = 5.25; p >.05; see Table 5). In post-test, there was no significant main effect for Group, either, of Concept Content-total variables interaction (L(3) = 5.75; p >.05; see Table 6).

No significant main effect was found for Group in Concept Content-variety variables interaction in pre-test (L(3) = 3.38; p >.05; see Table 5). In post-test, there was no significant main effect for Group, either, of Concept Content-variety variables interaction (L(3) = 3.49; p >.05; see Table 6).

The MANOVA showed no significant main effect for Group in Concept Sophistication variables interaction in pre-test (L(3) = 6.78; p >.05, see Table 5). In contrast, in post-test, there was a significant main effect for Group in Concept Sophistication variables interaction (L(3) = 9.25; p <.05). Follow-up univariate analysis of Concept Sophistication variables in post-test (Table 6) showed significant differences between experimental and control groups in Goal Concepts Level 2 (p <.05) and Action Concepts Level 3 (p <.01) with higher values in the experimental group.

No significant main effect was found for Group in Concept Structure variables interaction in pre-test (L(2) = 1.27; p >.05; see Table 5). In contrast, in post-test, there was a significant main effect for Group in Concept Structure variables interaction (L(2) = 7.23; p <.05). Follow-up univariate analysis of Concept Structure variables in post-test (Table 6) showed significant differences between experimental and control groups in number of linkages (p <.05) and triple concepts (p <.01) with higher values in the experimental group.

Decision-making

For decision making, a 2×2 Mixed ANOVA was conducted out. Multivariate analysis shows a significant effect in the interaction of Test-time and Group (Wilks Lambda = .318; F(1,9) = 19.318; p = .002; $\eta_p^2 = .682$). Univariate analysis showed no significant differences between experimental and control groups in pre-test (F(1,9) = 2.261; p = .167; $\eta_p^2 = .201$). In Post-test there was a significant difference between experimental and control groups (F(1,9) = 6.017; p = .037; $\eta_p^2 = .401$) with significant higher values of decision-making in the experimental group (Table 7 and Appendix S1).

Discussion

The hypothesis of our study suggested that the application of a tactical-cognitive training programme based on video-feedback and questioning would have a positive effect on the tactical

Table 5. Mean, standard deviation, mean rank and univariate contrast in planning strategy variables for pre–test.

Variables	**Control group (n=6)**			**Experimental group (n=5)**			$L_{(1)}$	p	**Diff. 95% CI [LO,HI]**
	M	**SD**	**MR**	**M**	**SD**	**MR**			
Concept Content (total)									
Total concepts	36.50	7.29	6.75	34.00	4.30	5.10	0.68	>.05	[-2.9,6.2]
Total goals	20.17	4.71	6.17	19.40	7.89	5.80	0.03	>.05	[-4.4,5.1]
Total conditions	7.83	5.46	6.75	5.80	4.09	5.10	0.70	>.05	[-2.9,6.1]
Total actions	8.00	3.85	7.17	5.60	3.65	4.60	1.69	>.05	[-1.7,6.9]
Total regulatory	1.00	1.26	6.25	0.80	1.09	5.70	0.09	>.05	[-3.8,4.9]
Concept Content (variety)									
Variety goals	6.67	1.86	6.33	6.20	1.48	5.60	0.14	>.05	[-3.9,5.4]
Variety conditions	3.50	2.26	6.42	3.20	1.64	5.50	0.21	>.05	[-3.8,5.6]
Variety actions	4.17	1.83	6.92	2.80	1.92	4.90	1.05	>.05	[-2.4,6.5]
Variety regulatory	0.83	0.98	6.58	0.40	.55	5.30	0.50	>.05	[-2.9,5.5]
Concept sophistication									
Goal hierarchies									
1-Selves & opponent	5.50	4.18	5.00	8.00	2.74	7.20	1.23	>.05	[-6.6,2.2]
2-Win attributes	4.83	2.64	6.17	4.40	2.70	5.80	0.03	>.05	[-4.3,5.1]
Condition qualities									
2-Appropriate-one feature	3.50	2.17	7.17	2.20	.84	4.60	1.68	>.05	[-1.7,6.9]
3-Appropriate-two features	1.17	1.17	6.17	1.00	1.00	5.80	0.04	>.05	[-4.2,4.9]
Action qualities									
2-Appropriate-one feature	4.50	1.64	6.92	3.20	1.79	4.90	1.07	>.05	[-2.4,6.4]
3-Appropriate-two features	0.67	0.82	6.00	0.60	0.55	6.00	0.00	>.05	[-4.3,4.3]
Concept structure									
N° linkages	17.33	4.55	6.92	15.20	3.27	4.90	1.01	>.05	[-2.5,6.5]
Double-concept linkages	7.17	1.60	6.42	6.60	1.52	5.50	0.22	>.05	[-3.7,5.5]
Triple-concept linkages	4.33	2.66	6.58	3.80	1.64	5.30	0.42	>.05	[-3.3,5.9]

MR = Mean Rank.

knowledge of tennis players, in content, sophistication and structure. Moreover, an improvement of athletes' cognitive expertise will produce an increase of decision-making skills with a higher percentage of successful decision-making in real game play.

Effects produced on conceptual content show that in both problem representation and strategy planning, players who took part in the video-feedback and questioning programme have modified this conceptual content, verbalising more concepts. Experimental group players get closer to an expert profile, with greater knowledge, where approaches to sport situations carried out in a global manner (typical of a lower level of expertise) are being substituted by more tactical approaches, producing a greater number of adaptations in LTM [6,22].

In the experimental group, significant differences with a higher quantity of regulatory concepts in problem representation show a greater and more varied evaluation of their actions and greater self-evaluation capacity, related to players with a higher level of expertise [19,50]. These regulatory concepts, already developed, will help increase athletes' comprehension of factors that have an influence on their performance [9] and also help to make more accurate decisions [24].

With reference to conceptual sophistication, it is possible to find a significantly larger number of goals related to the opponent, both in problem representation and in strategy planning. The greater number of references to the opponent in verbalisations shows that there is a development of tactical knowledge and cognitive skills related to higher levels of expertise, by means of tactics related to the opponent, and permitting a high specialisation of cognitive skills [12,51].

In condition sophistication, the experimental group develops a significantly larger number of concepts with two or more features, both in problem representation and in strategy planning. In quality of actions (level 3), these significant differences can only be found in strategy planning. Once again, tennis players from the experimental group get closer to the expert profile by developing more sophisticated concepts, because a more detailed problem representation is a characteristic feature of expert performance, especially in condition and action concept quality [9,22,52–53]. Thus, there is a more in-depth interpretation and with more tactical aspects, based on evaluations about the opponent, tendencies or more detailed weakness [13,53]. On the other hand, less concept sophistication in the control group shows that they continue to make more global approaches to sport situations with less interpretation of the environment [53], whilst the experimental group shows signs of change, from a superficial processing of the environment (related to lower levels of expertise) towards deep and tactical processing [13,54].

Table 6. Mean, standard deviation, mean rank and univariate contrast in planning strategy variables for post–test.

Variables	Control group (*n*=6)			Experimental group (*n*=5)			$L_{(1)}$	*p*	Diff. 95% CI [LO,HI]
	M	SD	MR	M	SD	MR			
Concept Content (total)									
Total concepts	35.50	8.41	4.00	51.80	9.20	8.40	**4.80**	**<.05**	[-7.9, -0.9]
Total goals	20.50	4.32	4.42	29.00	10.30	7.90	3.02	>.05	[-7.4,0.5]
Total conditions	6.17	5.64	5.00	10.00	2.12	7.20	1.22	>.05	[-6.7,2.3]
Total actions	8.50	2.88	4.92	11.80	4.60	7.30	1.44	>.05	[-6.8,2.0]
Total regulatory	0.17	0.41	5.83	0.40	0.89	6.20	0.07	>.05	[-3.6,2.8]
Concept Content (variety)									
Variety goals	6.83	1.17	5.00	7.80	1.64	7.20	1.26	>.05	[-6.6,2.2]
Variety conditions	3.50	2.88	4.92	5.20	2.59	7.30	1.43	>.05	[-6.8,2.0]
Variety actions	4.00	1.09	6.75	3.40	1.14	5.10	0.74	>.05	[-2.7,6.0]
Variety regulatory	0.17	0.41	5.92	0.20	0.45	6.10	0.02	>.05	[-3.4,3.0]
Concept sophistication									
Goal hierarchies									
1-Selves & opponent	7.83	3.06	4.17	14.00	5.61	8.20	**4.11**	**<.05**	[-7.6, -0.4]
2-Win attributes	4.17	2.48	7.00	2.60	1.14	4.80	1.25	>.05	[-2.2,6.6]
Condition qualities									
2-Appropriate-one feature	3.67	3.33	5.33	4.80	2.28	6.80	0.56	>.05	[-6.0,3.1]
3-Appropriate-two features	0.67	1.21	4.42	1.80	0.84	7.90	3.24	>.05	[-7.3,0.3]
Action qualities									
2-Appropriate-one feature	6.00	2.37	6.17	6.20	3.35	5.80	0.03	>.05	[-4.3,5.1]
3-Appropriate-two features	1.00	1.09	3.67	5.60	2.88	8.80	**8.61**	**<.01**	[-6.7, -3.6]
Concept structure									
N° linkages	17.50	4.76	3.83	29.60	5.18	8.60	**5.66**	**<.05**	[-7.9, -1.6]
Double-concept linkages	8.50	2.95	6.83	6.80	3.42	5.00	0.84	>.05	[-2.7,6.4]
Triple-concept linkages	3.33	2.42	3.58	7.80	1.09	8.90	**7.20**	**<.01**	[-7.8, -2.8]

MR = Mean Rank.

Within the conceptual structure, similar changes have been achieved, as the total number of connections, and the number of triple verbalised concepts, both in problem representation and in strategy planning by the experimental group is significantly higher. Results show once again that these players get closer to the expert profile, developing a greater interrelation of knowledge and concept association, and with a structural complexity that is more typical of players with greater expertise [9,20]. Likewise, this greater structuring of knowledge shows how concepts unite to form more complex profiles that are developed in the LTM and reflect a higher level of expertise, because these adaptations and improvements, exemplified in greater structures of the LTM, will favour better decisions [6,12–13].

Differences found here enable us to observe how experimental group players developed a higher problem representation, where the use of tactical knowledge is greater and will be more effective when trying to solve a game situation. They also developed a greater, more elaborated and more sophisticated, strategy planning, which will be used to plan subsequent actions based on relevant information for different game situations [6,13,19–21]. These adaptations will enable us to carry out continuous and

Table 7. Mean, standard deviation and differences analysis in decision-making.

Test-time	Control Group (*n*=6)		Experimental Group (*n*=5)		Mean diff.	Typical Error	$F_{(1,9)}$	*p**	η_p^2	Diff 95% CI [LO,HI]
	M	SD	M	SD						
Pre-test	58.65	2.46	55.54	4.31	3.10	2.06	2.26	.167	.201	[-1.5,7.7]
Post-test	54.95	4.25	61.20	4.15	-6.25	2.55	6.01	**.037**	**.401**	[-12.0, -0.5]

*Bonferroni adjust for multiple comparisons.

dynamic coding that will favour the athlete in order to anticipate events, to predict results and to develop proactive behaviours [17].

After the tactical-cognitive training programme, and when they get closer to the expert profile, the experimental group players make more successful decisions.

These improvements in decision-making skills show a higher quality of decision-making because the use of specific strategies enables them to take better decisions and make strategically better selections [24]. This improvement is due to the fact that the decisions made will take into account a larger number of conditions produced in the game context (i.e.: court position, opponent's position, or the scoreboard), as it reflects the results in tactical knowledge. They will also interpret tendencies, strengths and weaknesses in a more sophisticated manner, taking their opponents into account as well as their own features. And furthermore, they will take into account the different contextual conditions that may have an influence on shot selection [19,22,24].

Our results also show how the knowledge base of those players who have been exposed to the tactical-cognitive training programme based on video-feedback and questioning have evolved towards characteristics typical of a higher level of expertise, where: conditions and weak actions change into tactical and associated concepts; global approaches to sporting situations turn into tactical approaches with the presence of relevant information; and where the superficial processing of events of the environment is replaced with a deep processing of information [13,26].

The development of adaptations in the LTM such as current event profiles and action plan profiles require several years of experience [6,12], but by means of formative strategies such as the video-feedback and questioning programme, it can be developed faster and more effectively. These profiles will enable players to code, update and modify the relevant conditions for decision-making in the competition [55,56]. The development of these adaptations in the LTM also explains these improvements in decision-making. The video feedback and questioning tools develop adaptations in the action plan profiles and current event profiles. This improvement of tactical knowledge will permit the improvement of decision-making capacities because knowledge (i.e., problem representations) guides decision-making [9,45].

It is critical for athletes to gain an intellectual understanding of the implications of their behaviour to develop their decision-making skills and to get opportunities to practice these new skills [11]. An explicit learning strategy, like the programme shown in this work, could be effective for highly complex situations (like the ones that occur in tennis), and that are related to deliberate decision-making [35,36].

Furthermore, developing cognitive processes for deliberate decision-making may be the basis for processing information faster and using intuitive processes [11,57], as well as for prioritising information in situations involving time pressure and choosing the best option via simple heuristics [58]. Time pressure can determine which decisions are taken via deliberate processes and which are taken via intuitive and heuristic processes (e.g., "Take-the-first"), as intuitive and deliberate processes seem to be used in the various stages of the decision-making process in sports [36].

Therefore, this type of decisional training would not only be useful for deliberate decision-making but it may also be the basis of intuitive decision-making. Furthermore, when the expertise level increases, the time pressure to take decisions is also greater for athletes [59]. In this sense, the level of expertise may be a decisive factor to choose the most adequate decisional training processes, as explicit decisional learning processes may be more effective at lower levels of expertise, whilst implicit decisional learning processes (e.g., based on ecological dynamics and manipulation of task constraints; for a review in tennis, see [60]) may be more effective for higher levels of expertise.

With reference to the application of similar programmes, results of this study set out the effectiveness of tactical-cognitive training based on video-feedback and questioning on several cognitive variables, in the same way as in other studies developed in team sports [40,41]. It is also possible to confirm the effectiveness of video-feedback and questioning as useful tools for cognitive training, together with the help of an expert or supervisor to direct attention towards some signs [31,34]. It would be interesting to consider future studies with placebo group, or applying these tools separately, where the contribution of each tool to decisional learning can be assessed more directly, or if really by combining video-feedback and questioning greater effects are obtained.

One of the limitations of the study is the small number of participants, which limits the capacity to extrapolate the results. However, the reduced number of individuals has enabled us to study both the tactical knowledge and decision-making in tennis players in greater depth and detail, as well as to try to identify the underlying processes in cognitive expertise and in their training process. On the other hand, the need is raised to continue investigating into the relationships between cognitive variables and performance variables, both in tennis and in other sports.

Finally, we would like to highlight the effect produced on different variables related to cognitive expertise and decision-making, and the need to promote programmes focused on improving cognitive areas (by means of video-feedback, questioning or by some other tactical-decisional training tools) because of their importance during athletes' formative stages and the very strong relationship between cognition and performance in sport. To this end, it would be important for future studies to incorporate variables that may be direct performance indicators (e.g. through notational analysis) and verify the effect of decisional training on performance.

Supporting Information

Figure S1 Overall procedure and research design. Distribution of the 18 matches played, decision-making pre- and post-test, tactical knowledge pre- and post-test, on-court sessions in both groups, and intervention sessions in experimental group.

Appendix S1 Value graphics of variables with significant differences. Graphic 1. Values of percentage of decision-making for pre- and post-test in each player. DM = Decision-making; C1 = Control Player 1; C2 = Control Player 2; C3 = Control Player 3; C4 = Control Player 4; C5 = Control Player 5; C6 = Control Player 6; E1 = Experimental Player 1; E2 = Experimental Player 2; E3 = Experimental Player 3; E4 = Experimental Player 4; E5 = Experimental Player 5. **Graphic 2.** Values of total concepts in problem representation for pre- and post-test in each player. Tot Concept = Total of concepts; PR = Problem Representation; Abbreviations in X-axis are described in Graphic 1. **Graphic 3.** Values of total regulatory concepts in problem representation for pre- and post-test in each player. Tot Reg = Total regulatory concepts; PR = Problem Representation; Abbreviations in X-axis are described in Graphic 1. **Graphic 4.** Values of variety of regulatory concepts in problem representation for pre- and post-test in each player. Var Reg = Variety of regulatory concepts; PR = Problem Representation; Abbreviations in X-axis are described in Graphic 1. **Graphic 5.** Values of goal level 1 concepts in problem representation for pre- and post-test in each player. Goal-1 = Goal Level 1 concepts; PR = Problem Representation; Abbreviations in X-axis are described in Graphic 1. **Graphic 6.** Values of condition level 3 concepts in problem representation for pre- and post-test in each player. Cond-3 = Condition Level 3 concepts; PR = Problem Representation; Abbreviations in X-axis are described in Graphic 1. **Graphic 7.** Values of action level 3 concepts in problem representation for pre- and post-test in each player. Act-3 = Action Level 3 concepts; PR = Problem Representation; Abbreviations in X-axis are described in Graphic 1. **Graphic 8**. Values of number of linkages in problem representation for pre- and post-test in each player. PR = Problem Representation; Abbreviations in X-axis are described in Graphic 1. **Graphic 9.** Values of triple concepts in problem representation for pre- and post-test in each player. Triple = Triple concepts; PR = Problem Representation; Abbreviations in X-axis are described in Graphic 1. **Graphic 10.** Values of total concepts in planning strategy for pre- and post-test in each player. Tot Concept = Total Concepts; PS = Planning strategy; Abbreviations in X-axis are described in Graphic 1. **Graphic 11.** Values of goal level 1 concepts in planning strategy for pre- and post-test in each player. Goal-1 = Goal Level 1; PS = Planning strategy; Abbreviations in X-axis are described in Graphic 1. **Graphic 12.** Values of action level 3 concepts in planning strategy for pre- and post-test in each player. Act-3 = Action Level 3 concepts; PS = Planning strategy; Abbreviations in X-axis are described in Graphic 1. **Graphic 13.** Values of number of linkages in planning strategy for pre- and post-test in each player. PS = Planning strategy; Abbreviations in X-axis are described in Graphic 1. **Graphic 14.** Values of triple concepts in planning strategy for pre- and post-test in each player. Triple = Triple concepts; PS = Planning strategy; Abbreviations in X-axis are described in Graphic 1.

Acknowledgments

We want to acknowledge the participation of tennis players and coaches involved in this study.

Author Contributions

Conceived and designed the experiments: LGG MPM AM AG FdV. Performed the experiments: LGG AM AG. Analyzed the data: LGG MPM AM AG. Contributed reagents/materials/analysis tools: LGG MPM AM FdV. Wrote the paper: LGG MPM AM AG FdV.

References

1. Moran A (2012) Thinking in action: Some insight from cognitive sport psychology. Thinking Skills and Creativity 7: 85–92. doi:10.1016/j.tsc.2012.03.005
2. Williams AM, Ericsson KA (2005) Some considerations when applying the expert performance approach in sport. Hum Movement Sci 24: 283–307. doi:10.1016/j.humov.2005.06.002
3. Williams AM, Ford PR, Eccles DW, Ward P (2011) Perceptual-cognitive expertise in sport and its acquisition: implications for applied cognitive psychology. Appl Cognitive Psych 25: 432–442. doi:10.1002/acp.1710
4. Hodges NJ, Starkes JL, MacMahon C (2006) Expert performance in sport: A cognitive process. In: Ericsson KA,Charness N, Feltovich PJ, Hoffman RR, editors. The Cambridge handbook of expertise and expert performance. Cambridge, NY: Cambridge University Press. pp. 471–488.
5. Köppen J, Raab M (2009) Knowledge of athletes as cues for simple choices. In: Araújo D, Ripoll H, Raab M, editors. Perspectives on Cognition and Action in Sport New York:Nova Science Publishers. pp. 108–117.
6. McPherson SL, Kernodle MW (2007) Mapping two new points on the tennis expertise continuum: Tactical skills of adult advanced beginners and entry-level professionals during competition. J Sport Sci 25(8): 945–959. doi:10.1080/02640410600908035
7. Starkes JL, Helsen W, Jack R (2001). Expert performance in sports and dance. In: Singer RN, Hausenblas HA, Janelle CM, editors.. Handbook of sport psychology (3rd edition). New York: John Wiley & Sons. pp. 174–201.
8. Williams AM, Davids K, Williams JG (1999) Visual perception and action in sport. London: E & FN Spon. 451 p.
9. MacMahon C, McPherson SL (2009) Knowledge base as a mechanism for perceptual-cognitive tasks: Skills is in the details! Int J Sport Psychol 40: 565–579.
10. Harteis C, Koch T, Morgenthaler B (2008). How intuition contributes to high performance: An educational perspective. USA-China Educ Rev 5(1): 68–80.
11. Hogarth RM (2001) Educating intuition. Chicago: The University of Chicago Press. 335 p.
12. McPherson SL (2008) Tactics: Using knowledge to enhance performance. In: Farrow D, Baker J, MacMahon C, editors. Developing sport expertise: researchers and coaches put theory into practice. London: Routledge. pp. 155–167.
13. McPherson SL, Kernodle MW (2003) Tactics, the neglected attribute of expertise: Problem representations and performance skills in tennis. In: Starkes JL, Ericsson KA, editors. Expert performance in sports: Advances in research on sport expertise. Champaign, IL: Human Kinetics. pp. 137–168.
14. Rulence-Pâques P, Fruchart E, Dru V, Mullet E. (2005) Decision-making in soccer game: a developmental perspective. Eur Rev Appl Psychol 55: 131–136. doi:10.1016/j.erap.2004.05.003
15. Ericsson KA, Kintsch W (1995). Long-term working memory. Psychol Rev 102: 211–245. doi:10.1037//0033-295X.102.2.211
16. Ericsson KA, Patel V, Kintsch W (2000) How experts' adaptations to representative task demands account for the expertise effect in memory recall: Comment on Vicente and Wang (1998). Psychol Rev 107: 578–592. doi:10.1037//0033-295X.107.3.578
17. Williams AM, North JS (2009) Some constraints on recognition performance in soccer. In: Araújo D, Ripoll H, Raab M, editors. Perspectives on Cognition and Action in Sport. New York: Nova Science Publishers. pp. 95–107.
18. Williams AM, Ericsson KA (2008) From the guest editors: How do experts learn? J Sport Exerc Psychol, 30, 653–662.
19. McPherson SL (1999) Expert-novice differences in performance skills and problem representations of youth and adults during tennis competition. Res Quart Exerc Sport, 70, 233–251.
20. McPherson SL (1999) Tactical differences in problem representations and solutions in collegiate varsity and beginner women tennis players. Res Quart Exerc Sport 70: 369–384.
21. McPherson SL (2000) Expert-novice differences in planning strategies during collegiate singles tennis competition. J Sport Exerc Psychol 22: 39–62.
22. García-Gonzalez L, Moreno A, Moreno MP, Iglesias D, Del Villar F (2012) Tactical knowledge in tennis: a comparison of two groups with different levels of expertise. Percept Motor Skill 115(2): 567–580.
23. Overney LS, Blanke O, Herzog MH (2008) Enhanced Temporal but Not Attentional Processing in Expert Tennis Players. PLOS ONE 3(6): e2380. doi:10.1371/journal.pone.0002380
24. Nielsen TM, McPherson SL (2001) Response selection and execution skills of professionals and novices during singles tennis competition. Percept Motor Skill 93: 541–555. doi:10.2466/PMS.93.6.541-555
25. Elferink-Gemser MT, Kannekens R, Lyons J, Tromp EJY, Visscher C (2010) Knowing what to do and doing it: Difference in self assessed tactical skills o regional, sub-elite, and elite youth field hockey players. J Sport Sci 28: 521–528. doi:10.1080/02640410903582743
26. McPherson SL (1994) The development of sport expertise: Mapping the tactical domain. Quest 46: 223–240.
27. Lorains M, Bal K, MacMahon C (2013) Expertise differences in a video decision-making task: Speed influences on performance. Psychol Sport Exerc 14: 293–297. doi:10.1016/j.psychsport.2012.11.004
28. Baker J, Côté J, Abernethy B (2003) Learning from the experts: practice activities of expert decision-makers in sport. Res Quart Exerc Sport 74: 342–347.
29. Deakin JM, Cobley S (2003) An examination of the practice environments in figure skating and volleyball: a search for deliberate practice. In: Starkes JL, Ericsson KA, editors. Recent advances in the study of sport expertise. Champaigne, IL: Human Kinetics. pp. 115–135.
30. Raab M (2007) Think SMART, not hard-a review of teaching decision making in sport from ecological rationality perspective. Phys Educ Sport Pedago 12(1): 1–22.
31. Vickers JN (2007) Perception, Cognition, and Decision Training. The Quiet Eye in Action. ChampaingIL:Human Kinetics. 273 p.
32. Vickers JN, Reeves MA, Chambers KL, Martell S (2004) Decision training. Cognitive strategies for enhancing motor performance. In: Williams AM, Hodges NJ, editors. Skill acquisition in sport: research, theory and practice. London: Routledge. pp. 103–120.
33. Nelson LJ, Potrac P, Groom R (2011) Receiving video-based feedback in elite ice-hockey: a player's perspective. Sport Educ Soc. doi:10.1080/13573322.2011.613925
34. Vickers JN, Livingston L, Umeris S, Holden D (1999) Decision training: The effects of complex instruction, variable practice and reduced delayed feedback on the acquisition and transfer of a complex motor skill. J Sport Sci 17: 357–367. doi:10.1080/026404199365876
35. Raab M (2003) Implicit and explicit learning of decision making in sports is affected by complexity of situation. Int J Sport Psychol 34: 273–288.

36. Raab M, Johnson M (2008) Implicit learning as a means to intuitive decision making in sports. In: Plessner H, Betsch T, Betsch C, editors. Intuition in Judgment and Decision Making. New York: Lawrence Erlbaum Associates. pp.119–134.
37. Hogarth RM (2008) On the Learning of Intuition. In: Plessner H, Betsch T, Betsch C, editors. Intuition in Judgment and Decision Making. New York: Lawrence Erlbaum Associates. pp.91–105.
38. Hodges NJ, Chua R, Franks IM (2003) The role of video in facilitating perception and action of a novel coordination movement. J Motor Behav 35: 247–260. doi:10.1080/00222890309602138
39. Raab M, Masters RSW, Maxwell JP (2005) Improving the "how" and "what" decisions of elite table tennis players. Hum Movement Sci 24: 326–344. doi:10.1016/j.humov.2005.06.004
40. Moreno A, Del Villar F, García-González L, Gil A, Moreno M.P. (2011). Intervention in decision-making in volleyball players' formative stage. Rev Psicol Deporte 20(2): 785–800.
41. Moreno MP, Moreno A, Ureña A, Iglesias D, Del Villar F (2008) Application of mentoring through reflection in female setters of the Spanish national volleyball team. A case study. Int J Sport Psychol 39: 59–76.
42. McPherson SL, Thomas JR (1989) Relation of knowledge and performance in boys tennis: age and expertise. J Exp Child Psychol 48: 190–211. doi:10.1016/0022-0965(89)90002-7
43. Travassos B, Araújo D, Davids K, O'Hara K, Leitao J et al. (2013) Expertise effects on decision-making in sport are constrained by requisite response behaviours – A meta-analysis. Psychol Sport Exerc 14: 211–219. doi:10.1016/j.psychsport.2012.11.002
44. Fleiss J, Levin B, Paik M (2003) Statistical methods for rates and proportions. NY: John Wiley & Sons. 800 p.
45. Del Villar F, García-González L, Iglesias D, Moreno MP, Cervelló EM (2007). Expert-novice differences in cognitive and execution skills during tennis competition. Percept Motor Skill 104: 355–365.
46. Thomas JR, Nelson JK, Thomas KT (1999) A generalized rank-order method for nonparametric analysis of data from exercise science: a tutorial. Res Quart Exerc Sport 70(1): 11–23.
47. Thomas JR, Thomas KT (2002) Physical activity data: odd distributions yield strange answers. In: Welk GJ, editor. Physical activity assessments for health-related research. Champaign, IL:Human Kinetics. pp. 73–80.
48. Puri ML, Sen PK (1985) Nonparametric methods in general linear models. New York: Wiley.
49. Thomas JR, Nelson JK, Silverman SJ (2011). Research Methods in Physical Activity (6th Ed). Champaign, IL: Human Kinetics.
50. Ruiz LM, Sánchez M, Durán J, Jiménez C (2006) The study and analysis of sport experts: a psychological approach. An Psicol 22(1): 132–142.
51. Gorecki J, French KE (2003) Expert-novice comparison in the use of tactical knowledge during the game play of volleyball. Res Quart Exerc Sport 74 (1): A100.
52. Afonso J, Garganta J, McRobert A, Williams AM, Mesquita I (2012) The perceptual cognitive processes underpinning skilled performance in volleyball: Evidence from eye-movements and verbal reports of thinking involving an in situ representative task. J Sport Sci Med 11: 339–345.
53. McPherson SL (1993) The influence of player experience on problem solving during batting preparation in baseball. J Sport Exerc Psychol 15: 304–325.
54. Schack T, Mechsner F (2006) Representation of motor skills in human long-term memory. Neurosci Lett 391: 77–81. doi:10.1016/j.neulet.2005.10.009
55. Calmeiro L, Tenenbaum G (2011) Concurrent Verbal Protocol Analysis in Sport: Illustration of Thought Processes during a Golf-Putting task. J Clin Sport Psychol 5(3): 223–236.
56. McRobert AP, Ward P, Eccles DW, Williams AM (2011) The effect of manipulating context-specific information on perceptual-cognitive processes during a simulated anticipation task. Brit J Psychol 102: 519–534. doi:10.1111/j.2044-8295.2010.02013.x
57. Goldberg E. (2005), The Wisdom Paradox: How Your Mind Can Grow Stronger as Your Brain Grows Older. New York: Gotham Books. 337 p.
58. Bar-Eli M, Plessner H, Raab M (2011) Judgement, decision making and success in sport. Oxford: Wiley-Balckwell. 192 p.
59. Mann DTY, Williams AM, Ward P, Janelle CM (2007) Perceptual-cognitive expertise in sport: a meta-analysis. J Sport Exerc Psychol 29: 457–464.
60. Carvalho J, Araújo D, García-González L, Iglesias D (2011) Decision-making training in tennis: What Scientific principles can be applied to training programmes? Rev Psicol Deporte 20(2): 767–783.

21

Proximity to Sports Facilities and Sports Participation for Adolescents in Germany

Anne K. Reimers[1,2*], Matthias Wagner[1], Seraphim Alvanides[3], Andreas Steinmayr[4], Miriam Reiner[2], Steffen Schmidt[2], Alexander Woll[2]

1 Department of Sport Science, University of Konstanz, Konstanz, Germany, **2** Institute of Sport and Sport Sciences, Karlsruhe Institute of Technology, Karlsruhe, Germany, **3** Department of Geography and the Built Environment, Northumbria University, Ellison Building, Newcastle-upon-Tyne, United Kingdom, **4** Swiss Institute for Empirical Economic Research (SEW), University of St. Gallen, St. Gallen, Switzerland

Abstract

Objectives: To assess the relationship between proximity to specific sports facilities and participation in the corresponding sports activities for adolescents in Germany.

Methods: A sample of 1,768 adolescents aged 11–17 years old and living in 161 German communities was examined. Distances to the nearest sports facilities were calculated as an indicator of proximity to sports facilities using Geographic Information Systems (GIS). Participation in specific leisure-time sports activities in sports clubs was assessed using a self-report questionnaire and individual-level socio-demographic variables were derived from a parent questionnaire. Community-level socio-demographics as covariates were selected from the INKAR database, in particular from indicators and maps on land development. Logistic regression analyses were conducted to examine associations between proximity to the nearest sports facilities and participation in the corresponding sports activities.

Results: The logisitic regression analyses showed that girls residing longer distances from the nearest gym were less likely to engage in indoor sports activities; a significant interaction between distances to gyms and level of urbanization was identified. Decomposition of the interaction term showed that for adolescent girls living in rural areas participation in indoor sports activities was positively associated with gym proximity. Proximity to tennis courts and indoor pools was not associated with participation in tennis or water sports, respectively.

Conclusions: Improved proximity to gyms is likely to be more important for female adolescents living in rural areas.

Editor: Reury F. P. Bacurau, University of Sao Paulo, Brazil

Funding: This study was funded by a project grant from the German Bundesministerium für Bildung und Forschung (Federal Ministry of Education and Research) and by the German Bundesministerium für Gesundheit (Federal Ministry of Health) (grant number: 01ER0810). The content of this article reflects only the authors' views and the funders were not liable for any use that may be made of the information contained therein. The contribution of AKR was funded by a grant scholarship of the Brigitte Schlieben-Lange-Programm from the Ministry of Science of the German State of Baden-Württemberg. The funders had no role in study design, data collection and analysis, decision to publish, or preparation of the manuscript.

Competing Interests: The authors have declared that no competing interests exist.

* E-mail: anne.reimers@uni-konstanz.de

Introduction

Despite considerable evidence on the health benefits of regular physical activity [1,2], few adolescents worldwide as well as in Germany engage in sufficient levels of physical activity [3,4]. Individual-level socio-demographic disparities in physical activity participation have been well-established. Adolescents from families with low socioeconomic status [5–8] and non-native ethnic background [9–11] appear to be less active than those with medium or high socioeconomic status and native adolescents, respectively.

In addition to individual characteristics, environmental factors are assumed to explain disparities in physical activity participation [12,13]. On a theoretical basis, ecological models highlight the importance of the environment in relation to physical activity behavior [14–16]. These models posit that the neighborhood or community environment exhibits several features such as recreational facilities, aesthetic design and public spaces that hinder or promote the residents' physical activity [15,17,18]. Proximity to sports facilities is one important environmental resource that may predict participation in physical activity [19]. Two theoretical processes may determine the relationship between availability or proximity and utilization of sports facilities [20]. First, the absence of nearby sports facilities in the community increases the effort of residents to participate in physical activities that require these facilities or makes it impossible to participate in such activities when one is unable to reach a more distant facility. Thus, limited availability or low proximity to sports facilities may discourage their usage. This is particularly the case for adolescents because they are more independent from their parents than younger children and may be expected to organize their leisure-time by themselves [21]. The second theoretical process postulates that proximity to sports facilities may generate new demand for their use. Adolescents living close to a sports facility may see it on a daily basis and this familiarity could generate demand for individual visits, as well as for partaking in organised sports club activities taking place in these facilities.

In the geographical literature a distinction has been established between the terms availability and proximity [22]. Proximity is related to the concept of accessibility, in other words how easy it is to access a specific destination, in relation to physical distance or cost in general (e.g. financial or time resources). Availability, on the other hand, is referring to the number or density of destinations and has been utilized as a measure of "exposure" to resources in physical activity studies [23]. There are also methodological differences in the way the physical proximity aspects of accessibility can be measured (e.g. by street network or straight line distance), but these are likely to have very little impact for the relatively short distances examined here, as demonstrated by Burgoine and colleagues [24]. In the current study we implement the concept of accessibility to (rather than availability of) potential destinations by calculating and applying a measure of physical proximity to the nearest sports facilities.

Since the relationship between physical activity and the physical environment is assumed to be context- and behavior-specific [25], proximity to specific sports facilities is assumed to influence sport activities taking place in such facilities. For example, the proximity to indoor pools is supposed to influence water sports activities taking place in indoor pools such as leisure-time swimming or playing water polo for a sports club. Some evidence suggests that adolescents having better availability of or proximity to sports facilities are more likely to be physically active than adolescents with poor availability of sports facilities. Results from studies conducted in the U.S. [26,27], Hong Kong [28], Australia [29] and the Netherlands [30–32] showed that availability of sports facilities was associated with physical activity participation in adolescents. For Greenlandic adolescents, availability of indoor sports facilities showed a positive association with vigorous physical activity, but was negatively associated with moderate-to-vigorous physical activity [33]. For children in Germany, while in rural areas distance to the nearest sports facility was negatively associated with sports activities, no relationship was found in urban areas [34].

To date there are no studies of adolescents linking proximity to specific facilities with the corresponding sports activities that normally take place in such facilities. Additionally, the relationship between proximity to sports facilities and sports participation has not been studied in German adolescents. Thus, the aim of this study was to assess the relationship between proximity to specific sports facilities and participation in the corresponding sports activities for adolescents in Germany. It was hypothesized that proximity to specific sports facilities is positively related to participation in the corresponding leisure-time sports activities.

It is important to note here the distinction between a sports club and a sports facility in the German context. Sports clubs (translated from the German term "Vereine") are associations or unions which offer exercise programs (often for competitive sports), and refer to the administrative aspect of organised sports. Sports facilities are referring to the physical infrastructure (e.g. swimming pools, tennis cours and gyms) where sports clubs offer a range of competitive sports. In Germany there are roughly 90 000 sports clubs, which are particularly important settings for being physically active [35,36] and a substantial proportion of adolescents' physical activity takes place in organized sports [35]. Thus, the current study focuses on sports activity participation in sports clubs, in relation to proximity to sports facilities.

Additionally, physical activity in sports clubs contributes the highest proportion of vigorous physical activity compared to other leisure activities and school physical education [37] and as a result may have a higher impact on health [1]. Hence, investigating the association between proximity to sports facilities and sports activities in sports clubs is particularly important for our understanding of area-based disparities in adolescents' physical activity in Germany.

Materials and Methods

Sampling and participants

The study data set was collated from the Motorik Modul (MoMo Study) [38] and the German Health Interview and Examination Survey for Children and Adolescents (KiGGS). The MoMo Study is a nationwide study on physical fitness and physical activity habits for children and adolescents in Germany and is part of the KiGGS [37,39]. To ensure a diverse sample of children and adolescents between 4 and 17 years old a nationwide stratified multi-stage probability sample with three evaluation levels was drawn for both studies [39–41]. First, a systematic sample of 167 primary sampling units was selected from an inventory of German communities stratified according to the BIK classification system [42] that measures the level of urbanization and the geographic distribution of the population [39]. The probability of any community being picked was proportional to the number of inhabitants younger than 18 years. Second, an age stratified sample of randomly selected children and adolescents was drawn from the official registers of local residents for the KiGGS. Third, a subsample of the KiGGS was randomly assigned to the MoMo Study. The MoMo Study includes complete data sets from 1828 adolescents. The sample used here was further restricted to the participants selected from 161 communities (out of the 167 primary sampling units) for which data sources on sports facilities were available, resulting in a total of 1768 adolescents.

The KiGGS and the MoMo Study were approved by the Charité/Universitätsmedizin Berlin ethics committee and the Federal Office for the Protection of Data and were conducted according to the Declaration of Helsinki [43].

Data sources

The MoMo baseline data was collected between 2003 and 2006 [38]. Parents and adolescents were invited to the examination rooms located at central locations of the 167 cities and municipalities (primary sampling units) that were within close proximity of their homes. Parents and adolescents gave written informed consent and the adolescents answered the questionnaires in the presence of a qualified interviewer on site [41]. Socio-demographic characteristics were assessed using a parent questionnaire and information on sports activities was assessed using an adolescent self-report questionnaire. Furthermore, objective data on socioeconomic environments was drawn from another database, the INKAR database (Indikatoren und Karten zur Raum- und Stadtentwicklung; indicators and maps on spatial development) which is provided by the Federal Office for Building and Regional Planning. INKAR contains a wide range of regional variables, for instance regarding the composition of population, employment rates, levels of education, production and wages [44]. The INKAR data is available for several geographical levels and for the current study the community level was chosen.

Distances to the nearest sports facilities were objectively measured using a Geographical Information System (GIS) [34]. The address and type of different sports facilities were collected from various sources for 161 out of the 167 primary sampling units of the MoMo-Study. The main source of information was the official municipal websites, where most municipalities provide registers of available facilities. These were complemented with addresses from websites of local sports associations as well as from Google Maps. For communities where the relevant information could not be accessed online, lists of sports facilities were requested from the municipal administration. The home addresses of the survey participants and those of the sports facilities were geocoded using Microsoft MapPoint Europe 2010 in combination with IC-Tools, a MapPoint AddIn for Microsoft Excel. For addresses where MapPoint was not able to determine the exact coordinates, Google Maps and Bing Maps were used instead. Linear distances between home addresses and facilities were calculated using the STATA module globdist.

Measures

Proximity to sports facilities within the community. To determine proximity to sports facilities within the community, for each participant the linear distance from their home address to the nearest sports facility within the community was calculated. Thus, three proximity variables were created reflecting the distances to the nearest gym, tennis court, and indoor pool.

Participation in sports activities. Participation in specific activities in sports clubs was measured using the MoMo-PAQ [45]. In this questionnaire sports club membership was measured using one item: "Are you a member of a sports club?" (Responses: (1) Yes, I am currently a member of one sports club. (2) Yes, I am currently a member of several sports clubs. (3) I used to be a member of a sports club, but not anymore. (4) No, I have never been a member of a sports club). This measure was dichotomized and the new variable discriminates between members (combining response options 1 and 2) and non-members (response options 3 and 4). Furthermore, participants were asked to report at most four different sports they engage in at a sports club. Based on these items three new variables were computed that differentiate between non-members of sports clubs and members of sports clubs that (1) engage in sports taking place in gyms (e.g. gymnastics, handball, volleyball etc.); (2) engage in water sports taking place in indoor pools (e.g. swimming, water polo); (3) engage in tennis.

Covariates. Individual-level socioeconomic status was calculated separately for both parents combining their responses on educational and professional status and total household income [46]. These three aspects (income, educational and professional status) were scored on a scale from 1 to 7 and a sum score was created (range: 3–21) and categorized into low (3–8), medium (9–14) or high (15–21) socioeconomic status [47]. The higher score for either of the parents was used and adolescents with separated parents were assigned the socioeconomic status of the parent they lived with. Migration background was assumed if the adolescent had immigrated to Germany, or at least one parent was not born in Germany, or if both parents immigrated to Germany or had non-German nationality [39,48]. Level of urbanization is an area-level variable describing the population size of the community (rural area or small town: ≤19,999 residents; urban area: ≥20,000 residents) and was assigned to the primary sample units according to the BIK classification system [39]. Unemployment rate is also an area-level variable assigned to the primary sample units and calculated as the percentage of unemployed inhabitants of employable age. This variable was selected as an indicator of the community-level socioeconomic environment from the INKAR data set [44].

Statistical analysis

The associations of distances with specific sports facilities and leisure-time sports activities in sports clubs were analyzed using logistic regression analyses separately for both genders. In order to account for the hierarchical structure of the data with subjects nested within communities (primary sample units) multilevel analysis with community and individual as levels was considered [49]. However, since no significant clustering in communities was found in the unconditional (null) models (boys: $z = 1.506$, $p = 0.132$; girls: $z = 1.332$, $p = 0.183$), we decided to conduct single-level logistic regression analyses for individuals without adjustments for clustering at the sample point level of communities. We calculated four models, with model 1 disclosing the relationship of the covariates (age, socioeconomic status, migration background, unemployment rate, level of urbanization) with the outcome variable and model 2 disclosing the unadjusted effects of distances to specific sports facilities on the respective sports activities. Model 3 is the full model with both the covariates and the distances as predictors. In model 4 we included the interaction term of "distance * level of urbanization" because Steinmayr and colleagues [34] showed that the strength of the relationship of distances to the nearest sports facility and sports activity differed between rural and urban areas. In order to prevent multicollinearity in the interaction models, continuous variables were mean centered in the logistic regression analysis. To decompose significant interaction terms the PROCESS macro from Hayes [50] was run.

All analyses were carried out in IBM Statistical Package for Social Science (SPSS) version 20 (IBM, New York, USA)

Results

Description of the sample

Descriptive data of individual and community-level correlates and straight line distances to the nearest sports facilities are presented in Table 1. The sample consisted of 865 girls and 903 boys, with a mean age 14.21 (SD = 1.94). Approximately half of the sample had medium socioeconomic status and one out of four had either high or low socioeconomic status, respectively. Nearly 11% of the participants had migration background, while 56.0% resided in rural and 44.0% in urban areas. 47.9% of girls and 59.2% of boys participated in sports club activities. The shortest mean distance was to the nearest gym (1.26 km; SD = 1.53), followed by the mean distance to the nearest tennis court (2.13 km; SD = 2.18). The mean distance to the nearest indoor pool was the longest at 4.12 km (SD = 5.01).

Relationship between proximity to specific sports facilities and participation in the corresponding sports activities

Descriptives on participation in specific sports activities are presented in Table 2. The logisitic regression analysis showed that distances (in kilometers) to the nearest tennis court and to the nearest indoor pool were not significantly related to the respective sports activites (tennis playing, swimming or polo) for girls or for boys in any of the Models 2–4 (data not shown here). Concerning the distances to the nearest gym, regression analysis revealed that girls having longer distances were less likely to do sports activities that require access to a gym (Table 3). The distance to the nearest gym was negatively associated with participation in sports activities in the unadjusted regression model (Model 2) and the multiple regression model (Model 3) indicating that an increase of one standard deviation (= 1.43 km) in distance to the nearest gym reduces the odds of participating in sports activities in sports clubs by 24%. Model 4 revealed that distance to the nearest gym significantly interacted with level of urbanization. The PROCESS macro from Hayes [50] that was run to better interpret this

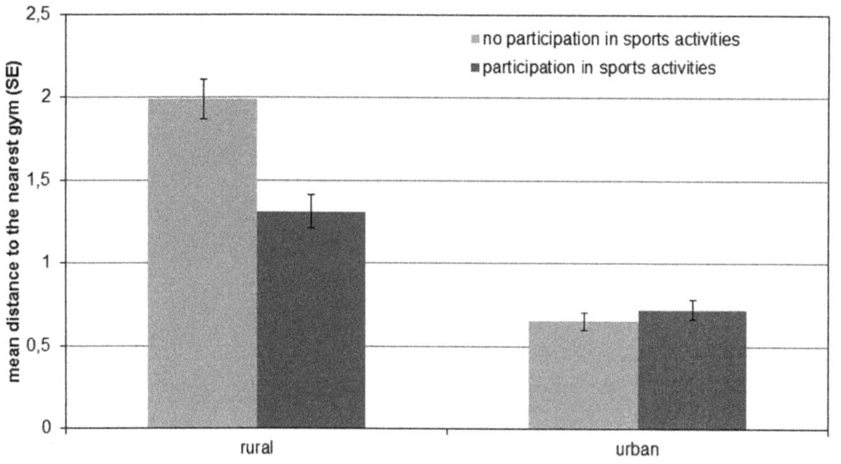

Figure 1. Visual presentation of the interaction of distances to the nearest gym and level of urbanization on leisure-time sports activities taking part in gyms in girls.

interaction term showed a negative association of distance and participation in sports activities for girls living in rural areas ($p<0.001$) but no significant relationship for girls living in urban areas ($p = 0.393$) (Figure 1). For boys, distances to the nearest gym were not associated with leisure-time sports activities that require access to a gym (Table 4).

Discussion

This nationwide study provides empirical evidence that girls from rural areas with better gym availability were more likely to participate in leisure-time indoor sports activities (e.g. dancing, volleyball, gymnastics, etc.).

Concerning the relationship between proximity to sports facilities and participation in sports clubs, only for adolescent girls from rural areas was gym proximity positively related to participation in indoor sports activities. The proximity to gyms was not associated with indoor sports activities for adolescent boys and no association was found between proximity to tennis courts and indoor pools and respective sports activities for either gender. Previous studies that do not distinguish the different types of sports

Table 1. Sample description.

	girls (n = 865)	**boys (n = 903)**	**total (n = 1768)**
Individual-level correlates n (%)			
Socioeconomic status			
low	238 (27.9)	220 (24.7)	458 (26.3)
medium	416 (48.8)	453 (50.9)	869 (49.9)
high	198 (23.2)	217 (24.4)	415 (23.8)
Migration background			
no	758 (87.7)	818 (90.6)	1576 (89.2)
yes	106 (12.3)	85 (9.4)	191 (10.8)
Participation in sports club activities			
no	450 (52.1)	367 (40.8)	817 (46.4)
yes	413 (47.9)	532 (59.2)	945 (53.6)
Community-level correlates			
Level of urbanization n (%)			
rural	477 (55.1)	513 (56.8)	990 (56.0)
urban	388 (44.9)	390 (43.2)	778 (44.0)
Unemployment rate M±SD	7.3 ±4.0	7.2 ±3.9	7.2 ±3.9
Straight line distances (in kilometers) to the closest sports facilities M±SD			
straigt line distance to gym	1.21 ±1.43	1.31 ±1.61	1.26 ±1.53
straight line distance to tennis court	2.17 ±2.12	2.09 ±2.25	2.13 ±2.18
straigt line distance to indoor pool	3.96 ±4.84	4.28 ±5.17	4.12 ±5.01

Note: numbers may not add to the full sample sizes due to missing values.

Table 2. Descriptive data on sports participation and distances (in kilometers) to the nearest sports facilities.

	no sports	indoor sports	tennis	water sports
Girls n (% of female sample)	466 (53.9)	366 (42.3)	30 (3.5)	51 (5.9)
Straigt line distance to gym M±SD	1.33 ±1.56	1.07 ±1.22	1.42 ±1.82	0.81 ±0.86
Straight line distance to tennis court M±SD	2.33 ±2.22	2.03 ±2.04	1.76 ±2.32	1.56 ±1.51
Straigt line distance to indoor pool M±SD	4.06 ±5.09	3.97 ±4.78	5.81 ±7.18	3.64 ±4.14
Boys n (% of male sample)	380 (42.1)	483 (53.5)	42 (4.7)	48 (5.3)
Straigt line distance to gym M±SD	1.33 ±1.62	1.26 ±1.57	1.10 ±0.89	1.27 ±1.45
Straight line distance to tennis court M±SD	2.10 ±2.18	2.09 ±2.32	1.80 ±2.15	1.97 ±1.76
Straigt line distance to indoor pool M±SD	4.44 ±5.26	4.33 ±5.31	4.17 ±4.92	3.28 ±3.06

Note: numbers may not add to the full sample sizes due to missing values.

facilities have been conflicting. While two studies conducted in Australia [29] and in the Netherlands [31] found no association between availability of sports facilities and sports participation, other studies from Europe [30,33], the U.S. [26,27] and Hong Kong [28] revealed positive relationships. The conflicting findings are likely to occur because availability of certain types of facilities may have an impact on sports participation while the availability of others may have no impact, as shown in the current study. Furthermore, no study has associated proximity to specific sports facilities with respective sports activities that normally take place in these facilities. Adolescents having low proximity to a specific type of facility might have compensated by engaging in other sports activities for which they can use other facilities available to them. Thus, overall sports participation may not be associated with proximity to a specific type of facility. In the current study proximity to indoor pools and tennis courts was not associated with the respective sports activities (e.g. tennis, swimming, water polo) which are in any case less common in Germany (<10%). Thus, adolescents choosing to participate in these activities may have strong preferences leading to this decision (e.g. for water sports), which could result in engaging with these sports irrespective of constraints in reaching the respective sports facilities.

The association between gym availability and indoor sports participation was only significant for girls from rural areas, but not for boys or for girls from urban areas. Powell and colleagues [26] also showed in a study conducted in the U.S. that only for female adolescents was proximity to commercial physical activity-related facilities associated to physical activity. Low proximity to sports facilities could be a barrier of participation in sports activities, especially in adolescent girls, because they tend to depend on others for their daily mobility and therefore experience more difficulty in reaching sports facilities further away from their home. Distinguishing between rural and urban areas may be appropriate in samples from countries with distinct rural-urban differences like Germany. To the best of our knowledge urban-rural differences have not been assessed in other studies, in the context of this research, but some studies were only based on participants from larger cities [28–30]. Although in Hong Kong [28] and Rotterdam/Netherlands [30] positive relationships were observed for availability of sports activities and physical activity, a stronger association may occur in rural areas. Since in rural areas public transport and infrastructure tend to be poorer, available facilities can be less accessible and sports participation may depend more on proximity to sports facilities. Furthermore, because in urban areas there is a higher density of sports facilities such as gyms, tennis courts and indoor pools, adolescents living there may have adequate proximity to sports facilities in general; thus, no association of proximity to sports facilities and sports participation can be observed in urban areas. Nevertheless, parents of middle school youth living in both urban and rural areas have commented

Table 3. Associations of socio-demographic variables and distances to the nearest gym with participation in leisure-time indoor sports for girls (N = 754).

	Model 1 OR (95%CI)	Model 2 OR (95%CI)	Model 3 OR (95%CI)	Model 4 OR (95%CI)
unemployment rate	.91 (.87; .94)		.91 (.87; .95)	.91 (.87; .95)
rural[a]	1.04 (.75; 1.43)		1.25 (.89; 1.76)	1.07 (.74; 1.54)
low SES[b]	.43 (.27; .66)		.44 (.29; .69)	.45 (.29; .70)
medium SES[b]	.87 (.60; 1.27)		.91 (.62; 1.33)	.91 (.62; 1.33)
no migration background[c]	1.84 (1.11; 3.02)		1.95 (1.18; 3.23)	2.03 (1.23; 3.37)
age	.90 (.83; .97)		.89 (.83; .97)	.89 (.82;.96)
distance to gym[d]		.82 (.70; .96)	.76 (.64; .91)	1.22 (.71; 1.93)
distance to gym[d] * level of urbanization				.58 (.35; .95)
Nagelkerkes Pseudo-R^2	.104	.012	.120	.128

Note: [a] reference = urban; [b] reference = high; [c] reference = migration background; [d] means centered; OR = Odds ratio, CI = confidence interval; bold values represent statistically significant associations (p≤0.05); italic values show significant interaction terms (p≤0.10).

Table 4. Associations of socio-demographic variables and distances to the nearest gym with participation in leisure-time indoor sports for boys (N = 815).

	Model 1 OR (95%CI)	Model 2 OR (95%CI)	Model 3 OR (95%CI)	Model 4 OR (95%CI)
unemployment rate	.90 (.86;.93)		.90 (.86; .93)	.90 (.86; .93)
rural[a]	1.06 (.78; 1.45)		1.08 (.77; 1.50)	1.14 (.80; 1.61)
low SES[b]	.41 (.26; .63)		.41 (.26; .63)	.41 (.26; .63)
medium SES[b]	.65 (.45; .94)		.65 (.45; .95)	.65 (.45; .95)
no migration background[c]	1.49 (.88; 2.52)		1.50 (.89; 2.54)	1.52 (.90; 2.58)
age	.88 (.81;.95)		.88 (.81;.95)	.88 (.85;.95)
distance to gym[d]		.96 (.83; 1.10)	.98 (.84; 1.15)	.81 (.52; 1.26)
distance to gym[d] * level of urbanization				1.25 (.78; 1.20)
Nagelkerkes Pseudo-R2	.108	.001	.108	.109

Note: [a] reference = urban; [b] reference = high; [c] reference = migration background; [d] means centered; OR = Odds ratio, CI = confidence interval; bold values represent statistically significant associations (p≤0.05).

that distance to sports facilities is one of the primary barriers to physical activity [51].

Strengths and limitations

The strengths of the current study are that it is based on objective measures of distances to the nearest sports facilities and on a nationwide diverse sample of adolescents encompassing a broad age range. Additionally, in this study we collected data on different types of sports facilities and were able to associate the proximity to specific sports facilities with respective sports activities usually taking place in such facilities. However, the results of this study should be interpreted with caution because of some limitations. First, this is a cross-sectional study that does not allow for causal inferences of relationships. Second, participation in specific leisure-time sports activities has been assessed using a self-report questionnaire which might question the validity of the measure. Third, we did not collect information matching the specific facilities used by each sports club that provides sports programs for adolescents. Thus, we cannot assume that sports club activity programs for adolescents were offered at the nearest sports facility. Furthermore, we cannot be certain that the adolescents participating in specific leisure-time sports activities use the nearest sports facility or another facility. Finally, we did not assess other attributes of the sports facilities, such as size or attractiveness that may also influence sports participation.

Conclusions

The results of the current study show that improved gym availability is likely to be more important for female adolescents living in rural areas. Although this study did not aim to fully explain community variance for adolescents' participation in specific leisure-time sports activities in sports clubs, there was unexplained community-level variance in the regression models. Additional community-level factors could be relevant in explaining sports participation, such as geographical distance and monetary or time costs. We suggest that in order to understand community-level influences on sports participation, the impact of, for example, accessibility to sports facilities should be investigated in further studies.

Acknowledgments

We thank all adolescents who participated in this study.

Author Contributions

Conceived and designed the experiments: AKR MOW AS AW. Performed the experiments: MOW AW. Analyzed the data: AKR MR SS. Contributed reagents/materials/analysis tools: AKR MOW AS MR SS AW. Wrote the paper: AKR. Provided comments and edited the manuscript: SA.

References

1. Janssen I, Leblanc AG (2010) Systematic review of the health benefits of physical activity and fitness in school-aged children and youth. International Journal of Behavioral Nutrition and Physical Activity 7: 40.
2. Biddle SJ, Asare M (2011) Physical activity and mental health in children and adolescents: a review of reviews. Br J Sports Med 45: 886–895.
3. Hallal PC, Andersen LB, Bull FC, Guthold R, Haskell W, et al. (2012) Global physical activity levels: surveillance progress, pitfalls, and prospects. Lancet 380: 247–257.
4. Jekauc D, Reimers A, Wagner MO, Woll A (2012) Prevalence and socio-demographic correlates of the compliance with the physical activity guidelines in children and adolescents in Germany. BMC Public Health 12: 714.
5. Brodersen NH, Steptoe A, Boniface DR, Wardle J (2007) Trends in physical activity and sedentary behaviour in adolescence: ethnic and socioeconomic differences. British Journal of Sports Medicine 41: 140–144.
6. Hanson MD, Chen E (2007) Socioeconomic status and health behaviors in adolescence: A review of the literature. Journal of Behavioral Medicine 30: 263–285.
7. Yang X, Telama R, Laakso L (1996) Parents' physical activity, socioeconomic status and education as predictors of physical activity and sport among children and youth – A 12-year follow-up study. International Review for the Sociology of Sport 31: 273–294.
8. Telama R, Laakso L, Nupponen H, Rimpela A, Pere L (2009) Secular Trends in Youth Physical Activity and Parents' Socioeconomic Status From 1977 to 2005. Pediatric Exercise Science 21: 462–474.
9. Brug J, van Stralen MM, Chinapaw MJ, De Bourdeaudhuij I, Lien N, et al. (2012) Differences in weight status and energy-balance related behaviours according to ethnic background among adolescents in seven countries in Europe: the ENERGY-project. Pediatr Obes 7: 399–411.
10. Owen CG, Nightingale CM, Rudnicka AR, Cook DG, Ekelund U, et al. (2009) Ethnic and gender differences in physical activity levels among 910-year-old children of white European, South Asian and AfricanCaribbean origin: the Child Heart Health Study in England (CHASE Study). International Journal of Epidemiology 38: 1082–1093.
11. Sagatun A, Kolle E, Anderssen SA, Thoresen M, Sogaard AJ (2008) Three-year follow-up of physical activity in Norwegian youth from two ethnic groups: associations with socio-demographic factors. Bmc Public Health 8: 419.

12. Ball K, Timperio AF, Crawford DA (2006) Understanding environmental influences on nutrition and physical activity behaviors: where should we look and what should we count? Int J Behav Nutr Phys Act 3: 33.
13. Macintyre S (2007) Deprivation amplification revisited; or, is it always true that poorer places have poorer access to resources for healthy diets and physical activity? International Journal of Behavioral Nutrition and Physical Activity 4: 32.
14. Sallis JF, Owen N, Fisher EB (2008) Ecological models of health behavior. In: Glanz K, Rimer BK, Viswanath K, editors. Health behavior and health education: theory, research, and practice. 4th ed. San Francisco, Calif.: Jossey-Bass.
15. Swinburn B, Egger G, Raza F (1999) Dissecting obesogenic environments: The development and application of a framework for identifying and prioritizing environmental interventions for obesity. Preventive Medicine 29: 563–570.
16. Spence JC, Lee RE (2003) Toward a comprehensive model of physical activity. Psychology of Sport and Exercise 4: 7–24.
17. Owen N, Leslie E, Salmon J, Fotheringham MJ (2000) Environmental determinants of physical activity and sedentary behavior. Exerc Sport Sci Rev 28: 153–158.
18. Pikora T, Giles-Corti B, Bull F, Jamrozik K, Donovan R (2003) Developing a framework for assessment of the environmental determinants of walking and cycling. Soc Sci Med 56: 1693–1703.
19. Grow HM, Saelens BE, Kerr J, Durant NH, Norman GJ, et al. (2008) Where Are Youth Active? Roles of Proximity, Active Transport, and Built Environment. Medicine and Science in Sports and Exercise 40: 2071–2079.
20. Jones A, Panter J (2010) Availability and accessibility in physical activity environments. In: Lake AA, Townshend TG, Alvanides S, editors. Obesogenic environments: complexities, perceptions and objective measures. Chichester, West Sussex: Wiley-Blackwell. pp. 41–61.
21. Davison KK, Jago R (2009) Change in Parent and Peer Support across Ages 9 to 15 yr and Adolescent Girls' Physical Activity. Medicine and Science in Sports and Exercise 41: 1816–1825.
22. Thornton LE, Pearce JR, Kavanagh AM (2011) Using Geographic Information Systems (GIS) to assess the role of the built environment in influencing obesity: a glossary. International Journal of Behavioral Nutrition and Physical Activity 8: 71.
23. Roux AVD, Evenson KR, McGinn AP, Brown DG, Moore L, et al. (2007) Availability of recreational resources and physical activity in adults. American Journal of Public Health 97: 493–499.
24. Burgoine T, Alvanides S, Lake AA (2013) Creating 'obesogenic realities'; do our methodological choices make a difference when measuring the food environment? Int J Health Geogr 12: 33.
25. Giles-Corti B, Timperio A, Bull F, Pikora T (2005) Understanding physical activity environmental correlates: increased specificity for ecological models. Exerc Sport Sci Rev 33: 175–181.
26. Powell LM, Chaloupka FJ, Slater SJ, Johnston LD, O'Malley PM (2007) The availability of local-area commercial physical actlivity-related facilities and physical activity among adolescents. American Journal of Preventive Medicine 33: S292–S300.
27. Gordon-Larsen P, Nelson MC, Page P, Popkin BM (2006) Inequality in the built environment underlies key health disparities in physical activity and obesity. Pediatrics 117: 417-424.
28. Wong BYM, Cerin E, Ho SY, Mak KK, Lo WS, et al. (2010) Adolescents' physical activity: Competition between perceived neighborhood sport facilities and home media resources. International Journal of Pediatric Obesity 5: 169–176.
29. Prins RG, Ball K, Timperio A, Salmon J, Oenema A, et al. (2011) Associations between availability of facilities within three different neighbourhood buffer sizes and objectively assessed physical activity in adolescents. Health & Place 17: 1228–1234.
30. Prins RG, Oenema A, van der Horst K, Brug J (2009) Objective and perceived availability of physical activity opportunities: differences in associations with physical activity behavior among urban adolescents. International Journal of Behavioral Nutrition and Physical Activity 6: 70.
31. Prins RG, Mohnen SM, van Lenthe FJ, Brug J, Oenema A (2012) Are neighbourhood social capital and availability of sports facilities related to sports participation among Dutch adolescents? International Journal of Behavioral Nutrition and Physical Activity 9: 99.
32. Prins RG, van Empelen P, Velde SJT, Timperio A, van Lenthe FJ, et al. (2010) Availability of sports facilities as moderator of the intention-sports participation relationship among adolescents. Health Education Research 25: 489–497.
33. Niclasen B, Petzold M, Schnohr CW (2012) The association between high recreational physical activity and physical activity as a part of daily living in adolescents and availability of local indoor sports facilities and sports clubs. Scandinavian Journal of Public Health 40: 614–620.
34. Steinmayr A, Felfe C, Lechner M (2011) The closer the sportier? Children's sports activity and their distance to sports facilities. European Review of Aging and Physical Activity 8: 67–82.
35. Jekauc D, Reimers AK, Wagner MO, Woll A (2013) Physical activity in sports clubs of children and adolescents in Germany: Results from a nationwide representative survey. Journal of Public Health DOI 10.1007/s10389-013-0579-2.
36. Brettschneider WD (2001) Effects of sport club activities on adolescent development in Germany. European Journal of Sport Science 1.
37. Woll A, Kurth BM, Opper E, Worth A, Bös K (2011) The 'Motorik-Modul' (MoMo): physical fitness and physical activity in German children and adolescents. Eur J Pediatr 170: 1129–1142.
38. Wagner MO, Bös K, Jekauc D, Karger C, Mewes N, et al. (2014) Cohort Profile: The Motorik-Modul (MoMo) Longitudinal Study - Physical Fitness and Physical Activity as Determinants of Health Development in German Children and Adolescents. International Journal of Epidemiology. In press.
39. Kurth BM, Kamtsiuris P, Hölling H, Schlaud M, Dolle R, et al. (2008) The challenge of comprehensively mapping children's health in a nation-wide health survey: design of the German KiGGS-Study. BMC Public Health 8: 196.
40. Kamtsiuris P, Lange M, Schaffrath Rosario A (2007) [The German Health Interview and Examination Survey for Children and Adolescents (KiGGS): sample design, response and nonresponse analysis]. Bundesgesundheitsblatt - Gesundheitsforschung - Gesundheitsschutz 50: 547–556.
41. Hölling H, Kamtsiuris P, Lange M, Thierfelder W, Thamm M, et al. (2007) [The German Health Interview and Examination Survey for Children and Adolescents (KiGGS): Study management and conduct of fieldwork]. Bundesgesundheitsblatt - Gesundheitsforschung - Gesundheitsschutz 50: 557–566.
42. BIK Aschpurwis und Behrens GmbH (2001) BIK Regionen: Ballungsräume, Stadtregionen, Mittel-/Unterzentrengebiete. Methodenbeschreibung zur Aktualisierung 2000. Hamburg.
43. Kurth BM (2007) [The German Health Interview and Examination Survey for Children and Adolescents (KiGGS): an overview of its planning, implementation and results taking into account aspects of quality management]. Bundesgesundheitsblatt - Gesundheitsforschung - Gesundheitsschutz 50: 533–546.
44. Federal Office for Building and Regional Planning (2012) Informationen aus der Forschung des BBSR. Bonn: BBSR.
45. Jekauc D, Wagner MO, Kahlert D, Woll A (2013) [Reliability and Validity of MoMo-Physical-Activity-Questionnaire for Adolescents (MoMo-AFB)]. Diagnostica 59: 100–111.
46. Lampert T, Schenk L, Stolzenberg H (2002) [Conceptualization and operationalization of social inequality in The Child and Adolescent Health Survey]. Gesundheitswesen 64 Suppl 1: S48–52.
47. Winkler J, Stolzenberg H (2009) [Adjustment of the Social Class Index for application in the German Health Interview and Examination Survey for Children and Adolescents (KiGGS)]. Wismar: HWS-Hochschule Wismar.
48. Schenk L, Ellert U, Neuhauser H (2007) [Children and adolescents in Germany with a migration background. Methodical aspects in the German Health Interview and Examination Survey for Children and Adolescents (KiGGS)]. Bundesgesundheitsblatt - Gesundheitsforschung - Gesundheitsschutz 50: 590–599.
49. Goldstein H (1995) Multilevel statistical models. London: Edward Arnold.
50. Hayes AF (2012) PROCESS: A versatile computational tool for observed variable mediation, moderation, and conditional modeling.
51. Moore JB, Jilcott SB, Shores KA, Evenson KR, Brownson RC, et al. (2010) A qualitative examination of perceived barriers and facilitators of physical activity for urban and rural youth. Health Education Research 25: 355–367.

Effects of the Racket Polar Moment of Inertia on Dominant Upper Limb Joint Moments during Tennis Serve

Isabelle Rogowski[1]*, Thomas Creveaux[1], Laurence Chèze[2], Pierre Macé[3], Raphaël Dumas[2]

1 Université de Lyon, Université Claude Bernard Lyon 1, Centre de Recherche et d'Innovation sur le Sport - EA 647, UFRSTAPS, Villeurbanne, France, **2** Université de Lyon, Université Claude Bernard Lyon 1, IFSTTAR, UMR_T9406, LBMC Laboratoire de Biomécanique et Mécanique des Chocs, Bron, France, **3** Babolat VS, Lyon, France

Abstract

This study examined the effect of the polar moment of inertia of a tennis racket on upper limb loading in the serve. Eight amateur competition tennis players performed two sets of 10 serves using two rackets identical in mass, position of center of mass and moments of inertia other than the polar moment of inertia (0.00152 vs 0.00197 kg.m^2). An eight-camera motion analysis system collected the 3D trajectories of 16 markers, located on the thorax, upper limbs and racket, from which shoulder, elbow and wrist net joint moments and powers were computed using inverse dynamics. During the cocking phase, increased racket polar moment of inertia was associated with significant increases in the peak shoulder extension and abduction moments, as well the peak elbow extension, valgus and supination moments. During the forward swing phase, peak wrist extension and radial deviation moments significantly increased with polar moment of inertia. During the follow-through phase, the peak shoulder adduction, elbow pronation and wrist external rotation moments displayed a significant inverse relationship with polar moment of inertia. During the forward swing, the magnitudes of negative joint power at the elbow and wrist were significantly larger when players served using the racket with a higher polar moment of inertia. Although a larger polar of inertia allows players to better tolerate off-center impacts, it also appears to place additional loads on the upper extremity when serving and may therefore increase injury risk in tennis players.

Editor: Robert J. van Beers, VU University Amsterdam, Netherlands

Funding: This study was supported by the "Agence Nationale pour la Recherche" and the "pôle de Compétitivité Sporaltec" [ANR ACE n°2010-BLANC-901] (www.agence-nationale-recherche.fr). The funders had no role in study design, data collection and analysis, decision to publish, or preparation of the manuscript.

Competing Interests: One author is employed by the commercial company BABOLAT VS.

* Email: isabelle.rogowski@univ-lyon1.fr

Introduction

Since the 1980s, the physical characteristics of the tennis racket have been changed drastically by modern designs and materials. The most obvious of the substantial changes in the racket frame is an increase in head size, which accommodates more efficient off-center impacts [1]. To control for advancements in racket design, the international Tennis Federation limited the frame size, i.e. length and racket head area [2]. Nowadays, alterations in the racket's inertial parameters are mainly obtained by manually adding mass to specific locations on the frame [3].

An overly light racket may be counterproductive as the transfer of energy to the ball becomes less effective [2]; but deliberate distribution of mass allows the maneuverability, power and control specifications of the racket to be modified [3]. Indeed, adding mass in the handle results in a racket that is easier to swing rapidly than when mass is added at the tip of the frame [3]. Adding mass symmetrically on both sides at mid-height of the racket head increases the polar moment of inertia (Figure 1) and the racket becomes more resistant to the long-axis twisting motions that occur when the ball is impacted on the lateral portions of the racket face [1]. Therefore, players who find it difficult to consistently impact the ball in the center of the racket face may be able to increase the efficiency of their racket-ball collision by using rackets with larger polar moments of inertia [2]. In addition, the increase in game speed reduces the time available for players to intercept the ball and execute groundstrokes, thus increasing the likelihood of off-center impacts. As a consequence, an increased polar moment of inertia may counteract the reduction in ball control that accompanies suboptimal impact locations. However, there is a paucity of information on the effects of racket specifications, in particular increased racket polar moment of inertia, on upper limb joint loads under playing conditions.

Creveaux at al. [4] found no influence of polar moment of inertia on upper limb loads during the tennis forehand drive. There may be several reasons for this. During ground strokes, the elbow and wrist joints are stabilized by upper arm and forearm muscles, and the upper arm appears as a rigid extension of the racket [5]. Conversely, the tennis serve motion requires extensive shoulder external rotation at the end of the backswing [6], followed by rapid shoulder internal rotation, elbow pronation [7,8] and wrist flexion during the forward swing, and shoulder horizontal flexion and adduction during the follow through [9]. Such large ranges of motion, combined with the high velocities observed during the tennis serve, increase the stress on the upper limb. Dynamic analysis shows excessive joint dynamics [6], notably, peak moment values in excess of 50 N.m [10,11]. Such loads applied on the upper limb joints are considered components

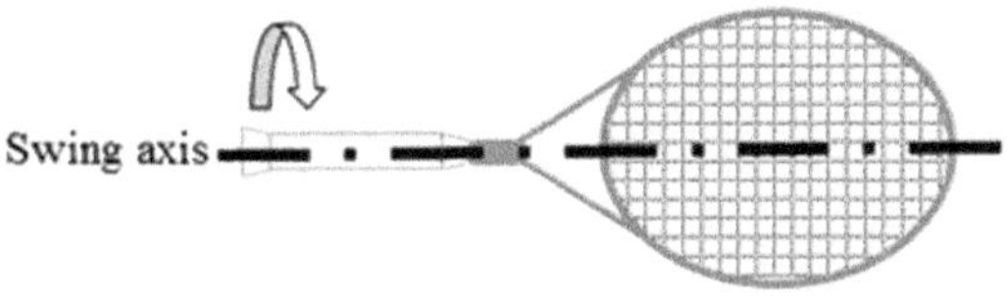

Figure 1. The polar moment of inertia of a tennis racket.

of injury risk, in particular when the motion is repeated frequently [10]. Tennis players play approximately 60 matches per year and hit between 50–150 serves per match, without counting serves during training sessions [6]. Although an increased polar moment improves racket-head stability during off-center impacts (especially for ground strokes), the added inertia also makes it more difficult to rotate the racket along its long axis during the serve. Given that the tennis serve is a potentially injurious stroke, changes in the racket polar moment of inertia could be a factor in upper limb joint overloads during the tennis serve.

The aim of this study was therefore to compare upper limb joint loads from serves using two different rackets, distinguished by their polar moment of inertia. It was hypothesized that increased polar moment of inertia of the tennis racket would lead to increased upper limb joint loads during the serve motion.

Methods

Eight male tennis players (mean ± SD: age = 26.7±4.9 years; height = 1.79±0.04 m; mass = 76.5±6.6 kg; skill = International Tennis Number 3) participated in this study, which was approved by the ethical committee 'Sud-Est II' (Lyon, France). All participants employed a full backswing as part of their service action and gave their written informed consent to participate in this study. No player reported having experienced an injury in the six-month period prior to testing. According to the International Tennis Federation (2004, http://www.tennisplayandstay.com/media/131802/131802.pdf), ITN 3 describes a player who "has good shot anticipation and frequently has an outstanding shot or attribute around which a game may be structured. He can regularly hit winners and force errors off short balls, and can put away volleys and smashes and has a variety of serves to rely on."

After warming-up, each player performed two sets of ten serves on an indoor acrylic tennis court, randomly using two rackets (noted I_L and I_H). The polar moment of inertia of both rackets was adjusted by adding mass (Scotch Brand Tape Core Series 591, 3 M Company, St. Paul, USA) to appropriate parts of the racket frame. After the rackets were strung (250 N), grip tape applied and video markers pasted on the racket frame, the polar moment of inertia was 0.00152 kg.m^2 for I_L and 0.00197 kg.m^2 for I_H; both rackets were identical in mass (0.327 kg), position of center of mass (0.336 m) and swingweight moment of inertia (0.0339 kg.m^2). The specifications of the racket were measured using a Racket Diagnostic Center (Babolat VS, Lyon, France). I_L was typical of the rackets used by male amateur competition tennis players, corresponding to Babolat Drive Z Lite, while I_H raised the polar moment of inertia beyond that of commercially available rackets. Each player was instructed to hit flat serves, i.e. with a minimal amount of spin, from the deuce service court with similar post-impact ball velocity and T-direction for both rackets. A radar gun (Stalker Pro II, Stalker Radar, Plano, TX, USA) was placed two meters behind the player at a height of 1.70 m, to measure the ball velocity after impact and give the player feedback on ball speed.

Fourteen spherical reflective markers (16 mm diameter) were attached to the player and racket to define the segment coordinate systems of the thorax, upper arm, forearm, hand and racket. The markers were affixed to the xiphoid process, incisura jugularis, 7th cervical vertebra, 8th thoracic vertebra, and, on the dominant side, angulus acromialis, medial and lateral humeral epicondyles, radial and ulnar styloid processes, and 2nd and 5th metacarpal heads, as recommended by the International Society of Biomechanics [12]. Two markers were placed symmetrically on both sides at mid-height of the racket head to determine the center of the racket face and one marker was placed on the top end of the handle to define the longitudinal axis of the racket [13]. Retro-reflective tape was placed around the ball to detect the ball–racket impact [13]. Two additional markers were located on the non-dominant shoulder and wrist to detect the beginning of the serve, defined as when the height of the wrist marker was higher than that of the shoulder marker. An eight-camera Eagle motion analysis system (Motion Analysis Corp., Santa Rosa, CA, USA) collected the 3D trajectories of markers during serves at a sampling rate of 500 Hz. Net joint moments and powers were computed as described by Creveaux et al. [13]. Briefly, the net joint moments were computed by a 3D inverse dynamic method [14]. Inputs for the computation were upper limb kinematics, mass, position of center of mass and matrix of inertia of each body segment [15] and the racket. Segment coordinate systems of each upper limb segment were constructed according to International Society of Biomechanics recommendations [12]. Outputs of the computation were the net joint moments acting at the three upper limb joints (wrist, elbow, shoulder) as well as the body segment angular velocities in the global coordinate system. The joint powers were computed as the dot product of net joint moments and the difference between distal and proximal segment angular velocities. The net joint moments were then expressed using the joint coordinate systems [16]. In other words, the net joint moments were projected on the same axes as the axes of the Euler angles computation (Figure 2). The sequences were XZ'Y" for the shoulder [17], ZX'Y" for the elbow [12] and ZY'X" for the wrist joint [18]. To facilitate comparison between the two rackets, the peak of net joint moments and joint powers were normalized. They were divided by the product of player body weight by height, and then multiplied by 100 [10].

For each racket, the three serves with the most similar post-impact ball speed and that landed in the serve box were used for subsequent analysis. For the purpose of this study, the serve was divided into three phases [7,19]. The cocking phase began at the ball toss and lasted until the maximal shoulder external rotation was reached. The forward swing initiated from maximal shoulder external rotation to the frame prior to impact (−0.002 s); the follow-through was from the frame after impact (+0.002 s) to the racket lowest height after impact. The impact frame was determined according to Creveaux et al. [13]. For the statistical analysis, the normalized moment extrema on each rotation axis of each joint, as well as the mean negative and positive powers at each joint, were extracted during each phase of the tennis serve, yielding 72 parameters characterizing the joint loads. First, to detect potential significant differences related to racket characteristics, multivariate analyses were performed. Twelve datasets composed of 16 lines (8 players * 2 rackets) and six columns (peak normalized moment of both orientations on each rotation axis and mean negative and positive power of one joint for all phases of the serve) were built. Then, Principal Component Analyses (PCA) [20] were performed to determine which variables (dynamic parameters) in each dataset contributed to the main principal components calculation, and how the rackets were located relative to the main

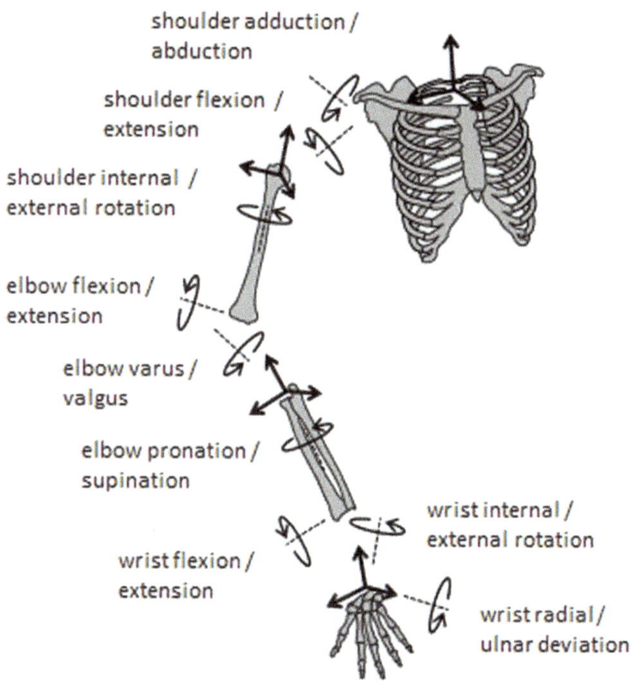

Figure 2. Convention for dynamic measurements.

principal components. Finally, paired t-tests were performed to test for significant differences between rackets in each parameter selected from the PCAs. Where statistical differences were found, effect sizes for pairwise samples (d) were calculated and interpreted according to Cohen's scale [21]. All statistical tests were performed using software SPSS 11.0.1. (Chicago, IL, USA), and level of significance was set at $p \leq 0.05$. The values for pre-impact racket resultant velocity, post impact ball velocity, phase duration, and peak normalized moments, as well as mean negative and positive shoulder, elbow, and wrist joint normalized powers during each phase of the tennis serve for both rackets are presented as mean ± standard error (SE).

Results

The mean pre-impact racket resultant velocities were 22.1 ± 0.4 $m.s^{-1}$ for racket I_L, and 21.8 ± 0.6 $m.s^{-1}$ for I_H, and the mean post-impact ball velocities were 37.5 ± 1.4 $m.s^{-1}$ for both rackets. No significant differences between rackets were observed for either velocity. The duration of the three phases did not significantly differ between rackets. On average, the duration was 0.97 ± 0.04 s for the cocking, 0.09 ± 0.01 s for the forward swing, and 0.23 ± 0.01 s for the follow-through of the serve.

From the Principal Component Analysis performed on the twelve datasets (shoulder flexion/extension, shoulder adduction/abduction, shoulder internal/external rotation, shoulder positive/negative power, elbow flexion/extension, elbow varus/valgus, elbow pronation/supination, elbow positive/negative power, wrist flexion/extension, wrist radial/ulnar deviation, wrist internal/external rotation, and wrist positive/negative power; see File S1 for the raw data), only the results of the peak shoulder flexion/extension moments for the three phases of the serve (Figure 3) are presented in detail here (see File S2 for the other PCA results). The first and second principal components (PC1, PC2) were considered, accounting for 71% of the total variance of the dataset. Figure 3 displays the location of the peak joint normalized moments in each serve phase (black markers), and the location of the players with each racket (grey markers) in the PC1/PC2 axis system. The peak shoulder flexion moment for the three serve phases and the peak extension moment for the forward swing and follow-through phases contributed to the first component calculation, and the peak shoulder extension moment of the cocking phase to the second. The location of each individual (player and racket) is summarized on figure 3 by the supplementary individuals (white markers). The vertical downward orientation from racket I_L to racket I_H followed the orientation of PC2, hence suggesting that increased polar moment of inertia of the racket may influence the peak shoulder extension moment during the cocking phase. As a consequence, among the six parameters describing the peak shoulder flexion/extension moment for the three phases of the serve, only the peak extension moment during the cocking phase was used for pairwise comparison. This procedure was applied for each of the eleven remaining datasets, and reduced the original dataset to 10 peak moments and 2 joint power parameters, which are presented in bold in Tables 1 and 2. The polar moment of inertia was deemed to have no effect on the remaining moments/powers.

Regarding peak shoulder moments (Table 1), significantly higher peak extension and abduction moments during the cocking ($d = 0.68$, medium-to-large effect, $p = 0.04$, and $d = 0.80$, large effect, $p = 0.03$, respectively), and significantly lower peak adduction moment during the follow-through were found for I_H than for I_L ($d = 0.84$, large effect, $p = 0.02$). At the elbow joint, significantly higher peak extension, valgus and supination moments during the cocking ($d = 1.21$, large effect, $p = 0.005$; $d = 0.78$, large effect, $p = 0.03$, and $d = 0.80$, large effect, $p = 0.03$, respectively), and significantly lower peak pronation moments during the follow-through ($d = 0.85$, large effect, $p = 0.02$) were observed for I_L than for I_H (Table 1). At the wrist joint, significantly higher peak extension and radial deviation moments during the forward swing ($d = 0.81$, large effect, $p = 0.03$, and $d = 1.43$, large effect,

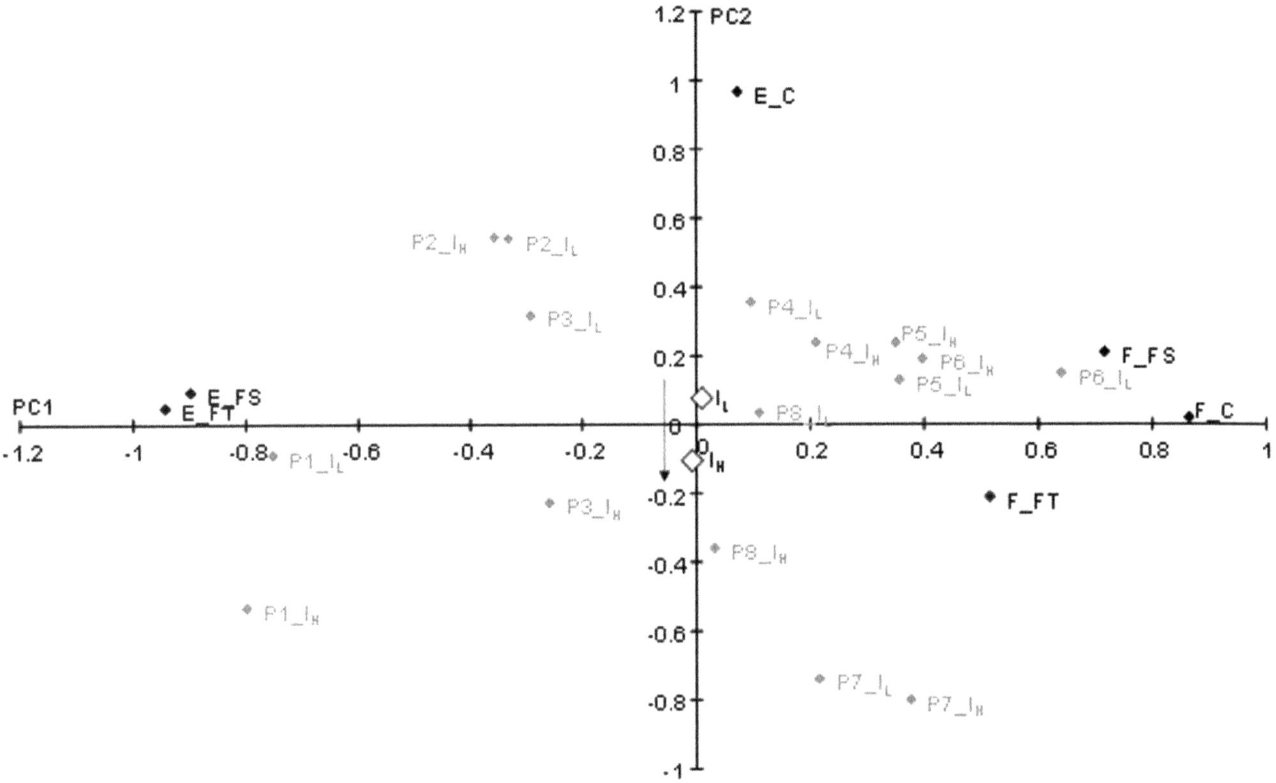

Figure 3. Principal Component 1 (PC1)/Principal Component 2 (PC2) axis system diagram of the peak shoulder extension (E_)/ flexion (F_) normalized moments (black markers) during the cocking (C), forward swing (FS) and follow-through (FT) phases. PC1 explains 54% of the dataset variance and PC2 17%. The individuals are represented by grey markers with PX_I_L and PX_I_H (X ranged from 1 to 8 according to each player), and the supplementary individuals, summarizing the behavior of I_L and I_H, are represented by white markers, I_L being the racket with a low polar moment of inertia and I_H the racket with a high polar moment of inertia. The arrow indicates the main orientation from I_L to I_H.

$p = 0.002$, respectively), and significantly lower peak external rotation moments during the follow-through ($d = 0.66$, medium-to-large effect, $p = 0.05$) were observed for I_L than for I_H (Table 1).

Concerning joint powers (Table 2), mean negative elbow and wrist normalized powers were significantly lower for I_L compared with I_H (Table 2) during the forward swing phase ($d = 1.18$, large effect, $p = 0.006$, and $d = 0.77$, large effect, $p = 0.03$, respectively).

Discussion

The aim of this study was to investigate the effects of the racket polar moment of inertia on dominant upper limb joint loads during the tennis serve. The main results show that, during the cocking phase, the peak shoulder extension and abduction, as well as elbow extension, valgus and supination normalized moments significantly increased when the racket polar moment of inertia increased. During the forward swing phase, the peak wrist extension and radial deviation normalized moments significantly increased with an increase in polar moment of inertia. During the follow-through phase, the peak shoulder adduction, elbow pronation and wrist external rotation normalized moments significantly decreased with an increase in polar moment of inertia. Finally, during the forward swing phase, the elbow and wrist negative normalized joint powers were significantly greater when the racket with a high polar moment of inertia was used. These findings provide coaches, players and scientists with new insights on the relationship between racket specifications and upper limb loads, which may be helpful in improving serve performance and for injury prevention.

The racket pre-impact resultant velocities and ball post-impact velocities were slightly lower than those reported in the literature for amateur competition male tennis players [6,22,23]. These differences may be explained by our experimental instructions, aiming to achieve similar post-impact ball velocities whatever the racket conditions, while players were instructed to serve at maximal ball velocity in previous studies [6,22,23]. Methodological differences could also explain the lower velocities in our study. Indeed, Reid et al. [22] reported the resultant velocity of the marker on the racket tip, which is faster than the resultant velocity of the center of the racket face, calculated in this study. Nevertheless, ball and racket velocities were similar in the two racket conditions, indicating both that the tennis players involved in this study complied with the experimental instructions, and that altering the polar moment of inertia has no effect on racket/ball velocity. Moreover, the duration of the serve phases was in line with those reported by the literature [24], and remained similar in the two racket conditions. The similarities in velocities and phase durations imply that the kinematic patterns remained stable whatever the racket used in the tennis serve. Furthermore, the peak normalized moments (Table 1) were close to those reported by Elliott et al. [10] for peak shoulder internal rotation, elbow varus and flexion normalized moments, while they remained well below those of Martin et al.'s study [6]. For the other orientations and joints, our moment values are difficult to compare to those of the literature. Firstly, in accordance with the recommendations of

Table 1. Mean (± Standard Error) peak shoulder, elbow and wrist normalized moments (Nm) for rackets with low (I_L) and high (I_H) polar moment of inertia during the three phases of the tennis serve, with * for significant difference at $p \leq 0.05$, and ** for significant difference at $p \leq 0.01$.

		Cocking		Forward Swing		Follow-through	
		I_L	I_H	I_L	I_H	I_L	I_H
Shoulder	Flexion	2.8±0.4	2.8±0.4	5.2±0.7	5.4±0.7	1.2±0.4	1.0±0.3
	Extension	**0.8±0.4**	**1.5±0.5****	7.6±0.9	7.9±0.8	7.7±1.0	7.6±0.8
	Adduction	1.6±0.5	1.5±0.3	6.1±0.7	5.9±0.7	**3.4±0.6**	**2.5±0.5***
	Abduction	**2.3±0.5**	**4.0±0.8***	2.7±0.3	2.3±0.4	4.7±0.5	4.2±0.4
	Internal rotation	4.3±0. 2	4.2±0.2	5.8±0.3	5.9±0.3	1.6±0.4	1.0±0.6
	External rotation	0.7±0.2	1.0±0.4	1.9±0.3	1.9±0.3	4.3±0.7	3.6±0.2
Elbow	Flexion	0.8±0.1	1.1±0.2	1.6±0.5	1.2±0.5	2.2±0.4	1.9±0.3
	Extension	**1.5±0.3**	**1.7±0.2****	1.8±0.2	1.9±0.2	1.6±0.4	1.2±0.2
	Varus	4.4±0.3	4.2±0.2	6.0±0.4	6.1±0.4	1.0±0.3	0.6±0.3
	Valgus	**0.9±0.3**	**2.0±0.6***	4.9±0.6	5.1±0.6	5.3±0.5	5.3±0.5
	Pronation	0.9±0.1	0.9±0.1	1.2±0.2	1.0±0.2	**1.1±0.2**	**0.7±0.1***
	Supination	**0.6±0.1**	**1.1±0.2***	0.8±0.2	0.7±0.2	1.2±0.2	1.0±0.1
Wrist	Flexion	1.6±0.3	1.6±0.4	2.9±0.5	2.9±0.5	0.9±0.2	0.5±0.1
	Extension	0.5±0.1	1.1±0.4	**2.8±0.6**	**3.3±0.6***	3.6±0.4	3.9±0.4
	Radial deviation	1.5±0.3	1.8±0.3	**2.1±0.4**	**2.5±0.4****	2.0±0.3	1.8±0.5
	Ulnar deviation	0.8±0.1	0.9±0.1	1.0±0.3	0.7±0.4	1.3±0.2	1.1±0.2
	Internal rotation	1.6±0.1	1.7±0.2	2.1±0.1	2.2±0.1	1.2±0.2	1.1±0.3
	External rotation	0.5±0.1	0.9±0.3	0.2±0.2	0.3±0.2	**1.5±0.2**	**1.2±0.1***

Table 2. Mean (± Standard Error) shoulder, elbow and wrist normalized positive and negative powers (W) for rackets with low (I_L) and high (I_H) polar moment of inertia during the three phases of the tennis serve, with * for significant difference at $p \leq 0.05$, and ** for significant difference at $p \leq 0.01$.

		Cocking		Forward swing		Follow-through	
		I_L	I_H	I_L	I_H	I_L	I_H
Shoulder	positive power	3.4±0.7	3.6±0.8	27.7±6.3	26.8±5.6	16.7±0.9	16.8±1.5
	negative power	1.3±0.1	1.5±0.1	23.5±2.9	24.6±3.5	6.6±2.2	4.5±1.2
Elbow	positive power	0.8±0.2	0.9±0.2	9.2±2.5	9.8±2.6	3.5±0.7	4.2±1.0
	negative power	1.1±0.1	1.2±0.1	**17.9±1.8**	**19.6±1.9****	5.7±0.8	4.6±0.9
Wrist	positive power	0.8±0.1	0.9±0.2	23.7±3.2	25.4±1.6	12.5±1.2	12.8±0.5
	negative power	0.2±0.1	0.2±0.1	**22.6±2.9**	**24.2±2.7***	2.1±0.5	1.2±0.3

Bonnefoy et al. [17], the peak shoulder moments in this study were expressed using a different decomposition (XZY) to that used by Elliott et al. [10]. This methodological choice facilitated the clinical and anatomical interpretation of the joint moment components [25,26]. Secondly, previous work delimited the analyses of net joint moments to a particular axis, joint or phase of the serve. In order to provide a more comprehensive description of the effects of the racket's polar moment of inertia on upper limb loading, it was necessary to examine all of the degrees of freedom at each joint throughout the entire duration of the service action. As such, the Principal Components Analyses were helpful to find the axes, joints and serves phases of interest.

The tennis serve has been known to cause both pain and injury to tennis players of all levels of skill [27]. This potential for musculoskeletal injury is related to the power and acceleration required in a very short time [11], the repetitive nature of these overhead mechanics [10], and the considerable joint loads, especially at the upper limb joints [10,11,28]. Net joint moments during the tennis serve are used to predict potentially injurious behavior by associating peak joint moments and overuse injury [6]. It might appear obvious that racket characteristics, especially the polar moment of inertia, are key to minimizing peak joint moments, and thus reducing the potential for injury of the tennis serve; yet no previous study has focused on the effects of the racket polar moment of inertia during the tennis serve. During the terminal point of the cocking phase, shoulder external rotation is driven by inertial lag and stores elastic energy in the passive structures of the shoulder [7]. The elbow flexes to position the racket parallel to and pointing down the spine. This phase is known to generate high values for shoulder internal rotation and horizontal adduction moments, elbow varus and wrist flexion moments [6,10]. Here, these particular joint moments were unaffected by changes in the polar moment of inertia of the tennis racket. However, the increased polar moment of inertia resulted in larger shoulder extension and abduction moments, as well as elbow extension and supination moments (Table 1). It could therefore be hypothesized that these increased joint moments and the large number of repetitions may contribute to muscular fatigue. In particular, when serving with a racket characterized by a high polar moment of inertia, the shoulder abduction moment could apply additional loads on the supraspinatus muscle in order to abduct the upper limb, and thus to maintain the congruence between the humeral head and glenoid cavity of the scapula. When extended to the whole of the upper limb, the increase in mean joint power coupled with an increased polar moment of inertia could reflect an additional muscular demand so as to maintain the racket in optimal position during the cocking phase (Table 2). However, as no significant differences were observed between the two rackets, this hypothesis remains to be confirmed. During the cocking phase, the elbow valgus moment also appears to increase with the racket's polar moment of inertia (Table 1). This may apply additional internal loads on the osseous and ligamentous structures of the elbow joint, which could contribute to the abutment of the posteromedial olecranon on the medial wall of the olecranon fossa. Specifically, the increased polar moment of inertia of the racket could exacerbate valgus extension overload mechanisms, known to lead to medial elbow injuries [29].

During the forward swing phase of the tennis serve, the dominant upper arm internally rotates vigorously [10], then the forearm pronates and finally the wrist flexes prior to impact [7]. The acceleration of the racket head requires large internal rotation and horizontal adduction moments at the shoulder joint, predominantly generated by the pectoralis major and rotator cuff muscles [11]. Additionally, the high elbow valgus moment can induce damage of the ulnar collateral ligament [11]. At the wrist, most pain occurs because of the repetitive loads induced by internal/external rotation moments [6]. Interestingly, our results showed that the peak moments at the shoulder and elbow joints during the forward swing phase of the serve were unaffected by the increased racket polar moment of inertia (Table 1). However, the increased polar moment of inertia generated significantly higher loads on wrist extension and radial deviation components (Table 1), as well as greater negative joint power at the elbow and wrist (Table 2). This implies that the increase in polar moment of inertia of the tennis racket placed greater demands on the extensor and abductor muscles in order to counteract the movements of wrist flexion and ulnar deviation. A higher polar moment of inertia may then be expected to contribute to overuse injuries in the wrist extensor muscles during the forward swing phase of the tennis serve, which is known to cause lateral epicondylitis pain [11]. Finally, during the follow-through phase of the tennis serve, the racket continues the up- and out- trajectory before it swings across the body [27] to decelerate the shoulder internal rotation, elbow extension and pronation. The deceleration of the racket-upper limb complex generates high horizontal abduction [6] and external rotation moments [22] at the shoulder joint, and places large loads on the rotator cuff muscles in order to maintain the humeral head in the glenoid cavity [11]. According to our results (Table 1), these moment components remained similar in both racket conditions. Additionally, an increased polar moment was associated with decreased peak shoulder adduction and elbow pronation moments, suggesting a reduced need for these deceleration actions. As this reduction was not concomitant with decreased joint power (Table 2) and as the wrist external rotation moment was also reduced in the condition featuring a high polar moment of inertia, it could be hypothesized that increasing the polar moment of inertia may reduce the loads applied on the osseous and ligamentous structures of the upper limb during the follow-through phase of the tennis serve. However, this beneficial effect should be nuanced, because the peak moment values attained during the follow-through remained low compared with those observed during the cocking and forward swing phases (Table 1).

This study presents some limitations that warrant discussion. Aside from the traditional issues relating to motion capture, the small sample size limits the immediate generalizability of these findings, which are also limited to male players and cannot be extended to specific serve types. Another limitation is the lack of markers on the player's lower limbs, making it impossible to break the cocking phase down into a preparation phase and a lower limb propulsion phase. However, the findings remain informative, as this study is the first to examine how the racket's polar moment of inertia affects upper extremity loading in tennis players.

The current findings suggest that a racket with a larger polar moment of inertia induces greater loads on five peak moment components at the shoulder and elbow joints during the cocking phase, and on two components at the wrist joint during the forward swing phase, of the tennis serve. Conversely, a higher racket polar moment of inertia resulted here in reduced loads on three moment components at the three joints of the dominant upper limb that are associated with decelerating the upper limb – racket complex during the follow-through phase of the tennis serve. Although the etiology of overuse injuries is multifactorial, the findings of this study suggest that an increased racket polar moment of inertia could contribute to excessive joint moments in the upper limb joints during the tennis serve, in particular during the cocking and forward swing phases. Therefore, although rackets with a larger polar moment of inertia may better accommodate off-center impacts, they appear more likely to increase loading at the upper extremity joints and increase injury risk therein. Future work should attempt to replicate and confirm these findings, extending the investigation to the temporal patterns of peak moment occurrence. It would also be interesting to investigate whether modifications to either (1) other racket parameters (e.g. mass, strings, or other inertial characteristics), or (2) mechanics (e.g. lower limb drive, grip, ball toss etc.) can offset the increases in upper extremity loading noted in this study.

Supporting Information

File S1 Raw data.

File S2 Results of Principal Component Analysis for peak shoulder abduction/adduction, shoulder internal/external rotation, elbow flexion/extension, elbow varus/valgus, elbow pronation/supination, wrist flexion/extension, wrist radial/ulnar deviation, wrist internal/external rotation normalized moments, as well as mean shoulder, elbow and wrist joint power.

Author Contributions

Conceived and designed the experiments: IR TC LC PM RD. Performed the experiments: IR TC LC PM RD. Analyzed the data: IR TC LC PM RD. Contributed reagents/materials/analysis tools: IR TC LC PM RD. Wrote the paper: IR TC LC PM RD.

References

1. Kotze J, Mitchell SR, Rothberg SJ (2000) The role of the racket in high-speed tennis serves. Sports Eng 3: 67–84.
2. Miller S (2006) Modern tennis rackets, balls, and surfaces. Br J Sports Med 40: 401–405.
3. Cross R (2001) Customising a tennis racket by adding weight. Sports Eng 4: 1–14.
4. Creveaux T, Dumas R, Chèze L, Macé P, Rogowski I (2013) Influence of racket polar moment on joint loads during tennis forehand drive. Comput Meth Biomech Biomed Eng 16: S99–101.
5. Morris M, Jobe F, Perry J, Pink M, Healy B (1989) Electromyographic analysis of elbow function in tennis players. Am J Sports Med 17: 241–247.
6. Martin C, Bideau B, Ropars M, Delamarche P, Kulpa R (2013) Upper limb joint kinetic analysis during tennis serve: Assessment of competitive level on efficiency and injury risks. Scand j Med Sci Sports DOI: 10.1111/sms.12043.
7. Bahamonde RE (2000) Changes in angular momentum during the tennis serve. J Sports Sci 18: 579–592.
8. Durovic N, Lozovina V, Mrduljas D (2008) New biomechanical model for tennis serve. Acta Kinesiol 2: 45–49.
9. Marshall RN, Elliott BC (2000) Long-axis rotation: the missing link in proximal-to-distal segmental sequencing. J Sports Sci 18: 247–254.
10. Elliott B, Fleisig G, Nicholls R, Escamilla R (2003) Technique effects on upper limb loading in the tennis serve. J Sci Med Sport 6: 76–87.
11. Abrams GD, Sheets AL, Andriacchi TP, Safran MR (2011) Review of tennis serve motion analysis and the biomechanics of three serve types with implications for injury. Sports Biomech 10: 378–390.
12. Wu G, van der Helm FCT, Veeger HEJ, Makhsous M, Van Roy P, et al. (2005) ISB recommendation on definitions of joint coordinate systems of various joints for the reporting of human joint motion–Part II: shoulder, elbow, wrist and hand. J Biomech. 38: 981–992.
13. Creveaux T, Dumas R, Hautier C, Macé P, Chèze L, et al. (2013) Joint kinetics to assess the influence of the racket on a tennis player's shoulder. J Sport Sci Med 12: 259–266.
14. Dumas R, Aissaoui R, de Guise JA (2004) A 3D generic inverse dynamic method using wrench notation and quaternion algebra. Comput Methods Biomech Biomed Eng 7: 159–166.
15. Dumas R, Cheze L, Verriest JP (2007) Adjustments to McConville et al. and Young et al. body segment inertial parameters. J Biomech 40: 543–553.

16. Desroches G, Cheze L, Dumas R (2010) Expression of joint moment in the joint coordinate system. J Biomech Eng 132: 114503.
17. Bonnefoy-Mazure A, Slawinski J, Riquet A, Lévêque J-M, Miller C, et al. (2010) Rotation sequence is an important factor in shoulder kinematics. Application to the elite players' flat serves. J Biomech 43: 2022–2025.
18. Baker R (2003) Letter to the editor. J Biomech 36; 300–302.
19. Ryu R, McCormick J, Jobe F, Moynes D, Antonelli D (1988) An electromyographic analysis of shoulder function in tennis player. American Journal of Sports Medicine 16: 481–485.
20. Kettaneh N, Berglund A, Wold S (2005) PCA and PLS with very large data sets. Comput Stat Data Anal 1: 69–85.
21. Cohen J (1988) Statistical Power Analysis for the Behavioral Sciences. Hillsdale, NJ: Lawrence Erlbaum Associates. 567 p.
22. Reid M, Elliott BC, Alderson J (2007) Shoulder joint loading in the high performance flat and kick tennis serves. Br J Sports Med 41: 884–889.
23. Sheets A, Abrams G, Corazza S, Safran M, Andriacchi T (2011) Kinematics differences between the flat, kick, and slice serves measured using a markerless motion capture method. Ann Biomed Eng 39: 3011–3020.
24. Seeley M, Uhl T, McCrory J, McGinn P, Kibler B, et al. (2008) A comparison of muscle activations during traditional and abbreviated tennis serves. Sports Biomech 7: 248–259.
25. Desroches G, Dumas R, Pradon D, Vaslin P, Lepoutre F-X, et al. (2010) Upper limb joint dynamics during manual wheelchair propulsion. Clin Biomech 25: 299–306.
26. Morrow MM, Hurd WJ, Kaufman KR, An KN (2009) Upper-limb joint kinetics expression during wheelchair propulsion. J Rehabil Res Dev 46: 939–44.
27. Elliott B (1988) Biomechanics of the serve in tennis. A biomedical perspective. Sports Med 6: 285–294.
28. Bahamonde RE (2005) Review of the biomechanical function of the elbow joint during tennis strokes. Int SportMed J 6: 42–63.
29. Aguinaldo AL, Chambers H (2009) Correlation of throwing mechanics with elbow valgus load in adult baseball pitchers. Am J Sports Med 37: 2043–2048.

Hamstring Muscle Fatigue and Central Motor Output during a Simulated Soccer Match

Paul W. M. Marshall[1]*, Ric Lovell[1], Gitte K. Jeppesen[2], Kristoffer Andersen[2], Jason C. Siegler[1]

1 School of Science and Health, University of Western Sydney, Sydney, Australia, **2** School of Medicine and Health, Aalborg University, Aalborg, Denmark

Abstract

Purpose: To examine changes in hamstring muscle fatigue and central motor output during a 90-minute simulated soccer match, and the concomitant changes in hamstring maximal torque and rate of torque development.

Method: Eight amateur male soccer players performed a 90-minute simulated soccer match, with measures performed at the start of and every 15-minutes during each half. Maximal torque (Nm) and rate of torque development (RTD; $Nm.s^{-1}$) were calculated from maximal isometric knee flexor contractions performed at 10° of flexion. Hamstring peripheral fatigue was assessed from changes in the size and shape of the resting twitch (RT). Hamstring central motor output was quantified from voluntary activation (%) and normalized biceps femoris (BF) and medial hamstrings (MH) electromyographic amplitudes (EMG/M).

Results: Maximal torque was reduced at 45-minutes by 7.6±9.4% ($p<0.05$). RTD in time intervals of 0–25, 0–50, and 0–75 ms post-contraction onset were reduced after 15-minutes in the first-half between 29.6 to 46.2% ($p<0.05$), and were further reduced at the end of the second-half ($p<0.05$). Maximal EMG/M was reduced for biceps femoris only concomitant to the time-course of reductions in maximal torque ($p = 0.007$). The rate of EMG rise for BF and MH was reduced in early time periods (0–75 ms) post-contraction onset ($p<0.05$). No changes were observed for the size and shape of the RT, indicating no hamstring peripheral fatigue.

Conclusion: Centrally mediated reductions in maximal torque and rate of torque development provide insight into factors that may explain hamstring injury risk during soccer. Of particular interest were early reductions during the first-half of hamstring rate of torque development, and the decline in maximal EMG/M of biceps femoris in the latter stages of the half. These are important findings that may help explain why the hamstrings are particularly vulnerable to strain injury during soccer.

Editor: François Hug, The University of Queensland, Australia

Funding: This study was supported by the NSW Sports Research and Injury Prevention Scheme. http://www.sportinginjuries.nsw.gov.au/ The funders had no role in study design, data collection and analysis, decision to publish, or preparation of the manuscript.

Competing Interests: The authors have declared that no competing interests exist.

* Email: p.marshall@uws.edu.au

Introduction

Examining mechanisms that contribute to muscular fatigue can provide insight into limitations to human sport and exercise performance, as well as the potential causation of musculoskeletal injuries in which fatigue is cited as a primary contributory factor [1–3]. Muscular fatigue is often identified as a risk factor linked to the high incidence of hamstring strain injuries observed across all levels of soccer [4–6], with injury typically observed in the latter stages of training and each half of competitive matches [1–3]. Studies have reported reductions in knee flexor maximal torque during and after actual and simulated soccer match play [7–10], with reductions most pronounced in the latter stages of each half [8,10]. No study has examined whether hamstring fatigue during soccer is mediated by peripheral or central mechanisms.

Mechanisms of fatigue are generally considered from peripheral factors associated with maintaining muscle contraction (e.g. blood flow, oxygen delivery, contraction efficiency), and factors associated with maintaining central motor output to the muscle from the nervous system (e.g. cortical and motoneuron output) [11,12]. Two studies have examined peripheral muscle fatigue and central motor output 30 to 40 minutes following soccer match play [13,14]. Both studies reported peripheral muscle fatigue, measured from reductions in the resting twitch elicited from stimulation of the quadriceps [14] and calf muscles [13] respectively, and reduced central motor output measured from declines in voluntary activation. However, neither study performed measurements within the time-course of the match to examine the interaction between peripheral muscle fatigue and central motor output.

Recent evidence from prolonged locomotor activity (e.g. cycling) suggests that increased peripheral feedback into the nervous system (e.g. group III/IV afferent feedback) provides an inhibitory stimulus that reduces central motor output to the muscle during exercise in order to restrict peripheral muscle fatigue and maintain performance [15,16]. Reduced central motor output to the hamstrings during soccer match play in order to offset peripheral muscle fatigue may explain reductions in knee flexor torque at the end of each half. However, an important consequence of any reductions in central motor output to the hamstrings is the likelihood of concomitant reductions in the ability to rapidly generate knee flexor torque [17].

Reductions in rate of torque development may be important for understanding hamstring injury risk during soccer, particularly at the end of each half. Knee angular velocities during sprinting have been estimated as high as 600 to 700°.s^{-1}, thus necessitating rapid hamstring torque development to decelerate knee extension during the terminal swing phase [18–20] where hamstring strain injury risk is greatest [21,22]. To our knowledge one study has reported reduced hamstring rate of torque development following soccer match play with concomitant reductions in the hamstring electromyogram as an estimate of central motor output [9]. However this study [9] did not use stimulation based methods to allow examination of twitch contractile properties as a measure of peripheral muscle fatigue that may also have contributed to declines in hamstring explosive torque [23]. Moreover, this study [9] did not profile the time-course of the change in hamstring rapid torque development during the soccer match. Examining the time-course of changes in rate of torque development during a simulated soccer match may provide greater insight why the hamstrings are vulnerable to fatigue associated injury in the latter stages of each half.

Therefore we designed this study to address critical gaps in the literature pertaining to the understanding of hamstring muscle fatigue and central motor output during soccer and the concomitant changes in hamstring maximal torque and rate of torque development. We used a soccer-specific aerobic field test (SAFT^{90} [8]) to replicate the distances and intensity distribution of elite level players during match play. This provided a controlled experimental context compared to open-field match play where within-game measures are difficult to perform [8], and the within- and between-match locomotor profile is highly variable [24,25]. We hypothesized that reductions in hamstring central motor output would occur prior to peripheral muscle fatigue during the SAFT^{90}. Moreover we hypothesized that reductions in hamstring central motor output would contribute to reductions in both maximal torque and rate of torque development, with the greatest reductions exhibited in the latter stages of each half.

Materials and Methods

Subjects

Participants received both verbal and written information concerning the experiment, and all participants gave their written informed consent prior to testing. The study was approved by the University of Western Sydney human research ethics committee, and carried out in accordance with the declaration of Helsinki. Eight healthy male amateur soccer players (age; 22.4 years±4.8, height; 181.2 cm±6.3, body mass; 76 kg±9.9) without any previous hamstring injuries within the last 6 months, participated in the study. The study was carried out during the off-season. On average, the players weekly amount of training during the off-season was 5.1±1.9 h, and included running and strength training.

General procedures

Participants reported to the temperature controlled laboratory on two occasions where they took part in a familiarization session and one experimental session, which were separated by a minimum of two days. In the 24 h period prior to the testing session participants performed no vigorous exercise or exercise they were unaccustomed to, and refrained from consuming any caffeine or alcohol. Additionally, participants were told to be hydrated upon arrival, and not to consume large quantities of food within 2 h prior to testing. At a preliminary visit to the laboratory, participants were thoroughly familiarized with procedures used to assess knee flexor maximal voluntary isometric torque (isokinetic dynamometer, KinCom 125, Version 5.32, Chattanooga, USA), and peripheral muscle fatigue and central motor output based on the interpolated twitch technique. Participants were also familiarized with the 90-minutes soccer-specific aerobic field test (SAFT^{90}), as they completed one 15-minute segment of the protocol [8].

In the experimental session participants completed the SAFT^{90}, during which maximal voluntary torque (MVT) measurements with supramaximal stimulation were obtained prior to SAFT^{90} (T_0), and every 15-minutes during each half of the protocol (T_{15}, T_{30}, T_{45} during each half), in addition to a measurement at the end of half-time. The half-time interval was conducted as a passive 15-minute rest and participants remained seated throughout the break. During the experimental session participants were allowed to drink water ad libitum before, at half-time, and after the SAFT^{90}. The SAFT^{90} is based on time-motion analysis data from English Championship level match play acquired during the 2007 season [8], and simulates the activity demands and physiological responses of soccer match play [10,26]. Players navigate around a 20 m agility course (Figure 1) in an intermittent fashion via standing (0 km.h^{-1}), walking (~5.5 km.h^{-1}), jogging (~10.7 km.h^{-1}), striding (~15 km.h^{-1}) or sprinting (Maximal effort). The players cover 11.1 km in total, 18.5% of this distance (2.04 km) is performed at high-speed (≥15 km.h^{-1}) with 1269 changes in speed (every 4.3 s), and 888 changes in direction (180 degrees) and 444 cutting manoeuvres over the 90 minutes (1332 directional changes). The protocol is divided into equivalent 15-minute activity profiles and was performed on an indoor running surface. The type of movement activity and intensity is controlled using verbal signals from an audio MP3 file [8]. Before commencing the SAFT^{90} participants performed a 15-minute standardized warm-up protocol, which consisted of 12 different soccer specific warm-up exercises. After the warm-up participants rested for 12-minutes before commencing the SAFT^{90}, to resemble the pre-match routine of a professional soccer match [27]. Sprint performance was assessed (Swift, Speedlight, Australia) as the average of three maximal 10 m sprints with a 3 m rolling start performed within each 15-minute block of the SAFT^{90}.

Maximal voluntary torque (MVT)

MVT with superimposed supramaximal stimulation was measured at the start of each half, and at 15-minute time intervals during the SAFT^{90}. Prior to the start of the first-half, two baseline maximal contractions (T_0) were performed with 1-minute rest between attempts prior to the 15-minute standardized warm-up protocol. The baseline trial with the highest torque was used for data analysis purposes as the start of the first-half. During all maximal contractions, surface electromyographic (EMG) data were simultaneously recorded.

All voluntary and evoked contractions were performed with the subject lying prone on an adjustable bed. Contractions were performed on the right leg in 10° knee flexion (0° corresponding to

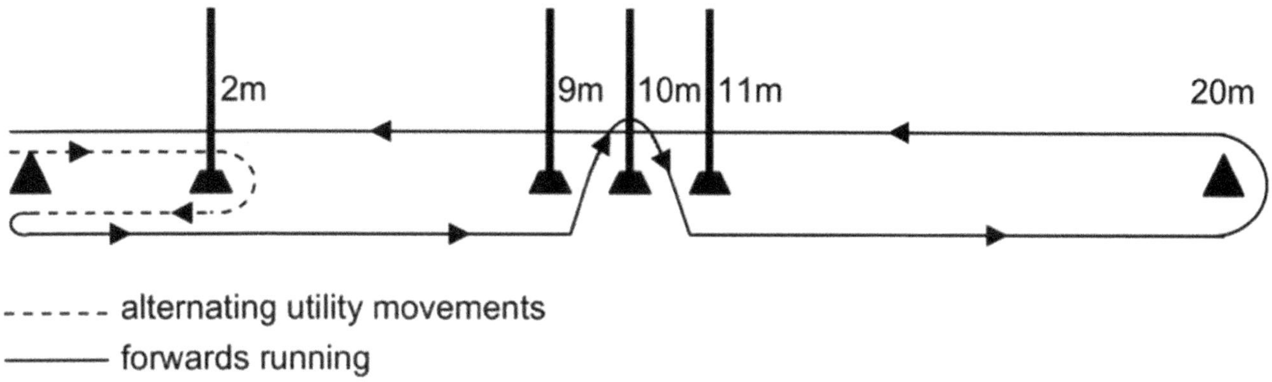

Figure 1. Schematic representation of the SAFT^{90} multidirectional running course.

full knee extension). The 10° knee flexion angle was selected to provide measurement at an extended muscle length where injury is typically reported to occur during the swing phase of sprinting [21,22]. The centre of rotation of the dynamometer lever arm was aligned with the femoral condyle of the right knee. The lever arm of the dynamometer was firmly strapped to the lower leg approximately 2 cm superior to the lateral malleolus. Participants were firmly strapped across the hip during contractions to restrict movement. Torque signals were recorded at 2000 Hz using an analog to digital converter (Powerlab 16/35, ADI instruments, Australia; 16-bit analog to digital conversion), and all measurements were corrected for the gravitational effect of the limb. Torque signals were smoothed during offline analysis by a 4th order digital 10 Hz low-pass filter. Each contraction was sustained for 3–4 s. Participants were instructed to flex their knee "as fast and forceful as possible", and strong verbal encouragement was provided by two investigators during each trial. Prior to baseline measurements (T_0), participants performed two sub-maximal contractions each at 25, 50 and 75% of self-perceived MVT. During the SAFT^{90} MVT was always measured within 30 s of completing each 15-minute segment.

Electromyography

Hamstrings electromyograms (EMG) were recorded from the right biceps femoris (BF) and medial hamstrings (MH) using pairs of Ag/AgCl surface electrodes (Maxsensor, Medimax Global, Australia). BF and MH electrodes (10 mm diameter, 10 mm inter-electrode distance) were applied to each muscle after careful skin preparation including removal of excess hair, abrasion with fine sandpaper and cleaning the area with isopropyl alcohol swabs. Placement over BF and MH was in accordance with previous recommendations [28]. The superior electrode was placed longitudinally 35% along a line from the ischial tuberosity to the lateral aspect of the popliteal cavity and 36% along a line from the ischial tuberosity to the medial side of the popliteal cavity for BF and MH respectively. A ground electrode (20 mm contact diameter) was placed on the right fibula head after careful skin preparation. Electrodes were firmly taped to the participant to ensure they remained in place during the SAFT^{90}. EMG signals were recorded using the ML138 BioAmp (common mode rejection ratio >85 dB at 50 Hz, input impedance 200 MΩ) with 16-bit analog-to-digital conversion, sampled at 2,000 Hz (ADI instruments, Sydney, Australia). Raw signals were filtered with a fourth-order Bessel filter between 20 and 500 Hz.

Hamstring muscle stimulation

Direct muscle stimulation was applied to the hamstrings with surface-stimulating electrodes constructed in the laboratory from aluminum foil, and coated with conduction gel. The width of the stimulating electrodes was 4 cm, and the length (range 11 to 15 cm for cathode, 6 to 8 cm for anode) was sufficient to encase the width of the muscle of both BF and MH. The anode was placed just superior to the popliteal fossa, and the cathode was placed beneath the gluteal fold. Stimulating electrodes were carefully taped down during the SAFT^{90}. Stimulation was delivered by a high-voltage stimulator (Digitimer DS7AH, Welwyn Garden City, UK), and consisted of a doublet using two 400-V rectangular pulses (pulse duration 1 ms) with an inter-pulse duration of 10 ms (100 Hz stimulation). During each experimental session, stimulation was initially delivered while participants lay passive and relaxed on the bed, in order to establish the stimulation intensity used during testing. Current was gradually increased in 10 mA increments until a plateau in twitch torque and maximal M-waves (M_{max}) for BF and MH were achieved. M-wave amplitude was calculated from the peak-to-peak amplitude of the first evoked M-wave in the EMG signals elicited following stimulation after initial bandpass filtering only (figure 2). This intensity was then used to establish the supramaximal stimulation intensity (130%) that was applied during all maximal contractions in the experimental session (average intensity 176.4 mA±26.9, range; 156–234 mA; between-session reliability for stimulus intensity ICC r-value = 0.98).

For the interpolated twitch technique, one doublet was evoked and superimposed on the maximal contraction when torque had reached a visible plateau. One potentiated doublet was evoked 3–4 s after the maximal contraction was stopped and the participant was relaxed to elicit the resting potentiated twitch (RT). The superimposed twitch (SIT) was calculated as the peak twitch torque in the time period immediately post stimulation subtracted from the average torque 100 ms prior to stimulation. The torque trace resolution was increased to a time epoch 100 ms prior and up to 250 ms post stimulation for careful inspection of a visible evoked twitch as compared to a normal increase in voluntary torque. The SIT was always calculated manually from careful selection and inspection of the respective time periods before and after stimulation. Peak torque of the potentiated twitch was recorded (RT). Voluntary activation (VA) was calculated according to the following equation: $VA\ (\%) = [1-(SIT/RT)] \times 100$.

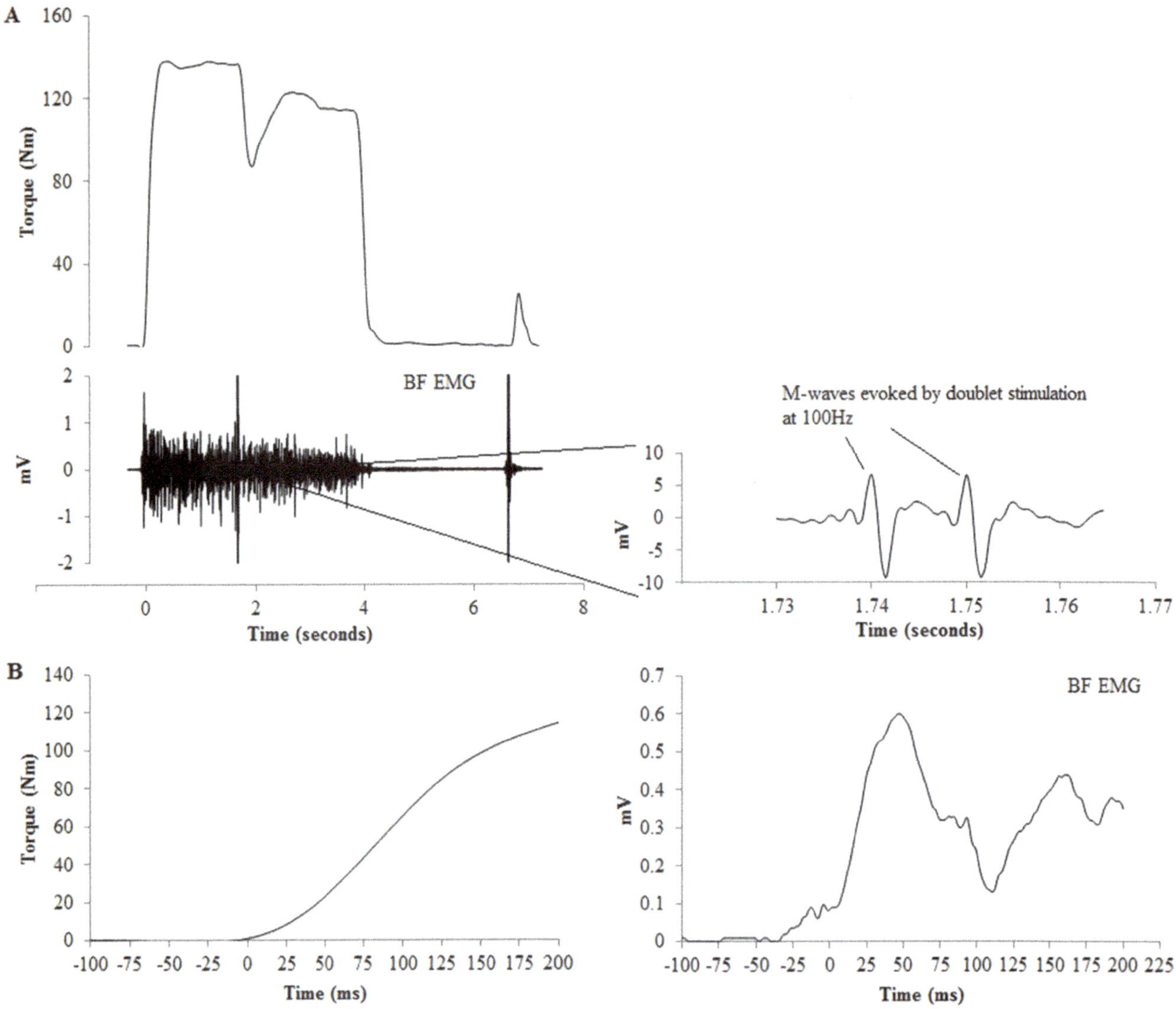

Figure 2. A (top trace), torque and raw electromyography signals recorded during a maximal isometric contraction of the hamstrings. BF, biceps femoris. Time = 0 corresponds to the onset of torque as determined by the integrated profile method. Also displayed are the two evoked M-waves during the maximal contraction, with the peak-to-peak amplitude of the first M-wave calculated for data analysis. B (bottom trace) are the torque and filtered EMG signals (4th order 100 Hz low pass Savitzky-Golay filter) for the same trial as A, in the time period −100 to + 200 ms around contraction onset.

Data analysis

The onsets of the torque and EMG signals were determined using the integrated profile (IP) method [29]. Onsets were identified within a physiologically relevant window from 75 ms prior to EMG activity (determined visually) and ending 200 ms after EMG onset. The following parameters were identified from each maximal contraction for analysis of the torque signal; 1) the maximal voluntary torque recorded during the contraction prior to stimulation (MVT, Nm), 2) rate of torque development (RTD) was calculated as the average slope of the torque-time curve (Δtorque/Δtime) during the time periods 0–25 ms, 0–50 ms, 0–75 ms and 0–100 ms post contraction onset, 3) maximum RTD was calculated as the greatest average 10 ms slope throughout the contraction.

Prior to EMG data processing signals from BF and MH were digitally smoothed and rectified using a 4th order 100 Hz low pass Savitzky-Golay filter. The following parameters were identified from each MVT trial for BF and MH EMG signals following filtering and onset identification; 1) the rate of EMG rise for BF and MH calculated from the average slope of the EMG-time curve during the time periods 0–25 ms, 0–50 ms, 0–75 ms and 0–100 ms post contraction onset, 2) maximal rate of EMG rise, calculated from the greatest average 10 ms slope throughout the initial 100 ms of the contraction, 3) maximal EMG of BF and MH was calculated as the greatest 250 ms activity throughout the maximal contraction prior to stimulation. All EMG variables were normalized to the respective M-waves elicited during each contraction for data analysis (EMG/M, %).

Using the same onset detection methodology as voluntary torque and EMG analysis, the following parameters were calculated from the resting potentiated twitch; 1) the amplitude of the peak twitch torque, 2) average slope of the torque-time curve during the time periods 0–25 ms, 0–50 ms, 0–75 ms and 0–100 ms post onset of the twitch, 3) maximal twitch RTD based on the greatest average 10 ms slope throughout the twitch, 4) the time to peak twitch, and 5) the half-relaxation time, defined as the time elapsed from the peak twitch torque to 50% peak twitch torque.

Reliability

From the familiarization session mean within-day, within-subject coefficients of variation for MVT were 2.7±1.9 (range 0.6 to 5.3), VA 1.3±0.7 (range 0.3 to 2.2), and RT 4.9±5.9 (range 0.4 to 14.1). Mean between-day, within-subject coefficients of variation for MVT were 10.4±8.8 (range 0.5 to 25.0), VA 2.4±2.0 (range 0 to 4.5), and RT 7.9±4.7 (range 1.1 to 16.6). No variable was significantly different between testing days. Within- and between-day intra-class correlation coefficients (ICC r-values) were >0.90 for all torque variables including evoked responses, and >0.85 for EMG variables.

Statistical analyses

All statistical analyses were performed using SPSS statistical software (IBM© SPSS© Statistics, version 22). Data were normally distributed, as assessed by inspection of skewness and kurtosis values and performance of Kolmogorov-Smirnov tests. Repeated-measures analysis of variance procedures (ANOVA) were used to analyze variables over time, with 4 levels of time and 2 levels of half (e.g. T_0, T_{15}, T_{30}, T_{45} for each half, where T_0 for the start of the second half was recorded at the end of half-time). In the event of a significant F ratio, post hoc comparisons were made using a Bonferroni correction. Unless otherwise stated, data are mean ± SD. Two-tailed statistical significance was accepted at $p \leq 0.05$.

Results

Maximal torque, voluntary rate of torque development, and sprint performance

For MVT, no time by half interaction was observed ($p = 0.41$). A main effect of half was observed with MVT averaged for the first half 15.7 Nm higher than the second half ($p = 0.025$). A significant time effect was observed (table 1; $p<0.001$), with MVT at 45-minutes reduced from all other time points ($p<0.05$; figure 3). The mean reduction at 45-minutes was 7.6%.

Time by half interaction effects were observed for RTD across the time intervals 0–25, 0–50, and 0–75 ms post contraction onset (table 1, figure 4; $p<0.05$). At 15-minutes in the first half, RTD 0–25, 0–50, and 0–75 ms were reduced from the start of the half by 46.2%, 37.6%, and 29.6% respectively ($p<0.05$). No reductions from the start of the half were observed at 15-minutes into the second half. At the end of each half RTD 0–25, 0–50, and 0–75 ms were reduced from the start of the half by 29.5%, 21.3%, and 16.0% respectively (table 1, $p<0.05$). No main effects of time, half, or time by half interactions were observed for RTD 0–100 ms and maximum RTD (table 1).

No main effects of time, half, or time by half interactions were observed for average sprint times within each 15-minute segment of the trial (first 15-minutes, 1.58±0.06 s; last 15-minutes of trial 1.69±0.20 s).

Central motor output

Voluntary activation at the start of the trial was 97.1±2.2%. No changes were observed for voluntary activation throughout the trial (table 2). A time effect only was observed for BF EMG/M from the maximal torque trials (figure 3; $p = 0.007$). On average BF EMG/M at 45-minutes was reduced by 20.7% from the start of each half ($p = 0.007$). In contrast no time, half, or time by half interaction effects were observed for MH EMG/M values (table 2).

For BF rate of EMG rise in the time period 0–50 ms, a significant time by half effect was observed (figure 5; $p = 0.019$). In the first half values were reduced by 66.5% at 15-minutes ($p = 0.032$), and remained reduced for the rest of the first half. No changes were observed during the second half. A main effect of time was observed for the rate of EMG rise from 0–75 ms ($p = 0.009$) and maximal BF rate of EMG rise ($p = 0.009$). The mean reduction at 45-minutes for EMG rate of rise 0–75 ms and the maximal rate were 30.4% ($p = 0.048$) and 97.9% ($p = 0.023$) respectively.

Main time effects only were observed for MH EMG rate of rise (figure 6) in time intervals 0–25 ms ($p = 0.05$) and 0–50 ms ($p = 0.027$) post-contraction onset. For 0–25 ms, the mean

Table 1. Absolute values for maximal voluntary torque (MVT) and voluntary rate of torque development (RTD) in time intervals post contraction onset throughout the simulated soccer match ($SAFT^{90}$).

		RTD ($Nm.s^{-1}$)				
First-half (minutes)	**MVT (Nm)**	**0–25 ms**	**0–50 ms**	**0–75 ms**	**0–100 ms**	**RTD Max**
0	104.8±18.1	346.7±151.3	469.8±174.9	558.9±168.9	570.1±163.4	790.4±228.3
15	103.8±16.3	177.6±124.5*†	288.8±178.5*†	391.1±218.6*†	450.9±224.2	735.9±288.4
30	101.2±14.4	214.4±108.7	325.9±139.0	427.3±154.0	484.9±152.5	741.9±188.6
45	94.1±9.7*	162.2±116.0*	260.5±155.5*	354.9±187.2*	415.2±179.1	720.1±222.3
Second-half (minutes)						
0	85.1±12.9	171.3±104.5	239.3±145.1	300.0±171.9	333.3±170.1	535.7±163.0
15	89.1±11.2	188.1±132.4	297.2±164.2	397.7±187.6	452.9±190.9	697.9±235.9
30	87.3±8.0	176.9±107.2	267.1±145.3	353.2±160.7	408.7±142.8	664.3±147.9
45	79.5±13.2*	83.5±70.2*	136.3±98.4*	199.1±121.9*	258.9±132.5	542.4±211.0

*is $p<0.05$ from the start of the half,
†is $p<0.05$ for difference between halves for the reduction from the start of the half. Data are mean ± SD.

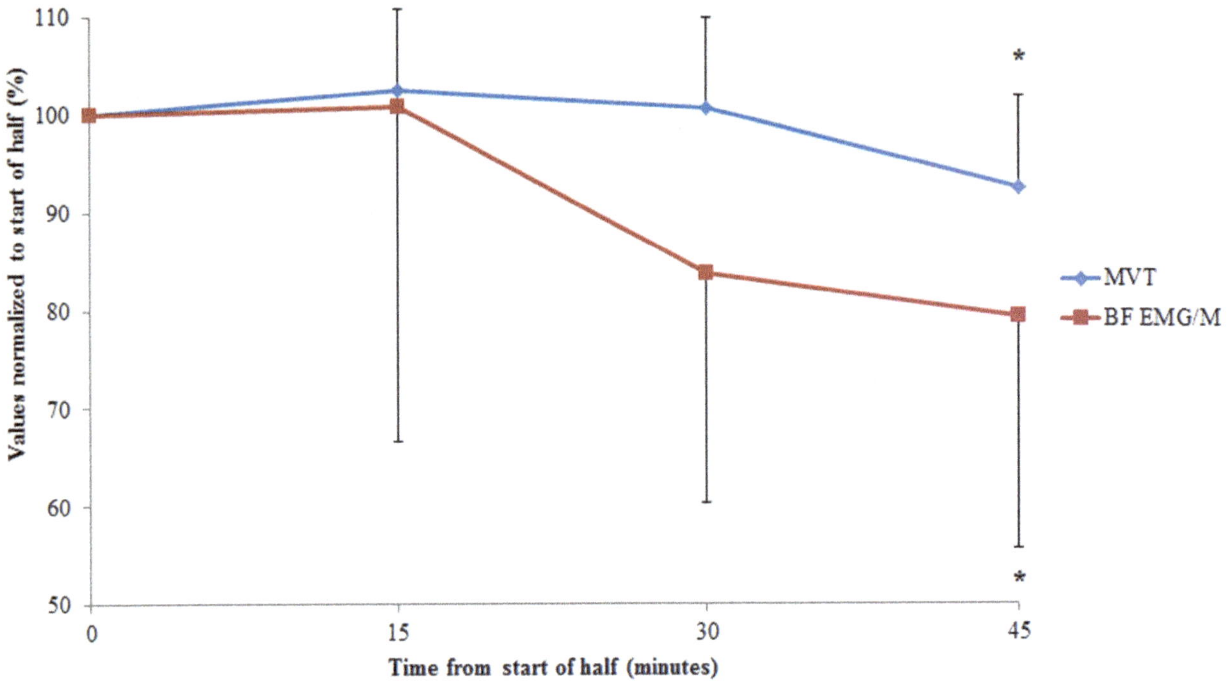

Figure 3. Changes in hamstring maximal voluntary torque (MVT) and biceps femoris (BF) EMG/M values, collapsed across each half at the different time points. Absolute data for each variable (MVT and EMG/M) are normalized to the value recorded before the start of each half. *indicates a significant reduction from the start of the half ($p<0.05$). Data are mean and SD.

reduction at 15-minutes during each half was 34.3% from the start of the half ($p=0.043$). For 0–50 ms, the mean reduction at 45-minutes was 48.6% from the start of the half ($p=0.019$).

Hamstring twitch properties

Maximal M-waves for BF and MH at the start of the trial were 18.1±1.6 mV and 17.0±2.1 mV respectively, and did not change throughout the experiment. The maximal amplitude of the resting potentiated twitch, time to peak twitch, and half-relaxation time of the twitch did not change (table 2). There were no changes observed for the RTD of the potentiated twitch in time intervals of 0–25, 0–50, 0–75, 0–100 ms, and the maximal RTD of the potentiated twitch (table 3).

Discussion

Summary of main findings

We examined changes in hamstring peripheral muscle fatigue and central motor output during a 90-minute simulated soccer match, in addition to changes in maximal torque and rate of torque development. The main results of this study were 1) on average, maximal voluntary torque decreased at the end of the half concomitant to reductions in central motor output to the biceps femoris, 2) no hamstring peripheral muscle fatigue was observed, based on the absence of changes in the size and shape of the resting twitch evoked from the hamstrings, 3) early rate of torque development (0–25, 0–50, 0–75 ms) declined after the first 15-minutes of the first-half concomitant to reduced hamstring muscle central motor output, and thereafter was reduced from the start of each half at 45-minutes.

Reduced central motor output

For the first time it has been observed that reductions in knee flexor maximal torque and rate of torque development during a simulated soccer match are associated with reduced central motor output to the hamstrings and not peripheral muscle fatigue. The findings of this study conflict with previous reports for reductions in both central motor output and the resting twitch of the quadriceps and plantarflexor muscles 30 to 40-minutes after actual soccer match play [13,14]. Differences between the studies may, in part, be explained by the use of different muscle groups, and the use of different stimulation methods.

The quadriceps and plantarflexor muscles are prime movers in knee extension and ankle plantarflexion, and thus are involved in many of the explosive movements exhibited in soccer match play (e.g. acceleration, kicking, jumping) and laboratory based simulations (e.g. acceleration, high-speed agility components, change of direction). In comparison, the hamstrings act to decelerate the forward movement of the lower leg during kicking and running motions [18–20]. Thus the functional involvement and demands placed on different muscle groups of the lower limb may explain the differences between studies, with the hamstrings lacking the overall contribution to many explosive movements required in the $SAFT^{90}$ that may contribute to peripheral muscle fatigue. Future studies should examine whether similar reductions of the peripheral quadriceps and calf twitch occur following the $SAFT^{90}$ compared to match play findings to validate the demands of the simulation performed in this study, and improve the generalizability of findings reported here.

Differences between studies in the stimulation method applied may also explain why we observed no reduction in the resting twitch. We used direct muscle stimulation to elicit twitch responses from the hamstrings, compared to direct motor nerve stimulation of the femoral [14] and posterior tibial nerves [13]. Comparison of

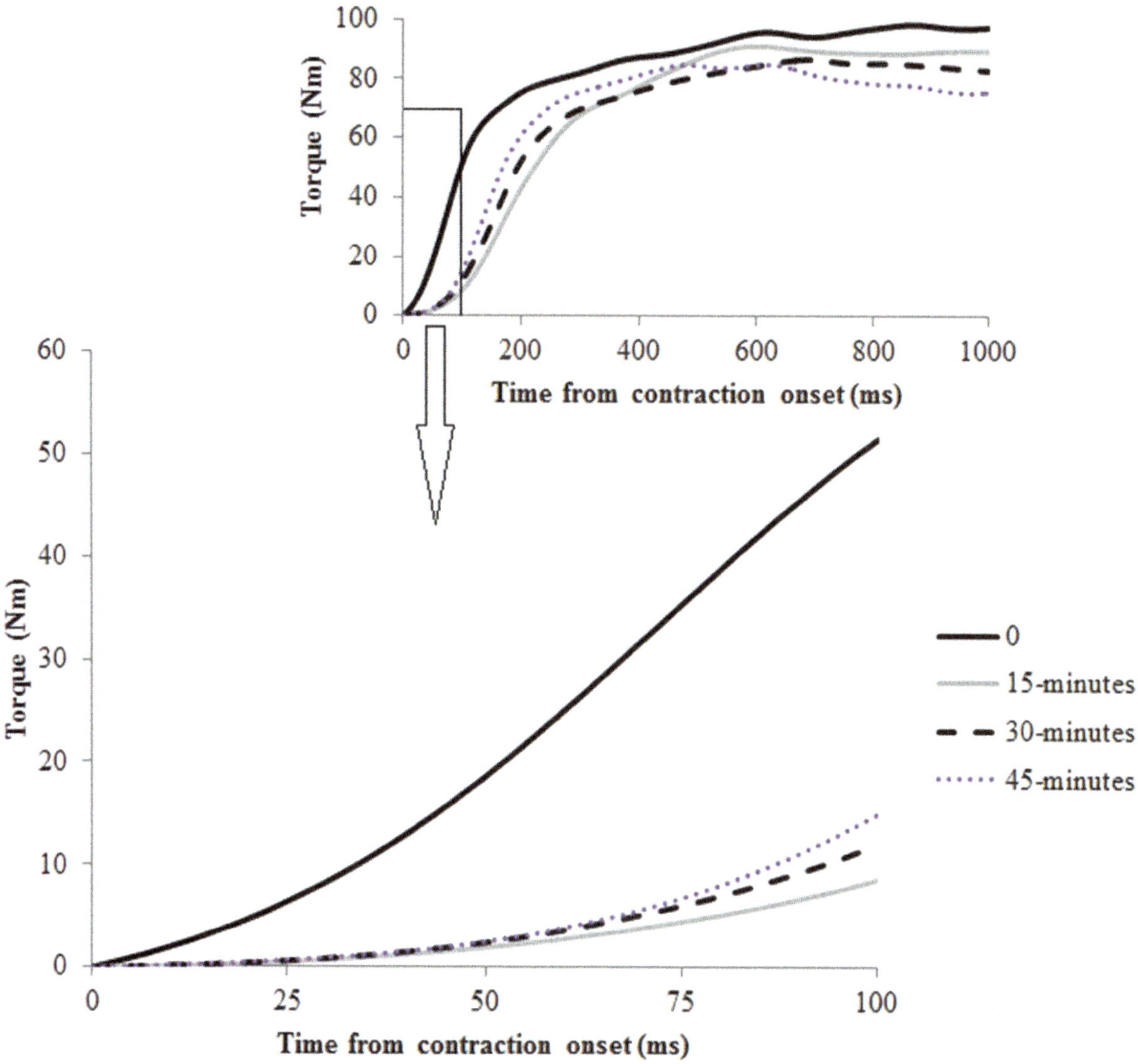

Figure 4. Single subject representation of the typical rate of torque development curves observed during the first-half of the SAFT[90]. Torque data is presented from the point of contraction onset, as defined using the integrated profile method.

voluntary activation and evoked twitch responses during maximal contractions between different stimulation methods (i.e. direct muscle vs motor nerve) revealed no differences [30], therefore we do not believe the use of direct muscle stimulation explains differences between the studies. A more plausible reason for between study differences in resting twitch changes in the frequency of stimulation used. One study reported reductions in the size and shape of evoked quadriceps twitch responses 40-minutes after soccer match play using single pulses and doublets at 10 Hz, whereas responses elicited with a doublet at 100 Hz similar to this study did not change [14]. While not explicit within the methods, it appears single pulses were used in the recent study that observed reductions in the resting twitch elicited from the calf 30-minutes following match play [13]. In contrast we only used a 100 Hz doublet to elicit twitches based on recommendations for measuring voluntary activation during maximal contractions [31,32]. The absence of a single pulse or doublet at 10 Hz means we may have profiled the high-frequency component of muscle fatigue, rather than the low-frequency component which has been previously reported following soccer match play [13,14].

An interesting finding in this study was that reductions in maximal torque at the end of each half occurred concomitant to reduced maximal biceps femoris muscle activity, but not medial hamstrings. This observation may be important because imaging studies of acute hamstring strain injuries in normal and athletic populations report that greater than 80% of injuries are from the biceps femoris [33–35]. The biceps femoris, particularly the long-head of the muscle, undergoes the greatest lengthening of all the hamstring muscles during sprinting [36]. Moreover, based on fine-wire EMG findings, the long-head of biceps femoris is more active than all the hamstring muscles at extended knee joint angles [37]. The surface site used in this study probably best represents the activity of the long-head of biceps femoris [37]. Therefore we appear to have observed a muscle specific reduction in central motor output owing to the greater demands placed on the long-head of biceps femoris during the SAFT[90] at the extended joint angle tested in this study. We are unable to identify the specific mechanism for this finding. While speculative, exercise induced muscle damage following soccer [38,39] is a stimulant for increased group III and IV afferent feedback [40,41]. Group III

Table 2. Absolute values for voluntary activation (%), biceps femoris (BF) and medial hamstrings (MH) normalized electromyograms (EMG/M, %), the amplitude of the resting potentiated twitch (RT), time to peak twitch (TPT), and half-relaxation time of the resting twitch (1/2 RT) during the SAFT[90].

First-half (minutes)	VA (%)	BF EMG/M (%)	MH EMG/M (%)	RT (Nm)	TPT (ms)	½ RT (ms)
0	97.1±2.2	5.2±1.8	4.7±2.1	26.8±5.9	110.1±8.2	63.0±11.2
15	98.0±3.2	4.2±1.5	4.9±2.4	25.3±6.6	104.9±9.2	65.0±19.5
30	98.4±2.6	3.5±0.8	4.3±2.1	25.6±6.1	108.3±11.0	68.4±20.8
45	96.5±3.5	3.6±1.2*	4.4±2.3	25.3±5.9	105.4±10.1	67.6±20.0
Second-half (minutes)						
0	97.6±3.2	3.4±1.3	4.1±2.0	23.3±5.3	102.8±10.1	65.9±14.1
15	95.7±2.4	3.7±1.3	4.2±1.7	24.6±6.5	104.0±10.6	70.3±21.7
30	96.5±3.4	3.2±1.4	4.2±2.2	24.9±6.6	105.3±13.3	69.4±22.6
45	96.8±2.9	2.9±1.1*	3.9±2.7	24.6±7.6	108.3±14.1	71.5±23.4

*is $p<0.05$ for the main effect of time for a reduction from the start of the half. Data are mean ± SD.

and IV afferent feedback is thought to provide an inhibitory stimulus to central motor output during prolonged locomotor type activity [15,16]. It may be likely that the combination of greater lengthening during sprinting and higher activity at extended knee joint angles makes the biceps femoris particularly vulnerable to exercise induced muscle damage during soccer. Future studies could examine muscle specific damage after an actual or simulated soccer match to explore the validity of this suggestion.

Rate of torque development

The results of this study support and extend previous findings for reductions in hamstring rate of torque development during soccer [9]. Reductions in early rate of torque development (0–25, 0–50, 0–75 ms) were observed after only 15-minutes of the first-half. These reductions were maintained through to the end of the second-half, where further decreases were observed. The early first-half reductions in rate of torque development were a surprising finding that do not mirror reported patterns for injury

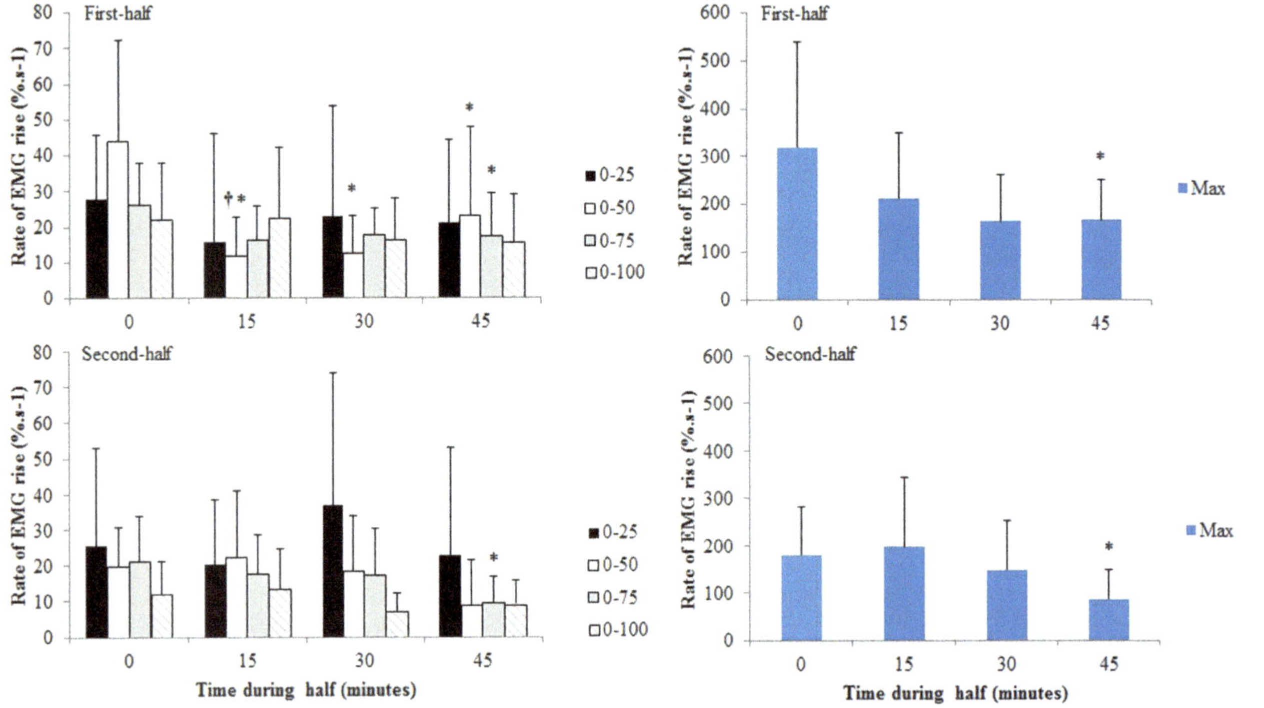

Figure 5. Rate of rise in the biceps femoris EMG signal (EMG/M, %.s^{-1}) in time intervals of 0–25, 0–50, 0–75, 0–100 ms, post contraction onset, and maximal rate of rise during the first and second half of the trial. *denotes a significant difference from the start of the half ($p<0.05$). † is $p<0.05$ for difference between halves for the reduction from the start of the half. Data are mean and SD.

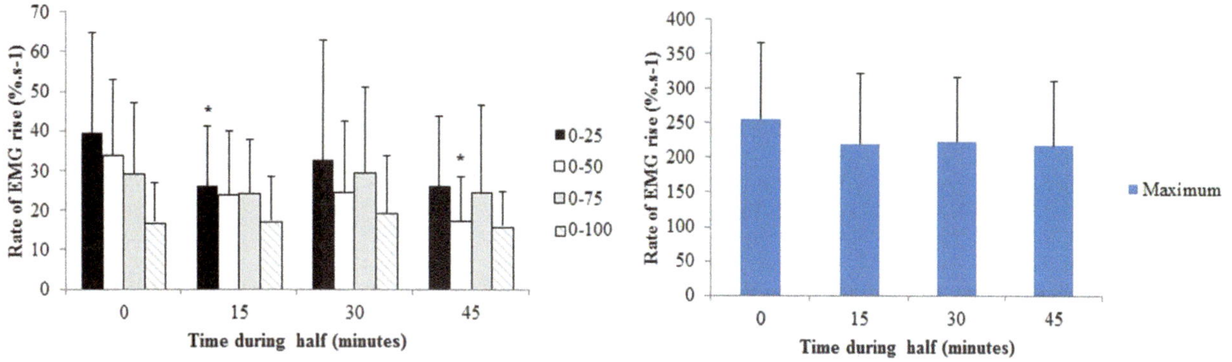

Figure 6. Rate of rise in the medial hamstrings EMG signal (EMG/M, %.s^{-1}) in time intervals of 0–25, 0–50, 0–75, 0–100 ms, post contraction onset, and maximal rate of rise at different time points during the half. Data are collapsed across the first and second half. *denotes a significant difference from the start of the half ($p<0.05$). Data are mean and SD.

occurrence in the latter stages of each half [1–3]. This finding may suggest that reductions in hamstring rate of torque development are not a predisposing factor to hamstring strain injury. Alternatively the early loss of hamstring rapid torque production could be the first mechanistic change that, when combined with the loss of maximal biceps femoris activity and torque output in the latter stage of the half, are the predisposing factors to increased injury risk.

Reductions in rate of torque development were associated with concomitant reductions in central motor output to both hamstring muscles measured in this study. The first-half results for rate of torque decreases were best matched by reductions in early activation of the biceps femoris, which again provides mechanistic insight into why this muscle seems most susceptible to strain injury [33–35]. Central motor output is thought to be one of the primary contributory mechanisms to rate of torque development in the early time periods post contraction onset [42]. The results of this study support recent research which suggests that fatigue induced reductions in central motor output have an earlier and more pronounced effect on the ability to rapidly generate torque compared to maximal torque output [17].

The reductions in knee flexor rate of torque development has important implications for the design of sports specific exercise training programs. Current injury prevention and muscle specific conditioning programs in soccer, as well as other team-sports, tend to neglect the development and within-game maintenance of explosive force producing capability. Typically training programs, such as the FIFA-11 [43,44], concentrate upon the development of eccentric hamstring strength to attenuate the high incidence rate of hamstring muscle strains. The large and early reductions in rate of torque development suggest that intervention strategies to maintain hamstring muscle explosive force generating capacity across soccer match-play should be investigated and applied. To facilitate the design of intervention programs, future research should examine whether hamstring muscle low frequency fatigue occurs. Identification of peripheral contributions to the loss of explosive torque observed in this study could provide a more direct target of training compared to the goal of attenuating declines in early central motor output.

Table 3. Absolute values for rate of torque development (RTD) of the resting potentiated twitch in time intervals post contraction onset throughout the simulated soccer match (SAFT^{90}).

	RTD (Nm.s^{-1})				
First-half (minutes)	**0–25 ms**	**0–50 ms**	**0–75 ms**	**0–100 ms**	**RTD Max**
0	219.8±67.6	260.0±88.8	278.5±73.6	241.0±60.7	392.8±79.1
15	181.8±98.4	256.1±112.9	274.3±94.6	232.0±65.1	382.5±118.8
30	191.4±99.8	260.1±118.2	276.1±100.9	231.8±62.2	388.4±116.3
45	195.0±89.8	265.4±102.1	280.7±84.5	232.9±56.4	385.3±105.4
Second-half (minutes)					
0	189.8±87.6	234.6±92.2	244.1±78.6	198.7±58.8	336.5±96.9
15	182.5±96.0	249.9±116.0	263.6±101.1	220.1±65.6	376.1±113.1
30	210.9±89.4	276.1±101.1	281.2±86.2	225.1±65.9	384.0±110.8
45	178.9±91.4	246.4±110.9	262.7±103.7	217.4±79.0	371.6±124.9

No main effects of time, half, or time by half interactions were observed.

Methodology considerations

The absence of change in voluntary activation in addition to the observed reduction in normalized EMG/M for biceps femoris may contradict conclusions that central motor output was reduced. However voluntary activation is measured from the evoked torque during the plateau phase of the maximal contraction, and is thus a summation of the additional torque contributions following stimulation of all of the hamstring muscles (short and long-head bicep femoris, semi-membranosus and semi-tendinosus for the medial hamstrings). Thus the measure of voluntary activation should be considered a net estimate of maximal hamstrings central motor output that does not appear to have been compromised during this study.

Conclusion

Our findings suggest that reductions in knee flexor maximal torque and rate of torque development during a simulated soccer match occurs concomitant to reductions in central motor output to the hamstrings. Of particular interest is that reductions in central motor output manifest as earlier and greater reductions in early rate of torque development compared to reductions in maximal torque. Early rate of torque was reduced after only 15-minutes of the soccer simulation, whereas maximal torque was reduced from the start of each half after 45-minutes. These findings have important implications for understanding injury risk to the hamstrings during soccer.

Author Contributions

Conceived and designed the experiments: PM RL JS. Performed the experiments: PM GJ KA. Analyzed the data: PM GJ KA. Contributed to the writing of the manuscript: PM RL GJ KA JS. Interpreted the data: PM RL JS. Performed required reanalysis of data following reviewer feedback: PM. Final approval: PM RL GJ KA JS.

References

1. Opar DA, Williams MD, Shield AJ (2012) Hamstring strain injuries. Sports Med 42: 209–226.
2. Woods C, Hawkins RD, Maltby S, Hulse M, Thomas A, et al. (2004) The Football Association Medical Research Programme: an audit of injuries in professional football - analysis of hamstring injuries. Br J Sports Med 38: 36–41.
3. Ekstrand J, Hägglund M, Waldén M (2011) Injury incidence and injury patterns in professional football: the UEFA injury study. Br J Sports Med 45: 553–558.
4. Steffen K, Myklebust G, Olsen OE, Holme I, Bahr R (2008) Preventing injuries in female youth football-a cluster-randomized controlled trial. Scand J Med Sci Sports 18: 605–614.
5. Arnason A, Andersen TE, Holme I, Engebretsen L, Bahr R (2008) Prevention of hamstring strains in elite soccer: an intervention study. Scand J Med Sci Sports 18: 40–48.
6. Petersen J, Thorborg K, Nielsen MB, Budtz-Jørgensen E, Hölmich P (2011) Preventive effect of eccentric training on acute hamstring injuries in men's soccer: a cluster-randomized controlled trial. Am J Sports Med 39: 2296–2303.
7. Delextrat A, Gregory J, Cohen D (2010) The use of the functional H:Q ratio to assess fatigue in soccer. Int J Sports Med 31: 192–197.
8. Small K, McNaughton L, Greig M, Lovell R (2010) The effects of multidirectional soccer-specific fatigue on markers of hamstring injury risk. J Sci Med Sport 13: 120–125.
9. Thorlund JB, Aagaard P, Madsen K (2009) Rapid muscle force capacity changes after soccer match play. Int J Sports Med 30: 273–278.
10. Lovell R, Midgley AW, Barrett S, Carter D, Small K (2013) Effects of different half-time strategies on second half soccer-specific speed, power and dynamic strength. Scand J Med Sci Sports 23: 105–113.
11. Allen DG, Lamb GD, Westerblad H (2008) Skeletal muscle fatigue: cellular mechanisms. Physiol Rev 88: 287–332.
12. Gandevia SC (2001) Spinal and supraspinal factors in human muscle fatigue. Physiol Rev 81: 1725–1789.
13. Nybo L, Girard O, Mohr M, Knez W, Voss S, et al. (2013) Markers of muscle damage and performance recovery after exercise in the heat. Med Sci Sports Exerc 45: 860–868.
14. Rampinini E, Bosio A, Ferraresi I, Petruolo A, Morelli A, et al. (2011) Match-related fatigue in soccer players. Med Sci Sports Exerc 43: 2161–2170.
15. Amann M (2011) Central and peripheral fatigue: interaction during cycling exercise in humans. Med Sci Sports Exerc 43: 2039–2045.
16. Sidhu SK, Cresswell AG, Carroll TJ (2013) Corticospinal responses to sustained locomotor exercises: moving beyond single-joint studies of central fatigue. Sports Med 43: 437–449.
17. Buckthorpe M, Pain MTG, Folland JP (2014) Central fatigue contributes to the greater reductions in explosive than maximum strength with high intensity fatigue. Exp Physiol.
18. Kuitunen S, Komi PV, Kyrolainen H (2002) Knee and ankle joint stiffness in sprint running. Med Sci Sports Exerc 34: 166–173.
19. Yu B, Queen RM, Abbey AN, Liu Y, Moorman CT, et al. (2008) Hamstring muscle kinematics and activation during overground sprinting. J Biomech 41: 3121–3126.
20. Chumanov ES, Heiderscheit BC, Thelen BJ (2007) The effect of speed and influence of individual muscles on hamstring mechanics during the swing phase of sprinting. J Biomech 40: 525–532.
21. Heiderscheit BC, Hoerth DM, Chumanov ES, Swanson WC, Thelen BJ, et al. (2005) Identifying the time of occurrence of a hamstring strain injury during treadmill running: a case study. Clin Biomech 20: 1072–1078.
22. Schache AG, Wrigley TV, Baker R, Pandy MG (2009) Biomechanical response to hamstring muscle strain injury. Gait Posture 29: 332–338.
23. Andersen L, Aagaard P (2006) Influence of maximal muscle strength and intrinsic muscle contractile properties on contractile rate of force development. Eur J Appl Physiol 96: 46–52.
24. Rampinini E, Coutts A, Castagna C, Sassi R, Impellizzeri F (2007) Variation in top level soccer match performance. Int J Sports Med 28: 1018–1024.
25. Gregson W, Drust B, Atkinson G, Salvo V (2010) Match-to-match variability of high-speed activities in premier league soccer. Int J Sports Med 31: 237–242.
26. Lovell R, Knapper B, Small K (2008) Physiological responses to SAFT90: a new soccer-specific match simulation. Coach Sports Sci 3: 46.
27. Towlson C, Midgley AW, Lovell R (2013) Warm-up strategies of professional soccer players: practitioners' perspectives. J Sports Sci 31: 1393–1401.
28. Rainoldi A, Melchiorri G, Caruso I (2004) A method for positioning electrodes during surface EMG recordings in lower limb muscles. J Neuroscience Methods 134: 37–43.
29. Allison GT (2003) Trunk muscle onset detection technique for EMG signals with ECG artefact. J Electromyogr Kinesiol 13: 209–216.
30. Scaglioni G, Martin A (2009) Assessment of plantar flexors activation capacity: nerve versus muscle stimulation by single versus double pulse. Eur J Appl Physiol 106: 563–572.
31. Behm D, St-Pierre D, Perez D (1996) Muscle inactivation: assessment of interpolated twitch technique. J Appl Physiol 81: 2267–2273.
32. Shield A, Zhou S (2004) Assessing voluntary muscle activation with the twitch interpolation technique. Sports Med 34: 253–267.
33. Koulouris G, Connell D (2003) Evaluation of the hamstring muscle complex following acute injury. Skeletal Radiol 32: 582–589.
34. Koulouris G, Connell DA, Brukner P, Schneider-Kolsky M (2007) Magnetic resonance imaging parameters for assessing risk of recurrent hamstring injuries in elite athletes. Am J Sports Med 35.
35. Verrall GM, Slavotinek JP, Barnes PG, Fon GT (2003) Diagnostic and prognostic value of clinical findings in 83 athletes with posterior thigh injury: comparison of clinical findings with magnetic resonance imaging documentation of hamstring muscle strain. Am J Sports Med 31: 969–973.
36. Thelen DG, Chumanov ES, Hoerth DM, Best TM, Swanson SC, et al. (2005) Hamstring muscle kinematics during treadmill sprinting. Med Sci Sports Exerc 37: 108–114.
37. Onishi H, Yagi R, Oyama M, Akasaka K, Ihashi K, et al. (2002) EMG-angle relationship of the hamstring muscles during maximum knee flexion. J Electromyogr Kinesiol 12: 399–406.
38. Andersson H, Raastad T, Nilsson J, Paulsen G, Garthe I, et al. (2008) Neuromuscular fatigue and recovery in elite female soccer: effects of active recovery. Med Sci Sports Exerc 40: 372–380.
39. Magalhaes J, Rebelo A, Oliveira E, Renato Silva J, Marques F, et al. (2010) Impact of Loughborough intermittent shuttle test versus soccer match on physiological, biochemical and neuromuscular parameters. Eur J Appl Physiol 108: 39–48.
40. Murase S, Terazawa E, Querne F, Ota H, Matsuda T, et al. (2010) Bradykinin and nerve growth factor play pivotal roles in muscular mechanical hyperalgesia after exercise (delayed-onset muscle soreness). J Neurosci 20: 3752–3761.
41. von During M, Andres KH (1990) Topography and ultrastructure of group III and IV nerve terminals of cat's gastrocnemius-soleus muscle. In: Zenker W, Neuhuber WL, editors. The Primary Afferent Neuron: A Survey of Recent Morpho-functional Aspects. New York: Plenum. 35–41.
42. Van Cutsem M, Duchateau J, Hainaut K (1998) Changes in single motor unit behaviour contribute to the increase in contraction speed after dynamic training in humans. J Physiol 513: 295–305.

43. Bizzini M, Impellizzeri FM, Dvorak J, Bortolan L, Schena F, et al. (2013) Physiological and performance responses to the "FIFA 11+" (part 1): Is it an appropriate warm-up? J Sports Sci 31: 1481–1490.

44. Impellizzeri FM, Bizzini M, Dvorak J, Pellegrini B, Schena F, et al. (2013) Physiological and performance responses to the FIFA 11+ (part 2): A randomised controlled trial on the training effects. J Sports Sci 31: 1491–1502.

24

Influence of the Mechanical Properties of Third-Generation Artificial Turf Systems on Soccer Players' Physiological and Physical Performance and Their Perceptions

Javier Sánchez-Sánchez[1,2]*, Jorge García-Unanue[2], Pedro Jiménez-Reyes[1], Ana Gallardo[1], Pablo Burillo[2,3], José Luis Felipe[2,4], Leonor Gallardo[2]

1 School of Sport Sciences, UCAM, Universidad Católica San Antonio, Murcia, Spain, **2** IGOID Research Group, University of Castilla-La Mancha, Toledo, Spain, **3** Sport Sciences Institute, Camilo José Cela University, Villafranca del Castillo, Madrid, Spain, **4** School of Sport Sciences, European University, Villaviciosa de Odón, Madrid, Spain

Abstract

The aim of this research was to evaluate the influence of the mechanical properties of artificial turf systems on soccer players' performance. A battery of perceptive physiological and physical tests were developed on four different structural systems of artificial turf (System 1: Compacted gravel sub-base without elastic layer; System 2: Compacted gravel sub-base with elastic layer; System 3: Asphalt sub-base without elastic layer; System 4: Asphalt sub-base with elastic layer). The sample was composed of 18 soccer players (22.44±1.72 years) who typically train and compete on artificial turf. The artificial turf system with less rotational traction (S3) showed higher total time in the Repeated Sprint Ability test in comparison to the systems with intermediate values (49.46±1.75 s *vs* 47.55±1.82 s (S1) and 47.85±1.59 s (S2); $p<0.001$). The performance in jumping tests (countermovement jump and squat jump) and ball kicking to goal decreased after the RSA test in all surfaces assessed ($p<0.05$), since the artificial turf system did not affect performance deterioration ($p>0.05$). The physiological load was similar in all four artificial turf systems. However, players felt more comfortable on the harder and more rigid system (S4; visual analogue scale = 70.83±14.28) than on the softer artificial turf system (S2; visual analogue scale = 54.24±19.63). The lineal regression analysis revealed a significant influence of the mechanical properties of the surface of 16.5%, 15.8% and 7.1% on the mean time of the sprint, the best sprint time and the maximum mean speed in the RSA test respectively. Results suggest a mechanical heterogeneity between the systems of artificial turf which generate differences in the physical performance and in the soccer players' perceptions.

Editor: Alejandro Lucia, Universidad Europea de Madrid, Spain

Funding: The authors have no support or funding to report.

Competing Interests: The authors have declared that no competing interests exist.

* Email: jssanchez@ucam.edu

Introduction

Soccer is a sport defined by periods of high intensity, with phases of recovery in which there are interspersed actions such as jumps, runs and kicks with frequent accelerations and direction changes [1–4]. The international impact of this sport has resulted in a high number of studies concerning the player's internal factors which have an impact on their performance. Thus, physical parameters [5–7], physiological parameters [8,9] and psychological parameters [10] have been demonstrated as being influential in the internal variables of soccer players' performance. On the other hand, the effect of external variables such as nutritional supplements [11], recovery treatment [12], the temperature [13] or the situational variables are increasingly studied.

One of these external variables that has an influence on the game is the sports surface. It has been seen that the condition of the playing field is also a factor which affects the soccer player's performance [14]. The surface–player interaction has been linked to the association between the different kinds of surfaces and sports footwear [15–18]. The first comparative studies between surfaces focused on the lower injury rates associated with natural grass compared to those associated with artificial turf [19,20]. However, the artificial surface has undergone qualitative improvement and injury rates between the two surfaces have been levelled [21,22]. Nonetheless, professional players still perceive there to be a higher risk of injury on artificial turf [23]. Despite this, a longer fibre, an improvement of the mechanical properties of the infill and the perfection of the structural component of support, have been enough to gain the backing of the Fédération Internationale de Football Association (FIFA) and the European Committee for Standardization (CEN) for these kind of surfaces to be used for playing soccer, through the corresponding quality control test adjusted to rigorous requirements [24–26].

The controversy provoked between the use of natural or artificial surfaces in soccer led to studies about their effects on the athlete's performance [14,27–32]. In sprint actions, these researches revealed similar times and speeds on both surfaces [14,27,29,30], or even better on artificial turf [31]. Furthermore, isolated exercises on artificial turf do not induce higher fatigue or a delay in recovery [14,32]. Nevertheless, despite this, some studies have shown a higher perceived physical effort by players when they play on artificial turf [27,33,34], as well as a higher level of lactate and heart rate in sub-maximum runs [28]. On the other hand, technical parameters in matches played on artificial turf evidenced a decrease in the incidences of slipping and an increase in the number of short passes [27]. The impact speed of the ball is another technical variable affected by the type of surface. [35]. Brito, Krustrup and Rebelo [36] extended the study framework to sand, asphalt and artificial turf surfaces. This work found a higher physical load in the sand compared to the artificial turf and the asphalt, due to a lower capacity to run at high speed on this surface [37]. These studies were undertaken due to the differences between the mechanical properties of each kind of surface and their effect on the performance. In fact, the increment of the traction coefficient between the footwear and the surface of up to 0.82 has demonstrated an improvement in the soccer player's performance in lineal accelerations and circular sprints [38]. Similar researches show that a higher energy restitution associated with a higher rigidity contributes to an improvement in the economy of running [39,40]. Lastly, McGhie and Etemma [41] highlight force reduction as an important factor in an athlete's performance and security due to the reduction of the impact peaks during the sports practice.

As a result, the evolution that has taken place in artificial turf pitches has led to a high heterogeneity in the construction structures of third-generation artificial turf surfaces [42]. In fact, Potthast, Verhelst, Hughes, Stone and De Clercq [35] showed that the differences between various systems of artificial turf can be even higher than those between natural grass and artificial turf. Recent studies have demonstrated the influence of the structural component on the mechanical properties of an artificial turf soccer field, showing differences in levels of force reduction, standard vertical deformation and rotational traction according to the system installed [43,44]. Despite this, no research has yet compared the effect of this mechanical variability in artificial turf pitches on the players' performance and physiological responses. Therefore, the aim of this research is to establish the influence of the mechanical properties of artificial turf pitches with different structures on the physical performance, physiological responses and perceptions of amateur soccer players.

Methods

Subjects

Eighteen amateur soccer players from the same team (regional competitions) participated in the study (Mean: 22.44 SD: ±1.72 years; 73.74±8.47 kg; 175±6 cm; 14.74±4.15% of body fat). All of them have at least five years (6.28±2.13 years) previous experience as soccer players on artificial turf and they train two hours per day, three to four days per week, with one weekly competition, currently. None of the participants had any known cardiopulmonary disease or took any medicine during the study. Moreover all of them confirmed they had passed the medical examination required to play soccer.

At the beginning, the sample was composed of 20 players, but the two goalkeepers were rejected due to the difference in their movement with the outfield players. The rest of the players completed every test. All players were informed about the possible risk associated with this study, and they signed the informed consent form to be able to participate in the study. The Clinical Research Ethical Committee of Castilla-La Mancha Health Service (Spain) approved this study (n.13/10) basing on the last version of the Helsinki Declaration.

Experimental design

A pilot test was conducted on an artificial turf pitch in order to guarantee that players became accustomed to the different tests included in the study protocol. Each player repeated the test on each of the four systems of third-generation artificial turf selected, following the sequence set up by the numeration of the surface (from System 1 to System 4). The four artificial turf pitches selected (located in Madrid and Castilla-La Mancha, which are central regions of Spain) had differences in their structural components of support (sub-base and elastic layer). Table 1 shows the characteristic of the artificial turf systems selected.

The mechanical properties related to the surface–player interaction were assessed in the four artificial turf systems selected for this study. *In situ* tests were conducted on the four surfaces which were followed by the protocols and specifications presented in norm EN 15330-1:2014 and previous studies [43,44]. The analyzed variables were force reduction (*FR-%*), standard vertical deformation (*StV-mm*), energy restitution (*ER-%*) and rotational traction (*RT-N·m*). The first three variables are related with the surfaces' response to an impact, and they were evaluated using an Advanced Artificial Athlete (Deltec Metaal, Duiven, Holland), under the procedures stipulated by the norm EN 14808:2005 and EN 14809:2005. A mass with an incorporated spring, weighing in total 20 kg, was dropped on the surfaces. The acceleration of the mass from the output until after surface impact was transmitted through a data acquisition box (data acquisition device case) to a laptop with an informatics software (G-Force v.3.03, DeltecMetaal, Duiven, Holland) to extrapolate the collected data to the variables evaluated. This procedure was repeated two more times at intervals of 60±10 s, resulting in a total of three impacts. For the statistical analysis, the mean value between the second and the third impact was registered. In turn, this was done inside the five zones specified by the regulations EN 15330-1:2014 (Figure 1) in two different testing positions separated by more than 100 mm.

The last variable informed about the resistance offered by the surface to perform a spin measured in Newton per meter (N·m). For this test, a Rotational Resistance Tester (Deltec Metaal, Duiven, Holland) was used, following the procedure indicated by the regulation EN 15301-1:2014. The test zones were those indicated by the norms EN 15330-1:2014 (Figure 1). A mass of 46 kg with a base of soccer cleats was dropped to the surface from a height of 60±5 mm. Once the base was anchored on the surface, a dynamometric key was turned 45° at a nominal rotation speed of 12 r/min. This procedure was repeated five times in each of the zones shown in Figure 1, with a distance of at least of 50 mm between each test point.

The geographical proximity of the four soccer pitches with artificial turf guaranteed similar climatic conditions in each of the trials. A period of 72 h was established between the different sessions in order to guarantee the total recovery of the players. Tests were carried out under climatic conditions of 18–22.5°C temperature and 20–35% humidity, during May.

Experimental protocol

The day before the experimental test, it was recommended to the players to not carry out any kind of exhausting activity, as well as to maintain similar eating habits; they were also advised to use the same footwear in all four systems being assessed. Players arrived at the test soccer pitches at 09:00 a.m. A Global Positioning System (GPS, Spi Pro X, GPSports, Australia) was

Table 1. Characteristics of the artificial turf selected.

Characteristics	System 1	System 2	System 3	System 4
Fibre				
Fibre material	Polyethylene	Polyethylene	Polyethylene	Polyethylene
Fibre type	Monofilament	Monofilament	Monofilament	Monofilament
Pile height	60 mm	45 mm	60 mm	45 mm
Dtex	12000	12000	12000	12000
Infill				
Sand material	Quartz	Quartz	Quartz	Quartz
Granulometry	0.3–0.8 mm	0.3–0.8 mm	0.3–0.8 mm	0.3–0.8 mm
Quantity	20 Kg/m^2	15 Kg/m^2	20 Kg/m^2	15 Kg/m^2
Rubber material	SBR	SBR	SBR	SBR
Granulometry	0.5–2.5 mm	0.5–2.5 mm	0.5–2.5 mm	0.5–2.5 mm
Quantity	13 Kg/m^2	8 Kg/m^2	13 Kg/m^2	8 Kg/m^2
Support structure				
Sub-base material	Compacted Gravel	Compacted Gravel	Asphalt	Asphalt
Elastic layer	No	Yes	No	Yes
Elastic layer thickness	-	23 mm	-	12 mm

incorporated on each soccer player's back. Before the beginning of the different tests, participants carried out a standard warm-up which had exercises such as 5 min of continuous run, 5 min of exercises of articulation mobility and three sprints of 30 m, increasing the intensity, with a recovery process of 2 min between each test. Stretching exercises were not carried out during the warm-up. At 10:00 a.m. players started the different performance tests, while they were verbally instructed to apply the maximum effort during the tests.

Repeated sprint ability test (RSA)

Players performed three maximum sprints of 30 m with intermediate measurement points at 5 and 10 m before carrying out the RSA test. The best time achieved in these sprints was selected for the analysis.

Players carried out the RSA test after 15 min of recovery. The test consisted of six 40 m sprints (20+20 m) [45]. Participants sprinted 20 m, then they turned on one line and then ran back to the starting line at maximum intensity. The deceleration took place one metre after passing the starting line. After 20 s of active recovery, players repeated the same procedure. There had to be a gap of 5 seconds before the start of the next sprint, and the researcher carried out the countdown. A system of four pairs of photocells (Microgate, Bolzano, Italy) was placed along the sprint zone, which collected time at 5, 10, 20, 30 and 40 m with a sensibility of 0.001 s. If the time of the first sprint of the RSA test was higher (increment higher than 5%) than the best individual sprint done before the beginning of the test, it was not considered valid [5,46,47], therefore players had to repeat the test after 5 min of recovery. The best time of sprint (RSA_{BEST}), the mean time (RSA_{MEAN}), the total time (RSA_{TT}), the percentage of decreasing (%Dec) and the difference between the best and worst sprint during the RSA test (%Diff) were calculated [45,46,48]. The %Dec ((mean time/best time$\times$100) $-$100) has been identified as the most valid and reliable method for assessing fatigue in these kinds of tests [12,48], while recent studies have demonstrated a high correlation with the %Diff [46]. The maximum peak of speed (V_{MAX}), the maximum mean speed of run (V_{MEAN}) and the heart rate of players during the RSA were monitored by GPS of 10 HZ, which has been demonstrated as being a valid and reliable tool in the collection of these variables [1,49].

A minute after finishing the RSA test, a specialized researcher took a sample of 5-μL of blood lactate from the fingertip of the participants using a portable device (Lactate Scout, SensLab GmbH, Leipzig, Germany). This procedure was repeated 3 minutes after finishing the RSA test.

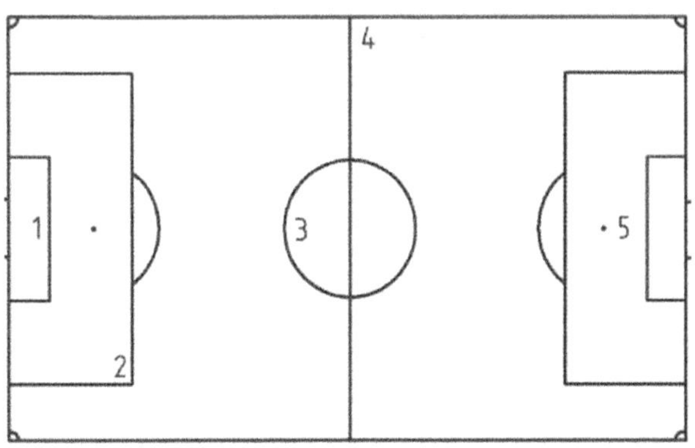

Figure 1. Test zones according to regulation EN 15330-1: 2014.

Vertical jumping

Countermovement jumps (CMJ) and squat jumps (SJ) were done before and after the RSA test, using an infrared system (Optojump Next, Microgate, Bolzano, Italy). Participants had to keep their hands on their hips to eliminate the influence of arm movement on jump performance. Every player did two jumps in each modality before (with 2 min of recovery between jumps) and after the RSA test. The best of them was selected for the statistical analysis.

In the same way, players carried out the fifteen seconds maximal jump test to assess the performance deterioration in their jumping action. For this test, participants had to stand upright with feet apart at shoulder width and with their hands on their hips in the same way as in the CMJ. At the start signal, subjects flexed their knees and carried out a maximum performance of jumps for 15 s, landing with both feet at the same time. The maximum height in cm, % Dec (100–(mean jump/best jump × 100)) [12] and the output power [(62.5 × 50.3 × jump height+body mass)–2184.7] × number of jumps] [50] were calculated for this test.

Kicking from goal

Players had to kick, at the fastest speed possible, a stationary ball placed on the penalty point at 11 m from the goal. The ball used for this test had the FIFA-approved certification and a level of pressure according to the standards established by the organisation. Players kicked twice before and after the RSA test, with a rest of 1 min between each kick. The fastest kick in each round was selected for the statistic analysis. The ball speed (Km/h) was collected by means of a Stalker ATS System TM radar (Radar Sales, MN, US) placed behind the goal and pointing at the ball.

Visual analogue scale

The perceived effort and the fatigue experience on each artificial turf system were evaluated by means of a visual analogue scale (VAS) questionnaire used in previous studies [27,36]. The questionnaire included six questions and it was applied once the session on each artificial turf system was finished. Players answered on a horizontal line of 100 mm where 0 was "nothing, hard/tired/comfortable" and 100 was "very hard/tired/comfortable." The questions were: "How can you classify the effort made during this session?" (VAS1); "How tired are you at this moment?" (VAS2); "How difficult have you found it to do a turn or change direction?" (VAS3); "How did you feel during the jumps?" (VAS4); "How did you feel during the run?" (VAS5); "In general, how have you felt during the session?" (VAS6).

Statistical analysis

Results are presented as mean and standard deviation (SD). The verification of the normality and homogeneity of the variances was assumed by means of the Kolmogorov–Smirnov test and the Leven's statistic. The influence of artificial turf systems on the selected variables was assessed through a variance analysis (ANOVA) and the differences between means were identified using a post hoc Bonferroni procedure. The comparison between results collected in the vertical jumping test and kicking ball tests before and after the RSA test were developed through a two-way ANOVA test (artificial turf system × time). A lineal regression analysis was used for the mechanical properties of the artificial turf systems as independent variables and the results from the different performance test as dependent variables. The *StV* was omitted due to its high correlation with *FR* ($r = 0.99$; $p < 0.0001$), deleting possible problems of multicollinearity. Data were analyzed with the statistic software SPSS v 20.0. The level of significance was established at $p < 0.05$.

Results

Mechanical properties of the surface

Table 2 shows the mechanical differences between the four selected systems of artificial turf. System 2 (composed of a compacted gravel sub-base and elastic layer) presented the highest value of *FR* (69.83±1.18%) and *StV* (6.56±0.37 mm) in comparison with the rest of the systems ($F = 451.63$ y

Table 2. Mechanical properties of the selected artificial turf systems.

	System 1 (a)		System 2 (b)		System 3 (c)		System 4 (d)		*F*	*p*
FR (%)	51.30	(2.52)^{b,c}	69.83	(1.18)	60.10	(2.04)^{b}	48.07	(3.67)^{a,b,c}	451.63	<0.001
StV (mm)	3.53	(0.43)^{b,c}	6.56	(0.37)	4.68	(0.45)^{b}	3.43	(0.48)^{b,c}	326.92	<0.001
ER (%)	42.63	(1.50)^{c,d}	42.07	(1.46)^{c,d}	43.90	(1.45)^{d}	50.50	(2.19)	161.26	<0.001
RT (N·m)	45.56	(2.84)^{b,c,d}	42.44	(3.14)^{a,d}	41.72	(2.81)^{a,d}	54.60	(4)	83.81	<0.001

System 1: Compacted gravel sub-base without elastic layer; System 2: Compacted gravel sub-base with elastic layer; System 3: Asphalt sub-base without elastic layer; System 4: Asphalt sub-base with elastic layer.
FR = Force Reduction; *StV* = Standard Vertical Deformation; *ER* = Energy Restitution; *RT* = Rotational Traction.
^{a,b,c,d}Significant differences with the system indicated ($p < 0.05$).

$F = 326.92$; $p<0.001$). The highest results of *ER* and *RT* were identified in System 4 (50.50±2.19% y 54.60±4 N·m, respectively) which incorporated an asphalt sub-base and elastic layer.

Repeated sprint ability test

The global performance analysis done in the RSA test (Table 3) on the four artificial turf systems revealed a significantly lower RSA_{MEAN} of sprint and RSA_{TT} ($F = 4.214$ and $F = 4.216$; $p<0.01$) in Systems 1 and 2 in comparison with System 3, which presented the lowest level of *RT*. On the other hand, the time of the best sprint was 7.38±0.35 s on System 1 and 7.74±0.29 s on System 3 ($F = 4.002$; $p<0.05$). Speed parameters of run and heart rate during the RSA test were not affected by the system of artificial turf. Also the performance deterioration in the RSA test was similar in all four artificial turf systems.

In the analytic comparison per number of sprints, the times achieved in the four first sprints of the RSA test were significantly higher on the system with an asphalt sub-base and elastic layer (System 3) than on Systems 1 and 2 (Figure 2: $p<0.05$). Therefore, the maximum speed achieved in the fourth sprint was 23.23±0.78 km/h on System 3 and 24.32±1.05 km/h on System 1 ($F = 3.552$; $p<0.05$). The absence of significant differences in the variables of %Diff and %Dec indicates that the game surface has no additional influence on the development of fatigue during the RSA test ($p<0.05$).

The split-distance RSA test revealed superior times on System 3 compared to the other artificial turf systems. These differences were more significant from the 20 m ($p<0.001$; Figure 3). The direction changes presented significantly lower times in Systems 1 and 2, which evidenced intermediate values of *RT*, than Systems 3 and 4 with traction values in the lower and upper end of the sample, respectively (4.35±0.34 s y 4.38±0.27 s *vs* 4.59±0.34 s y 4.50±0.32 s; $F = 11.553$; $p<0.001$). Once again, the fatigue index (%Diff and %Dec) did not significantly differ between the evaluated systems of artificial turf ($p>0.05$), negating the influence of the game surface on this variable.

Lactate values in blood after the RSA test were not affected by the game surface. The collected samples at 1 minute (S1: 12.92±2.27 $mmol \cdot L^{-1}$; S2: 12.44±2.42 $mmol \cdot L^{-1}$; S3: 11.04±2.31 $mmol \cdot L^{-1}$; S4: 11.80±2.53 $mmol \cdot L^{-1}$) and 3 min after the ending of the RSA (S1: 12.98±2.51 $mmol \cdot L^{-1}$; S2: 12.97±2.98 $mmol \cdot L^{-1}$; S3: 11±1.86 $mmol \cdot L^{-1}$; S4: 11.06±2.46 $mmol \cdot L^{-1}$) test were similar for the four analyzed systems ($p>0.05$).

Vertical jumping

The system of artificial turf did not generate any influence upon either the jumping height or the power generated in the CMJ and SJ test and the 15 s test ($p>0.05$; Table 4). After the RSA test a significant deterioration in the jumping height and the power generated in the CMJ and SJ was detected in all the evaluated artificial turf systems ($p<0.05$). The interaction between the artificial turf system and the performance deterioration reveals significant differences in the fatigue index (%Diff) in the ANOVA test of the CMJ ($F = 2.942$; $p<0.05$) and the SJ test ($F = 3.539$; $p<0.05$). Results showed a higher fatigue index in the systems with higher levels of *FR* and *StV*. However, the post hoc analysis did not confirm the significant differences between pairs ($p>0.05$). On the other hand, in the 15 s jumping test, players confirmed a significantly greater deterioration in the height of the jump on the system with the biggest *ER* (System 4; $F = 3.188$; $p<0.05$). Finally, the variation percentage of the applied power (%Diff Power output) in the CMJ and SJ test after the RSA test was not affected by the type of artificial turf system ($p>0.05$).

Goal kicking

The RSA test generated a significant deterioration of the kicking speed of the ball in each of the four systems of artificial turf (S1: 7.34±5.18%; S2: 11.62±7.67%; S3: 11.79±6%; S4: 7.55±6; $p<0.05$). However, there was no significant interaction between the game surface and the kicking speed of the soccer players ($p>0.05$), which showed a mean between the four systems of 102.54±8.87 km/h before the RSA test and 92.85±8.96 at the end of the test.

VAS

Once the session was ended, the perception of players regarding the effort parameters (VAS1), fatigue (VAS2), difficulty in direction changes (VAS3), jumps (VAS4) and run (VAS5) showed no differences between the systems of artificial turf ($p>0.05$; Figure 4). In contrast, at a general level, players reported a higher sense of comfort during the session developed on the system with fewer *FR* and *StV*, as well as with the highest levels of *ER* and *RT* (System 4), compared to System 2, which presented the biggest *FR* and *StV* and the lowest *ER* of the four systems (VAS6: 70.83±14.28 *vs* 54.24±19.63, respectively; $F = 3.413$; $p<0.05$).

The lineal regression analysis evidenced a significant influence of the mechanical properties of the systems of artificial turf on the performance in the RSA test ($p<0.05$; Table 5). In particular, the *ER* presented a positive influence on the RSA_{MEAN}, RSA_{TT} y RSA_{BEST} ($p<0.001$) and a negative one on the maximum mean speed in this test ($p<0.05$). Moreover, the *RT* showed a negative influence on the RSA times ($p<0.01$). Therefore, this highlights the fact that the evaluated mechanical properties (*FR, ER and RT*) had a significant influence of 16.5%, 15.8% y 16.5% on RSA_{MEAN}, RSA_{BEST} and RSA_{TT}, respectively. Lastly, a higher *FR* was associated by players with a lower perceived comfort on the respective different artificial turf systems ($p<0.05$).

Discussion and Conclusions

This research exposes the influence of the mechanical heterogeneity of the artificial turf system on the sport performance, which is evaluated through specific tests. With regards to physical tests, this study included a combination of performance measures and physiological responses similar to recent researches that compared artificial turf with natural grass [14,32]. However, this is the first research which applies these measures on several different systems of artificial turf. Previous studies defend a lack of connection between the mechanical devices and the mechanical properties perceived by the players, due to the lack of the human movement auto-regulation [51,52]. The surface with a compacted gravel sub-base and elastic layer had the highest levels of *FR* and *StV*, coinciding with previous studies which assessed the influence of the structural components of support on the mechanical properties of the surface [44], in spite of this; this system met the regulation requirements. The inclusion of the *ER* and *RT* provides more details about hardness, the capacity of absorption and turn resistance from the surface, respectively. This property presents an inverse relationship with the impact reduction ($r = -0.665$; $p<0.01$) and this differs depending on the system of artificial turf introduced, due to the heterogeneity and the state of conservation of the structural components used [52–55].

The results of the current research show differences between the systems of artificial turf in the performance of the RSA test. The mean, total and best times identified as the main indicators of the performance in this test [56–58], show significant differences based on the surface assessed. The systems with intermediate values adapted to the normative requirement specified for *RT*, presented

Table 3. Time speed and heart rate values in the RSA test in the four artificial turf systems.

	System 1 (a)		System 2 (b)		System 3 (c)		System 4 (d)		*F*	*p*
Time										
RSA_{MEAN} (s)	7.93	(0.30)[c]	7.97	(0.26)[c]	8.24	(0.29)	8.02	(0.25)	4.214	0.009
RSA_{BEST} (s)	7.38	(0.35)[c]	7.50	(0.26)	7.74	(0.29)	7.51	(0.32)	4.002	0.011
RSA_{TT} (s)	47.55	(1.82)[c]	47.85	(1.59)[c]	49.46	(1.75)	48.14	(1.48)	4.216	0.009
% sprint Dec 40 m	7.44	(1.74)	6.40	(2.45)	6.53	(2.10)	6.90	(2.85)	0.681	0.567
% sprint Diff 40 m	13.42	(2.99)	12.20	(4.63)	11.37	(3.87)	12.08	(4.03)	0.782	0.508
Speed										
V_{MAX} (km/h)	26.84	(1.06)	27.13	(1.66)	26.69	(2.28)	26.72	(1.22)	0.267	0.849
V_{MEAN} (km/h)	24.78	(0.71)	24.67	(1.06)	24.19	(0.72)	24.44	(0.78)	1.635	0.190
% speed Dec	7.62	(2.55)	8.94	(3.29)	9.02	(4.62)	8.45	(2.24)	0.649	0.586
% speed Diff	14.52	(3.48)	15.99	(4.80)	15.71	(5.36)	15.39	(4.14)	0.342	0.795
Heart rate										
Peak HR (b.p.m)	184.00	(12.90)	185.18	(12.48)	183.13	(13.19)	184.78	(11.72)	0.083	0.969

System 1: Compacted gravel sub-base without elastic layer; System 2: Compacted gravel sub-base with elastic layer; System 3: Asphalt sub-base without elastic layer; System 4: Asphalt sub-base with elastic layer.
RSA = Repeated Sprint Ability.
[a,b,c,d]Significant differences with the indicated system ($p<0.05$). Data are presented as mean (SD) in 18 soccer players.

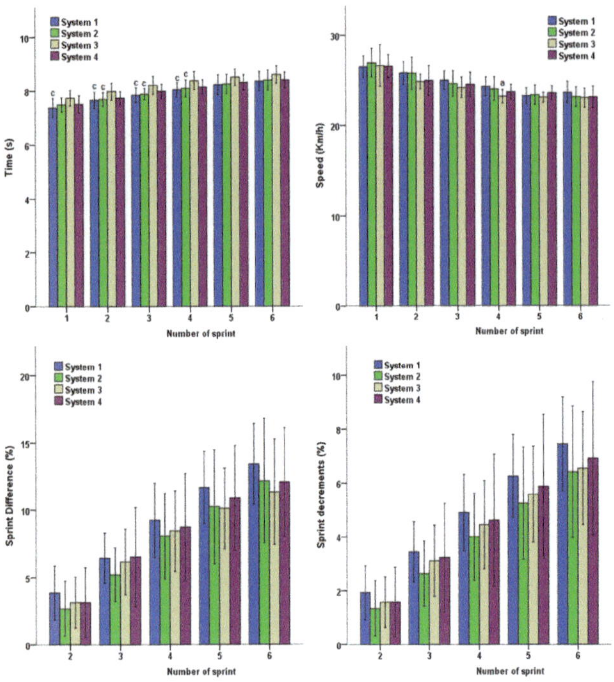

Figure 2. Time, speed and performance deterioration profile in the sprints (%Diff and %Dec) of the RSA test (6×40 m) on different artificial turf systems.

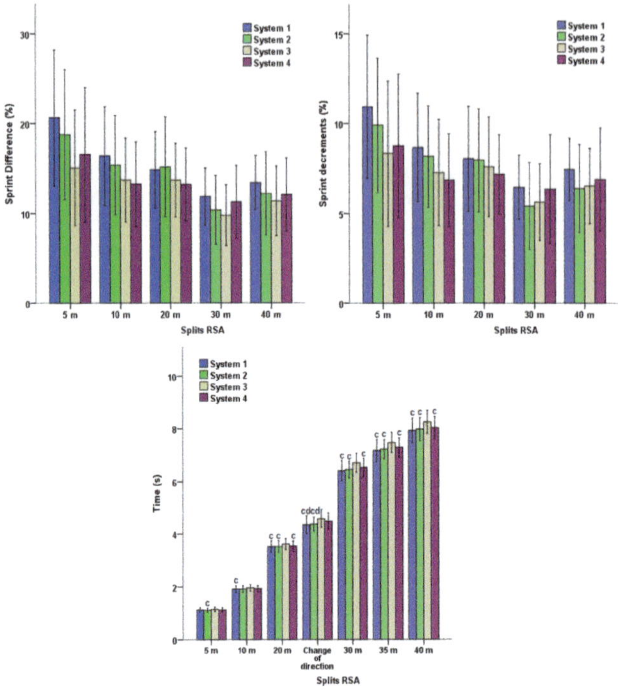

Figure 3. Performance and deterioration of times and percentage (%Dec and %Diff) in sprints of the RSA test specified by distance splits on different artificial turf systems.

faster sprint times (mean, total and best) than the system with a lower index of *RT* and System 4, which is over the limit of 50 N·m according to the regulations. Similarly, Luo and Stefanyshyn [38] concluded that increases in the traction levels up to a certain threshold came from systematic advantages in the performance of sprints and accelerations, but these improvements were not detected in the performance from a certain threshold as it is observed with System 4 in this work. Moreover, higher levels of *RT* constitute a risk injury factor in the lower limbs of the players [59]. The inclusion of a direction change of 180° and the split analysis in the RSA test demonstrated that optimum levels of *RT* improve the lineal performance in the sprints, and also facilitate the capacity to change direction, because the differences between the artificial turf systems became more evident from the turns of 180°. Previous researches explained this improvement as being a result of less slipping by players on a surface with adequate rotational traction [29,60,61]. Gains et al. [30] found similar sprint speeds between artificial turf and natural grass, but found direction changes to be faster on artificial surfaces. Data from this work show the same tendency in third-generation systems of artificial turf in the times collected for the direction change in the RSA test, which presented significant differences between them, while changes in the speed were not observed. However, the lineal regression analysis revealed a negative influence of the *ER* of the surface on the V_{MEAN}. In addition, the sum of the mechanical properties analyzed in the current study has demonstrated a effect of the 7.1% on the V_{MEAN} achieved by players during the RSA test. This analysis allows quantifying the limited influence of the mechanical properties of the surface on the maximum speed, discovered in previous studies that compared artificial turf with natural grass [14]. McGhie and Etemma [41] evidenced an influence of different types of artificial turf on the impact forces and the time of contact on soccer players in two run tests, but they did not take into account the traction properties of the surface. The comparison with these kinds of studies shows that the differences between natural grass and artificial turf are similar to the differences found between the different systems of third-generation artificial turf.

The lineal regression also shows the influence of *ER* on the performance in the RSA test. The analysis reveals that if the rigidity is excessive, it provokes an increase in the times of this test. However, the *FR* did not constitute a determinant variable on the performance in the repetitive sprints. This suggests that the percentages of *FR* were not high enough to generate an increase in the times derived from the reduction of the reaction forces as a result of the partial absorption of the energy applied [62]. The lack of differences in the performance, fatigue and physiological response in the RSA test between the systems of artificial turf with higher and lower impact-damping capacities, negates the hypothesis that softer surfaces require a greater exertion of energy [63,64]. This is probably due to the limited magnitude of the differences in the force reduction between systems. The studies which explain a lower muscle-sinew efficiency [65] or a higher hip and knee flexion [66] as being indicative of a higher energy outlay on surfaces with a higher impact reduction, were performed on a sand surface with a much higher level of impact reduction than that detected on artificial turf. Current studies regarding artificial and natural grass present mixed results. Hughes et al. [14] did not detect any differences in the lactate levels in blood and heart rate after a simulated match. However, Di Michele et al. [28] evidenced differences in these parameters in a run test. In our case, the lactate samples in blood were collected after the RSA test, therefore results have to be compared cautiously, because several authors have demonstrated that lactate concentration is influenced by the activity done immediately before to the sampling [67]. The physiological load, which is similar between the systems of artificial turf, contrasts with the players' perceptions on ending the session. In terms of general perceived effort, players reported higher

Table 4. Valuation of the jumping tests CMJ, SJ and 15 s cn the different artificial turf systems.

	System 1 (a)		System 2 (b)		System 3 (c)		System 4 (d)		*F*	*p*
CMJ										
CMJ_{PRE} height (cm)	36.53	(4.40)*	35.46	(5.38)*	36.36	(5.72)*	36.92	(5.11)*	0.249	0.862
CMJ_{POST} height (cm)	28.31	(4.46)	26.03	(4.87)	26.53	(5.21)	30.09	(5.85)	2.248	0.091
% Diff CMJ height	22.49	(7.45)	26.12	(10.67)	27.05	(7.62)	18.47	(11.26)	2.942	0.040
Power $output_{PRE}$ (W)	3809.35	(515.98)*	3697.76	(491.98)*	3852.28	(553.17)*	3832.01	(528.95)*	0.294	0.830
Power $output_{POST}$ (W)	3295.37	(527.67)	3108.42	(492.59)	3237.83	(547.07)	3404.92	(577.83)	0.919	0.437
% Diff Power output	13.66	(5.13)	15.91	(7.14)	16.09	(5.24)	11.25	(7.10)	2.286	0.087
SJ										
SJ_{PRE} height (cm)	28.49	(4.39)*	29.69	(4.03)*	29.30	(5.46)*	29.60	(4.55)*	0.238	0.869
SJ_{POST} height (cm)	24.57	(4.28)	23.22	(4.35)	23.14	(4.69)	25.09	(3.53)	0.922	0.436
% Diff SJ height	13.74	(7.50)	21.71	(9.86)	20.72	(9.85)	14.66	(8.50)	3.539	0.019
15 s Test										
Mean jump height (cm)	28.68	(3.66)	28.25	(4.51)	28.55	(4.92)	29.34	(3.65)	0.211	0.888
Número de saltos (n)	17.18	(2.13)	15.53	(1.33)	16.56	(2.10)	15.94	(1.80)	2.554	0.063
Power output (W)	57030.07	(11577.78)	50598.42	(9234.74)	55574.10	(10710.92)	53522.08	(9962.71)	1.218	0.310
% jump Dec	10.58	(2.84)	10.37	(2.86) ^{d}	11.57	(3.93)	13.66	(4.26)	3.188	0.030

System 1: Compacted gravel sub-base without elastic layer; System 2: Compacted gravel sub-base with elastic layer; System 3: Asphalt sub-base without elastic layer; System 4: Asphalt sub-base with elastic layer.
CMJ = Counter Movement Jump; SJ = Squat Jump; 15 s Test = Fifteen seconds maximal jump test.
Data are presented as mean (SD) in 18 soccer players.
*Significant differences between pre- and post-RSA ($p<0.05$).
^{a,b,c,d}Significant differences with the indicated system ($p<0.05$).

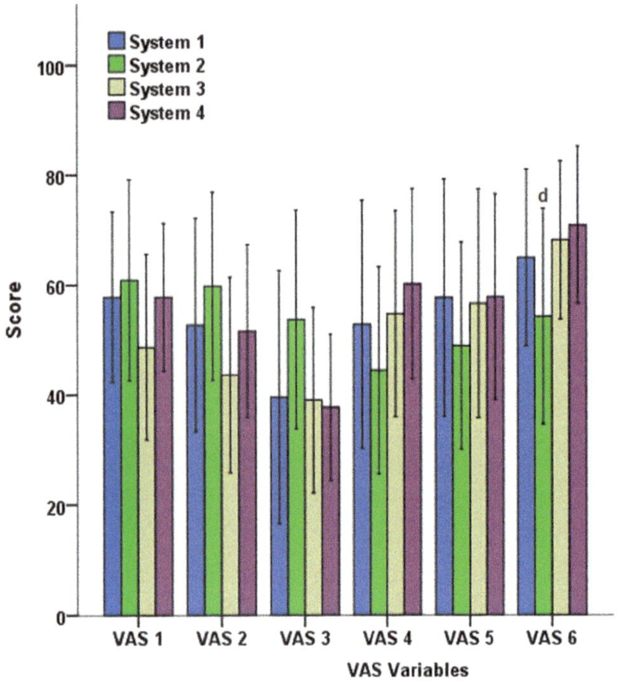

Figure 4. Results of the visual analogue scale (VAS) after the session on the artificial turf systems.

comfort on the system with lower levels of *FR* with respect to the system with the biggest capacity for cushioning. Moreover, the regression demonstrated that the *FR* was the only variable which significantly influenced the users' perception. The negative influence observed suggests that the softer surfaces seemed less comfortable for players during the different actions performed on the surface, in spite of the fact that there are no differences between the systems in the physiological answers from participants. This discovery coincides with Brito et al. [36] who show that the perceived demand is more related to the difficulty in running (external load) than to the physiological responses (internal load), even though the activity performed prior to the evaluation of the players' perception was different in both studies. Similarly, Nédélec et al. [32] turn to the protocol used and the familiarisation with artificial turf in order to justify the lack of differences in the players' perception of natural grass and artificial turf which was found in other studies [27]. However, in the current study every player was familiar with this surface and they showed different levels of perceived comfort regarding the artificial turf system. Regardless of the perceived effort, the mechanical properties evaluated showed an influence of 16.5%, 15.8% and 16.5%, on the RSA_{MEAN}, RSA_{BEST} and RSA_{TT} respectively. These results highlight the importance of including the *ER* as a measurable parameter of the functionality of artificial turf soccer pitches, as well as the requirement of assessing the mechanical properties of the different surfaces in comparative studies.

The kicking ball to goal speed did not present differences in the four analysed systems. In all of them, players showed a significant deterioration of kicking speed after the RSA test. Nevertheless, the lack of interaction between the surface and the kick moment indicates that the artificial turf system has no additional influence on fatigue development. On the contrary, Potthast [68] found differences between two systems of artificial turf in the speed, accuracy and biomechanics parameters of kicking a ball. The

Table 5. Lineal regression analysis of the effect of the mechanical properties of the artificial turf system on the jump, sprint and perception parameters.

	CMJ (cm)	Fatigue CMJ	SJ (cm)	Fatigue SJ	Power output 15 s (W)	% Jump Dec 15 s	RSA_{MEAN} (s)	RSA_{BEST} (s)	RSA_{TT} (s)	% Sprint Dec	V_{MAX} RSA (km/h)	V_{MEAN} RSA (Km/h)	% Speed Dec	VAS6
FR (%)	-0.075	-0.025	0.071	0.277	-513.887	-0.029	-0.013	-0.009	-0.079	-0.044	0.032	0.020	0.042	-1.001*
	(0.142)	(0.260)	(0.127)	(0.246)	(285.729)	(0.097)	(0.008)	(0.008)	(0.046)	(0.064)	(0.044)	(0.023)	(0.090)	(0.455)
ER (%)	0.136	0.843	0.160	1.299	321.772	0.570	0.114***	0.120**	0.684***	-0.191	-0.110	-0.217*	0.341	3.247
	(0.611)	(1.120)	(0.547)	(1.060)	(1229.840)	(0.418)	(0.033)	(0.036)	(0.196)	(0.276)	(0.190)	(0.098)	(0.386)	(1.997)
RT (N·m)	-0.102	-1.189	0.008	-0.930	-851.791	-0.167	-0.093**	-0.093**	-0.558**	0.091	0.094	0.159	-0.191	-2.528
	(0.510)	(0.935)	(0.456)	(0.885)	(1027.172)	(0.349)	(0.027)	(0.030)	(0.164)	(0.230)	(0.159)	(0.082)	(0.323)	(1.653)
Constant	39.199*	42.006	17.627	-13.480	108482.935**	-4.629	7.981***	6.992***	47.882***	13.704	25.660***	25.742***	-0.397	93.033
	(16.119)	(29.543)	(14.417)	(27.956)	(32440.648)	(11.028)	(0.864)	(0.952)	(5.183)	(7.278)	(5.019)	(2.598)	(10.190)	(52.703)
R^2	0.012	0.121	0.011	0.142	0.054	0.130	0.165	0.158	0.165	0.031	0.012	0.071	0.030	0.144

CMJ = Counter Movement Jump; SJ = Squat Jump; 15 s = Fifteen seconds maximal jump test; RSA = Repeated Sprint Ability; VAS = Visual Analogue Scale.
FR = Force Reduction; *ER* = Energy Restitution; *RT* = Rotational Traction.
Significant influence *$p<0.05$ **$p<0.01$ ***$p<0.001$.

utilization of two different systems of infill (rubber, or rubber and sand) in this research [68] may be the main reason for this discrepancy, because in the current study, the type of superficial structural components (fibre and infill) was identical in all four systems. Despite this, many more studies with biomechanical parameters are required to establish the determinant factors in ball kicking.

Finally, the different jumping tests (CMJ and SJ) performed before and after the RSA test evidence a significant deterioration in performance on the four systems with no interaction between the system of surface and the jump moment. This suggests a lower jumping capacity after a succession of sprints, regardless of the third-generation artificial turf system of employed to perform. This conclusion is similar to the results attained in other studies after applying a simulated protocol of soccer on natural grass and artificial turf [14]. The jumping test of 15 s evidenced a higher deterioration of performance (%Dec) on the system with harder and more rigid artificial turf. This system presented mechanical properties which were a long way from meeting the regulation requirements; therefore these results highlight the importance of meeting the regulations in order to guarantee optimum parameters of sport functionality. On the other hand, there are not any systems which exceed the regulation specifications established for the properties of the cushioning of surfaces. This suggests that the disadvantages offered by a soft surface [36,63,64,66] are not apparent until a particular limit, in a similar way to the *RT*, although more studies on the influence of the surface on the repetitive jumping capacity are required to accept this hypothesis.

The variety of perceptual, physiological and physical tests included in the current study has permitted a comparison of the influence of different artificial turf systems and their mechanical properties on the players' performance. Tests have focused on the main actions performed during a soccer match, such as repetitive sequences of explosive movements, sprints with direction changes and maximum jumps [12,47]. However, in order to confirm whether the results collected are translatable to a real match these variables would need to be checked during a real-life game. Future studies regarding artificial turf systems should include more variability of artificial turf systems based on the superficial components as well as the different rates of mechanical properties so as to know the exact point in which the deterioration of performance begins and the risk of injury increases.

One of the possible limitations of this research was the implementation of an only data collection for each one of the artificial turf systems. The repetition of the test battery (with the same sample of players) in more selected fields with these characteristics will increase the consistency of the obtained results.

In conclusion, the different systems of artificial turf selected, based on their structural components of support, evidenced a mechanical heterogeneity which had influence on the physical parameters implicated in soccer performance. This mechanical variability placed artificial turf systems at different levels of compliance with specified regulatory requirements for artificial turf soccer pitches. The physical performance in sprint and jumps actions was influenced by the parameters of traction, stiffness and force reduction of the artificial turf systems. However, the physiological load remains invariable between the different systems, in spite of players' perceived less comfort on the softer surfaces. The differences between artificial turf systems are similar to the variability between natural grass and artificial turf, so that control of the mechanical properties of the game surface is essential to ensure adequate sport functionality. The coaches must take into account that the practice of football on different structures of artificial turf does not modify the physiological parameters of the players, although differences are obtained in physical performance. This research provides the bases to ensure favourable conditions of the game that encourage sports participation at the community level. Future studies should incorporate technical and biomechanical parameters of different systems to complement the findings of this study.

Author Contributions

Conceived and designed the experiments: JSS LG PB. Performed the experiments: JSS JLF LG PJR PB AG. Analyzed the data: JSS JGU. Contributed reagents/materials/analysis tools: JSS JLF JGU PB. Contributed to the writing of the manuscript: JSS JGU JLF PB LG.

References

1. Barbero-Álvarez JC, Coutts A, Granda J, Barbero-Álvarez V, Castagna C (2009) The validity and reliability of a global positioning satellite system device to assess speed and repeated sprint ability (RSA) in athletes. J Sci Med Sport 13: 232–235.
2. Bloomfield J, Polman R, O'Donoghue P (2007) Physical demands of different positions in FA Premier League soccer. J Sports Sci Med 6: 63.
3. Carling C, Bloomfield J, Nelsen L, Reilly T (2008) The role of motion analysis in elite soccer. Sports Med 38: 839–862.
4. Chamari K, Chaouachi A, Hambli M, Kaouech F, Wisløff U, et al. (2008) The five-jump test for distance as a field test to assess lower limb explosive power in soccer players. J Strength Cond Res 22: 944–950.
5. Castagna C, Abt G, Manzi V, Annino G, Padua E, et al. (2008) Effect of recovery mode on repeated sprint ability in young basketball players. J Strength Cond Res 22: 923–929.
6. Figueiredo AJ, Gonçalves CE, Coelho e Silva MJ, Malina RM (2009) Characteristics of youth soccer players who drop out, persist or move up. J Sports Sci 27: 883–891.
7. Rebelo A, Brito J, Maia J, Coelho-e-Silva MJ, Figueiredo AJ, et al. (2013) Anthropometric characteristics, physical fitness and technical performance of under-19 soccer players by competitive level and field position. Int J Sports Med 34: 312–317.
8. Kalapotharakos VI, Strimpakos N, Vithoulka I, Karvounidis C, Diamantopoulos K, et al. (2006) Physiological characteristics of elite professional soccer teams of different ranking. J Sports Med Phys Fit 46: 515–519.
9. Rampinini E, Impellizzeri FM, Castagna C, Abt G, Chamari K, et al. (2007) Factors influencing physiological responses to small-sided soccer games. J Sports Sci 25: 659–666.
10. Greig M, Marchant D, Lovell R, Clough P, McNaughton L (2007) A continuous mental task decreases the physiological response to soccer-specific intermittent exercise. Br J Sports Med 41: 908–913.
11. Goedecke JH, White NJ, Chicktay W, Mahomed H, Durandt J, et al. (2013) The effect of carbohydrate ingestion on performance during a simulated soccer match. Nutrients 5: 5193–5204.
12. Buchheit M (2010) Performance and physiological responses to repeated-sprint and jump sequences. Eur J Appl Physiol 110: 1007–1018.
13. Mohr M, Nybo L, Grantham J, Racinais S (2012) Physiological responses and physical performance during football in the heat. PLoS One 7: e39202.
14. Hughes MG, Birdsey L, Meyers R, Newcombe D, Oliver JL, et al. (2013) Effects of playing surface on physiological responses and performance variables in a controlled football simulation. J Sports Sci 31: 878–886.
15. De Clercq D, Debuyck G, Gerlo J, Rambour S, Segers V, et al. (2014) Cutting performance wearing different studded soccer shoes on dry and wet artificial turf. Footwear Sci 6: 81–87.
16. Hennig EM (2014) Plantar pressure measurements for the evaluation of shoe comfort, overuse injuries and performance in soccer. Footwear Sci 6: 119–127.
17. Kuhlman S, Sabick M, Pfeiffer R, Cooper B, Forhan J (2010) Effect of loading condition on the traction coefficient between shoes and artificial turf surfaces. Proc Inst Mech Eng Part P J Sport Eng Technol 224: 155–165.
18. Müller C, Sterzing T, Lange J, Milani TL (2010) Comprehensive evaluation of player–surface interaction on artificial soccer turf. Sports Biomech 9: 193–205.
19. Ekstrand J, Hägglund M, Fuller CW (2011) Comparison of injuries sustained on artificial turf and grass by male and female elite football players. Scand J Med Sci Sports 21: 824–832.
20. Ekstrand J, Timpka T, Hägglund M (2006) Risk of injury in elite football played on artificial turf versus natural grass: a prospective two-cohort study. Br J Sports Med 40: 975–980.

21. Dragoo JL, Braun HJ (2010) The effect of playing surface on injury rate. Sports Med 40: 981–990.
22. Fuller CW, Dick RW, Corlette J, Schmalz R (2007) Comparison of the incidence, nature and cause of injuries sustained on grass and new generation artificial turf by male and female football players. Part 1: match injuries. Br J Sports Med 41: i20–i26.
23. Poulos CCN, Gallucci J, Gage WH, Baker J, Buitrago S, et al. (2014) The perceptions of professional soccer players on the risk of injury from competition and training on natural grass and 3rd generation artificial turf. BMC Sports Sci Med Rehabil 6: 11.
24. Comité Européen de Normalisation (2014) EN 15330-1: 2014. Surfaces for sports areas –synthetic turf and needle-punched surfaces primarily designed for outdoor use. Bruselas: CEN.
25. FIFA (2012a) Quality concept for football turf. Handbook of test method. FIFA: Zurich.
26. FIFA (2012b) Quality concept for football turf. Handbook of requirements. FIFA: Zurich.
27. Andersson H, Ekblom B, Krustrup P (2008) Elite football on artificial turf versus natural grass: movement patterns, technical standards, and player impressions. J Sports Sci 26: 113–122.
28. Di Michele R, Di Renzo AM, Ammazzalorso S, Merni F (2009) Comparison of physiological responses to an incremental running test on treadmill, natural grass, and synthetic turf in young soccer players. J Strength Cond Res 23: 939–945.
29. Ford KR, Manson NA, Evans BJ, Myer GD, Gwin RC, et al. (2006) Comparison of in-shoe foot loading patterns on natural grass and synthetic turf. J Sci Med Sport 9: 433–440.
30. Gains GL, Swedenhjelm AN, Mayhew JL, Bird HM, Houser JJ (2010) Comparison of speed and agility performance of college football players on field turf and natural grass. J Strength Cond Res 24: 2613–2617.
31. Kanaras V, Metaxas TI, Mandroukas A, Gissis I, Zafeiridis A, et al. (2014) The effect of natural and artificial grass on sprinting performance in young soccer players. Am J Sport Sci 2: 1–4.
32. Nédélec M, McCall A, Carling C, Le Gall F, Berthoin S, et al. (2013) Physical performance and subjective ratings after a soccer-specific exercise simulation: comparison of natural grass versus artificial turf. J Sports Sci 31: 529–536.
33. Burillo P, Gallardo L, Felipe JL, Gallardo AM (2014) Artificial turf surfaces: perception of safety, sporting feature, satisfaction and preference of football users. Eur J Sport Sci 14: S437–S447.
34. Zanetti E (2009) Amateur football game on artificial turf: Players' perceptions. App Erg 40: 485–490.
35. Potthast W, Verhelst R, Hughes M, Stone K, De Clercq D (2010) Football-specific evaluation of player–surface interaction on different football turf systems. Sport Technol 3: 5–12.
36. Brito J, Krustrup P, Rebelo A (2012) The influence of the playing surface on the exercise intensity of small-sided recreational soccer games. Hum Mov Sci 31: 946–956.
37. Giatsis G, Kollias I, Panoutsakopoulos V, Papaiakovou G (2004) Biomechanical differences in elite beach-volleyball players in vertical squat jump on rigid and sand surface. Sports Biomech 3: 145–158.
38. Luo G, Stefanyshyn D (2011) Identification of critical traction values for maximum athletic performance. Footwear Sci 3: 127–138.
39. Kerdok AE, Biewener AA, McMahon TA, Weyand PG, Herr HM (2002) Energetics and mechanics of human running on surfaces of different stiffnesses. J Appl Physiol 92: 469–478.
40. Schrier NM, Wannop JW, Lewinson RT, Worobets J, Stefanyshyn D (2014) Shoe traction and surface compliance affect performance of soccer-related movements. Footwear Sci 6: 69–80.
41. McGhie D, Ettema G (2013) Biomechanical analysis of surface–athlete impacts on third-generation artificial turf. Am J Sports Med 41: 177–185.
42. Burillo P, Gallardo L, Felipe JL, Gallardo AM (2012) Mechanical assessment of artificial turf football pitches: the consequences of no quality certification. Sci Res Essays 7: 2457–2465.
43. Alcántara E, Gámez J, Rosa D, Sanchis M (2009) Analysis of the influence of rubber infill morphology on the mechanical performance of artificial turf surfaces for soccer. Proc Inst Mech Eng Part P J Sport Eng Technol 223: 1–9.
44. Sánchez-Sánchez J, Felipe JL, Burillo P, del Corral J, Gallardo L (2014) Effect of the structural components of support on the loss of mechanical properties of football fields of artificial turf. Proc Inst Mech Eng Part P J Sport Eng Technol: 1754337114527276.
45. Bravo DF, Impellizzeri FM, Rampinini E, Castagna C, Bishop D, et al. (2008) Sprint vs. interval training in football. Int J Sports Med 29: 668–674.
46. Chaouachi A, Manzi V, Wong DP, Chaalali A, Laurencelle L, et al. (2010) Intermittent endurance and repeated sprint ability in soccer players. J Strength Cond Res 24: 2663–2669.
47. Spencer M, Bishop D, Dawson B, Goodman C (2005) Physiological and metabolic responses of repeated-sprint activities. Sports Med 35: 1025–1044.
48. Fitzsimons M, Dawson B, Ward D, Wilkinson A (1993) Cycling and running tests of repeated sprint ability. Australian J Sci Med Sport 25: 82–82.
49. Varley MC, Fairweather IH, Aughey RJ (2012) Validity and reliability of GPS for measuring instantaneous velocity during acceleration, deceleration, and constant motion. J Sports Sci 30: 121–127.
50. Lara AJ, Abián J, Alegre LM, Jiménez L, Aguado X (2006) Assessment of power output in jump tests for applicants to a sports sciences degree. J Sports Med Phys Fitness 46: 419.
51. Dixon SJ, Stiles VH (2003) Impact absorption of tennis shoe–surface combinations. Sports Eng 6: 1–9.
52. Allgeuer T, Torres E, Bensason S, Chang A, Martin J (2008) Study of shockpads as energy absorption layer in artificial turf surfaces. Sport Technol 1: 29–33.
53. Naunheim R, Parrott H, Standeven J (2004) A comparison of artificial turf. J Trauma Acute Care Surg 57: 1311–1314.
54. Severn KA, Fleming PR, Dixon N (2010) Science of synthetic turf surfaces: player–surface interactions. Sport Technol 3: 13–25.
55. Villwock MR, Meyer EG, Powell JW, Fouty AJ, Haut RC (2009) The effects of various infills, fibre structures, and shoe designs on generating rotational traction on an artificial surface. Proc Inst Mech Eng Part P J Sport Eng Technol 223: 11–19.
56. Oliver JL (2009) Is a fatigue index a worthwhile measure of repeated sprint ability? J Sci Med Sport 12: 20–23.
57. Pyne DB, Saunders PU, Montgomery PG, Hewitt AJ, Sheehan K (2008) Relationships between repeated sprint testing, speed, and endurance. J Strength Cond Res 22: 1633–1637.
58. Spencer M, Fitzsimons M, Dawson B, Bishop D, Goodman C (2006) Reliability of a repeated-sprint test for field-hockey. J Sci Med Sport 9: 181–184.
59. Villwock MR, Meyer EG, Powell JW, Fouty AJ, Haut RC (2009) Football playing surface and shoe design affect rotational traction. Am J Sports Med 37: 518–525.
60. Livesay GA, Reda DR, Nauman EA (2006) Peak torque and rotational stiffness developed at the shoe–surface interface The effect of shoe type and playing surface. Am J Sports Med 34: 415–422.
61. Pérez Soriano P, Llana Belloch S, Cortell Tormo JM, Pérez Turpin JA (2009) Biomechanical factors to be taken into account to prevent injuries and improve sporting performance on artificial turf. J Hum Sport Exerc 4: 78–92.
62. Bishop D (2003) A comparison between land and sand-based tests for beach volleyball assessment. J Sports Med Phys Fit 43: 418–423.
63. Hardin EC, Van Den Bogert AJ, Hamill J (2004) Kinematic adaptations during running: effects of footwear, surface, and duration. Med Sci Sports Exerc 36: 838–844.
64. Pinnington HC, Lloyd DG, Besier TF, Dawson B (2005) Kinematic and electromyography analysis of submaximal differences running on a firm surface compared with soft, dry sand. Eur J Appl Physiol 94: 242–253.
65. Lejeune TM, Willems PA, Heglund NC (1998) Mechanics and energetics of human locomotion on sand. J Exp Biol 201: 2071–2080.
66. Pinnington HC, Dawson B (2001) The energy cost of running on grass compared to soft dry beach sand. J Sci Med Sport 4: 416–430.
67. Krustrup P, Bangsbo J (2001) Physiological demands of top-class soccer refereeing in relation to physical capacity: effect of intense intermittent exercise training. J Sports Sci 19: 881–891.
68. Potthast W (2010) Motion differences in goal kicking on natural and artificial soccer turf systems. Footwear Sci 2: 29–35.

25

The Effect of Online Violent Video Games on Levels of Aggression

Jack Hollingdale[1]*, Tobias Greitemeyer[2]

1 School of Psychology, University of Sussex, Brighton, United Kingdom, **2** Institute of Psychology, University of Innsbruck, Innsbruck, Austria

Abstract

Background: In recent years the video game industry has surpassed both the music and video industries in sales. Currently violent video games are among the most popular video games played by consumers, most specifically First-Person Shooters (FPS). Technological advancements in game play experience including the ability to play online has accounted for this increase in popularity. Previous research, utilising the General Aggression Model (GAM), has identified that violent video games increase levels of aggression. Little is known, however, as to the effect of playing a violent video game online.

Methods/Principal Findings: Participants ($N = 101$) were randomly assigned to one of four experimental conditions; neutral video game—offline, neutral video game—online, violent video game—offline and violent video game—online. Following this they completed questionnaires to assess their attitudes towards the game and engaged in a chilli sauce paradigm to measure behavioural aggression. The results identified that participants who played a violent video game exhibited more aggression than those who played a neutral video game. Furthermore, this main effect was not particularly pronounced when the game was played online.

Conclusions/Significance: These findings suggest that both playing violent video games online and offline compared to playing neutral video games increases aggression.

Editor: Cheryl McCormick, Brock University, Canada

Funding: This research was supported by grant P23809 from the Austrian Science Fund. The funder had no role in study design, data collection and analysis, decision to publish, or preparation of the manuscript.

Competing Interests: The authors have declared that no competing interests exist.

* Email: jack.hollingdale@live.co.uk

Introduction

The video game industry is now the largest entertainment industry in the UK. 2011 industry figures have identified that game sales, including platform and digital, have exceeded both music and video sales [1]. Violent video games have previously been identified to be the most popular video games played by consumers [2]. Research into the effect of violent video games on levels of aggression has led to concerns that they may pose a public health risk [3]. Indeed, cross-sectional studies have found positive correlations between violent video game play and real-life aggression [4–6]. Longitudinal studies showed that habitual violent video game play predicts later aggression even after controlling for initial levels of aggressiveness [7–9]. Finally, experimental studies have revealed that playing violent video games is a causal risk factor for increased aggression [10–12]. It should be noted, however, that there is other research showing no evidence that engagement with violent video games leads to increases in aggression or reductions in prosocial behaviour [13–16], warranting the need for further research in this area. On balance however, evidence from meta-analyses confirm that exposure to violent video games increases aggressive cognitions, aggressive affect and aggressive behaviour, and decreases empathy and prosocial behaviour [17,18].

Much of the research that has provided evidence to indicate the negative effects of violent video games has utilised the General Aggression Model (GAM) [19]. A widely accepted model for understanding media effects, the GAM posits that cognition, affect and arousal mediate an individual's perception of a situation. Thus, in the short term a violent video game may temporarily increase aggression through the activation of one or more of these domains. In the long term aggressive scripts can develop and become more readily available [4]. Therefore the GAM can explain how properties of a video game can affect players' thoughts, feelings, physiological arousal and subsequent behaviour. Technological developments have afforded such games, and subsequent gaming experience, to expand beyond the realms of the console, and computer programmed opponents (offline gaming), and now allow players to engage in video game play with multiple players from all over the world via the internet (online gaming). Schubert, Regenbrecht and Friedmann [20] found that players who interact with other human players experience a heightened sense of being part of the action. Significant differences in physiological arousal and evaluations of game experience, including presence and likability, have also been found when video game opponents are controlled by other humans [21]. In regards to the negative effects, increases in aggressive thoughts and hostile expectations have been found when playing human opponents in a violent video game [22,23]. Further to this, Wei [24] found, from a survey of 312 Chinese adolescents, that those who played violent video games online against human opponents expressed a greater tolerance of violence, a lower empathetic attitude and more aggressive behaviour than those who played against computer opponents. Based on previous studies, engagement with/against human opponents may strengthen gaming experiences and therefore, in accordance with the GAM, heighten their effects on players' thoughts, feelings and behaviour.

As noted above, violent content within violent video games has also been identified to increase levels of aggression. Within specific violent video games, progression through gaming levels achieved by engaging in violence poses an additional risk of increasing levels of aggression. Carnagey and Anderson [25] found that rewarding violence increased in-game violence and that rewards for killing other racing drivers and pedestrians, in the race-car video game *Carmageddon 2*, increased levels of hostile emotion, aggressive thinking and aggressive behaviour. Sherry [26] identified that video games that portray human violence were associated with increases in levels of aggression, potentially due to higher rates of action, and subsequent heightened nonspecific arousal. More specifically, increases in experience of perceived difficulty, enjoyment and action have yielded significant game effects on aggressive thoughts [27]. These findings lend support to the processes involved in the GAM.

One of the most popular violent gaming formats to date is the First Person Shooter (FPS), in which the gamer experiences the action through the eyes of the main protagonist, centred on a projectile weapon. Reports indicate that a specific franchise, utilising the FPS format, *Call of Duty*, a military war game, has broken all previous sales records. *Call of Duty: Modern Warfare 2*, made $550 m (£350 m) in the first five days of sale. This was surpassed by *Call of Duty: Black Ops* and *Call of Duty: Modern Warfare 3*, which made $650 m (£412 m) and $775 m (£490 m) in sales respectively [28]. FPSs have been found to significantly increase hostility and aggression from base line levels [29]. Based on anecdotal evidence much of the success of this franchise has been attributed to features of online game play.

Despite the popularity of the genre, to date, there is a lack of research that has attempted to investigate the effect of playing violent video games, specifically FPSs, online on levels of aggression.

Overview of the present research

In the present research, we examined whether playing a FPS online would exacerbate the negative effects of violent video game play on aggression. Further to this we examined the effect of particular game experiences including perceived difficulty, enjoyment and action, previously identified to be associated with increases in aggressive thoughts [27], on levels of behavioural aggression. To this end, participants played either a violent video game online or offline, or a neutral video game online or offline. Afterwards, aggressive behaviour was assessed. It was expected that playing a violent video game would increase aggression. It was also expected that participants who had played the violent video game online would show the highest levels of aggression (relative to the remaining three experimental conditions) due to the previously identified experiences specific to online game play. Finally, we examined whether these proposed effects would hold when controlling for perceived difficulty, enjoyment and action.

Ethical approval was given by the University of Sussex's School of Life Sciences Research Governance Committee (Ethical Approval Reference: RBJH0510). All relevant data are within the paper and its Supporting Information files.

Method

Within this paper the authors report how we determined our sample size, all data exclusions (if any), all manipulations, and all measures in the study. One hundred and one students (64 men and 37 women; ages range from 18 to 44: $M = 21.38$, $SD = 4.00$) from a UK University participated in the study in exchange for course credits or payment. After being welcomed by the examiner all participants were asked to complete a consent form. Participants were randomly assigned to one of four experimental conditions; 26 participants in a neutral video game offline, 26 participants in a neutral video game online, 23 participants in a violent video game offline and 26 participants in a violent video game online. Participants were advised that they would be undertaking two unrelated marketing surveys that had been combined for the economy of time. The first would ask for their views about a popular video game and the second would involve a marketing survey for a new recipe of hot chilli sauce.

The first task involved playing a video game for thirty minutes [29] either offline or online. In the offline condition participants were allowed to play against computer characters, subject to the video game's narrative. In the online condition participants played against human opponents via the internet, utilising randomly computer selected pre-existing levels, thus reducing the time spent navigating menus. In the online conditions, when appropriate, participants were requested to wait patiently whilst the server selected and loaded following levels. There was no opportunity for players to communicate with other human players via the internet in the online condition. The audio was turned off in all conditions to prevent participants being exposed to other players' attitudes or opinions in the online condition and to promote consistency. The gaming approach and engagement of online opponents was not recorded. All participants were initially introduced to a Playstation 3 computer console. The type of video game (violent and neutral) was identified using their Pan European Game Information (PEGI) ratings. Participants in the neutral video game condition were introduced to *LittleBigPlanet 2*, certificate 7, a game that would normally be rated suitable for all age groups but contains scenes that may be considered frightening for young children [30]. *LittleBigPlanet 2* allows players to create, explore, solve puzzles, and interact with fantasy environments which they can enjoy or share online with other gamers. All participants in the neutral condition played the initial training level and were then allocated to either the offline condition, subject to the game's narrative, or online condition, able to engage freely with the game's online content, for the remainder of the experiment. Participants in the violent video game condition were introduced to *Call of Duty: Modern Warfare*, certificate 18. *Call of Duty: Modern Warfare* is a FPS that sets gamers as soldiers tasked to kill the enemy in various environments. Games with a certificate 18 depict extreme violence including multiple, motiveless killing and violence towards defenceless people that may make the viewer experience a sense of revulsion [30]. All participants were asked to play the initial level, that introduces players to the gaming controls, and then were set up to play offline levels, following the narrative of the game, or online levels, during which the player played against other human operated opponents in free-for-all mode (Deathmatch). Having played for the allotted time participants were then asked to complete a number of questions about the game they had just played. This survey investigated their attitudes towards the games, including how violent they perceived the content and the

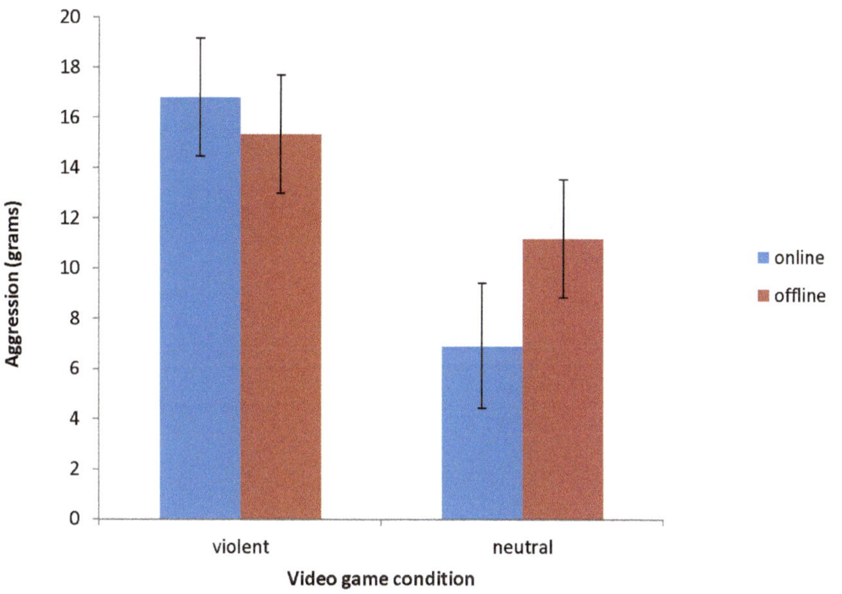

Figure 1. Mean grams of chilli sauce by experimental condition.

graphics to be. Among some filler items, participants indicated how difficult they perceived the game to be (using two items, $\alpha = .72$), to what extent they enjoyed the game (using two items, $\alpha = .79$), and how fast the action of the game was (using one item). All items were assessed on a Likert scale from 1 to 7.

Following this, some affective measures were employed. There were no significant effects on these measures so this is not considered further. Finally, participants completed a marketing survey investigating a new hot chilli sauce recipe. Participants were informed that they were not required to taste the hot chilli sauce but to prepare an amount of chilli sauce for a taste tester. During the instructions they were made aware that the taste tester 'couldn't stand hot chilli sauce' but was taking part due to good payment. They were presented with a hot chilli sauce, depicting three out of three chillies for hotness, a spoon and a plastic receptacle. The amount of chilli sauce was weighed in grams after the participant had left the experiment. The chilli sauce paradigm has been successfully used in previous studies to measure behavioural aggression in the laboratory environment [31]. All participants completed all parts of the experiment with none admitting to knowing the true purpose of the study, therefore all data was included within the study. At the conclusion of the experiment all participants were offered a comprehensive debrief form which included information as to the true purpose of the experiment.

Results

The manipulation check identified that participants in the violent video game condition reported that the violent video game *Call of Duty: Modern Warfare 2* ($M = 4.08$, $SD = 1.29$) depicted a more violent content and more violent graphics compared to the neutral video game *LittleBigPlanet 2* ($M = 1.41$, $SD = 0.89$), $F(1, 97) = 146.97$, $p < .001$, $\eta_p^2 = .60$.

A 2 (type of video game: violent vs. neutral) x 2 (setting: online vs. offline) analysis of variance (ANOVA) on the amount of chili sauce (aggression measure) revealed a significant main effect of type of video game, $F(1, 97) = 8.63$, $p = .004$, $\eta_p^2 = .08$. Participants who had played the violent video game were more aggressive ($M = 16.12$, $SD = 15.30$) than participants who had played the neutral video game ($M = 9.06$, $SD = 7.65$). The main effect of setting, $F(1, 97) = 0.35$, $p = .558$, $\eta_p^2 = .00$, and the interaction were not significant, $F(1, 97) = 1.44$, $p = .234$, $\eta_p^2 = .02$.

To test our specific prediction that aggressive behaviour, grams of chilli sauce dispensed by participants, would be particularly pronounced after playing a violent video game online, planned contrasts were performed, which are particularly adequate to answer such specific research questions [32,33]. In fact, participants who had played the violent video game online were more aggressive ($M = 16.81$, $SD = 16.57$; contrast weight: 3) compared to participants who had played the violent video game offline ($M = 15.35$, $SD = 14.04$; contrast weight: -1), participants who had played the neutral video game online ($M = 6.92$, $SD = 7.62$; contrast weight: -1), and participants who had played the neutral video game offline ($M = 11.19$, $SD = 7.20$; contrast weight: -1), $t(97) = 2.07$, $p = .041$ (Figure 1). Note, however, that the orthogonal contrast comparing the violent video game offline condition (contrast weight: 2) with the neutral video game online (contrast weight: -1) and the neutral video game offline (contrast weight: -1) condition was also significant, $t(97) = 2.09$, $p = .039$. Finally, the orthogonal contrast comparing the neutral video game online (contrast weight: 1) with the neutral video game offline (contrast weight: -1) condition was not significant, $t(97) = 1.28$, $p = .202$. This pattern of data suggests that both playing violent video games online and offline compared to playing neutral video games increases aggression.

The violent video game ($M = 4.11$, $SD = 1.48$) was perceived as being more difficult than the neutral game ($M = 2.71$, $SD = 1.18$), $F(1, 97) = 27.11$, $p < .001$, $\eta_p^2 = .22$. Participants also enjoyed the violent video game more ($M = 4.81$, $SD = 1.46$) than the neutral game ($M = 3.76$, $SD = 1.38$), $F(1, 97) = 13.34$, $p < .001$, $\eta_p^2 = .12$. The violent video game ($M = 5.00$, $SD = 1.47$) was also perceived as having faster action than the neutral video game ($M = 2.94$, $SD = 1.56$), $F(1, 97) = 46.06$, $p < .001$, $\eta_p^2 = .32$. Note, however, that in a multiple regression the effect of type of video game (violent vs. neutral) was still significant when controlling for these video game ratings, $\beta = .27$, $t(96) = 2.15$, $p = .034$. Moreover, none of the video game ratings received a significant regression weight, all $\beta s < .15$, all $ts < 1.29$, all $ps > .202$.

Discussion

The present study examined the effect of playing a violent video game online and the impact of game experience including perceptions of difficulty, enjoyment and action on levels of behavioural aggression. Supporting previous research, this study found that playing a violent video game in comparison to a neutral video game significantly increased levels of aggression [3–6]. However, this main effect was not particularly pronounced when the game was played online. That is, both playing the violent video game online and offline relative to playing a neutral video game increased levels of aggression.

It is important to note that the violent and the neutral video game differed in terms of perceived difficulty, enjoyment and action, with the violent game perceived as being more difficult, more enjoyable, and being faster. However, when controlling for these video game properties, there was still a significant influence of type of video game on aggression. To put it differently, the effect that playing the violent relative to the neutral video game increases aggression is *not* due to differences in perceived difficulty, enjoyment and action. It should be noted, however, that controlling for potential confounders within video game research should be viewed with caution [34].

It should be acknowledged that the violent and the neutral video game chosen for this study may differ in properties other than difficulty, pace of action, and enjoyment. For example, the first-person shooter game, even when played offline (alone), contains a great deal of competitive content (competing in shooting battles for survival against other computer-generated characters), whereas the neutral video game contains little to no competitive content. Importantly, previous research has demonstrated an effect of competitive video game content (i.e., competing against other computer-generated characters in a game) on aggressive behavior in the short-term [35] and long-term [36]. Unfortunately, we did not control for competitive content so it may well be that our finding that violent video games increase aggression can be (in part) accounted for by differences in how competitive the game is perceived to be. This is certainly an important endeavor for future investigations.

With the growing popularity and prevalence of online video gaming, more specifically the engagement with violent video games online, and evidence to suggest that playing against human opponents can heighten the gaming experience, we thought it an important endeavor to investigate whether violent video games played online would exacerbate any negative effects on aggression. As expected, online violent video game play relative to the three remaining experimental increased aggression. However, inasmuch as offline violent video game play relative to the neutral video game conditions also significantly increased aggression, we have to conclude that the violent video game affected aggression but that this effect was not further strengthened by playing the game online. Because this is the first study to have examined the effects of online violent video game play on aggression, we hasten to add that more research is needed before the conclusion is warranted that playing online vs. offline has no consequences on the player's social behavior. For instance, future research may address the effects of online violent video game play on behavioural aggression in the long term. Differences in perceived competition when playing video games online and offline should also be explored. Further to this, future research should investigate the properties of violent video games experienced online that impact on players' aggressive cognitions, affect, physiological arousal and behaviour.

Consideration could also be given to potential positive effects of playing prosocial video games online. Previous research has shown that playing a prosocial video game (where the main objective of the game is to benefit video game characters) increases prosocial behaviour [37–39] and empathy [40] and decreases the accessibility of aggressive thoughts [41] and reduces aggressive behaviour [42]. Likewise, playing cooperative team-player (relative to a single-player) video games increases cooperative behaviour and empathy and decreases aggressive cognitions and angry feelings [43–49]. It may well be that prosocial and antisocial outcomes are even more affected by prosocial and cooperative video games when played online.

It is important to acknowledge a limitation in regards to the video games selected in this study. The perspective of the FPS is specific, and the authors are unaware of a neutral video game that utilises the first person perspective. It may be possible, in the future, to identify a non-violent first person perspective video game and thus better match the characteristics of the violent and neutral video games. As a result, *LittleBigPlanet 2* was selected for its low PEGI rating and ease of operating the controls (unrelated to game difficulty). It should also be conceded that the two online conditions differed in that participants competed against human opponents in the first-person shooter game, whereas the neutral video game allowed players to play competitively and cooperatively. This possible confound might have led to increased aggression in the online/violent (relative to the offline/violent) video game condition and decreased aggression in the online/neutral (relative to the offline/neutral) video game condition (that is, an interaction between type of video game and setting). However, we did not find this interaction, but simply a main effect of type of video game. In fact, it is compelling that despite these differences in online/offline shooter games that they did not differ in their effect on aggression.

Further to this some concerns have been raised as to the suitability of the chilli sauce paradigm as an accurate measurement of behavioural aggression within the laboratory environment [50]. In addition the current sample size was relatively small and therefore limits the generalisability of the results. Future research should increase the experimental population and may examine the effects of violent video games online on other measures of aggression.

In conclusion this study has identified that increases in aggression are not more pronounced when playing a violent video game online in comparison to playing a neutral video game online. This is an important finding in relation to the growing online community and popularity of violent video games, specifically FPSs, and the potential for subsequent increases in aggression. We think there should be concern about the harmful effects of playing violent video games but it appears that playing the game online does not further exacerbate these effects.

Author Contributions

Conceived and designed the experiments: JH TG. Performed the experiments: JH. Analyzed the data: TG. Contributed reagents/materials/analysis tools: JH TG. Wrote the paper: JH TG.

References

1. Entertainment Retailers Association (2012) The voice of entertainment retailing. Available: http://www.eraltd.org/info-stats/overview.aspx. Accessed 2013 Jan 5.
2. Dill KE, Gentile DA, Richter WA, Dill JC (2005) Violence, sex, age and race in popular video games: A content analysis. In Cole E, Henderson-Daniel J, editors. Featuring females: Feminist analyses of media. Washington DC: American Psychological Association. pp. 115–130.
3. Anderson CA, Bushman BJ (2001) Effects of violent video games on aggressive behavior, aggressive cognition, aggressive affect, physiological arousal, and prosocial behavior: A meta-analytic Review of the scientific literature. Psychological Science 12: 353–359.
4. Anderson CA, Dill KE (2000) Video games and aggressive thoughts, feelings, and behavior in the laboratory and life. Journal of Personality and Social Psychology 78: 772–790.
5. DeLisi M, Vaughn MG, Gentile DA, Anderson CA, Shook JJ (2013) Violent video games, delinquency, and youth violence: New evidence. Youth Violence and Juvenile Justice 11: 132–142.
6. Krahé B, Möller I (2004) Playing violent electronic games, hostile attribution style, and aggression related norms in German adolescents. Journal of Adolescence 27: 53–69.
7. Anderson CA, Sakamoto A, Gentile DA, Ihori N, Shibuya A, et al. (2008) Longitudinal effects of violent video games on aggression in Japan and the United States. Pediatrics 122: e1067–e1072.
8. Möller I, Krahé B (2009) Exposure to violent video games and aggression in German adolescents: A longitudinal analysis. Aggressive Behavior 35: 75–89.
9. Willoughby T, Adachi PC, Good M (2012) A longitudinal study of the association between violent video game play and aggression among adolescents. Developmental Psychology 48: 1044–1057.
10. Anderson CA, Carnagey NL (2009) Causal effects of violent sports video games on aggression: Is it competitiveness or violent content? Journal of Experimental Social Psychology 45: 731–739.
11. Greitemeyer T (2014) Intense acts of violence during video game play make daily life aggression appear innocuous: A new mechanism why violent video games increase aggression. Journal of Experimental Social Psychology 50: 52–56.
12. Hollingdale J, Greitemeyer T (2013) The changing face of aggression: The effect of personalized avatars in a violent video game on levels of aggressive behavior. Journal of Applied Social Psychology 43: 1862–1868.
13. Williams D, Skoric M (2005) Internet fantasy violence: A test of aggression in an online game. Communication Monographs 72: 217–233.
14. Elson M, Ferguson CJ (2014) Twenty-five years of research on violence in digital games and aggression: Empirical evidence, perspectives, and a debate gone astray. European Psychologist 19: 33–46.
15. Tear MJ, Nielsen M (2013) Failure to demonstrate that playing violent video games diminishes prosocial behavior. PloS One 8: e68382.
16. Ferguson CJ, Rueda SM (2010) The Hitman study: Violent video game exposure effects on aggressive behavior, hostile feelings and depression. European Psychologist 15: 99–108.
17. Anderson CA, Shibuya A, Ihori N, Swing EL, Bushman BJ, et al. (2010) Violent video game effects on aggression, empathy, and prosocial behavior in Eastern and Western countries. Psychological Bulletin 136: 151–173.
18. Greitemeyer T, Mügge DO (2014) Video games do affect social outcomes: A meta-analytic review of the effects of violent and prosocial video game play. Personality and Social Psychology Bulletin 40: 578–589.
19. Anderson CA, Bushman BJ (2002) Human aggression. Annual Review of Psychology 53: 27–51.
20. Schubert T, Regenbrecht H, Friedmann F (2000, March 27–28)Real and illusory interactions enhance presence in virtual environments. Paper presented at Presence 2000—The Third International Workshop on Presence, Delft University of Technology, Delft, Netherlands.
21. Lim S, Reeves B (2010) Computer agents versus avatars: Responses to interactive game characters controlled by a computer or other player. International Journal of Human-Computer Studies 68: 57–68.
22. Eastin MS (2006) Video game violence and the female game player: Self- and opponent gender effects on presence and aggressive thoughts, Human Communication Research 32: 351–372.
23. Eastin MS, Griffiths RP (2006) Beyond the shooter game. Examining presence and hostile outcomes among male game players, Communication Research 33: 448–466.
24. Wei R (2007) Effects of playing violent video games on Chinese adolescents' pro-violence attitudes, attitudes towards others, and aggressive behavior. Cyberpsychology & Behaviour 10: 371–380.
25. Carnagey NL, Anderson CA (2005) The effects of reward and punishment in violent video games on aggressive affect, cognition, and behavior. American Psychological Science 16: 882–889.
26. Sherry JL (2001) The effects of violent video games on aggression: A meta-analysis. Human Communication Research 27: 409–431.
27. Anderson CA, Carnagey NL, Flanagan M, Benjamin AJ, Eubanks J, et al. (2004) Violent video games: Specific effects of violent content on aggressive thoughts and behaviour. Advances in Experimental Social Psychology 36: 199–249.
28. British Broadcasting Corporation (BBC) (2011) Call of Duty enjoys record sales despite retail woes. Available: http://www.bbc.co.uk/news/technology-15796585. Accessed 2013 Jan 5.
29. Barlett CP, Harris RJ, Baldassaro R (2007) Longer you play, the more hostile you feel: examination of first person shooter video games and aggression during video game play. Aggressive Behavior 33: 486–497.
30. Pan European Game Information (PEGI) (2013) What do the labels mean? Available: http://www.pegi.info/en/index/id/33/. Accessed 2013 Jan 5.
31. McGregor HA, Lieberman JD, Greenberg J, Soloman S, Arndt J, et al. (1998) Terror management and aggression: Evidence that mortality salience motivates aggression against worldview threatening others. Journal of Personality and Social Psychology 74: 590–605.
32. Rosenthal R, Rosnow RL (1985) Contrast analysis: Focused comparisons in the analysis of variance. Cambridge, United Kingdom: Cambridge University Press.
33. Steiger JH (2004) Beyond the F test: Effect size confidence intervals and tests of close fit in the analysis of variance and contrast analysis. Psychological Methods 9: 164–182.
34. Miller GA, Chapman JP (2001) Misunderstanding analysis of covariance. Journal of Abnormal Psychology 110: 40–48.
35. Adachi PJC, Willoughby T (2011) The effect of video game competition and violence on aggressive behavior: Which characteristic has the greatest influence? Psychology of Violence 1: 259–274.
36. Adachi PJC, Willoughby T (2013) Demolishing the competition: The longitudinal link between competitive video games, competitive gambling, and aggression. Journal of Youth and Adolescence 42: 1090–1104.
37. Greitemeyer T (2011) Effects of prosocial media on social behavior: When and why does media exposure affect helping and aggression? Current Directions in Psychological Science 20: 251–255.
38. Gentile DA, Anderson CA, Yukawa S, Ihori N, Saleem M, et al. (2009) The Effects of Prosocial Video Games on Prosocial Behaviors: International Evidence from Correlational, Experimental, and Longitudinal Studies. Personality and Social Psychology Bulletin 35: 752–763.
39. Greitemeyer T, Osswald S (2010) Effects of prosocial video games on prosocial behavior. Journal of Personality and Social Psychology 98: 211–221.
40. Prot S, Gentile DA, Anderson CA, Suzuki K, Swing E, et al. (2014) Long-term relations between prosocial media use, empathy, and prosocial behavior. Psychological Science 25: 358–368.
41. Greitemeyer T, Osswald S (2009) Prosocial video games reduce aggressive cognitions. Journal of Experimental Social Psychology 45: 896–900.
42. Greitemeyer T, Agthe M, Turner R, Gschwendtner C (2012) Acting prosocially reduces retaliation: Effects of prosocial video games on aggressive behavior. European Journal of Social Psychology 42: 235–242.
43. Eastin MS (2007) The influence of competitive and cooperative play on state hostility. Human Communication Research 33: 450–466.
44. Ewoldsen DR, Eno CA, Okdie BM, Velez JA, Guadagno RE, et al. (2012) Effect of playing violent video games cooperatively or competitively on subsequent cooperative behavior. Cyberpsychology, Behavior, and Social Networking 15: 277–280.
45. Greitemeyer T (2013) Playing video games cooperatively increases empathic concern. Social Psychology 44: 408–413.
46. Greitemeyer T, Cox C (2013) There's no "I" in team: Effects of cooperative video games on cooperative behavior. European Journal of Social Psychology 43: 224–228.
47. Greitemeyer T, Traut-Mattausch E, Osswald S (2012) How to ameliorate negative effects of violent video games on cooperation: Play it cooperatively in a team. Computers in Human Behavior 28: 1465–1470.
48. Schmierbach M (2010) "Killing Spree": Exploring the connection between competitive game play and aggressive cognition. Communication Research 37: 256–274.
49. Velez JA, Mahood C, Ewoldsen DR, Moyer-Gusé E (2014) Ingroup versus outgroup conflict in the context of violent video game play: The effect of cooperation on increased helping and decreased aggression. Communication Research 41: 607–626.
50. Ritter D, Eslea M (2005) Hot sauce, toy guns, and graffiti: A critical account of current laboratory aggression paradigms. Aggressive Behavior 31: 407–419.

Resting Energy Expenditure Prediction in Recreational Athletes of 18–35 Years: Confirmation of Cunningham Equation and an Improved Weight-Based Alternative

Twan ten Haaf[1], Peter J. M. Weijs[1,2,3]*

1 Department of Nutrition & Dietetics, School of Sports and Nutrition, Amsterdam University of Applied Sciences, Amsterdam, The Netherlands, 2 Department of Nutrition & Dietetics, Internal Medicine, VU University Medical Center, Amsterdam, The Netherlands, 3 EMGO+ Institute for Health and Care Research, VU University Medical Center, Amsterdam, The Netherlands

Abstract

Introduction: Resting energy expenditure (REE) is expected to be higher in athletes because of their relatively high fat free mass (FFM). Therefore, REE predictive equation for recreational athletes may be required. The aim of this study was to validate existing REE predictive equations and to develop a new recreational athlete specific equation.

Methods: 90 (53M, 37F) adult athletes, exercising on average 9.1±5.0 hours a week and 5.0±1.8 times a week, were included. REE was measured using indirect calorimetry (Vmax Encore n29), FFM and FM were measured using air displacement plethysmography. Multiple linear regression analysis was used to develop a new FFM-based and weight-based REE predictive equation. The percentage accurate predictions (within 10% of measured REE), percentage bias, root mean square error and limits of agreement were calculated.

Results: The Cunningham equation and the new weight-based equation $REE(kJ/d) = 49.940^{*} weight(kg) + 2459.053^{*} height(m) - 34.014^{*} age(y) + 799.257^{*} sex(M=1, F=0) + 122.502$ and the new FFM-based equation $REE(kJ/d) = 95.272^{*} FFM(kg) + 2026.161$ performed equally well. De Lorenzo's equation predicted REE less accurate, but better than the other generally used REE predictive equations. Harris-Benedict, WHO, Schofield, Mifflin and Owen all showed less than 50% accuracy.

Conclusion: For a population of (Dutch) recreational athletes, the REE can accurately be predicted with the existing Cunningham equation. Since body composition measurement is not always possible, and other generally used equations fail, the new weight-based equation is advised for use in sports nutrition.

Editor: Marià Alemany, Faculty of Biology, Spain

Funding: These authors have no support or funding to report.

Competing Interests: The authors have declared that no competing interests exist.

* Email: p.j.m.weijs@hva.nl

Introduction

An optimal balance between energy intake and energy expenditure is crucial for athlete performance. Determining resting energy expenditure (REE) is essential for nutrition and exercise professionals in providing nutritional advice for athletes, since REE contributes to 60–70% of daily energy expenditure [1]. REE is the maintenance energy cost of the body in rest under steady state conditions. This is different from the minimal energy cost. Energy expenditure can for example be lower during sleep or during undernutrition [2]. REE can be measured through indirect calorimetry or estimated using REE predictive equations. The gold standard to determine the REE is measurement by indirect calorimetry. However, nutrition and exercise professionals do not usually have the necessary equipment. Moreover, indirect calorimetry [3] is expensive and requires trained personnel to guarantee the reliability. Therefore, predictive equations are most often used to estimate the REE.

In general, REE predictive equations can be considered population specific [4–8]. Because of their relatively high fat free mass (FFM), REE in athletes is underestimated by the majority of the existing equations [9]. Only a few studies have validated predictive equations in a group of athletes [10,11]. Thompson and Manore [11] concluded that the Cunningham equation was the most accurate equation, while LaForgia et al. [10] indicated the equation of De Lorenzo as the most accurate predictive equation. However, it should be noted that both studies investigated a different set of equations.

Cunninghams equation was established using 239 healthy adult subjects from the studies of Harris and Benedict [12], but they excluded 16 male subjects because they were identified as trained athletes. Moreover, the only factor included in the equation is lean body weight, but body composition measurements are not always possible in sports practice. Factors in De Lorenzo's equation are weight and height, which are better applicable in sports practice.

Moreover, the De Lorenzo equation is actually based on athletes [13]. However, the De Lorenzo equation was developed using the REE from 51 male athletes exercising at least 3 hours/day. This equation may therefore only apply to (sub) elite athletes while it may less accurately predict the REE for recreational athletes, which represent a significant part of the society. Therefore, the aim of this study was to validate existing resting energy expenditure predictive equations (Table 1) and to develop 2 new equations, specifically for recreational athletes. One equation was developed using FFM, since the body composition of (recreational) athletes differs from that of the average population. In addition, an equation was developed without FFM, since this parameter cannot always be used in sport practice. It was hypothesized that a new equation specifically developed for recreational athletes would result in better estimations of the resting energy expenditure.

Methods

103 athletes (age 18–35 y), who participated in sports for at least 3 hours a week and 2 times a week, participated in the study. Subjects were of self-reported stable weight, did not suffer from any metabolic disorders and did not take any medications affecting metabolic rate. They did not perform vigorous exercise within 12 hours before the measurement, neither did they consume food or beverages (except water) within 4 hours before the measurement. Subjects were at least 30 minutes at rest in the laboratory before the start of the measurement. 9 participants were excluded from analysis because they were in the ovulation phase of the menstrual cycle [14] and 4 were excluded because their Respiratory Exchange Ratio (RER) was below 0.7 or above 1.0 [15]. Finally, 90 athletes (Characteristics: Table 2; Sport specifications: Table 3; Age and Activity level: Figure 1) were included for validation and development of REE predictive equations. Mean (±SD) age was 23.2±4.8 year and mean REE was 7.68±1.16 MJ/day (1837±278 kcal/day). The training hours were 9.1±5.0 hours/week and the training frequency spent on sports was 5.0±1.8 times/week. Written informed consent was obtained from all subjects and the study was approved by the medical ethical committee of the VU University Medical Center (2009/302).

REE was calculated by the manufacturer's software, using oxygen consumption and carbon dioxide production measured by indirect calorimetry with a ventilated hood system (Vmax Encore n29; Viasys Healthcare, Houten, Netherlands). Calibration of the equipment with 2 different standard gases and 1 standard volume was performed on a daily basis, before starting the measurements. Additionally, an automatic recalibration of the system was done every 5 minutes. The subjects remained lying down but awake. The measurement took 30 minutes. Only steady state periods of measurement were selected according to the procedures for the ventilated hood system (<10% CV). The first 5 minutes of the measurements were discarded.

Body weight, FFM, and fat mass (FM) were determined using air displacement plethysmography (BODPOD, Life Measurement Inc, Concord, CA). Total lung volume was measured (31 were estimated) with the BODPOD system to correct total body volume. The BODPOD was calibrated on a daily basis directly before use. Height was measured by using a stadiometer (Seca 222; Seca; Hamburg; Germany).

Statistical analysis was performed using SPSS 20. Multiple linear regression analysis was used to develop 2 new REE predictive equations. Firstly, a stepwise regression approach was used with the variables FFM, FM, age, sex and a constant to verify a possible FFM-based REE equation. Weight-based equations are usually most successful when predictors of active cell mass are entered, being body weight, height, age and sex [16]. Therefore, these variables and a constant were used in a regression analysis. In both regression analyses, variables were included when the p-value for the F-test was smaller than 0.05.

The predicted REE from the 2 developed equations and from other commonly used equations (Table 4) were compared with the measured REE. Firstly, accuracy was calculated as the percentage of accurate REE predictions (within 10% of the measured REE). Secondly, the bias was calculated as the relative deviation (%) of the predicted REE from the measured REE. Thirdly, the root mean squared error (RMSE) was calculated as the expected absolute deviation (MJ/d) of the predicted REE from the measured REE. Lastly, limits of agreement were calculated as the 95% confidence interval of the bias.

Results

Using the previously described regression analyses, the following new equations were obtained (in kJ and kcal) for weight-based:

Table 1. Equations evaluated in this study.

Equation	Sample size	Remarks on population
Cunningham [17]	M = 120 F = 103	Healthy adults, trained athletes were excluded
De Lorenzo [13]	M = 51	Athletes, exercising at least 3 hours a day
FAO [21]	N = 11000	Mainly based on Schofield data, also including group mean values also
FAO (height) [21]	N = 11000	Mainly based on Schofield data, also including group mean values
Harris-Benedict 1919 [21]	M = 136 F = 103	Mainly normal weight subject
Harris-Benedict 1984 [28]	M = 168 F = 169	Mainly normal weight subject
Mifflin [18]	M = 251 F = 247	Including obese subjects
Mifflin (FFM) [18]	M = 251 F = 247	Including obese subjects
Owen [19,20]	M = 60 F = 44	Including obese subjects
Owen (FFM) [19,20]	M = 60 F = 44	Including obese subjects
Schofield [29]	M = 3575 F = 1239	47% Italian subjects
Schofield (height) [29]	M = 3575 F = 1239	47% Italian subjects

Table 2. Subjects characteristics: mean ± standard deviation [range].

	Male (N = 53)		Female (N = 37)		Total (N = 90)	
Age (y)	23.1±4.7	[18–35]	23.5±5.0	[18–35]	23.2±4.8	[18–35]
Height (m)	1.82±.09	[1.63–2.05]	1.72±.05	[1.61–1.84]	1.78±.09	[1.61–2.05]
Weight (kg)	75.7±7.8	[62.1–100.3]	62.6±6.6	[52.8–78.3]	70.3±9.7	[52.8–100.3]
BMI (kg/m²)	22.8±2.0	[18.6–27.0]	21.3±1.9	[17.9–26.7]	22.2±2.1	[17.9–27.0]
FFM (%)	88.3±4.9	[73.7–98.5]	78.4±4.7	[67.8–88.8]	84.3±6.8	[67.8–98.5]
FM (%)	11.7±4.9	[1.5–26.3]	21.6±4.7	[11.2–32.2]	15.7±6.8	[1.5–32.2]
REE (kcal/d)	2007±206	[1562–2551]	1594±162	[1111–1832]	1837±278	[1111–2551]
REE (MJ/d)	8.40±0.86	[6.53–10.67]	6.67±0.68	[4.65–7.67]	7.69±1.16	[4.65–10.67]
Activity (h/week)	10.0±5.4	[3.0–28.0]	7.9±4.0	[3.0–18.0]	9.1±5.0	[3.0–28.0]
Activity (#/week)	5.3±1.8	[2–12]	4.5±1.7	[2–9]	5.0±1.8	[2–12]

BMI: Body mass index, FFM: Fat free mass, FM: Fat mass, REE: Resting energy expenditure.

$$\text{REE(kJ/d)} = 49.940^{*} weight(kg) + 2459.053^{*} height(m) - 34.014^{*} age(y) + 799.257^{*} sex(M=1, F=0) + 122.502$$

or,

$$\text{REE(kcal/d)} = 11.936^{*} weight(kg) + 587.728^{*} height(m) - 8.129^{*} age(y) + 191.027^{*} sex(M=1, F=0) + 29.279$$

and FFM-based:

$$\text{REE(kJ/d)} = 95.272^{*} FFM(kg) + 2026.161$$

or,

$$\text{REE(kcal/d)} = 22.771^{*} FFM(kg) + 484.264$$

The weight-based equation for resting energy expenditure included body weight (kilograms), body height (meters), age (years), sex (value 1 for male, value 0 for female) and a constant. The fat free mass based equation only included fat free mass (kilograms) and a constant. The predicted REE values are plotted against measured REE values (Figure 2).

The accuracy for all equations is depicted in Figure 3B. The Cunningham equation resulted in the highest percentage accurate predicted equations (M 84.9%; F 78.4%), followed by the weight-based equation (M 83.0%; F 75.7%) and the FFM-based equation (M 83.0%; F 72.3%). The De Lorenzo equation for elite male athletes (M 77.4%; F 59.5%) had an inferior accuracy compared to the weight-based equation. All other, generally used equations showed less than 50% accuracy.

Equal to the accuracy, lowest bias was observed for Cunningham, both new equations and De Lorenzo (Figure 3A). The low bias for De Lorenzo's equation was based on opposite bias (male: negative, female: positive). Since this is not a cross-validation study, the bias for the new equations approached zero.

The FFM-based equation resulted in the lowest RMSE (M 0.62 MJ/d; F 0.57 MJ/d), and Cunningham's and the weight-based equation resulted in a comparable RMSE (Figure 3C). The RMSE for De Lorenzo was higher (M 0.74 MJ/d; F 0.77 MJ/d).

Table 3. Description of sports activity.

	Male (N = 53)	Female(N = 37)	Total (N = 90)
Athletics Long distance	5	9	14
Athletics Sprint	3	2	5
Cycling	6	4	10
Gymnastics	4	5	9
Fitness	3	5	8
Rowing/canoeing	7	5	12
Swimming	2	1	3
Team sports*	17	4	21
Remaining sports**	6	2	8

* Hockey, korfball, soccer, volleyball.
** Dancing, martial arts, skating, tennis.

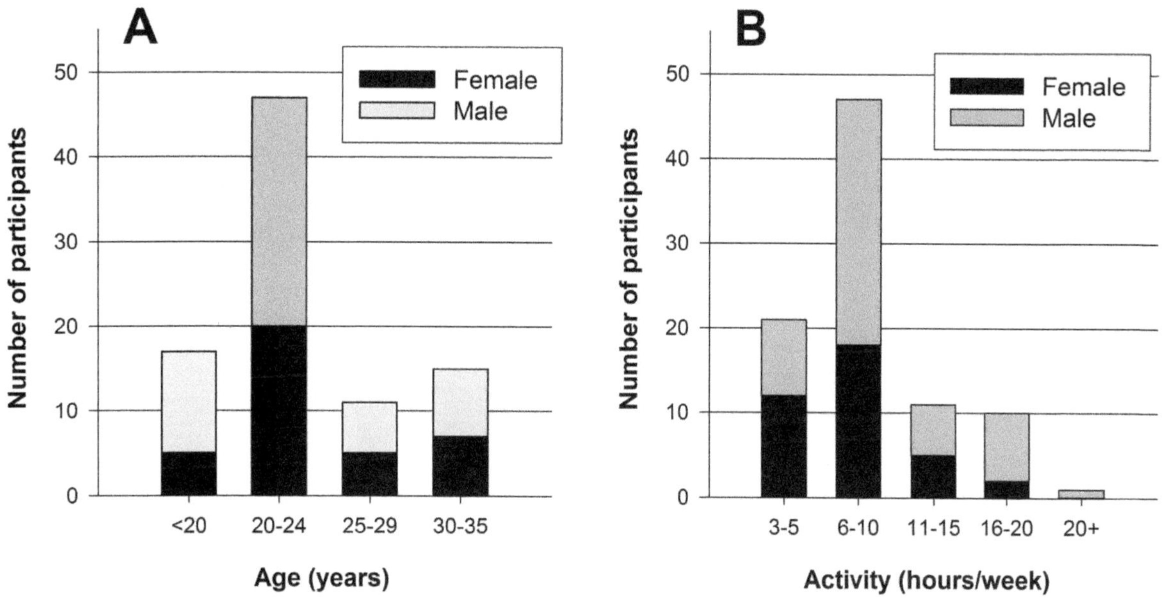

Figure 1. Description of the study participants (N = 90) for (A) age group and (B) activity level (hours per week).

The generally used equations all resulted in RMSE larger than 0.95 MJ/day.

In Figure 4 the errors are plotted against the individual measured REE for 6 equations. A negative proportional bias could be observed for all equations, meaning the equations tended to underestimate a higher REE.

Discussion

The purpose of this study was to validate existing predictive equations for REE and to develop and validate 2 new equations, specifically for recreational athletes. This study shows that the new FFM-based equation provides the best prediction of REE in recreational athletes. The weight-based equation and Cunningham's equation [17] performed equally well. De Lorenzo's equation [13] performed less, and can be improved by the new weight-based equation. The other generally used REE predictive equations have low accuracy in recreational athletes.

Although the Cunningham equation was developed in a general population, this equation performed better than the already existing equations. This suggests that FFM is an important predictor of REE for a population of recreational athletes. However, the FFM-based equations from Mifflin [18] and Owen [19,20] did perform worse than the new weight-based equation and De Lorenzo's equation [13], and not better than the other non-FFM equations. The difference of those equations with Cunningham [17] and the new FFM-based equation might be explained by the population that was used to develop the equations. Mifflin [18] and Owen [19,20] used lean and obese subjects. The mean BMI in Mifflin's study was 27.5±4.1 kg/m^2 for male and 26.2±4.9 kg/m^2 for female, with a maximum of 42 kg/m^2. In Owen's study, the BMI for male was 28.2±7.5 kg/m^2 and 27.8±8.6 kg/m^2 for female, with a maximum of 58.7 kg/m^2. Therefore, the better performance of the new FFM-based and Cunningham's equation over the weight and/or height based equations might result from the different body composition of (recreational) athletes compared with a general population.

De Lorenzo's equation [13] is the only equation which is actually based on a population of athletes. The accuracy was higher than the other generally used equations, but lower than Cunningham and the new developed equations. The participants in the study of De Lorenzo exercised at least 3 hours/day. The equation includes body weight and height and probably these factors do not predict resting energy expenditure well in recreational athletes due to a substantial different body composition. This emphasises the role of the specificity of the population. Other studies have pointed out that the accuracy of a prediction equation not only depends on activity level. For example, Henry [2] described the inaccuracy of the FAO equations [21] for many communities. The population used to develop the FAO equations consisted of a disproportional number of Italians, who seem to have a higher basal metabolic rate then people living in the tropical area, China or Australia. Another example of the specific accuracy of REE prediction equation is depicted by Weijs [5], who showed differences between US and Dutch obese adults. As a consequence of the specificity of a REE equation, a researcher always has to deal with a trade-off between internal and external validity (i.e. the more homogeneous the population, the more accurate the REE prediction but the less applicable to a heterogeneous population). Therefore, validation of the new equations in other cohorts is needed.

This study has some major limitations. Firstly, participants were instructed to not perform vigorous exercise within 12 hours before the measurement. However, Compher et al. [15] advised to perform no physical activity 14 hours prior to indirect calorimetry measurement to have energy expenditure returned to baseline levels. Physical activity will increase REE after exercise [22,23]. The time needed for REE to return to normal is called recovery time, which is dependent on the type of activity, intensity, duration and physical exercise level. In trained individuals, like in this study, recovery time is shorter than in untrained [15]. The study upon which the advice of 14 hours is based, included only 10 subjects [24]. Another small, but well designed study [25] used a 12 hour recovery time for different levels of activity, and showed no effect of physical activity on REE. Therefore, a period of 12 hours was selected for the present study.

Table 4. Resting energy expenditure prediction equations given in their original unit (kcal/day, except Schofield (MJ/day)).

Name	Equation
Cunningham	22(FFM) +500
De Lorenzo	9(wt) +1170(ht) –857
FAO	
Male (18–30 y)	15.3(wt) +679
Male (30–60 y)	11.6(wt) +879
Male (>60 y)	13.5(wt) +487
Female (18–30 y)	14.7(wt) +496
Female (30–60 y)	8.7(wt) +829
Female (>60 y)	10.5(wt) +596
FAO (height)	
Male (18–30 y)	15.4(wt) –27(ht) +717
Male (30–60 y)	11.3(wt) –16(ht) +901
Male (>60 y)	8.8(wt) + 1128(ht) –1071
Female (18–30 y)	13.3(wt) +334(ht) +35
Female (30–60 y)	8.7(wt) –25(ht) +865
Female (>60 y)	9.2(wt) + 637(ht) –302
Harris-Benedict 1919	
Male	13.75(wt) +500.33(ht) –6.76(age) +66.47
Female	9.56(wt) +184.96(ht) –4.68(age) +655.10
Harris-Benedict 1984	
Male	13.40(wt) +479.9(ht) –5.68(age) +88.36
Female	9.25(wt) +309.8(ht) –4.33(age) +477.59
Mifflin	9.99(wt) +625(ht) –4.92(age) +166(gender) –161
Mifflin (FFM)	19.7(FFM) +413
Owen	
Male	10.2(wt) +879
Female	7.18(wt) +795
Owen (FFM)	
Male	22.3(FFM) +290
Female	19.7(FFM) +334
Schofield	
Male (18–30 y)	63(wt) +2896*
Male (30–60 y)	48(wt) +3653*
Male (>60 y)	49(wt) +2459*
Female (18–30 y)	62(wt) +2036*
Female (30–60 y)	34(wt) +3538*
Female (>60 y)	38(wt) +2755*
Schofield (height)	
Male (18–30 y)	63(wt) –42(ht) +2953*
Male (30–60 y)	48(wt) –11(ht) +3670*
Male (>60 y)	49(wt) +4068(ht) –3491*
Female (18–30 y)	62(wt) +1148(ht) +411*
Female (30–60 y)	34(wt) +6(ht) +3530*
Female (>60 y)	38(wt) +1917(ht) +74*

FFM: Fat free mass (kg); wt: weight (kg); ht: height (m); age (y); gender (0: female, 1: male).
* Equation for values in MJ/day.

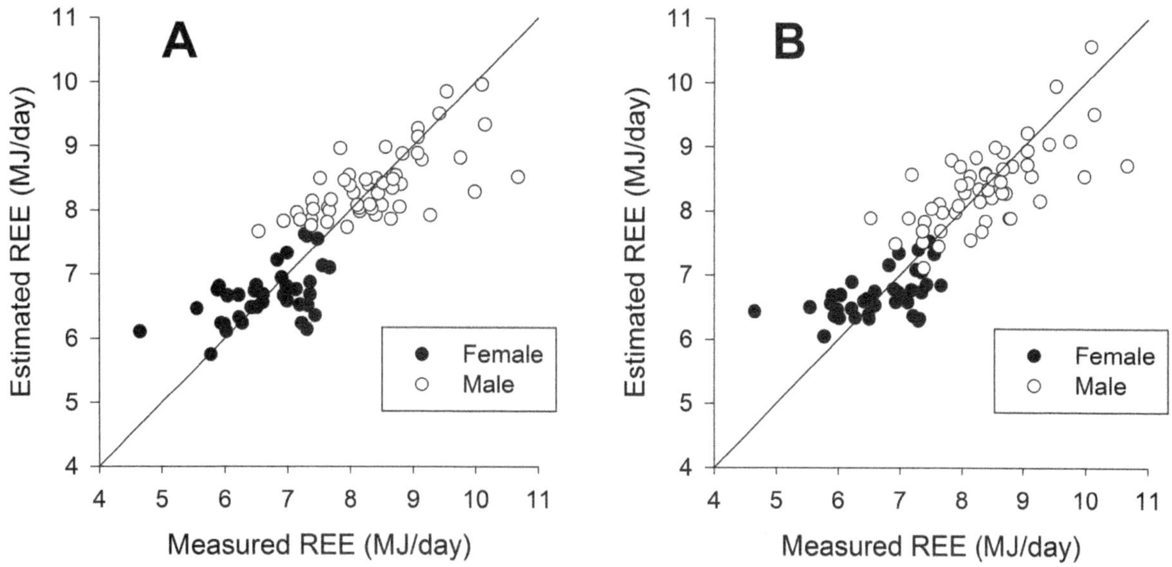

Figure 2. Predicted REE (MJ/day) plotted against REE (MJ/day) measured by indirect calorimetry for male (open dot) and female (filled dot). Graphs represent (A) the new weight-based and (B) the new FFM-based equation. The solid line is the line of identity.

Secondly, subjects were instructed to not eat within 4 hours prior to the measurement, while Compher et al. [15] recommended a minimal fast of 5 hours. However, they stated that for small meals a minimum fast of 4 hours is acceptable. Moreover, Weststrate [26,27] showed that the thermic effect of food could be nearly completed within 4 hour. The mean period of fasting by our subjects was on average 9.1±4.6 hours. Therefore, it is assumed that the thermic effect of food was negligible in this study.

Conclusions

In general, it is advised to use the REE prediction equation that is most specific for the target population. For a population of (Dutch) recreational athletes, the REE can accurately be predicted with the existing Cunningham equation. Since body composition measurement is not always possible, and other generally used equations fail, the new weight-based equation is advised for use in sports nutrition.

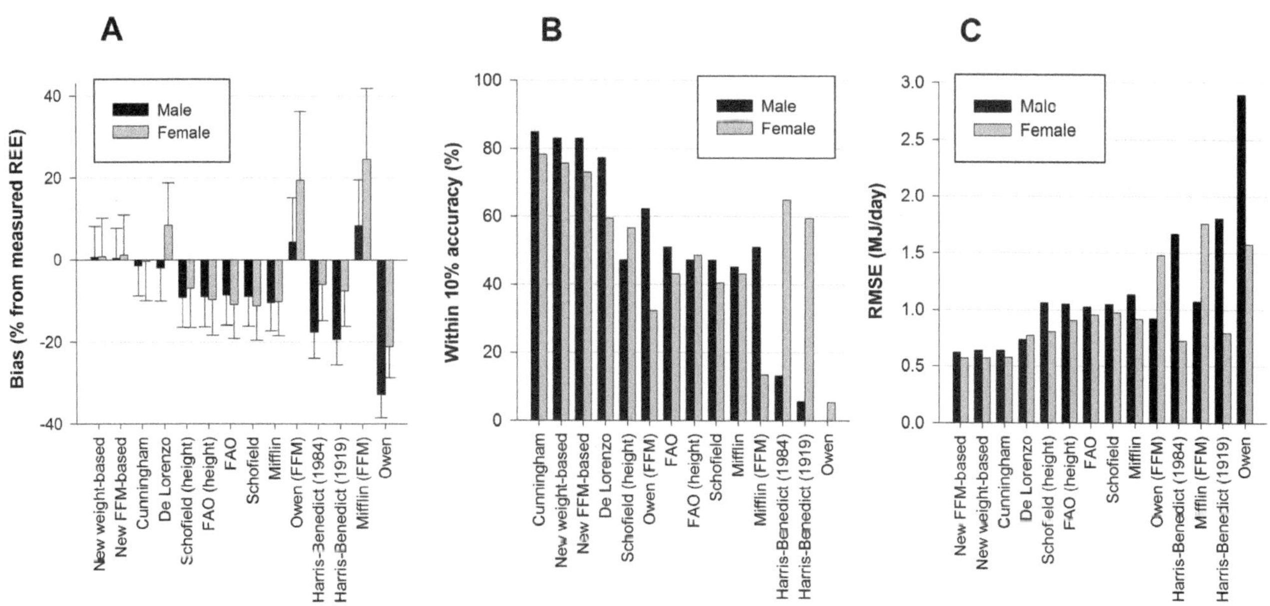

Figure 3. Outcome measures for the REE predictive equations for male (N = 53) and female (N = 37). The graphs represent (**A**) Percentage bias (±SD), (**B**) percentage accurate REE predictions and (**C**) Root mean squared error (MJ/day).

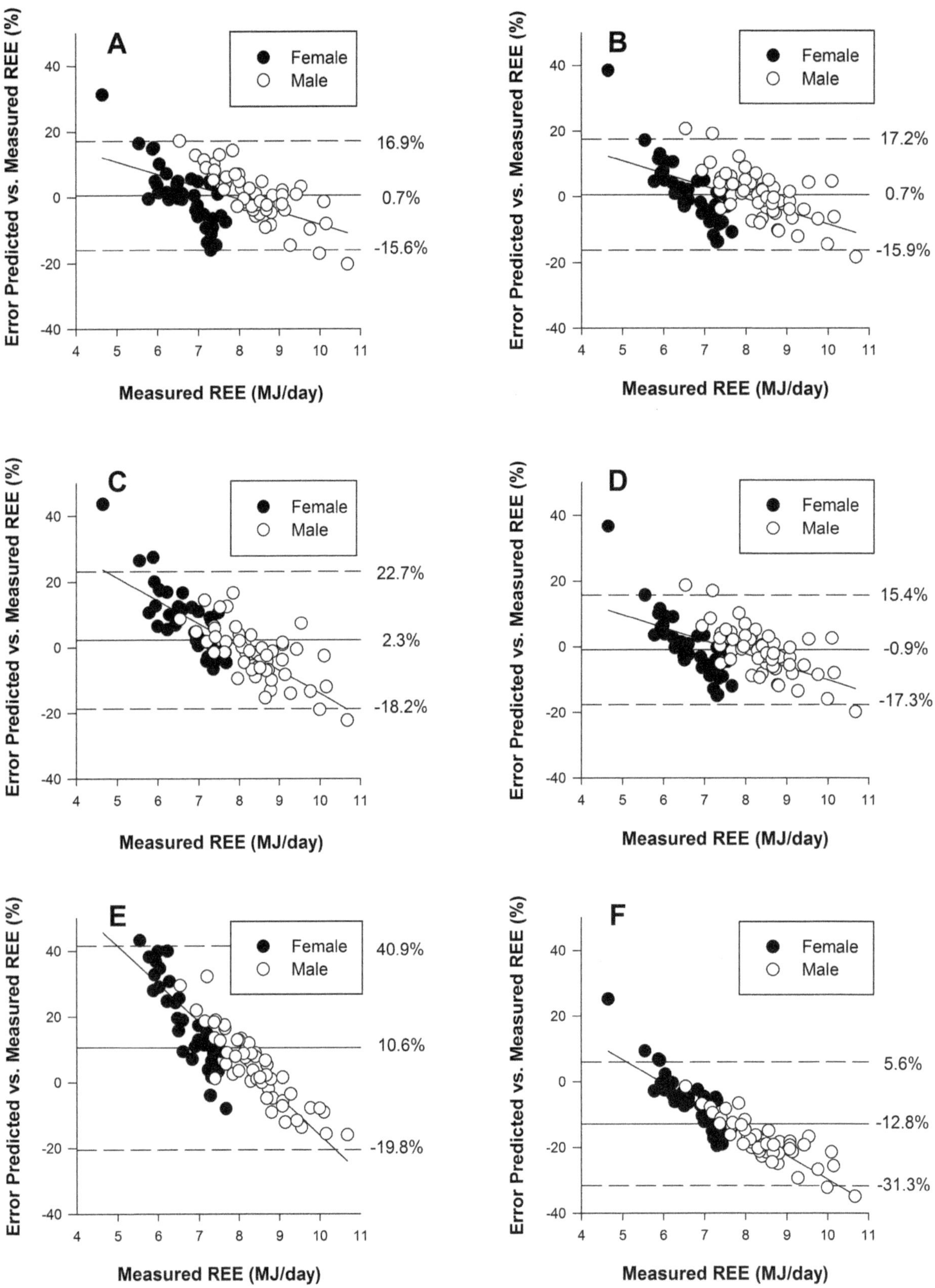

Figure 4. Limits of agreement analysis (bias: vertical solid line; 95% confidence interval: vertical dashed lines) for REE predictive equations versus measured REE (MJ/day) for male (open dot) and female (filled dot). Graphs represent equations of (**A**) new weight-based; (**B**) new FFM-based; (**C**) De Lorenzo; (**D**) Cunningham; (**E**) Owen FFM and (**F**) Harris-Benedict 1984.

Supporting Information

Dataset S1 Contains raw data used for development and testing of the prediction equations. The dataset contains information on gender; age; training volume; training frequency; weight; fat mass (%); fat mass (kg); fat free mass (kg); height; BMI; fat free mass (%) and measured REE (kJ) of the subjects.

Acknowledgments

We thank Marcel Hesseling for his help in the Nutritional Assessment Lab, all athletes for their participation, Anna Elisabeth van den Hoven, Jitske Spijker, Anne-Marijke Ambergen, Janine Reitsema, Jessica van Nieuwkerk, Maaike van Rijn, Astrid Schepers, Lisette van Wijk, Anneke Sman, Carine Bekenkamp, Antoinette Drexhage, Anousckha Severin and Martine Kampman for collecting part of the data, Amely Verreijen and Minse de Bos Kuil for their assistance.

Author Contributions

Conceived and designed the experiments: TtH PW. Analyzed the data: TtH PW. Wrote the paper: TtH PW.

References

1. Trexler ET, Smith-Ryan AE, Norton LE (2014) Metabolic adaptation to weight loss: implications for the athlete. J Int Soc Sports Nutr 11: 7–7.
2. Henry CJK (2005) Basal metabolic rate studies in humans: measurement and development of new equations. Public Health Nutr 8: 1133–1152.
3. Ferrannini E (1988) The theoretical bases of indirect calorimetry: A review. Metabolism 37: 287–301.
4. da Rocha EEM, Alves VGF, Silva MHN, Chiesa Ca, da Fonseca RBV (2005) Can measured resting energy expenditure be estimated by formulae in daily clinical nutrition practice? Curr Opin Clin Nutr Metab Care 8: 319–328.
5. Hofsteenge GH, Chinapaw MJ, Delemarre-van de Waal HA, Weijs PJ (2010) Validation of predictive equations for resting energy expenditure in obese adolescents. Am J Clin Nutr 91: 1244–1254.
6. Weijs PJM (2008) Validity of predictive equations for resting energy expenditure in US and Dutch overweight and obese class I and II adults aged 18–65 y. Am J Clin Nutr 88: 959–970.
7. Weijs PJM, Kruizenga HM, van Dijk AE, van der Meij BS, Langius JaE, et al. (2008) Validation of predictive equations for resting energy expenditure in adult outpatients and inpatients. Clin Nutr 27: 150–157.
8. Weijs PJM, Vansant GaaM (2010) Validity of predictive equations for resting energy expenditure in Belgian normal weight to morbid obese women. Clin Nutr 29: 347–351.
9. Dunford M (2006) Sports Nutrition. Chicago, USA: American Dietetic Association.
10. LaForgia J, Withers RT, Van der Ploeg GE, Gunn SM (2000) The accuracy of resting metabolic rate prediction equations in male athletes. Proc Nutr Soc Aust 24: 127–127.
11. Thompson J, Manore MM (1996) Predicted and measured resting metabolic rate of male and female endurance athletes. J Am Diet Assoc 96: 30–34.
12. Harris JA, Benedict FG (1919) A biometric study of basal metabolism in man. Washington DC: Carnegue Institution of Washington.
13. De Lorenzo A, Bertini L, Candeloro N, Piccinelli R, Innocente L, et al. (1999) A new predictive equation to calculate resting metabolic rate in athletes. J Sports Med Phys Fitness 39: 213–219.
14. Henry CJK, Lightowler HJ, Marchini J (2003) Intra-individual variation in resting metabolic rate during the menstrual cycle. Br J Nutr 89: 811–817
15. Compher C, Frankenfield D, Keim N, Roth-Yousey L (2006) Best practice methods to apply to measurement of resting metabolic rate in adults: A systematic review. J Am Diet Assoc 106: 881–903.
16. Korth O, Bosy-Westphal A, Zschoche P, Glüer CC, Heller M, et al. (2007) Influence of methods used in body composition analysis on the prediction of resting energy expenditure. Eur J Clin Nutr 61: 582–589.
17. Cunningham JJ (1980) A reanalysis of the factors influencing basal metabolic rate in normal adults. Am J Clin Nutr 33: 2372–2374.
18. Mifflin MD, St Jeor ST, Hill LA, Scott BJ, Daugherty SA, et al. (1990) A new predictive equation for resting energy expenditure in healthy individuals. Am J Clin Nutr 51: 241–247.
19. Owen OE, Holup JL, D'Alessio Da, Craig ES, Polansky M, et al. (1987) A reappraisal of the caloric requirements of men. Am J Clin Nutr 46: 875–885.
20. Owen OE, Kavle E, Owen RS (1986) A reappraisal of caloric requirements in healthy women. Am J Clin Nutr 44: 1–19.
21. FAO/WHO/UNU (1985) Energy and protein requirements: Report of a joint FAO/WHO/UNU expert consultation. Geneva, Switzerland. pp.1–206.
22. Horton TJ, Geissler CA (1994) Effect of habitual exercise on daily energy expenditure and metabolic rate during standardized activity. Am J Clin Nutr 59: 13–19.
23. Poehlman ET, Melby CL, Badylak SF (1988) Resting metabolic rate and postprandial thermogenesis in highly trained and untrained males. Am J Clin Nutr 47: 793–798.
24. Short KR, Wiest JM, Sedlock DA (1996) The effect of upper body exercise intensity and duration on post-exercise oxygen consumption. Int J Sports Med 17: 559–563.
25. Weststrate JA, Weys P, Poortvliet E, Deurenberg P, Hautvast JG (1990) Lack of a systematic sustained effect of prolonged exercise bouts on resting metabolic rate in fasting subjects. Eur J Clin Nutr 44: 91–97.
26. Weststrate JA (1993) Original Resting metabolic a methodological Communications rate and diet-induced thermogenesis. Am J Clin Nutr 58: 592–601.
27. Weststrate JA, Weijs PJ, Poortvliet EJ, Deurenberg P, Hautvast JG (1989) Diurnal variation in postabsorptive resting metabolic rate and diet-induced thermogenesis. Am J Clin Nutr 50: 908–914.

27

Pay Dispersion and Performance in Teams

Alessandro Bucciol[1], Nicolai J. Foss[2]*, Marco Piovesan[3]

1 Department of Economics, University of Verona, Verona, Italy, **2** Department of Strategic Management and Globalization, Copenhagen Business School, Frederiksberg, Denmark, **3** Department of Economics, University of Copenhagen, Frederiksberg, Denmark

Abstract

Extant research offers conflicting predictions about the effect of pay dispersion on team performance. We collected a unique dataset from the Italian soccer league to study the effect of intra-firm pay dispersion on team performance, under different definitions of what constitutes a "team". This peculiarity of our dataset can explain the conflicting evidence. Indeed, we also find positive, null, and negative effects of pay dispersion on team performance, using the *same data* but *different definitions of team*. Our results show that when the team is considered to consist of only the members who directly contribute to the outcome, high pay dispersion has a detrimental impact on team performance. Enlarging the definition of the team causes this effect to disappear or even change direction. Finally, we find that the detrimental effect of pay dispersion is due to worse individual performance, rather than a reduction of team cooperation.

Editor: Peter G. Roma, Institutes for Behavior Resources and Johns Hopkins University School of Medicine, United States of America

Funding: The authors received no specific funding for this work.

Competing Interests: The authors have declared that no competing interests exist.

* Email: njf.smg@cb.dk

Introduction

Does pay dispersion have a positive or negative effect on work and organizational performance [1–2]? Pay dispersion is a property of a pay distribution, which is the "array of compensation levels paid for differences in work responsibilities, human capital, or individual performance within a single organization" [3]. The literature presents mixed evidence on the relation between the level of pay dispersion within an organization and work performance [4–5]. From one perspective (mainly social psychology), pay dispersion is believed to cause perceptions of inequity and relative deprivation that are detrimental to cooperation [6]. From another perspective (economics), pay dispersion can motivate employees located near the bottom of the pay-distribution scale to work harder for a future reward—a higher salary [7–8] —particularly when the pay dispersion is viewed as legitimate [9]. Pay dispersion may also be beneficial for attracting and keeping talent [10] or for avoiding the loss of workers who are crucial to the firm's output [11]. To add to the already blurry picture, some research finds no significant relation between pay dispersion and work performance [12–14].

In this study we focus on teams because teams are fundamental, and increasingly common, units of organization [15–18]. Teams are adopted because of their potential synergies. Thus, "team production may expand production possibilities by utilizing collaborative skills" [19]. Research suggests that firms increasingly organize around teams [20–21]. At the same time, firms also increasingly differentiate rewards [22], such that the firm-level dispersion of pay is widening. The two trends may be related, as smaller organizational units (i.e., teams) are associated with smaller costs of measuring and, therefore, rewarding input and output performance [23]. Although pay dispersion may exist between teams, pay may also be differentiated within teams [24], especially within top-management [25] and professional sports teams [26]. This raises the issue of the effects of within-team pay dispersion on team performance.

The empirical evidence concerning the relation between pay dispersion within teams and performance is mixed and inconclusive. Some studies support the idea that pay dispersion has a beneficial effect on team performance [27–29]; other studies show that pay dispersion has a detrimental effect [30–33] further studies find no significant effect [34–36].

In this study we show that the estimates of the effect of pay dispersion vary when using different definitions of what constitutes a team. Pfeffer and Langton [37] note that "one of the more useful avenues for research on pay systems may be precisely this task of determining not which pay scheme is best but, rather, under what conditions salary dispersion has positive effects and under what conditions it has negative effects." We provide evidence that the effect of pay dispersion can be positive, null, or negative depending on the precision of the definition of team. Our dataset in fact allows us to measure pay dispersion by distinguishing between "active" and "passive" players. Both are part of the team, but only the former ones contribute to the team's performance.

Our dataset is drawn from two seasons of the men's major soccer league in Italy. Professional sports data represent a unique source of data for labor market research, and they are widely used because they provide detailed statistics about team performance, as well as the individual athletes' performances and salaries. Soccer is a particularly appropriate area of study for our research question for a number of reasons. First, it is a team sport where cooperation is crucial, although teams may also win (lose) because of extraordinarily good (bad) individual performance. Second, it is possible to identify each individual's participation (in terms of minutes played) and to obtain repeated measures of performance over time (multiple matches in one season). Third, these data are reliable, detailed, and reported with high precision. Our dataset contains information on the net salary of each team member, and statistics on each team, each team member, each head coach, and each match. Fourth, this sport is one of the best known and popular in the world, particularly in Italy, where it generates revenues of about 1,5 billion euros [38]. Given this popularity, players' salaries are highly publicized in the media. This means that each player is aware of the pay of his teammates, at least until the opening of a new session of the players' transfer market (each January).

Another important reason why we decided to use soccer data is that each team roster usually consists of around 25 to 30 athletes, but only 11 to 14 of them actually play a single match, with a moderate turnover from one match to another. Therefore, these data allow us to measure the effect of pay dispersion using various definitions of team and provide an explanation for why the previous literature has found mixed evidence. The existing literature cited above [39] looks at end-of-season data, comparing the wins-to-matches ratio with the pay dispersion of the entire team roster, paying no attention to individual contributions to team performance. To the best of our knowledge, our study is the first to compare the outcome of a single task (a match) with the pay dispersion of only those who contributed to the task. We believe our approach improves the precision of the comparison and can shed new light on our understanding on the effect of pay dispersion on work performance.

Our data show that the within-team variation of pay dispersion is related only to the number of injured and disqualified players, but not to the characteristics of the opponent team or whether the team plays at home or away. This suggests that pay dispersion is not chosen strategically by the coach and endogeneity does not seem to play a role in our dataset. As a further control, in our analysis we study the relation between team performance and pay dispersion, including in the specification several characteristics of the team, the head coach, the match and the opponent team. Repeating the analysis on a sub-sample of teams homogeneous in terms of pay size, age, and experience would even reinforce our results.

Our findings are clear-cut. Using the narrowest definition of a team, that is, considering only those who played the match and how long they played for, pay dispersion has an overall negative impact on team performance; this result is consistent with different robustness checks. However, that effect changes—and it may even become significantly positive—when we enlarge the definition of team to include the entire team roster. We interpret this result as the consequence of taking an approximation of the correct pay dispersion where a less precise definition can bias the estimates.

Different scenarios may explain the negative effect of pay dispersion on team performance.In particular, the effect may come about because high pay dispersion affect team performance through lack of cooperation among team members or it comes about through lack of individual effort. To understand which explanation is supported by data, we collected all (subjective) individual performance assessments for each match, for each team, and for each player reported by the three most popular Italian sports newspapers. Our results show that higher pay dispersion has a detrimental impact on individual performances, but has no significant effect on cooperation. There is, however, a third possibility that our data unfortunately does not allows us to satisfactorily address and resolve. Specifically, there is the possibility that pay dispersion reflects a dispersion of the skills, abilities and talents of players, and that the association between pay dispersion and decreased team performance comes about because a high disparity of skills, etc. makes the team play less well together. For example, more homogenous players coordinate efforts better.

Finally, our analysis controls for pay size and we use indicators of pay dispersion that are dimensionless. For this reason, our results can be extended to other work contexts, beyond the peculiar work environment of professional sports. Our findings may be able to help managers determine which type of pay distribution will be more effective within a firm and make the right decisions about which employees to hire. For example, should a firm hire one expensive superstar employee and two inexpensive employees, or three medium-priced employees? We provide numerical examples showing that managers should carefully take into account the hidden cost of hiring a superstar and its effect on team performance, while keeping constant the overall team quality.

Data and Estimation Methodology

Empirical Setting and Data

Our data cover the two seasons 2009–2010 and 2010–2011 of the men's major soccer league in Italy ("Serie A"). Every season 20 teams participate in the league, and each team plays against each other team twice (one time at the home stadium and one time away) for a total of 38 matches. After a match three points are assigned for a win, one point for a draw, and no points for a defeat. The ultimate goal of each team is to earn points and be classified as high as possible in the league's ranking in order to win it or at least be in the top six positions and in this way gain access to the European cups. Teams also want to avoid being placed in any of the bottom three positions, which would relegate them to the second division. In fact, at the end of each season, the three teams ranked last are replaced by the three teams ranked first in the second division.

Our dataset contains information on the outcome of each match (win, draw, or defeat), on who played every single match and for how many minutes, and his annual net pay, as well as other statistics on each player, on each team, on each head coach, and on each match. We collected this unique dataset by merging data from the three most popular Italian sports newspapers (*La Gazzetta dello Sport*, *Corriere dello Sport*, and *Tutto Sport*), and (for players' statistics) from the website www.tuttocalciatori.net.

In any season, each team consists of about 25 to 30 athletes (henceforth, the team roster) specializing in different roles (goalkeeper, defender, midfielder, forward). However, only 18 members are summoned for each match: 11 (starter players) start the game and the other 7 (substitutes) sit on the bench and can enter the match at any time after the beginning, replacing one of the starter players (who can no longer take further part in the match). During a match a maximum of three substitutions is allowed. Common reasons for substitutions include injury, tiredness, ineffectiveness, or a tactical switch. In the 2009–2010 season 462 players and in the 2010–2011 season 463 players played for at least one minute during our observation period. In most cases those who played in one season also played in the other one; however, from our perspective they are completely different players because they may earn different salaries in the two seasons. For this reason and for sake of simplicity and with a little abuse of terminology, we say that 925 team members have played overall. A similar argument can be made for teams: because those teams present in both seasons may have very different lists of team members, we treat them as different teams, so that our sample includes 40 teams. We know the salaries of only 874 of the 925 players (94.49%), while we impute the pay of the remaining 51. This imputation has a negligible impact on our statistics, because players for whom we needed to impute salaries have a marginal role in the team (on average they have played about 1% of the available time). Repeating our benchmark analysis without imputations (results available upon request) confirms our findings.

Our dataset includes the matches played between August 23, 2009, and December 20, 2009 (2009–2010 season), and between August 29, 2010, and December 19, 2010 (2010–2011 season), for a total of 666 observations. To be conservative and have a clean dataset, we decided to use only the matches played before the opening of the January players' transfer market, during which every team is allowed to trade players with other teams. We then ignored the remaining matches, for which we cannot be sure about the exact salaries of players transferred, especially the ones coming from foreign leagues. On average these players account for around 12% of the team members after the January market, and they usually take a relevant role in the team—playing most of the remaining matches. If we included these data, any guesses about the missing salaries would likely bias our estimates. However, there is relatively high correlation (0.589) between the number of points earned in the first 17 matches and the number of points earned in the remaining matches.

Variables and Estimation Method

Our unit of analysis is the team playing a match in a given season; in total we then have 40 teams, 20 for each season. Recall that the team may win, draw, or lose a match, earning respectively three, one, or no points. Our dependent variable, measuring team performance, is a dummy equal to 1 if the team wins the match (which happens in 37.24% of the cases); it is equal to 0 if the team draws or loses the match. We group draws and defeats together because the ultimate goal for a team is to win a match. In a robustness check, we repeat the analysis treating first both wins and draws as a positive outcome, and then each outcome separately. Our main results were confirmed (Supplementary material available upon request).

We perform a probit regression with panel-robust standard errors (clustered for each team in each season); this way we allow for possible correlation across observations referring to different matches of the same team. We opted for this model because our data show no evidence of team-specific panel effects (see the discussion at the end of Section 3.1); use of this model allows us to obtain more efficient estimates.

Our purpose is to obtain measures of pay dispersion, as well as other indicators, that are specific for each match of each team. For this purpose, the term *active team members* (ATMs) for a team in a given match refers to all team members who actually played at least one minute of the match. For such a match we then neglect all of the remaining members who did not contribute to the result of the match. As a consequence, the set of active team members for a team varies match by match.

The benchmark specification includes different variables that for clarity we group into six categories: *pay, team, coach, match, opponent*, and *time*. Our focus is on the first group of pay variables; the remaining ones serve as control variables. In the analysis, all of the variables concerning team composition are based solely on the ATMs, and the contribution of each member is weighted by the amount of time he actually played in the match. The variables in the *pay* and *team* categories thus refer to the ATMs of the team, whereas the variables in the *opponent* category refer to the ATMs of the opponent team. This means that *pay, team*, and *opponent* statistics differ match by match and that members who had no active role in the match are ignored. In what follows we discuss the variables used in the analysis.

Pay variables. We consider the logarithm of the average pay, and the logarithm of a dimensionless measure of pay dispersion. In all the cases we refer to annual salaries in thousands of euros net of taxes. Let us define $p_{i,x}$ as the pay of player $i, i=1,\ldots,I$ in team $x, x=1,\ldots,X$, where $m_{i,x,t}\in[0,90]$ represents the minutes of the match actually played by the same player in match $t, t=1,\ldots,T$. We treat $m_{i,x,t}$ as a weight to compute the average pay for team x in match t:

$$\bar{p}_{x,t}=\frac{1}{\sum_{i=1}^{I} m_{i,x,t}}\sum_{i=1}^{I} m_{i,x,t}p_{i,x}.$$

As a pay dispersion measure, we take the Theil index. This indicator belongs to the class of entropy indexes and is frequently used to measure economic inequality. The index is defined as the mean of the products between individual pay relative to average pay, and its logarithm is as follows:

$$T_{x,t}=\frac{1}{\sum_{i=1}^{I} m_{i,x,t}}\sum_{i=1}^{I} m_{i,x,t}\frac{p_{i,x}}{\bar{p}_{x,t}}\ln\left(\frac{p_{i,x}}{\bar{p}_{x,t}}\right).$$

The index is equal to 0 for the case of no pay dispersion (i.e., all salaries are identical); a higher index denotes higher pay dispersion. Notice that the indicator is dimensionless, which means that what matters to us is only the individual pay *relative to the average pay*; this allows us to compare pay distributions across teams and matches, disregarding the average pay level, which varies markedly (from 213,808 euros to 4,356,061 euros). As a robustness check, we repeated the analysis using the popular Gini index rather than the Theil index. In this case our main findings were qualitatively confirmed, and quantitatively even emphasized (Supplementary material available upon request).

Team variables. We use weighted average values in a given match for players' ages, the fraction of new players on the team, and the number of years (even if not consecutive) on the team and in the Italian first division; the last two variables serve to proxy players' experience.

Coach variables. For the coach we use the same set of information as for the team, that is: coach age, a dummy variable equal to 1 if he is in his first season with the team, and the number of years (even if not consecutive) on the team and in the Italian first division. Head coaches in soccer are often fired from one season to another, and even during the same season. We then also include in the analysis a dummy variable equal to one if the head coach has been replaced during the season.

Match variables. We use a dummy variable equal to 1 if the team plays a domestic (home) match. In addition, soccer players may be sanctioned with a yellow or red card for a specific misconduct; multiple yellow cards or one red card produce an automatic disqualification for at least one following match. We therefore use the number of disqualified players as well as the number of injured players. These variables are added because injuries and disqualifications may prevent a coach from using his preferred players during a match. However, we expect disqualifications to have a stronger effect because they usually involve team members who play more frequently.

Opponent variables. We consider the same variables as in the *pay* and *team* groups, but we base them on the ATMs of the opponent team. The purpose is to in this way capture the characteristics (in particular the strength) of the opposing team. An alternative would be to add as many dummy variables as the teams (40). Doing so, our main results would be confirmed. The shortcoming of such an approach, however, is the potential inefficiency of estimating many coefficients in a probit regression model; for this reason we prefer our benchmark specification.

Time variables. We use a dummy variable equal to 1 if the match was played during the 2010–2011 season, and dummy variables for the month if the match was played from August to December.

Summary Statistics

Table 1 lists all variables used in the analysis and reports some summary statistics. All statistics are calculated for the ATMs in the 666 observations of our sample. The purpose of using all of these variables is to control for the physical, social, and other characteristics of the team members, the coach, and the match.

From the table we learn that, for the median observation, the ATMs' average pay is 584 thousand euros, the Theil index is 0.093 (ranging from 0.006 to 0.497), on average the ATMs are around 27 years old, they already have accumulated two years of experience in the team and five years in the first division, and around 26% of them are in their first year with the team. In addition, 57% of the coaches are new to the team, 14% of them started managing the team after the beginning of the season, and they have little experience with the team and the first division. Finally, disqualifications and especially injuries are frequent, and sometimes they may force the coach to reshape the starting team formation (in fact, we observe a maximum of 4 disqualified players and 11 injured players). In our analysis we account for this when measuring the effect of pay dispersion; further statistics on pay dispersion are shown in the supplementary material (available upon request).

Table 2 lists the teams in our dataset (20 for each season) and some average statistics (age, experience, fraction of new players) for their ATMs in each match. Teams are listed according to the ranking at the end of each season, where the first team listed is the winner of the championship and the last three teams are eventually relegated to the second division.

First of all, we notice that the 17 teams enrolled in both seasons show marked differences over the two years. From the table we also observe wide heterogeneity across teams within the same season, with no clear pattern going from bottom to top teams. The last column of Table 2 shows the fraction of players that in our sample played at least for one minute. This fraction is between 0.69 and 0.96; note that it is always below 1. This indicates that some team members never play; usually those excluded are injured and homegrown players. Ignoring this, and treating all team members equally, the analysis on the effect of pay dispersion may generate different results, as we later clarify.

To stress this point, Figure 1 plots for each team the fraction of wins over the Theil index, using two different methods. In the top panel, the pay dispersion index is based on the whole team roster, disregarding players' involvement in the matches; this is the standard approach adopted in the literature. In the bottom panel, the index is the average over the matches, where for each match pay dispersion is based on the ATM; this approach is closer to the one followed in this paper. First of all, we notice that the index calculated in the top panel uses values that are on a higher scale than those of the index in the bottom panel; the reason is that this measure is inflated by the low pay of those members (usually the homegrown ones) who, although formal members of the team, do not contribute to the team's performance.

The figure also shows a line indicating the predicted winning probability for a given level of the Theil index. The prediction is obtained from a simple probit regression over 666 observations, where the dependent variable is equal to 1 if the team wins the

Table 1. Summary statistics (666 observations on 40 teams).

Variable	Median	Mean	Std. dev.	Minimum	Maximum
Pay					
Average pay (thousands of euros)	583.788	1039.801	998.699	213.808	4356.061
Theil index	0.093	0.114	0.077	0.006	0.497
Team					
Fraction of new players in the team	0.255	0.263	0.156	0	0.701
Years in the team	2.202	2.341	1.039	0.483	5.985
Years in first division	4.635	4.858	1.510	1.597	9.645
Average age	27.465	27.488	1.327	24.298	30.889
Coach					
New to the team	1	0.571	0.495	0	1
Replaced during season	0	0.144	0.351	0	1
Years in the team	0	0.685	0.982	0	4
Years in first division	3	4.372	3.686	0	14
Age	48	49.414	6.802	38	65
Match					
Injured players	3	3.081	1.798	0	11
Disqualified players	0	0.431	0.662	0	4
Home play	0.5	0.5	0.500	0	1

Note: For the "opponent" variables we consider the same variables as in the pay and team categories, but we base them on the ATM of the opposing team. We do not report summary statistics because they coincide with those in the pay and team categories.

Table 2. Team statistics.

a) 2009–2010 Season

Team	Fraction new to the team	Years on the team	Years in first division	Age	Fraction of players employed
FC Internazionale Milano	0.314	3.553	4.961	29.320	0.733
AS Roma	0.093	3.755	6.278	28.378	0.871
AC Milan	0.128	4.538	8.063	29.619	0.786
UC Sampdoria	0.265	1.862	5.751	26.639	0.778
US Città di Palermo	0.188	1.650	4.085	25.886	0.852
SSC Napoli	0.289	1.465	4.743	26.897	0.808
Juventus FC	0.239	3.056	5.838	28.460	0.929
Parma FC	0.535	0.847	6.160	27.604	0.808
Genoa CFC	0.359	1.527	4.421	27.760	0.786
AS Bari	0.435	1.507	2.836	26.267	0.774
ACF Fiorentina	0.110	2.695	7.519	27.818	0.750
SS Lazio	0.042	2.582	5.689	27.455	0.806
Catania Calcio	0.282	1.650	2.333	26.120	0.893
Cagliari Calcio	0.134	3.406	4.695	26.910	0.720
Udinese Calcio	0.131	2.370	4.312	25.502	0.733
AC Chievo Verona	0.199	2.647	4.622	29.198	0.852
Bologna FC	0.439	0.810	5.098	29.076	0.815
Atalanta Calcio	0.253	2.513	4.024	26.915	0.923
AS Siena	0.302	1.692	4.203	26.550	0.885
AS Livorno	0.310	1.552	3.689	27.437	0.800
AVERAGE	**0.252**	**2.280**	**4.962**	**27.491**	**0.834**

b) 2010–2011 Season

Team	Fraction new to the team	Years on the team	Years in first division	Age	Fraction of players employed
AC Milan	0.228	4.749	7.927	29.480	0.828
FC Internazionale Milano	0.108	3.786	5.430	29.308	0.862
SSC Napoli	0.166	1.766	5.393	27.573	0.917
Udinese Calcio	0.166	3.117	4.723	25.740	0.909
SS Lazio	0.196	2.130	4.479	27.918	0.846
AS Roma	0.188	4.001	7.135	29.506	0.963
Juventus FC	0.542	2.066	5.297	27.173	0.926
US Città di Palermo	0.308	1.555	3.299	24.939	0.692
ACF Fiorentina	0.124	2.960	7.440	27.659	0.929
Genoa CFC	0.499	1.550	4.310	27.718	0.846
AC Chievo Verona	0.434	2.065	3.594	27.916	0.880
Parma FC	0.311	1.358	5.315	27.914	0.769
Cagliari Calcio	0.077	3.281	4.391	26.090	0.760
Catania Calcio	0.083	2.255	2.887	27.144	0.889
Bologna FC	0.399	0.902	3.363	26.605	0.923
AC Cesena	0.494	1.703	4.168	28.302	0.852
US Lecce	0.401	2.446	2.529	27.306	0.926
UC Sampdoria	0.124	2.258	5.975	26.046	0.929
Brescia Calcio	0.383	2.446	4.015	28.541	0.960
AS Bari	0.236	2.322	3.679	27.012	0.929
AVERAGE	**0.274**	**2.401**	**4.755**	**27.484**	**0.873**

Note: Teams are listed according to their position at the end of the season; teams promoted from second division are highlighted. Averages for each team are based on the ATM of all of the matches (either 16 or 17) played by the team in a given season. Fraction of players employed: number of players employed at least for one minute over total number of players.

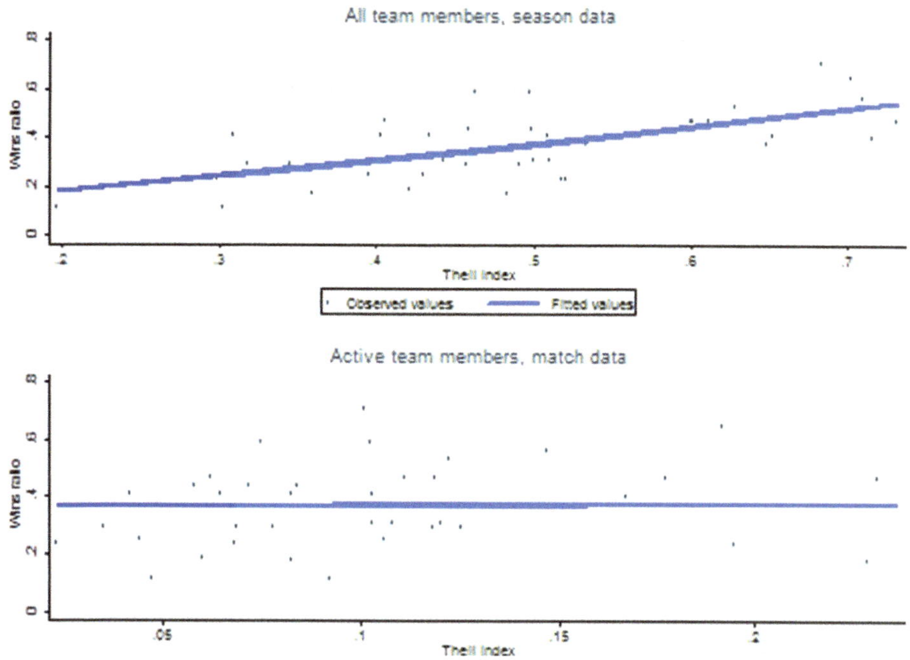

Figure 1. Team performance and pay dispersion (40 team observations).

match, and 0 otherwise; the specification includes just the constant and the Theil index, based on either the whole team roster (top panel) or the ATM of each match (bottom panel). Comparing the two panels, we see that pay dispersion positively affects team performance when considering the whole team roster (top panel), whereas it has no impact when considering the ATMs (bottom panel). This suggests that results may change depending on how pay dispersion is measured. This finding warns us that findings may change depending on our definition of what constitutes a "team."

We conclude this section with an exploratory analysis of the effect of pay dispersion on performance, which is our ultimate goal. Overall in the data, pay dispersion shows no significant difference (t test: 0.37; p value: 0.712) when the match is won (average: 0.116) or when the match is drawn/lost (average: 0.114). Pay dispersion is not even affected by the team performance of the previous match (t test: 0.607; p value: 0.544; average after a match won: 0.117; average after a match drawn/lost: 0.113). This suggests that the coach does not adjust it to keep the team compact in case of performance problems.

Table 3 then shows, separately for each team, the average pay, the average Theil index, and the wins ratio. Teams are listed as in Table 2, following their ranking at the end of the season. The first thing to note brings to mind the famous slogan "*The more you spend, the more you get.*" Indeed, teams that spend more (i.e., with a higher average pay) rank higher at the end of the season. In fact, our data exhibit a large Spearman's rank correlation (0.701) between average team pay and the wins ratio in the season. The data thus suggest that better players are also better paid, and for this reason we can interpret the average pay of a team as a proxy for the average skill in the team. In contrast, pay dispersion is much less highly correlated with the wins ratio (the rank correlation is 0.241), although the sign of this correlation is still positive.

A problem with this analysis is that it ignores the specific characteristics of each team. For this reason, we now compare, separately for each team, the wins ratio obtained in two groups of matches, where the Theil index is either below or above the median for the team. The last column of Table 3 shows that the wins ratio is higher in the matches with high pay dispersion in only 11 cases out of 40.

We have then found that, looking at the same data, one can interpret the relationship between team performance and pay dispersion as positive (considering all the team members: Figure 1, top panel), null (considering the ATMs: Figure 1, bottom panel), or negative (considering the ATMs separately for each team: Table 3). Our empirical exercise in the next section further analyzes the relationship considering the ATMs, each match separately, and controlling for the most relevant characteristics of the team, the coach, the match, and the opponent.

Pay Dispersion and Team Performance

In this section we summarize our main findings regarding the effect of pay dispersion on team performance. We then discuss some robustness checks around the definition of team members, and we report the results of a further analysis connecting pay dispersion with individual performance. Our benchmark estimates are shown in Table 4.

Benchmark Analysis

The first column of Table 4 reports the average marginal effects from our benchmark probit regression analysis. The column shows that pay dispersion has a *negative impact* on team performance: doubling pay dispersion, the probability of winning a match would reduce on average by 0.06. Panel (a) of Figure 2 plots the predicted winning probability, conditional on pay dispersion and the other explanatory variables (fixed to their average), computed using this probit regression. It shows that probability falls, from 0.56 when there is no pay dispersion, to 0.24 when the Theil index is $T = 0.50$.

Table 3. Pay and team performance.

a) 2009–2010 Season

Team	Average pay	Theil index	Wins ratio: average by matches			(2)–(1)>0
			All	Low disp.	High disp.	
				(1)	(2)	
FC Internazionale Milano	4115.021	0.101	0.706	0.875	0.556	NO
AS Roma	1718.652	0.232	0.471	0.375	0.556	YES
AC Milan	3250.733	0.147	0.563	0.750	0.375	NO
UC Sampdoria	724.647	0.393	0.412	0.750	0.111	NO
US Città di Palermo	658.497	0.083	0.412	0.500	0.333	NO
SSC Napoli	842.041	0.103	0.412	0.500	0.333	NO
Juventus FC	2673.181	0.123	0.529	0.625	0.444	NO
Parma FC	536.108	0.062	0.471	0.500	0.444	NO
Genoa CFC	817.235	0.058	0.438	0.500	0.375	NO
AS Bari	435.087	0.126	0.375	0.125	0.625	YES
ACF Fiorentina	1177.068	0.072	0.438	0.250	0.625	YES
SS Lazio	729.187	0.229	0.176	0.125	0.222	YES
Catania Calcio	413.871	0.048	0.118	0.125	0.111	NO
Cagliari Calcio	367.552	0.084	0.438	0.625	0.250	NO
Udinese Calcio	464.575	0.103	0.313	0.250	0.375	YES
AC Chievo Verona	380.442	0.042	0.412	0.500	0.333	NO
Bologna FC	523.939	0.106	0.250	0.375	0.125	NO
Atalanta Calcio	334.134	0.060	0.188	0.125	0.250	YES
AS Siena	436.847	0.083	0.176	0.250	0.111	NO
AS Livorno	358.900	0.125	0.294	0.500	0.111	NO

b) 2010–2011 Season

Team	Average pay	Theil index	Wins ratio: average by matches			(2)–(1)>0
			All	Low disp.	High disp.	
				(1)	(2)	
AC Milan	3590.499	0.191	0.647	0.750	0.556	NO
FC Internazionale Milano	3250.635	0.167	0.400	0.429	0.375	NO
SSC Napoli	918.736	0.102	0.588	0.625	0.556	NO
Udinese Calcio	568.033	0.065	0.412	0.500	0.333	NO
SS Lazio	1099.115	0.075	0.588	0.750	0.444	NO
AS Roma	2049.492	0.177	0.471	0.625	0.333	NO
Juventus FC	2034.127	0.119	0.471	0.500	0.444	NO
US Città di Palermo	576.675	0.111	0.471	0.500	0.444	NO
ACF Fiorentina	1024.088	0.108	0.313	0.250	0.375	YES
Genoa CFC	1128.980	0.236	0.375	0.500	0.250	NO
AC Chievo Verona	316.556	0.035	0.294	0.375	0.222	NO
Parma FC	559.824	0.068	0.235	0.250	0.222	NO
Cagliari Calcio	403.838	0.078	0.294	0.250	0.333	YES
Catania Calcio	447.094	0.069	0.294	0.250	0.333	YES
Bologna FC	555.712	0.119	0.294	0.125	0.444	YES
AC Cesena	223.423	0.044	0.250	0.250	0.250	=
US Lecce	300.007	0.023	0.235	0.375	0.111	NO
UC Sampdoria	897.708	0.121	0.313	0.250	0.375	YES
Brescia Calcio	359.365	0.195	0.235	0.250	0.222	NO
AS Bari	482.681	0.093	0.118	0.250	0.000	NO

Note: See note to Table 2. Average pay is in thousand euros. For each team we split matches in two groups based on whether the Theil index was below (low) or not below (high) the median value for the team.

An example will help the reader understand this figure. Suppose a team manager has to buy 11 new players who are expected to play all the next matches fully and on a regular basis. Your budget is limited, and you have to decide whether to buy (at the same total expenditure) either 1 top player and 10 average players, or instead 11 players with above-average skill. We assume their pays reflect their skill. Further, let us say that the average pay is 600 thousand euros (the actual pay size in our sample; however, this is irrelevant for the pay dispersion index) and that the manager can choose to pay all 11 players the same amount (600 thousand euros) or 1 top player much more (1.5 million euros as opposed to 510 thousand euros for the other ones). In the latter case the top player will earn 2.5 times the average pay, while each other player will earn 0.85 times the average pay; this pay distribution roughly corresponds to the median distribution in the sample. The resulting Theil index is $T = 0.083$, whereas it is $T = 0$ if all 11 players earn 600 thousand euros each. Hence, higher pay dispersion denotes higher variability of players' skills. Our estimates suggest that, everything else being equal, the differentiated pay distribution will make the probability of winning a match fall on average by 20%, from 0.56 to 0.36.

In our regression we also find significant evidence of a positive effect of average pay (doubling it would increase the probability of winning a match by around 0.15), replacing a coach during the season (the probability then increases by 0.12), and playing at home (0.25). In addition, we find significantly negative effects for the coach's experience with the team (one more year reduces the probability of winning a match by 0.03) and the opponent's average pay (doubling it would reduce the probability by 0.17). These results are not surprising: on average, the pay can be seen as a proxy for a player's skill (above we made an argument about this); replacement of a coach during the season may have a large psychological impact on the players; a team playing in its home stadium may benefit from the support of its fans; the longer a coach is on the team, the lower is the strength of his effort and the psychological impact on the players; and the opponent's average pay can also be seen as a proxy for its skill, which then lowers the winning probability of the team. No other explanatory variables—noticeably, those on the team characteristics and on the opponent's pay dispersion—are significantly different from 0, at least at a 5% significance level.

The "rho" coefficient, shown in the bottom part of Table 4, is the proportion of the total variance contributed by the team-level variance. This is statistically equal to 0, indicating that we can disregard the panel dimension of our data, and run our analysis with a probit regression on the pooled dataset. In what follows we then perform pooled probit regressions with team-clustered standard errors, because this approach is more efficient than using panel regression methods (fewer parameters have to be estimated).

In an additional analysis (Supplementary material, Section B.1; available upon request), we discuss the link between pay dispersion and the main characteristics of the match and the team opponent, showing positive correlation with the number of injured and disqualified players, but no correlation with the characteristics of the opponent team or whether the team plays at home or away. This suggests that match-by-match variations in pay dispersion are not driven by strategic reasons. The section then replicates our analysis on a sub-sample of teams homogeneous in terms of pay size, age and experience. In this case, the effect of pay dispersion on team performance would remain negative, but larger than in the benchmark analysis (-0.16 rather than -0.06). Section B.2 repeats the benchmark analysis, also treating draws as a positive outcome, and confirms our benchmark results. Moreover, Section B.3 reports the results of some robustness checks on the specification, where we substitute the Theil index with the Gini index (which actually shows a stronger significant effect: -0.13 rather than -0.06), or where we add an indicator of the symmetry of the pay distribution (eventually not significant), a quadratic polynomial on pay dispersion, or the interaction between the index and a dummy variable equal to 1 if the team played a match in December. In the latter two cases, the purpose is to understand whether the effect of pay dispersion is non-monotonic or if it changes as team members get to know each other better. In neither case are the added variables significantly different from 0. In addition Section 3.3 discusses, among other things, the relationship between team performance and different technologies of production.

Team Members

We repeat the analysis with the same regression specification as in the benchmark case, but this time we consider different definitions of team members. As we have already seen, the definition affects the computation of the variables on pay, team, and opponent statistics that are all match specific. The effect of pay dispersion on team performance may then change with the definition of group. The average marginal effects from the analysis are shown in columns (2), (3), and (4) of Table 4; the latest column is based on the broadest definition of team members.

Unweighted ATM. We first consider the ATM, as in the benchmark, but disregarding the amount of time they actually played. For instance, if the match started with 11 players and then 3 substitutes also took part in the match, we derive our pay and players statistics from the characteristics of 14 team members, without weights.

Our results are reported in column (2) of Table 4, and they are close to the benchmark case of column (1). In particular, pay dispersion is still associated with a negative marginal effect of -0.06, although the effect is now significant at only 10%. This suggests that ignoring the amount of time spent in the field may create noise in the estimates.

Potential players. We then consider as team members all 18 athletes who were potentially able to play in the match because they were either starter players or substitute players. In this manner we exclude injured players, disqualified players, or players who are out of the match as a result of a decision made by the coach. All members are given the same weight, disregarding the number of minutes they actually played in the match. This definition of team members is less precise than our benchmark definition of ATMs, because at least four of these members in each match make no contribution to team performance, but they still affect the pay, team, and opponent statistics.

Our results are shown in column (3) of Table 4. Most variables show effects that are in line with the benchmark results; however, the pay dispersion index is now associated with a coefficient insignificantly different from zero.

Entire team roster. We conclude the analysis by considering as team members all athletes enrolled on the team, that is, the entire team roster, thus including injured, disqualified, and homegrown players. Hence, we consider the same team composition in each match, disregarding who actually played. This implies that, in our regression equation, the variables on pay and team statistics are constant for a given team (they are then fixed "team effects"), and the variables on opponent statistics are constant for a given opponent team. Such an approach is similar to that of some previous works in the literature, because it does not pay attention to whether and how much each team member contributed to team performance.

Table 4. Team performance and pay dispersion (average marginal effects).

		(1)	(2)	(3)	(4)
Members:		**ATM**	**Unweighted**	**Potential**	**Roster**
Pay:	Log(average pay)	0.146***	0.142***	0.147***	0.076**
		(0.027)	(0.028)	(0.032)	(0.039)
	Log(pay dispersion index)	−0.061**	−0.058*	−0.046	0.167**
		(0.030)	(0.032)	(0.031)	(0.082)
Team:	Fraction of new players on the team	0.095	0.040	0.059	0.044
		(0.143)	(0.148)	(0.144)	(0.141)
	Years on the team	0.015	0.011	0.020	0.006
		(0.026)	(0.029)	(0.030)	(0.037)
	Years in first division	0.002	−0.004	−0.006	0.006
		(0.016)	(0.018)	(0.018)	(0.022)
	Age	0.001	0.014	0.005*	0.009
		(0.017)	(0.016)	(0.002)	(0.017)
Coach:	New to the team	−0.091*	−0.086*	−0.089*	−0.116**
		(0.050)	(0.050)	(0.047)	(0.046)
	Replaced during the season	0.119**	0.115**	0.120**	0.108**
		(0.051)	(0.054)	(0.056)	(0.048)
	Years on the team	−0.034**	−0.033**	−0.032**	−0.033**
		(0.015)	(0.016)	(0.015)	(0.016)
	Years in first division	0.010*	0.011**	0.011**	0.009*
		(0.006)	(0.006)	(0.005)	(0.005)
	Age	0.000	−0.000	0.000	−0.000
		(0.004)	(0.004)	(0.004)	(0.003)
Match:	Injured players	−0.006	−0.005	−0.004	−0.007
		(0.010)	(0.010)	(0.010)	(0.010)
	Disqualified players	0.040*	0.040*	0.040*	0.024
		(0.023)	(0.023)	(0.023)	(0.022)
	Home play	0.253***	0.250***	0.248***	0.256***
		(0.034)	(0.035)	(0.033)	(0.034)
Opponent:	Log(average pay)	−0.169***	−0.160***	−0.183***	−0.125***
		(0.029)	(0.032)	(0.035)	(0.037)
	Log(pay dispersion index)	0.030	0.018	0.015	−0.083
		(0.025)	(0.026)	(0.033)	(0.095)
	Fraction of new players on the team	0.139	0.206*	0.088	0.183
		(0.105)	(0.119)	(0.120)	(0.153)
	Years on the team	0.044*	0.048*	0.045	0.084**
		(0.022)	(0.027)	(0.029)	(0.041)
	Years in first division	0.001	0.004	0.012	−0.014
		(0.015)	(0.016)	(0.017)	(0.025)
	Age	0.004	−0.007	−0.003**	−0.019
		(0.015)	(0.017)	(0.001)	(0.020)
+ time dummy variables on month and year of the match					
	Log-likelihood	−371.461	−371.522	−370.738	−371.522
	McFadden R^2	0.155	0.155	0.157	0.155
	Count R^2	0.689	0.688	0.700	0.688
	Rho coefficient	0.000			

Table 4. Cont.

	(1)	(2)	(3)	(4)
Members:	**ATM**	**Unweighted**	**Potential**	**Roster**
LR test rho = 0	0.000			
	[0.496]			

Note: 666 observations on 40 teams (on average, 16.6 matches per team). The dependent variable is a dummy = 1 in case of win. Pay and team statistics are based on ATM players (column 1); ATM players, not weighted by the amount of time they actually played (column 2); all potential players (starter players and substitute players; column 3); whole team roster (column 4). Team-clustered standard errors are given in parentheses; p values in brackets.

**p<0.1;*

***p<0.05;*

****p<0.01.*

Our results are shown in column (4) of Table 4, and they are largely different from our benchmark analysis of column (1): we find a smaller effect of the team average pay (0.08 instead of 0.15), while the effect of pay dispersion is now even positive: according to these estimates, doubling pay dispersion would increase the probability of winning by 0.17. In contrast, the remaining variables, which have not changed relative to the benchmark case (they do not depend on the definition of team members), provide parameter estimates comparable with those of the benchmark case.

The results in Table 4 thus inform that, when broadening the definition of team (i.e., when going from column 1 to column 4), conclusions about the effects of pay dispersion change enormously: at a 5% level we may indeed find either a negative effect (column 1), a null effect (columns 2 and 3), or a positive one (column 4). Figure 2 plots the predicted winning probability, conditional on pay dispersion and the other explanatory variables (fixed to their average), computed separately from each of the four probit regressions in Table 4. From the figure it is clear that the direction of the effect goes from negative to positive as we use less information on the group definition, from panel (b) (where we ignore the amount of time actually played) to panel (c) (where we consider all starter and substitute players), and on to panel (d) (where we include the whole team roster).

This result is essentially a warning that the measurement of an effect can be biased if we do not consider a precise definition of

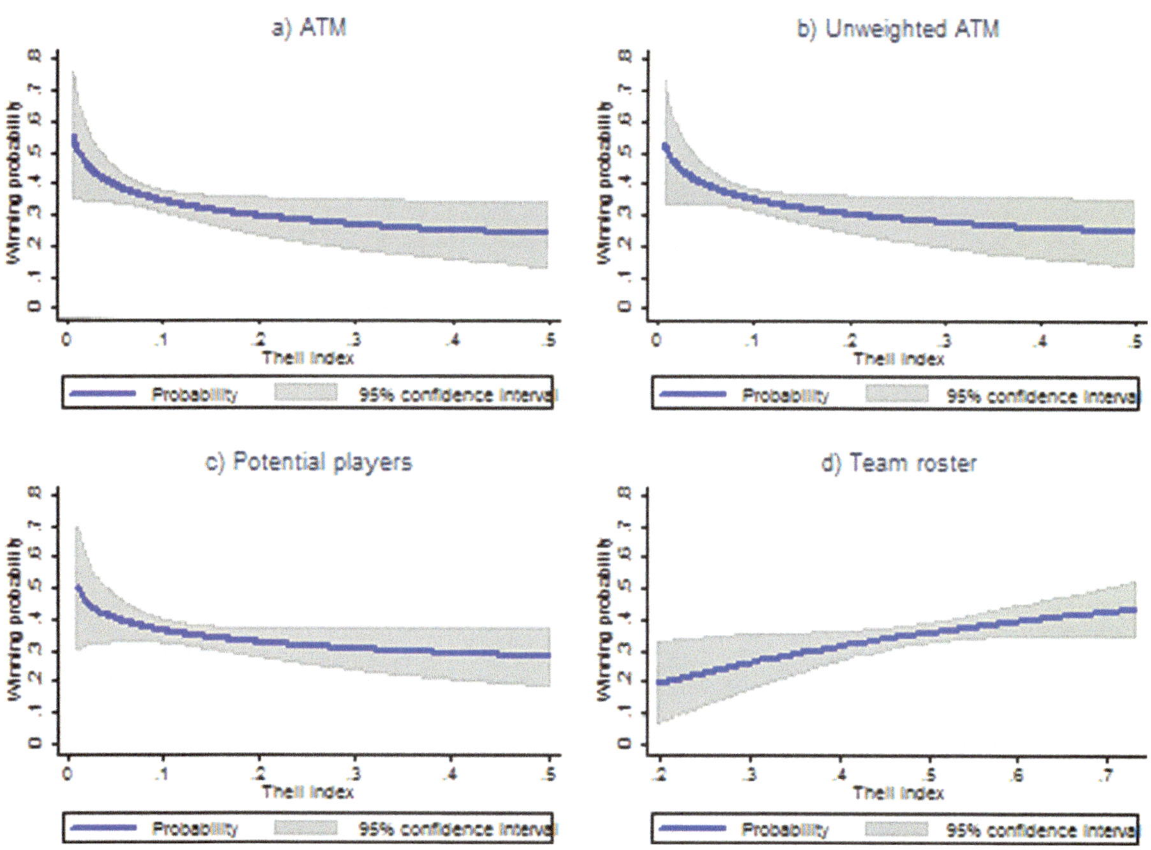

Figure 2. Predicted winning probability by pay dispersion. Note: Predictions are based on the average explanatory variables and the parameter estimates from Table 4.

what constitutes a "team." Notice in particular that we find a positive effect when we look at the most general definition (whole team roster). Those who play little or not at all usually earn less than those who play regularly. See supplementary material (available upon request), Section A.4, for details.

As a result, pay dispersion increases if we use a definition of team that incorporates them; in particular, considering the entire team roster, the index is on average 0.493, as opposed to 0.114 if we consider just the ATMs. Pay dispersion increases significantly more in the top 10 teams at the end of December of each season: the average difference between the pay dispersion index computed from the team roster and from the ATMs is on average 0.437 among the top teams, as opposed to 0.321 among the other teams (t test: 16.512; p value: 0.000). The pay dispersion index then captures part of the effect of the team skill; indeed, the correlation between average pay and pay dispersion is 0.722 using the whole team roster, whereas it is only 0.253 using the ATM. This correlation may explain why in column (4) of Table 4 the effect of pay dispersion is positive, and the effect of average pay is about half the effect found in the other three columns.

This suggests that our benchmark conclusions are not driven by a dataset with different features than others. Actually, our conclusions depend on the way we look at the data, and in particular on what we mean by "team members." This may explain why in the literature we observe different results, and it shows the importance of the precision of the definition of team to evaluate the effect of pay dispersion.

Individual Performance

So far the analysis has focused on objective indicators of team performance. Team performance, however, derives from individual performance and cooperation among team members. It is then possible that we observe poor team performance because there is *poor individual performance* or because there is *little cooperation*. For instance, in soccer, we can observe a poor team performance when each player tries to score without passing the ball to other players (lack of cooperation) or when each player prefers not to take the initiative but instead passes the ball to other players, thereby delegating to them the responsibility to score (the lack of effort). One may thus wonder what determines the detrimental effect of pay dispersion on team performance. Does pay dispersion work as a disincentive to individual effort? Alternatively, does pay dispersion merely decrease cooperation between players, leaving individual performance unchanged? These are the issues we want to address in this section.

Our data suggest that teams that win more often make significantly more passes during the match: the 20 teams winning more frequently on average make 410.47 passes, significantly more than the other teams making on average 383.52 passes (t test: 1.876; p value: 0.034). In Section B.2 of the supplementary material (available upon request), we report the output of a within-group panel regression analysis of the number of passes over the same specification as in the benchmark. We find no significant effect of pay dispersion. To the extent that the number of passes can be seen as a valid measure of team cooperation, the finding may be interpreted as an indication that team cooperation is not affected by pay dispersion. If our argument is correct, team performance is then affected solely by individual performance.

Obtaining an objective and thorough measurement of individual performance is impossible in our environment, because soccer is a team sport where few individual statistics are recorded compared to other sports such as baseball. (See, e.g., Scully (1974) for an analysis of the connection between individual performance and individual pay [40].) In addition, those few existing individual statistics record rare events (e.g., goals, assists, yellow cards) and are highly role specific (e.g., a forward player is more likely to score a goal than any other player). It would be difficult to use these statistics as measures of individual performance.

In Italy, however, it is quite common for journalists, when writing a newspaper report about a match, to assign a "mark" to each single player's performance. The mark is a number based on a scale from 0 to 10; a mark of 6 denotes fair performance and higher marks indicate good or excellent performance. This mark represents a *subjective individual performance assessment* (SIPA), because it is based only on the arbitrary opinion and taste of the journalist who attended the match. Still, it is a rough indicator of the individual performance of each team member and can be used to look at the effect of pay dispersion on individual team members. In this regard we collected all of the SIPAs for the players involved in the 333 matches considered in the main analysis, using the three major sport newspapers in Italy: *La Gazzetta dello Sport*, *Corriere dello Sport*, and *Tutto Sport*. To make SIPAs less heavily affected by the personal opinion of the journalists, we took an average SIPA from the three newspapers (the SIPAs from the three sources show a correlation of around 0.7). Overall we have 8,226 observations on 876 players (434 in the 2009–2010 season and 442 in the 2010–2011 season), who then played an average of 9.39 matches each. The number of players considered is smaller than the number of players who played at least for one minute, 925, because marks are given only to those who play a significant portion of the match. The decision on what is a "significant portion of the match" is subjective, and different journalists may have different opinions. In a separate analysis in the supplementary material (available upon request), Section B.4, we take the SIPAs from the major sport newspaper, *La Gazzetta dello Sport*, and add to the specification dummy variables on the journalist who made the SIPA. Our main conclusions are confirmed, both qualitatively and quantitatively.

Figure 3 plots the distribution of SIPAs in our sample. We see that SIPAs are concentrated between 4 and 9, with a peak around 6 (fair performance). Table 5 reports some summary statistics at the player level. First of all, we notice that SIPAs are generally higher when the team wins a match. However, low SIPAs are possible also in this case: players may indeed receive a SIPA of 4 even if their team wins the match. Moreover, the table lists some statistics about the main player's characteristics: his pay, his age, his past experience with the team and the first division, and his role (midfielder, forward, as opposed to goalkeeper or defender). We observe wide heterogeneity on these variables.

SIPAs show a weakly positive correlation with individual salaries (0.09) and team average pay (0.05), and a weakly negative correlation with pay dispersion (−0.05). It is also interesting to understand which "technology of production"—meant as a combination of individual SIPAs—determines team performance. If we regressed team performance over the minimum, mean, and maximum SIPAs of the team in the match (controlling for team, coach, match, opponent, and time characteristics), we would find all coefficients to be significant at 1%, suggesting that different technologies coexist. However, the average marginal effect of the mean SIPA is quantitatively much higher: 0.717, as opposed to −0.069 for the minimum SIPA and 0.129 for the maximum SIPA. This suggests that team performance depends on the individual effort of *all* players, more than on the effort of the best/worst ones.

The analysis in this section is meant to assist in understanding the link between individual performance and pay dispersion using an approach similar to our benchmark analysis. For this purpose we run a regression analysis, where the dependent variable is the individual SIPA, and the specification includes variables on the

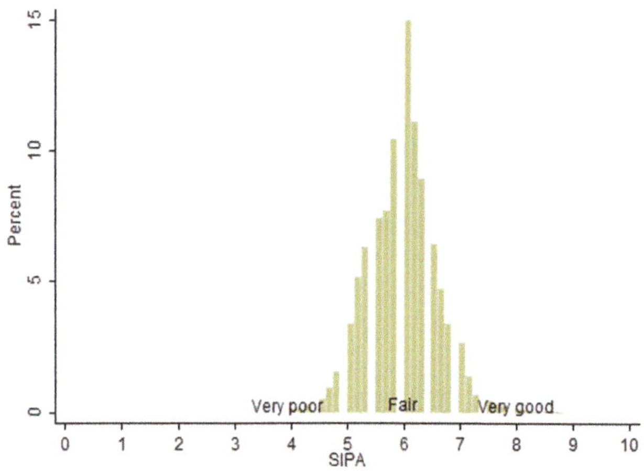

Figure 3. Distribution of individual SIPAs (8,226 observations).

player (pay relative to the average pay, age, experience, and role), as well as the same variables used in Table 4. We consider ATMs as team members to construct our statistics. Table 6 shows the output from this regression, where we estimate the coefficients using a pooled ordinary least squares (OLS) method with player-clustered standard errors (column 1), a random-effect (RE) panel GLS method (column 2), or a fixed-effect (FE) panel OLS method (column 3); the latter method does not allow us to separate the effect of match-invariant variables from the player-specific effect. The "rho" coefficient reported in the bottom part of the table suggests that, in this context, it is important to consider player-specific effects. Moreover, the statistical tests comparing the three models, reported at the end of the table, suggest that it is advisable to use a panel method.

Our main findings are as follows. In columns (1) and (2), where we can estimate the effects of match-invariant variables, we find positive effects for individual pay, years of experience with the team, and the midfield role of the player (a core role in soccer). The direction of all of these effects is intuitive. Notice in particular that a high relative pay seems to work as an incentive on individual performance; this result is in line with, for instance, the results of Pfeffer and Langton (1993) [41]. However, giving a disproportionately high pay to some is not necessarily an effective strategy. In fact, it may give rise to high pay dispersion, and in Table 6 we consistently find a negative effect for the team pay dispersion. In addition, we find positive effects for playing at home, number of disqualified players, and the opponent's pay dispersion, and a negative effect for the opponent's average pay.

In Section B.5 of the supplementary material (available upon request), we repeat the same analysis, adding into the specification variables that consider whether the player is a "superstar" (when he earns at least two times the average pay in the team) or a "regular player" (one of the 11 most frequent players in the first month of the season), alone and interacting with pay dispersion. Interestingly, we find that SIPA increases with regular players, and responds more negatively to pay dispersion among superstars. In particular the first result suggests that infrequent players, when they have "all eyes on them" during the match, are not able to perform as well as the regular players for whom they substitute.

Figure 4 reports the predicted SIPA conditional on pay dispersion and the average explanatory variables, using the estimates from column (2) of Table 6. We focus on this column, rather than column (3), because it shows a lower effect of pay dispersion (−0.08 instead of −0.14), and overall it provides more convincing estimates—in particular, because it shows significant effects as a result of the players' and team salaries. As its counterpart for team performance (panel [a] of Figure 2), the figure shows that the SIPA is the highest when there is no pay dispersion at all. This suggests that pay dispersion has a detrimental effect not just on team performance, but that it also negatively impacts individual performance.

To interpret this figure, we return to our previous example with the team manager. Suppose the manager has to choose whether to increase or decrease the current pay dispersion (where 1 player earns 2.5 times the average income, and each of the 10 remaining players earns 0.85 times the average income). The outcome of this choice is not trivial, because varying the distribution of pays affects not only pay dispersion, but also the average pay and the players' pay, which in turn have different implications on individual performance. To keep the situation simple, let us say that the

Table 5. Summary statistics, individual players (8,226 observations on 876 players).

Variable	Median	Mean	Std. dev.	Minimum	Maximum
SIPA					
If win	6.333	6.308	0.563	4	8.833
If draw	6	5.968	0.504	4	7.833
If defeat	5.667	5.631	0.531	4	7.833
OVERALL	6	5.966	0.611	4	8.833
Individual variables					
Pay (thousands of euros)	600	1029.200	1255.642	30	10500
Pay/average pay	0.920	0.997	0.496	0.010	4.348
New to the team	0	0.271	0.445	0	1
Years on the team	1	2.287	2.679	0	18
Years in first division	4	4.789	3.807	0	18
Age	27	27.429	3.954	17	41
Midfield role	0	0.399	0.490	0	1
Forward role	0	0.191	0.393	0	1

Table 6. Individual performance and pay dispersion (average marginal effects).

		(1)	(2)	(3)
Method:		**Pooled OLS**	**RE GLS**	**FE OLS**
Player:	Pay/average pay	0.105***	0.110***	−0.220
		(0.021)	(0.020)	(0.172)
	New to the team	−0.002	−0.004	
		(0.026)	(0.023)	
	Years on the team	0.014***	0.015***	
		(0.005)	(0.005)	
	Years in first division	−0.005	−0.005	
		(0.004)	(0.004)	
	Age	0.001	0.000	
		(0.003)	(0.003)	
	Midfield role	0.047**	0.050***	
		(0.019)	(0.019)	
	Forward role	−0.015	−0.014	
		(0.028)	(0.026)	
Pay:	Log(average pay)	0.082***	0.080***	−0.253
		(0.019)	(0.017)	(0.196)
	Log(pay dispersion index)	−0.064***	−0.080***	−0.139***
		(0.016)	(0.014)	(0.024)
Team:	Fraction of new players on the team	0.053	0.023	−0.007
		(0.073)	(0.071)	(0.115)
	Years on the team	−0.006	−0.012	−0.026
		(0.014)	(0.013)	(0.025)
	Years in first division	0.001	0.002	−0.007
		(0.010)	(0.010)	(0.018)
	Age	−0.009	−0.003	0.014
		(0.010)	(0.009)	(0.016)
Coach:	New to the team	−0.008	0.003	0.094
		(0.028)	(0.027)	(0.098)
	Replaced during the season	−0.016	0.012	0.134**
		(0.027)	(0.027)	(0.059)
	Years on the team	−0.011	−0.009	0.055*
		(0.014)	(0.013)	(0.033)
	Years in first division	0.007**	0.007**	−0.001
		(0.003)	(0.003)	(0.011)
	Age	0.001	0.002	0.004
		(0.002)	(0.002)	(0.007)
Match:	Injured players	−0.010**	−0.006	−0.000
		(0.005)	(0.004)	(0.005)
	Disqualified players	0.048***	0.056***	0.072***
		(0.011)	(0.011)	(0.012)
	Home play	0.144***	0.144***	0.140***
		(0.013)	(0.013)	(0.013)
Opponent:	Log(average pay)	−0.042***	−0.043***	−0.048***
		(0.014)	(0.013)	(0.013)
	Log(pay dispersion index)	0.055***	0.053***	0.053***
		(0.012)	(0.011)	(0.012)
	Fraction of new players on the team	0.035	0.058	0.120**
		(0.056)	(0.057)	(0.058)

Table 6. Cont.

	(1)	(2)	(3)
Method:	**Pooled OLS**	**RE GLS**	**FE OLS**
Years on the team	−0.001	0.003	0.011
	(0.010)	(0.010)	(0.010)
Years in first division	0.004	0.005	0.009
	(0.006)	(0.006)	(0.007)
Age	0.007	0.007	0.003
	(0.006)	(0.006)	(0.007)
Constant	5.443***	5.217***	7.126***
	(0.308)	(0.276)	(1.521)
+ time dummy variables on month and year of the match			
R^2	0.041	0.040	0.000
Rho coefficient		0.063	0.380
Test pooled vs. panel		276.810	1.930
		[0.000]	[0.000]

Note: 8,226 observations on 876 players (on average, 9.39 matches per player). The dependent variable is the average SIPA from three newspapers. Standard errors are given in parentheses; p values in brackets. In column 1 we report player-clustered standard errors.
**p<0.1;*
***p<0.05;*
****p<0.01.*

manager has a budget balance and he considers two alternatives that do not alter average pay: in plan A, the top player earns three times the average pay, and each remaining player earns 0.8 times the average pay; in plan B, the top player earns two times the average pay, and each remaining player earns 0.9 times the average pay. The corresponding Theil index goes from an initial level of $T = 0.083$ to either $T = 0.137$ in plan A or $T = 0.040$ in plan B.

We know from Table 6 that an increase in player's pay has a positive effect on individual performance, while an increase in pay dispersion has a negative effect. As a result, the direction of the effect on the top player is unclear *a priori*, while we already know that in plan A the performance of the lower-paid players will fall, and in plan B their performance will rise. With these numbers we find that, in plan A the SIPA of the top player will rise by 0.015 points, whereas the SIPA of each other player will fall by 0.046 points. In plan B, the SIPA of the top player will rise by 0.003 points (notwithstanding a reduction of his pay), while the SIPA of each other player will rise by 0.064 points. All in all, the effect on the top player is lower than that on the other players. Considered along with the fact that there is just one top player, but 10 other players, this suggests that plan B is preferable, because it increases the average SIPA by 0.058 points; in contrast, plan A reduces the average SIPA by 0.04 points.

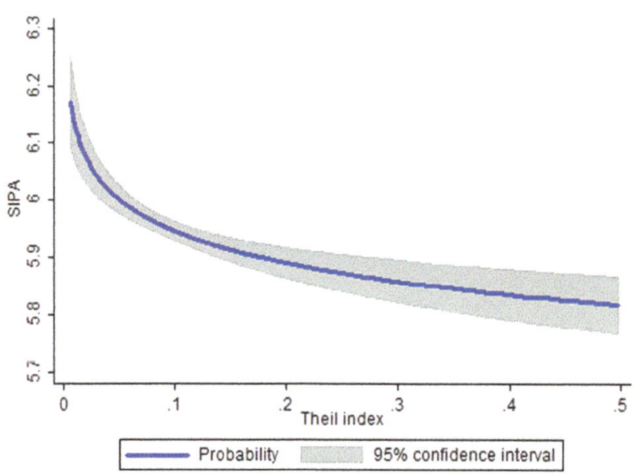

Figure 4. Predicted SIPA, by pay dispersion. Note: Predictions are based on the average explanatory variables and the parameter estimates from Table 6, column (3).

Conclusions

Relatively little is known about how the introduction of dispersed pay in teams influences team performance. However, teams are becoming increasingly widespread in organizations [42–43]. The same is true for performance-contingent pay on the individual level [44]. In fact, firms introduce dispersed pay in teams [45–46], but the effect of this managerial intervention on team performance has thus far been unclear. The broader literature on pay dispersion in organizations has resulted in very different, even contradictory, findings. In fact, the extant research suggests that the effect of pay dispersion on organizational performance can be positive, null, or negative [47].

In this study we collected and analyzed a unique dataset of matches played during two seasons of the men's major soccer league in Italy. This unique dataset allows us to measure the effect of pay dispersion according to different definitions of team. This peculiarity of our dataset is the crucial element that can explain the conflicting evidence. Indeed, we also find positive, null, and negative effects of pay dispersion on team performance, using the *same data* but *different definitions of team*. However, when we take the narrowest definition of a team—considering only the members who actually took part in the task and how long they played—pay dispersion has a detrimental impact on team performance: doubling pay dispersion decreases by 6% the probability of winning a match. This result is consistent with several robustness checks.

This negative effect of pay dispersion on team performance may be the reason why salaries are usually kept secret within a firm [48]. Employees do not like to earn less than their coworkers; as a result, pay dispersion can decrease cooperation within the team and it may affect individual performance. We investigate this issue in our environment by looking at the number of passes within a match and the (subjective) individual performance assessments reported by the three most important Italian sports newspapers. Our results show that higher pay dispersion has a detrimental impact on individual evaluations, whereas it does not have a significant effect on cooperation.

Our results hold for any level of pay given the dimensionless nature of our pay dispersion index. Therefore, the external validity of our analysis goes beyond this specific sports environment. Actually, the fact that in the sport environment salaries can be high is a strong feature of our dataset, because it allows us to study a large variety of pay dispersions.

One limitation of our analysis is that the association between pay dispersion and team performance is really driven by underlying differences in players skills, abilities and talents and that such differences cause both pay dispersion and team performance. We cannot resolve this issue, given our data. The proper way to address it arguably is by means of an experimental research design that allows the experimentalist to control talent-related as well as pay-related variables. We hope our study will inspire future research into this issue.

Author Contributions

Analyzed the data: AB NF MP. Contributed reagents/materials/analysis tools: AB NF MP. Wrote the paper: AB NF MP.

References

1. Lawler EE (1990) Strategic pay: Aligning organizational strategies and pay systems. San Francisco, CA: Jossey-Bass.
2. Shaw JD, Gupta N, Delery JE (2002) Pay dispersion and workforce performance: Moderating effects of incentives and interdependence. Strategic Management Journal 23: 491–512.
3. Milkovich GT, Newman JM (1996) Compensation. (5th ed.) Homewood IL: Irwin: 45.
4. Jirjahn W, Kraft K (2007) Intra-firm wage dispersion and firm performance – Is there a uniform relationship? Kyklos 60 2: 231–253.
5. Trevor CO, Reilly G, Gerhart B (2012) Reconsidering pay dispersion's effect on the performance of interdependent work: Reconciling sorting and pay inequality. Academy of Management Journal, 55: 585–610.
6. Martin J (1981) Relative deprivation: A theory of distributive injustice for an era of shrinking resources. In LL Cummings, BM Staw (eds.) Research in Organizational Behavior 3. Greenwich, CT: JAI Press.
7. Lazear EP, Rosen S (1981) Rank-order tournaments as optimum labor contracts. The Journal of Political Economy 89: 841–864.
8. Ramaswamy R, Rowthorn RE (1991) Efficiency pays and pays dispersion. Economica 58: 501–14.
9. Aime F, Meyer CJ, Humphrey SE (2010) Legitimacy of team rewards: Analyzing legitimacy as a condition for the effectiveness of a team incentive designs. Journal of Business Research 61: 60–66.
10. Milgrom P, Roberts J (1992) Economics, organization, and management, upper saddle river. NJ: Prentice Hall.
11. Ramaswamy R, Rowthorn RE (1991) Efficiency pays and pays dispersion. Economica 58: 501–14.
12. Avrutin BM, Sommers PM (2007) Work incentives and salary distributions in Major League Baseball. Atlantic Economic Journal, 35: 509–510.
13. Berri DJ, Jewell TR (2004) Pay inequality and firm performance: Professional basketball's natural experiment. Atlantic Economic Journal 32: 130–139.
14. Katayama H, Nuch H (2011) A game-level analysis of salary dispersion and team performance in the National Basketball Association. Applied Economics 43: 1193–1207.
15. Lazear EP, Shaw KL (2007) Personnel economics: the economist's view of human resources, Journal of Economic Perspectives 21: 91–114.
16. Stewart GL (2006) A meta-analytic review of relationships between team design features and team performance. Journal of Management 32: 29–54.
17. LePine AL, Piccolo RF, Jackson CL, Mathieu JE, Saul JR (2008) A meta-analysis of teamwork processes: Tests of a multidimensional model and relationships with team effectiveness criteria. Personnel Psychology 61: 273–307.
18. Park G, Spitzmuller M, DeShon RP (2013) Advancing our understanding of Team motivation – Integrating conceptual approaches and content areas. Journal of Management 39 5: 1339–1379.
19. Hamilton B, Nickerson JA, Owan H (2003) Team incentives and worker heterogeneity: An empirical analysis of the impact of teams on productivity and participation. Journal of Political Economy 111: 465–497.
20. Guzzo RA, Dickson MW (1996) Teams in organizations: Recent research on performance and effectiveness. Annual Review of Psychology 47 1: 307–338.
21. Zenger T, Hesterly W (1997) The disaggregation of corporations: Selective intervention, high-powered incentives, and molecular units. Organization Science 8 3: 209–222.
22. Davis SJ, Haltiwanger J (1991) Wage dispersion between and within U.S. manufacturing plants. In Baily M & Winston C eds., Brookings papers on Economic Activity, Microeconomics: 115–200.
23. Zenger T, Hesterly W (1997) The disaggregation of corporations: Selective intervention, high-powered incentives, and molecular units. Organization Science 8 3: 209–222.
24. Aime F, Meyer CJ, Humphrey SE (2010) Legitimacy of team rewards: Analyzing legitimacy as a condition for the effectiveness of a team incentive designs. Journal of Business Research 61: 60–66.
25. Fredrickson JW, Davis-Blake A, Sanders W (2010) Sharing the wealth: social comparisons and pay dispersion in the CEO's top team. Strategic Management Journal, 31: 1031–1053.
26. Bloom M (1999) The performance effects of pay dispersion on individuals and organizations. Academy of Management Journal 42: 25–40.
27. Becker BE, Huselid MA (1992) The incentive effects of tournament compensation systems. Administrative Science Quarterly, 37: 336–350.
28. Ehrenberg RG, Bognanno ML (1990) Do tournaments have incentive effects? The Journal of Political Economy 98: 1307–1324.
29. Marchand JT, Smeeding TM, Torrey BB (2006) Salary distribution and performance: Evidence from the National Hockey League, unpublished manuscript, Department of Economics and Center for Policy Research, Maxwell School of Citizenship and Public Affairs, Syracuse University and Population Reference Bureau.
30. Bloom M (1999) The performance effects of pay dispersion on individuals and organizations. Academy of Management Journal 42: 25–40.
31. Depken CA (2000) Pay disparity and team productivity: Evidence from Major League Baseball. Economics Letters 67: 87–92.
32. Jane W (2010) Raising salary or redistributing it: A panel analysis of major league baseball. Economics Letters, 107: 297–299.
33. Wiseman F, Chatterjee S (2003) Team payroll and team performance in Major League Baseball: 1985–2002. Economics Bulletin 1: 1–10.
34. Avrutin BM, Sommers PM (2007) Work incentives and salary distributions in Major League Baseball. Atlantic Economic Journal 35: 509–510.
35. Berri DJ, Jewell TR (2004) Pay inequality and firm performance: Professional basketball's natural experiment. Atlantic Economic Journal 32: 130–139.
36. Katayama H, Nuch H (2011) A game-level analysis of salary dispersion and team performance in the National Basketball Association. Applied Economics 43: 1193–1207.
37. Pfeffer J, Langton N (1993) The effect of wage dispersion on satisfaction, productivity, and working collaboratively: Evidence from college and university faculty. Administrative Science Quarterly 38: 382–407.
38. Deloitte (2011) Annual review of football finance 2011. Manchester, UK: Deloitte Touche Tohmatsu Limited.
39. Kahn LM (2000) The sports business as a labor market laboratory. Journal of Economic Perspectives 14: 75–94.
40. Scully GW (1974) Pay and performance in Major League Baseball. The American Economic Review 64: 915–930.
41. Pfeffer J, Langton N (1993) The effect of wage dispersion on satisfaction, productivity, and working collaboratively: Evidence from college and university faculty. Administrative Science Quarterly 38: 382–407.
42. Lazear EP, Shaw KL (2007) Personnel economics: the economist's view of human resources. Journal of Economic Perspectives 21: 91–114.
43. Stewart GL (2006) A meta-analytic review of relationships between team design features and team performance. Journal of Management 32: 29–54.
44. Davis SJ, Haltiwanger J (1991) Wage dispersion between and within U.S. manufacturing plants. In Baily M & Winston C eds., Brookings papers on Economic Activity. Microeconomics: 115–200.

45. Bloom M (1999) The Performance effects of pay dispersion on individuals and organizations. Academy of Management Journal 42: 25–40.
46. Fredrickson JW, Davis-Blake A,Sanders W (2010) Sharing the wealth: social comparisons and pay dispersion in the CEO's top team. Strategic Management Journal 31: 1031–1053.
47. Jirjahn W, Kraft K (2007) Intra-firm wage dispersion and firm performance – Is there a uniform relationship? Kyklos 60 2: 231–253.
48. Lawler EE (1990) Strategic Pay: Aligning organizational strategies and pay systems. San Francisco, CA: Jossey-Bass. 238–42.

PERMISSIONS

All chapters in this book were first published in PLOS ONE, by The Public Library of Science; hereby published with permission under the Creative Commons Attribution License or equivalent. Every chapter published in this book has been scrutinized by our experts. Their significance has been extensively debated. The topics covered herein carry significant findings which will fuel the growth of the discipline. They may even be implemented as practical applications or may be referred to as a beginning point for another development.

The contributors of this book come from diverse backgrounds, making this book a truly international effort. This book will bring forth new frontiers with its revolutionizing research information and detailed analysis of the nascent developments around the world.

We would like to thank all the contributing authors for lending their expertise to make the book truly unique. They have played a crucial role in the development of this book. Without their invaluable contributions this book wouldn't have been possible. They have made vital efforts to compile up to date information on the varied aspects of this subject to make this book a valuable addition to the collection of many professionals and students.

This book was conceptualized with the vision of imparting up-to-date information and advanced data in this field. To ensure the same, a matchless editorial board was set up. Every individual on the board went through rigorous rounds of assessment to prove their worth. After which they invested a large part of their time researching and compiling the most relevant data for our readers.

The editorial board has been involved in producing this book since its inception. They have spent rigorous hours researching and exploring the diverse topics which have resulted in the successful publishing of this book. They have passed on their knowledge of decades through this book. To expedite this challenging task, the publisher supported the team at every step. A small team of assistant editors was also appointed to further simplify the editing procedure and attain best results for the readers.

Apart from the editorial board, the designing team has also invested a significant amount of their time in understanding the subject and creating the most relevant covers. They scrutinized every image to scout for the most suitable representation of the subject and create an appropriate cover for the book.

The publishing team has been an ardent support to the editorial, designing and production team. Their endless efforts to recruit the best for this project, has resulted in the accomplishment of this book. They are a veteran in the field of academics and their pool of knowledge is as vast as their experience in printing. Their expertise and guidance has proved useful at every step. Their uncompromising quality standards have made this book an exceptional effort. Their encouragement from time to time has been an inspiration for everyone.

The publisher and the editorial board hope that this book will prove to be a valuable piece of knowledge for researchers, students, practitioners and scholars across the globe.

List of Contributors

Andrea Nicoló, Ilenia Bazzucchi, Jonida Haxhi, Francesco Felici and Massimo Sacchetti
Department of Human Movement, Social and Health Sciences, "Foro Italico" University, Rome, Italy

Kathrin Kienapfel
Department of Animal Ecology, Evolution and Biodiversity, Ruhr Universität Bochum, Bochum, Germany

Yvonne Link
Institute of Animal Breeding and Husbandry, Christian-Albrechts University of Kiel, Kiel, Germany

Uta König v. Borstel
Department of Animal Breeding and Genetics, Georg-August-Universität Göttingen, Göttingen, Germany

Pedro Silva and Júlio Garganta
CIFI2D - Centre for Research, Education, Innovation and Intervention in Sport, Faculdade de Desporto, Universidade do Porto, Porto, Portugal

Bruno Travassos
CIDESD, Department of Sport Sciences, Universidade da Beira Interior, Covilhã, Portugal

Lúıs Vilar
Faculty of Physical Education and Sports, Luśofona University of Humanities and Technologies, Lisboa, Portugal
CIPER, Faculdade de Motricidade Humana, Universidade de Lisboa, Cruz Quebrada Dafundo, Lisboa, Portugal

Paulo Aguiar
Centre for Mathematics, Faculdade de Ciências, Universidade do Porto, Porto, Portugal

Keith Davids
Centre for Sports Engineering Research, Sheffield Hallam University, Sheffield, United Kingdom
FiDiPro Programme, University of Jyväskylä, Jyvä skylä, Finland

Duarte Araújo
CIPER, Faculdade de Motricidade Humana, Universidade de Lisboa, Cruz Quebrada Dafundo, Lisboa, Portugal

Robert Trivers
Graduate Program in Ecology and Evolution, Rutgers University, New Brunswick, New Jersey, United States of America

Bernhard Fink
Courant Research Centre, Evolution of Social Behavior & Institute of Psychology, University of Göttingen, Göttingen, Germany

Mark Russell
Faculty of Health and Life Sciences, Northumbria University, Newcastle-upon-Tyne, United Kingdom

Kristofor McCarty
Department of Psychology, Faculty of Health and Life Sciences, Northumbria University, Newcastle-upon-Tyne, United Kingdom

Bruce James
MVP Track and Field Club, University of Technology, Kingston, Jamaica

Brian G. Palestis
Department of Biological Sciences, Wagner College, Staten Island, New York, United States of America

Michacl J. Wright
Centre for Cognition and Neuroimaging, Department of Psychology, Brunel University London, Uxbridge, United Kingdom

Robin C. Jackson
Centre for Sports Medicine and Human Performance, Department of Sport and Exercise Science, Brunel University London, Uxbridge, United Kingdom

Miroslav Petr and Eva Kohlíková Michal Šteffl
Department of Physiology and Biochemistry, Faculty of Physical Education and Sport, Charles University in Prague, Prague, Czech Republic

Petr Šťastný
Department of Sport Games, Faculty of Physical Education and Sport, Charles University in Prague, Prague, Czech Republic

Ondřej Pecha
Department of Kinanthropology and Humanities, Faculty of Physical Education and Sport, Charles University in Prague, Prague, Czech Republic

Ondřej Šeda
Institute of Biology and Medical Genetics, the First Faculty of Medicine, Charles University and the General Teaching Hospital, Prague, Czech Republic

Shaobin Huang and Yange Yang
College of Computer Science and Technology, Harbin Engineering University, Harbin, China

Tianyang Lv
College of Computer Science and Technology, Harbin Engineering University, Harbin, China
College of Computer Science and Technology, Tsinghua University, Beijing, China
Audit Research Institute, National Audit Office, Beijing, China

Xizhe Zhang and Chao Wen
College of Information Science and Engineering, Northeastern University, Shenyang, China

Weimin Zheng
College of Computer Science and Technology, Tsinghua University, Beijing, China

Juliana Antero-Jacquemin and François Deni Desgorces
Institut de Recherche bioMédicale et d'Epidemiologie du Sport (IRMES), Institut National du Sport de l'Expertise et de la Performance (INSEP), Paris, France
Université Paris Descartes, EA 7329, Sorbonne Paris Cité, Paris, France

Frédéric Dor, Adrien Sedeaud and Amal Haïda
Institut de Recherche bioMédicale et d'Epidemiologie du Sport (IRMES), Institut National du Sport de l'Expertise et de la Performance (INSEP), Paris, France

Philippe LeVan
Comité National Olympique et Sportif Franc¸ais (CNOSF), Medical Commission, Paris, France
Institut National du Sport de l'Expertise et de la Performance (INSEP), Medical Department, Paris, France

Jean-François Toussaint
Institut de Recherche bioMédicale et d'Epidemiologie du Sport (IRMES), Institut National du Sport de l'Expertise et de la Performance (INSEP), Paris, France
Université Paris Descartes, EA 7329, Sorbonne Paris Cité, Paris, France
Centre d'Investigations en Médecine du Sport, Hôpital Hôtel-Dieu, Assistance Publique-Hôpitaux de Paris, Paris, France

Christopher W. Herman, Andrew R. Burghardt and Stephen J. McGregor
Eastern Michigan University, Ypsilanti, Michigan, United States of America

Anna S. C. Conlonn and Melvyn Rubenfire
University of Michigan, Ann Arbor, Michigan, United States of America

Gregory S. Kolt, Emma S. George and Justin M. Guagliano
School of Science and Health, University of Western Sydney, Sydney, Australia

Chris Lonsdale
Institute for Positive Psychology and Education, Australian Catholic University, Sydney, Australia

Richard R. Rosenkranz
School of Science and Health, University of Western Sydney, Sydney, Australia
Department of Human Nutrition, Kansas State University, Manhattan, Kansas, United States of America

Anders Kilen, Tanja Hultengren Larsson, Majke Jørgensen and Nikolai B. Nordsborg
Department of Nutrition, Exercise and Sport, University of Copenhagen, Copenhagen, Denmark,

Lars Johansen and Susanne Jørgensen
Team Denmark, Copenhagen, Denmark

Florian Loffing and Norbert Hagemann
Institute of Sports and Sports Science, University of Kassel, Kassel, Germany

Florian Sölter
Institute of Sports and Sports Science, University of Kassel, Kassel, Germany
Institute of Sport and Exercise Sciences, University of Muenster, Muenster, Germany

Andreas Heuer and Oliver Rubner
Institute of Physical Chemistry, WWU Muenster, Muenster, Germany
Center of Nonlinear Science CeNoS, WWU Muenster, Muenster, Germany

Timothy N. Kruse
The University of Washington School of Medicine, 1959 N. E. Pacific Street, Seattle, WA, 98195, United States of America

Rickey E. Carter and Jordan K. Rosedahl
Department of Health Sciences Research, Mayo Clinic, 200 First Street SW, Rochester, MN, 55905, United States of America

Michael J. Joyner
Department of Anesthesiology, Mayo Clinic, 200 First Street SW, Rochester, MN, 55905, United States of America

Daniel M. V. Santos, Michele C. Souza, Thayse N. Gomes, Fernanda K. Santos and José A. R. Maia
Centre of Research, Education, Innovation and Intervention in Sport, Faculty of Sports, University of Porto, Porto, Portugal

Peter T. Katzmarzyk
Pennington Biomedical Research Center, Louisiana State University System, Baton Rouge, Louisiana, United States of America

Vincent P. Diego and John Blangero
Texas Biomedical Research Institute, San Antonio, Texas, United States of America

Duarte L. Freitas
Sport and Physical Education Department, University of Madeira, Funchal, Portugal

Raquel N. Chaves
Physical Education Department, Federal University of Technology - Parana, Campus Curitiba, Curitiba/PR, Brasil

Carlos Balsalobre-Fernández, Carlos Ma Tejero-González and Juan del Campo-Vecino
Department of Physical Education, Sport and Human Movement, Autonomous University of Madrid, Madrid, Spain

Zhi Jie Zhang
Department of Rehabilitation Sciences, The Hong Kong Polytechnic University, Hung Hom, Kowloon, Hong Kong
Guangdong-Hongkong Joint Sports Rehabilitation and Research Center, Guangdong Provincial Work Injury Rehabilitation Hospital, Guangzhou, China

Gabriel Yin-fat Ng, Wai Chun Lee and Siu Ngor Fu
Department of Rehabilitation Sciences, The Hong Kong Polytechnic University, Hung Hom, Kowloon, Hong Kong

Liam D. Harper, Daniel J. West, Emma Stevenson and Mark Russell
Health and Life Sciences, Northumbria University, Newcastle-upon-Tyne, United Kingdom

Miriam Chang Yi Lee, Jia Yi Chow and Clara Wee Keat Tan
Physical Education and Sports Science, National Institute of Education, Nanyang Technological University, Singapore, Singapore

John Komar
CETAPS, Faculty of Sports Sciences, University of Rouen, Rouen, France

Chris Button
School of Physical Education, Sport and Exercise Sciences, University of Otago, Dunedin, New Zealand

Michael W. Kraus
Department of Psychology, University of Illinois, Urbana-Champaign, Champaign, Illinois, United States of America

Christopher Oveis
Rady School of Management, University of California San Diego, San Diego, California, United States of America

Maria Logli Allison and Dacher Keltner
Department of Psychology, University of California, Berkeley, California, United States of America

Randall C. Young
Department of Psychology, Bridgewater College, Bridgewater, Virginia, United States of America

John Tauer
Department of Psychology, University of St. Thomas, Saint Paul, Minnesota, United States of America

Christopher R. Gagne and Sean P. MacEvoy
Department of Psychology, Boston College, Chestnut Hill, Massachusetts, United States of America

Isabelle Rogowski and Thomas Creveaux
Universitéde Lyon, UniversitéClaude Bernard Lyon 1, Centre de Recherche et d'Innovation sur le Sport - EA 647, UFRSTAPS, Villeurbanne, France

Laurence Chéze and Raphaël Dumas
Universitéde Lyon, UniversitéClaude Bernard Lyon 1, IFSTTAR, UMR_T9406, LBMC Laboratoire de Biomécanique et Mécanique des Chocs, Bron, France

Pierre Macé
Babolat VS, Lyon, France

Paul W. M. Marshall, Ric Lovell and Jason C. Siegler
School of Science and Health, University of Western Sydney, Sydney, Australia

Gitte K. Jeppesen and Kristoffer Andersen
School of Medicine and Health, Aalborg University, Aalborg, Denmark

Javier Sánchez-Sánchez
School of Sport Sciences, UCAM, Universidad Católica San Antonio, Murcia, Spain
IGOID Research Group, University of Castilla-La Mancha, Toledo, Spain

Jorge García-Unanue and Leonor Gallardo
IGOID Research Group, University of Castilla-La Mancha, Toledo, Spain

Pedro Jiménez-Reyes and Ana Gallardo
School of Sport Sciences, UCAM, Universidad Católica San Antonio, Murcia, Spain

Pablo Burillo
IGOID Research Group, University of Castilla-La Mancha, Toledo, Spain
Sport Sciences Institute, Camilo José Cela University, Villafranca del Castillo, Madrid, Spain

José Luis Felipe
IGOID Research Group, University of Castilla-La Mancha, Toledo, Spain
School of Sport Sciences, European University, Villaviciosa de Odón, Madrid, Spain

Xianchao Tang
School of Computer Science and Technology, Tianjin University, Tianjin, China,

Tao Xu and Xia Feng
School of Computer Science and Technology, Civil Aviation University of China, Tianjin, China
Information Technology Research Base of Civil Aviation Administration of China, Tianjin, China

Guoqing Yang
School of Computer Science and Technology, Tianjin University, Tianjin, China,
Information Technology Research Base of Civil Aviation Administration of China, Tianjin, China

Jack Hollingdale
School of Psychology, University of Sussex, Brighton, United Kingdom

Tobias Greitemeyer
Institute of Psychology, University of Innsbruck, Innsbruck, Austria

Twan ten Haaf
Department of Nutrition & Dietetics, School of Sports and Nutrition, Amsterdam University of Applied Sciences, Amsterdam, The Netherlands

Peter J. M. Weijs
Department of Nutrition & Dietetics, School of Sports and Nutrition, Amsterdam University of Applied Sciences, Amsterdam, The Netherlands
Department of Nutrition & Dietetics, Internal Medicine, VU University Medical Center, Amsterdam, The Netherlands
EMGO+ Institute for Health and Care Research, VU University Medical Center, Amsterdam, The Netherlands

Alessandro Bucciol
Department of Economics, University of Verona, Verona, Italy

Nicolai J. Foss
Department of Strategic Management and Globalization, Copenhagen Business School, Frederiksberg, Denmark

Marco Piovesan
Department of Economics, University of Copenhagen, Frederiksberg, Denmark

Index